Mechanical Ventilation

Mechanical Ventilation

Edited by

ROBERT R. KIRBY, M.D., Col USAF, M.C.

Chairman, Department of Anesthesiology
Wilford Hall USAF Medical Center
Lackland Air Force Base, Texas
Clinical Professor of Anesthesiology
The University of Texas Health Science Center
San Antonio, Texas
Tulane University School of Medicine
New Orleans, Louisiana

ROBERT A. SMITH, M.S., R.R.T.

Technical Director
Critical Care Medicine Research and Training Laboratory
Memorial Medical Center
Jacksonville, Florida

DAVID A. DESAUTELS, M.P.A., R.R.T.

Director, Hyperbaric Medicine Program
Hospital Information System Liaison to Operations
Shands Hospital at the University of Florida
Gainesville, Florida

Churchill Livingstone
New York, Edinburgh, London, and Melbourne 1985

The views expressed in this book are those of the authors and do not reflect the official policy or position of the Department of Defense or the US government

Acquisitions Editor: Lewis Reines
Copy Editor: Michael Kelley
Production Editor: Charlie Lebeda
Production Supervisor: Joe Sita
Compositor: Maryland Composition Company, Inc.
Printer/Binder: The Maple Vail Book Manufacturing Co.

Distributed in the United Kingdom by Churchill Livingstone, Robert Stevenson House, 1-3 Baxter's Place, Leith Walk, Edinburgh EH1 3AF and by associated companies, branches and representatives throughout the world.

First published in 1985

Printed in the U.S.A.

ISBN 0-443-08063-1

9 8 7 6 5 4 3 2 1

Library of Congress Cataloging in Publication Data
Main entry under title:
Mechanical ventilation.

Includes bibliographies and index.
1. Artificial respiration.   2. Respirators.
I. Kirby, Robert R.   II. Smith, Robert A.   R.R.T.
III. Desautels, David A. [DNLM: 1. Respiration,
Artificial.   2. Respirators.   3. Respiratory Therapy.
WF 26 M486]
RC87.9.M43 1984   615.8'36'028   84-17001

ISBN 0-443-08063-1

This book is dedicated to E. Trier Mörch, a true pioneer in the field of mechanical ventilation, to Forrest M. Bird and to John H. Emerson, re-sourceful, innovative, and creative geniuses who have taught us much of what we know. They have imparted a rich legacy of expert knowledge.

Contributors

Neel B. Ackerman, Jr., M.D., Major USAF, M.C.
Assistant Director Neonatal Nursery
Wilford Hall USAF Medical Center
San Antonio, Texas

Eduardo Bancalari, M.D.
Professor of Pediatrics
Director, Division of Neonatology
University of Miami/Jackson Memorial Medical Center
Miami, Florida

Michael J. Banner, M.Ed., R.R.T.
Assistant in Anesthesiology
Department of Anesthesiology
University of Florida College of Medicine
Gainesville, Florida

Roger C. Bone, M.D.
Professor and Chairman
Department of Internal Medicine
Rush Presbyterian-St. Luke's Medical Center
Chicago, Illinois

Robert A. deLemos, M.D., Col USAF, M.C.
Chairman, Division of Maternal Child Health
Wilford Hall USAF Medical Center
San Antonio, Texas

Robert R. Demers, B.S., R.R.T.
Chief Respiratory Therapist
Stanford University Hospital
Stanford, California

David A. Desautels, M.P.A., R.R.T.
Director, Hyperbaric Medicine Program
Hospital Information System Liaison to Operations
Shands Hospital at the University of Florida
Gainesville, Florida

Esther Eisler, B.A., R.R.T.
Co-ordinator, Respiratory Therapy Department
University of Miami/Jackson Memorial Medical Center
Miami, Florida

T. James Gallagher, M.D.
Associate Professor
Departments of Anesthesiology & Surgery
University of Florida College of Medicine
Gainesville, Florida

Richard S. Irwin, M.D.
Chief, Division of Pulmonary Medicine
Professor of Medicine
University of Massachusetts Medical School
Worcester, Massachusetts

Robert R. Kirby, M.D., Col USAF, M.C.
Chairman, Department of Anesthesiology
Wilford Hall USAF Medical Center
Lackland Air Force Base, Texas
Clinical Professor of Anesthesiology
The University of Texas Health Science Center
San Antonio, Texas
Tulane University School of Medicine
New Orleans, Louisiana

E. Trier Mörch, M.D., Ph.D., F.F.A.R.C.S.
Emeritus Professor of Anesthesiology
Rush University School of Medicine
Abraham Lincoln School of Medicine
Chicago, Illinois
Staff Anesthesiologist
Nassau General Hospital
Fernandina Beach, Florida

Donald M. Null, Jr., M.D., Col USAF, M.C.
Director, Neonatal Nursery
Wilford Hall USAF Medical Center
San Antonio, Texas

Howard G. Sanders, Jr., B.S., R.R.T.
Chairman, Department of Respiratory Therapy
School of Allied Health Professions
Loma Linda University
Loma Linda, California

Robert A. Smith, M.S., R.R.T.
Technical Director
Critical Care Medicine Research and Training Laboratory
Memorial Medical Center
Jacksonville, Florida

Charles B. Spearman, B.S., R.R.T.
Instructor, Department of Respiratory Therapy
School of Allied Health Professions
Loma Linda University
Loma Linda, California

Preface

For a long time we hesitated to embark upon the writing of this book. Several factors were responsible for this less than enthusiastic approach, not the least of which was the drudgery and monotony of ventilator performance analyses. More importantly, we were not convinced of the need for such a book, since many treatises on the subject of mechanical ventilation had already been prepared. In addition, we wondered whether this work would satisfy a need which existed or merely be a superfluous addition to a rather crowded field.

More recently, however, we became convinced that a book of this type does have some redeeming features which, although not social, may be useful:

(1) Most currently available references treat mechanical ventilators essentially in one of two ways. Either they are described in terms which are either so complex that a more than nodding acquaintance with physics and mathematics is required or so simple and concise that they provide little understanding of a fairly complicated subject. Furthermore, mechanical ventilators and ventilation are often covered by only a chapter or so in books which attempt to deal with the entire field of respiratory care. In such instances, regardless of the methodology employed, a less than satisfactory treatment of the subject results.

(2) In the early 1960s only a few unsophisticated (but surprisingly effective) ventilators were available in the United States. Since then, a bewildering assortment of makes, models, colors, and options have appeared, with an equally bewildering increase in cost. At this writing, one may pay in excess of $15,000 for a single ventilator with features which may or may not contribute to improved patient care. Costs of $12,000 to $15,000 are commonplace. The busy physician or respiratory therapist needs something more than a manufacturer's word to ascertain whether, for his/her purpose, certain features are necessary or desirable.

(3) For over three decades exciting advances in the understanding of normal and abnormal ventilation have been published. However, basic changes which incorporate much of this knowledge into ventilator design have been widespread for 10 to 15 years only. At the same time, practitioners must ponder other forms of support related to but not dependent upon the use of a ventilator, which must be appreciated by those who are caring for the patient with respiratory insufficiency.

Other areas of importance closely related to ventilator support are also included (cardiorespiratory monitoring, pulmonary hygiene, and airway maintenance), as well as specific types of pulmonary dysfunction (neonatal and adult respiratory distress syndrome). The subject of high frequency ventilation is discussed in some detail, not because of widespread clinical usefulness at this time, but because of the tremendous interest and research effort in defining its present and future roles in respiratory care. We have not dealt with ventilators manufactured outside the United States unless they are widely used here. Generally, we have neither access to such devices nor expertise in their use, so an attempt to include them would be a disservice to both their manufacturers and the reader.

Does this book meet both stated and unstated goals? We hope so but really don't know. One problem with almost any topic related to mechanical ventilators is that much opinion is often expressed without much scientifically documented fact. Almost any form of therapy employed in acute or chronic ventilatory insufficiency generates heated controversy—witness the subjects of intermittent mandatory ventilation (IMV) and ''super PEEP.'' One thing is certain: those who agree with us will applaud our efforts; those who do not will be encouraged to rebut what we say. In either event, more attention will be paid to topics which, in our estimation, have been treated previously in a somewhat perfunctory fashion.

It is customary to pay tribute to persons who are important to the development of a book. We are indebted and grateful to many individuals, but one who stands out particularly is Lew Reines, President of Churchill Livingstone. For many years he has cajoled, threatened, and encouraged us in this undertaking. Whether he (or we) will be glad he did remains to be seen. We also thank Mrs. Pat Smith and Ms. Esperanza Olivo who endured seemingly endless editing and rewrites prior to our acquisition of word-processing capabilities.

Robert R. Kirby, M.D.
Robert A. Smith, RRT
David Desautels, RRT

Contents

1

History of Mechanical Ventilation

E. Trier Mørch

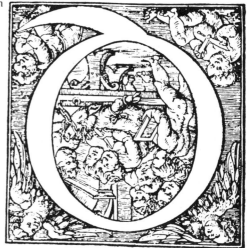

Quo vadis? Only history will tell

EARLY HISTORY OF RESUSCITATION

The illustrated letter ''O'' is copied from Andreas Wesele Vesalius' (1515–1564) *de Humani Corporis Fabrica*, printed in 1555. It depicts chubby cherubs performing a tracheostomy on a sow. In the *Fabrica*, Vesalius was the first to give a detailed report of ''modern'' resuscitation. He reported:

But that life may in a manner of speaking be restored to the animal, an opening must be attempted in the trunk of the trachea, into which a tube of reed or cane should be put; you will then blow into this, so that the lung may rise again and the animal take in air. Indeed, with the slight breath in the case of the living animal, the lung will swell to the full extent of the thoracic cavity, and the heart become strong . . . for when the lung, long flaccid, has collapsed, the beat of the heart and arteries appears wavy, creepy, twisting; but when the lung is inflated, it becomes strong again . . . And as I do this, and take care that the lung is inflated at intervals, the motion of the heart and arteries does not stop . . . .

It is impressive how well Vesalius understood the ''modern'' principles of resuscitation and how clearly he described the ventricular fibrillation he saw. Unfortunately, lack of human adaptability delayed extensive application of this same technique for 400 years.

Vesalius was an impetuous genius with an intense desire for correct knowledge and true reporting of anatomy. He was the first to base his anatomical studies on human dissections, which in those days were strictly prohibited by the Church. In so doing, he changed the very principles of the understanding of human anatomy.

The great Greek physician Galen, who lived during the second century A.D. based his knowledge of anatomy on dissections of the pig, ape, dog, and ox. He assumed that the structures he found in these animals were identical to those of the human body. For 13 centuries the human breastbone was thought to be segmented like that of the ape, and the liver to be divided into many lobes like that of the hog. The uterus supposedly consisted of two long horns as in the dog, and the hip bones were assumed to be flared as in the ox. Not even the number of bones in the body was accurately known, most often quoted at between 248 and 252, including the bone of Luz. The latter was supposed to be the indestructible nucleus, a sort of seed, from which the body was resurrected. The belief in the bone of Luz and in the missing rib of Adam persisted until Vesalius showed that both were myths. Galen's teaching, accepted by physicians and the Church, had acquired an authority like that of orthodox theology, undebated for 1300 years. To question Galen was heresy.

Vesalius' demand for truth in anatomy, his impatience, and his hot temper made him take some extreme risks. To obtain a human skeleton, he surreptitiously stole the body of a criminal who had been executed and hanged in chains on exhibit as a lesson to the people. He boiled the body and thus obtained the first complete human skeleton available for study. Had this theft been detected, he would have been executed.

At the age of 23 Vesalius was appointed Professor of Anatomy in Padua in northeastern Italy. During the next 6 years he secretly conducted painstaking dissections on a number of human cadavers. In 1543, before reaching the age of 29, he was ready to publish his great work on anatomy in seven volumes. The illustrations were exact and artistic, probably drawn by one of Titian's pupils.

Vesalius completely contradicted Galenic anatomy. The four abdominal muscles of the ape no longer graced man; the multilobed liver disappeared, as did the segmented sternum, the double bile duct, and the horned uterus. Even the bone of Luz, the resurrection bone, was proved a myth, and Adam's missing rib was restored.

The first correct demonstration of the anatomy of the human body was met with a storm of violent protests. Vesalius had dared to cast discredit on Galen—to discard galenic traditions, which were accepted like the Bible. No one had previously had the audacity to doubt them publicly. Intense indignation was aroused among physicians. Even his former teacher Sylvius called Vesalius' "an impious madman who is poisoning all of Europe with his vaporings."

To discredit his medical brethren was one thing. It was quite another to offend the clergy, who held strong opposition to dissections because of their belief in material resurrection—that only the whole body would be accepted in heaven. It is difficult to comprehend how much brutal suppression and how many sadistic and often fatal tortures were rampant during the Middle Ages. The Inquisition was instigated in 1235 by Pope Gregoire IX as a special tribunal court to examine and punish heretics. Repression of anyone who did not slavishly follow the rigorous medieval Catholic doctrines against sorcery, witchcraft, and magic was widespread. The Inquisition, which openly violated all ideas of freedom, left a legacy of ignorant, intolerant fanaticism (which was often to the political and financial advantage of the ruling monarch). Galen's work held a powerful influence over the clerics and physicians of the Middle

Ages. When Vesalius demonstrated that Galen's description of the flared hipbone was wrong, the excuse offered for his error was that man had changed his shape through wearing tight trousers! Even though Vesalius escaped it, the punishment for dissection was burning at the stake. Legend has it, however, that eventually he was forced to make a pilgrimage to the Holy Land to avoid horrible execution by the Inquisition. The judgment against him was that he performed an autopsy on a Spanish nobleman shortly after his exitus lethalis. Out of curiosity, he experimentally inflated the lungs through the trachea, and the nobleman's heart started to beat again. This only outraged his medical associates further. Vesalius died during the pilgrimage in a shipwreck on the island of Zante, west of Greece.

Vesalius' technique of resuscitation was the simplest form of intermittent positive-pressure breathing (IPPB), a form of support which has proven to be by far the most efficient means of artificial breathing for the last 400 years. One wonders why it has come in and out of vogue so many times. A series of detours have been interspersed, many of which were bizarre and bewildering though often amusing. Because it was hoped that strong and insulting stimulations would revive patients, they were rolled over barrels, loud bells were rung close to their ears, bright lights were shone into their eyes, they were burned with red-hot irons, or their anuses were dilated and tobacco smoke blown into their rectums. Often they were thrown stomach-down across a trotting horse. Limitless human ingenuity and stupidity of this sort was repeated to an impressive degree over the years.

For 100 years after Vesalius, no progress was made. In 1667 Robert Hooke of London (1635–1703) repeated Vesalius' experiment by fixing a pair of fireside bellows tightly into the cut trachea (aspera arteria) of a dog, keeping it alive by regular intermittent inflations.

Another century passed without any publications on resuscitation until in 1744 John Fothergill of England reported a successful case of mouth-to-mouth resuscitation:

A pair of bellows might possibly be applied with more advantage in these cases, than the blast of a man's mouth; but if any person can be got to try the charitable experiment by blowing, it would seem preferable to the other. . . .

Fothergill, one of the founders of the British Humane Society, was afraid of overdistension of the lungs. He also thought that the warmth of the rescuer's exhaled air might be more beneficial than cold air passing through a bellows.

Because there was a strong prejudice against touching the dead, particularly if the death was due to the criminal offense of suicide, no attempt was made to resuscitate people apparently dead from drowning or other causes of asphyxia until about 1750. Also, a prevalent theory held that drowned people died of apoplexy, and that the lungs collapsed. Therefore anyone taken from the water was deemed dead, and resuscitation was not attempted. Furthermore, if an unknown person was brought into a house and died there, the owner of the house might be liable for the expenses of the funeral.

THE HUMANE SOCIETY

More progressive times began in 1767. To the Dutch belongs the credit for the first serious attempt to take care of the unfortunate citizens who drowned in their many waterways. It was during that year that a group of wealthy merchants in Amsterdam formed a society called *Maatschappy tot Redding van Drenklingen* (The Society for the Rescue of Drowned Persons), also called The Humane Society. Similar societies were formed in England and Denmark, and soon in other European countries too.

The most important methods employed by members of the Dutch Humane Society were to keep the patient warm and provide mouth-to-mouth ventilation. By compress-ing the belly and chest with his free hand, the operator brought about an expiratory movement. Several unusual "accessory and useful means" were also recom-mended, e.g., fumigation by blowing to-bacco smoke into the great bowel (Fig. 1-1). Sometimes all the passengers on a Dutch canal boat might be summoned to assist the operator in administering this treatment if the special instrument, the "Fumigator," was not at hand: "Blood letting by opening the jugular vein" was assumed to be ben-eficial and particularly necessary as life re-turned. Vomiting produced by ipecacuanha wine or other emetics was popular, as were sneezing caused by "spirit of quick lime in a rag held in front of the nostrils" and in-ternal stimulants, such as "pouring a gill or two of warm wine into the gullet."

Mouth-to-mouth resuscitation oscillated in popularity with the use of fireside bel-lows. Other methods were soon con-demned, especially by the British and the Danish. In 1776 John Hunter of London ad-vocated the use of a double bellows which he had contrived, so that the first stroke blew fresh air into the lungs and the next stroke, from the other bellows, sucked out the "bad air." He also recommended ap-plying gentle pressure on the larynx against the esophagus to prevent air from going into the stomach (which might be called a "re-verse" Sellick maneuver). Hunter advised the use of "dephlogisticated air," or oxy-gen, and firmly stated that venesection, or blood-letting, should be forbidden.

In 1786 Edmund Goodwyn of London re-ceived the gold medal of the Humane Soci-ety for his dissertation on the connection between life and respiration. He speculated that respiration enabled a beneficial chem-ical substance to be transmitted to the blood.

Laymen were encouraged to use artificial respiration as a result of the efforts of Lord Cathcart in Scotland. The method was pub-lished, and rewards were offered. A half-crown would go to the messenger who in-formed the surgeon or minister when a body had been taken out of the water, two gui-

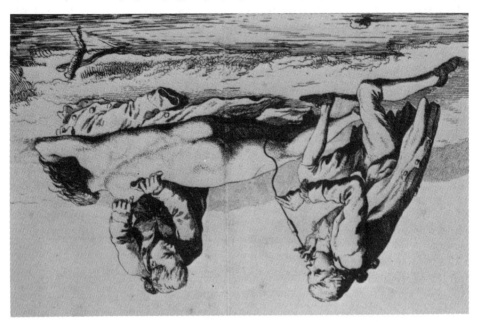

Fig. 1-1. Attempt at resuscitation from drowning by insufflation of tobacco smoke per rectum.

neas to anyone who used the advocated measures for 2 hours, and four guineas if the life was saved. Anyone whose house was used for the rescue was reimbursed all expenses plus one guinea for his trouble.

In 1796 the medical doctor John Daniel Herholdt and the botanist Carl Gottlob Rafn published *Life-Saving Measures for Drowning Persons* in Copenhagen. Together, they took up vital problems for critical analysis and evaluation, reported their findings in a clear and objective style, and pointed the way toward the methods of resuscitation used today (Fig. 1-2). The professor of medicine and physiology and the practical, versatile, scientific government official complemented each other in a way that could well serve as a model! Regretfully, their outstanding work was written in Danish and therefore for all practical purposes was buried until 1960, when Henning Poulsen of Aarhus, Denmark had it translated and pub-

lished to celebrate the tenth anniversary of the founding of the Scandinavian Society of Anaesthetists. It has since received wide acclaim and recognition.

E. Coleman from Ayreshine, Scotland, later veterinary professor in London, recommended tracheal intubation and used a silver catheter much wider than those previously employed. He suggested using a bellows for insufflation and added that oxygen would be beneficial. He also recommended that an electrical current be passed through the heart by means of electrodes placed over the apex and base.

In retrospect, one can only wonder why most of the excellent theories and methods of resuscitation used or advocated by some of the early European workers have been overlooked or completely forgotten, i.e., artificial respiration with tracheal intubation, chest compression, and electrical stimulation of the heart.

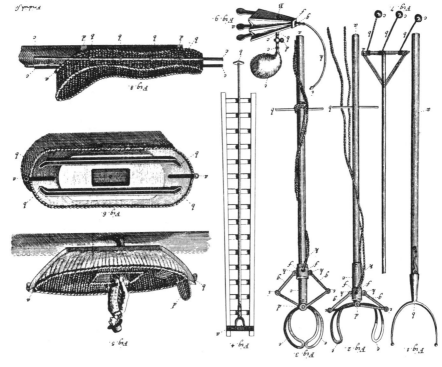

Fig. 1-2. Herholdt and Rafn included this illustration of equipment used to retrieve and resuscitate drowning victims during the late eighteenth century.

Discovery of Oxygen

Joseph Priestley, a dissenting minister, was an earnest inquirer into all wonders of nature and philosophy. In 1774 both he and the Swedish chemist Carl Wilhelm Scheele discovered oxygen independently of each other. Priestley called it "pure" or "vital air," or "dephlogisticated air," i.e., air from which "phlogiston" (nitrogen) had been removed. He knew that this gas could support life in mice and could cause a candle to burn more vigorously. He wrote: "who can tell but that in time, the pure air may become a fashionable article of luxury; hitherto only two mice and myself have had the privilege of breathing it."

The French chemist Laurent Antoine Lavoisier coined the term "oxygen" and destroyed the phlogiston theory. Simon de Laplace showed that metabolism based on oxidation formed water and carbon dioxide as by-products, and that the lungs take up oxygen and give off carbon dioxide. Lavoisier was condemned as an "enemy" of the people because of the prerevolutionary royal support of his laboratory. His life was ended on 8 May 1794 by one lightning stroke of the guillotine, and France lost her leading scientist in the prime of his creative career. Paradoxically, the discovery of oxygen contributed to the disuse of mouth-to-mouth resuscitation; in addition to the indelicacy of the method, it was believed that more oxygen could be given with a bellows than from exhaled air.

In 1827 Leroy d'Etiolle showed that incorrect use of the bellows could lead to emphysema and tension pneumothorax. Unfortunately, he forgot to emphasize the benefits when they were used correctly. His discovery led to the abandonment of the bellows.

Early in the nineteenth century Sir Benjamin Brodie and the Royal Humane Society discontinued attempts to revive drowned people by artificial ventilation. They postulated that no one survived after 4 to 5 minutes under water no matter what was done. Thus the correct ideas of resuscitation were discredited, discontinued, and then forgotten.

Again it took another hundred years before real progress evolved.

CONTRAPTIONS APPLYING NEGATIVE PRESSURE TO THE SURFACE OF THE HUMAN BODY

From the middle of the nineteenth century to the first quarter of the twentieth century, an unbelievable number of devices were introduced which applied subambient or "negative" pressure to the outside of the body. Most of them offered the patient only a brief prolongation of a miserable death.

Two excellent reviews of apparatus using negative pressure were published in England by C. H. W. Woolman in 1976. J. H. Emerson of Cambridge, Massachusetts, also published the interesting and informative pamphlet, *The Evolution of the "Iron Lung."*

Apparatus using negative pressure on the body surface can be classified in three groups: the tank respirator, or "iron lung"; the cuirass ventilators; and the "differential pressure chamber" of Sauerbruch.

Iron Lung

The iron lung was a rigid container big enough to house the entire patient except for the head, which protruded through a hole with an airtight collar around the patient's neck. Intermittent negative or alternating negative/positive pressure could be created by mouth, by hand, or by mechanical pumps.

Physicians believed it to be physiologically more beneficial to breathe for a patient by applying negative pressure to the outside of the lungs than to blow positive pressure into the airways. Although this belief is undoubtedly true from an academic (theoretical) point of view, the early machines did not prove it. They were large, cumbersome, awkward, and burdened by innumerable complications. Most of all, in their initial developmental stages they did not work.

In 1838 Dr. John Dalziel of Drumlanrig, Scotland described a body-enclosing respirator in which the patient sat upright with his head protruding from the top. A bellows created the pressure changes. A similar iron lung was described by Alfred F. Jones of Lexington, Kentucky in 1864. He obtained a patent (U.S. pat. no. 44 198) in which he postulated that when properly and judiciously applied it will ''cure paralysis, neuralgia, rheumatism, seminal weakness, asthma, bronchitis, and dyspepsia. Also, deafness . . . and . . . many other diseases.'' . . .

In 1876 Woillez of Paris built the first workable iron lung, called the ''Spirophore,'' which was very similar to the best of the later models (Fig. 1-3). One unique feature was a rod which rested lightly on the patient's chest and moved up and down, giving visual proof of chest movements.

Some of the other older devices were interesting, though useless. One was described in 1887 by Dr. Charles Breuillard of Paris (Fig. 1-4) in which the patient sat upright in a ''bath cabinet.'' Vacuum was created by a steam ejector, fed by a steam boiler, which was heated by a spirit lamp. The patient was supposed to operate a valve, alternately connecting the cabinet to

the vacuum for inhalation and to the atmosphere for exhalation.

In 1889 Dr. Egon Braun of Vienna described similar machines for resuscitation of asphyxiated children (Fig. 1-5). An infant was placed in a small wooden box supported by a plaster mold, his head was then extended so that the nose and mouth were pressed against a hole in a rubber closure. Pressure and suction were created by the doctor's own breath via a tube going into the box.

In 1905 Dr. William Davenport of London and Dr. Charles Morgan Hammond of Memphis, Tennessee designed iron lungs very similar to that of Woillez. In 1908 Peter Lord of Worchester, Massachusetts, patented a respirator room large enough to allow a nurse to work inside it. Melvin L. Severy of Boston patented an ingenious but

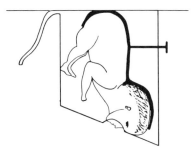

Fig. 1-5. Dr. Egon Braun of Vienna devised a small wooden box in 1889 in which pressure and suction were created by the doctor's own breath (via the tube at the right). This was employed for resuscitating asphyxiated children. Courtesy of J. H. Emerson Company.

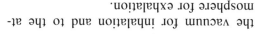

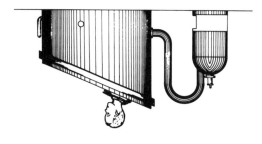

Fig. 1-4. Dr. Charles Breuillard of Paris patented a ''bath cabinet'' type of respirator in 1877. Courtesy of J. H. Emerson Company.

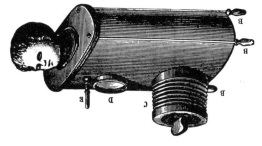

Fig. 1-3. ''Spirophore'' by Woillez of Paris built in 1876.

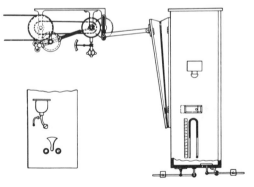

Fig. 1-6. Dr. Melvin L. Severy of Boston created an ingenious mechanical device for ventilation. However, the patient was obliged to stand, pressing his nose and mouth against a triangular aperture below two eye-windows. Courtesy of J. H. Emerson Company.

hopeless box in 1916 in which the patient had to stand up, pressing his nose and mouth against a triangular opening in the front wall (Fig. 1-6).

The ''Barospirator'' was introduced in 1920 by Dr. T. Thunberg of Lund, Sweden. The first design had the entire patient enclosed in a tank. Later, it was reconfigured into a room so large that the medical staff could be accommodated as well. It worked on a completely different principle from the rest, being based on the high compressibility of air. An enormously large, motor-driven piston cylinder caused the pressure to vary from 7 kPa (50 mm Hg) above atmospheric pressure to 7 kPa below it. When pressure increased, the volume of the air decreased and air flowed into the lungs; the reverse occurred as pressure decreased. By this ingenious technique, artificial respiration was obtained with no respiratory movements of the chest.

In 1926 Wilhelm Schwake of Oranienburg-Eden, Germany patented perhaps the most unusual pneumatic chamber in which the patient had to stand up and create pressure differences by moving a large bellows with his own hands. Schwake also postulated that ''negative pressure upon the skin . . . draws out . . . the gaseous by-products'' (Fig. 1-7).

The first truly workable iron lung to receive widespread clinical application was developed in 1928 at the Department of Ventilation, Illumination, and Physiology of the Harvard Medical School by engineer Philip Drinker, pediatrician Charles F. McKhann, and physiologist Louis Agassiz Shaw. This iron lung was comprised of a sheet metal cylinder sealed at one end. The patient's head and neck protruded through a hole with a rubber collar in the other end. The sides of the cylinder had portholes for observing the patient as well as numerous other small sealed outlets for manometers, blood pressure cuffs, stethoscopes, etc. The pumps ran continuously, producing alternating positive and negative pressure in the tank via a system of valves. This original tank respirator design was to undergo many changes over the succeeding 25 years.

During a visit to New York, the famous Danish physiologist August Krogh saw the Drinker respirator in use and was immediately impressed by its possibilities as a clinical tool. Upon his return to Copenhagen in

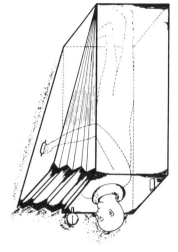

Fig. 1-7. William Schwake of Oranienburg-Eden, Germany, patented a ''pneumatic chamber'' in 1926. Courtesy of J. H. Emerson Company.

1931, he constructed the first Danish respirator designed especially for clinical use (Fig. 1-8). In principle, it was identical to the Drinker respirator but was improved and simplified. The motor was powered by water from the city pipelines. Reciprocating movements were created by leading the water alternatingly to the upper and lower compartments of a piston cylinder, which acted on a large spirometer bell. Among its worthwhile features were a water jacket for regulating the temperature inside the tank, maneuverability which allowed a 15-degree head-down position, and a hood which could be placed over the patient's head to supply him with oxygen or carbogen, a mixture of 95 percent oxygen and 5 percent carbon dioxide which at that time was a popular respiratory stimulant. Krogh also made an infant respirator version and a rocking stretcher.

The most important improvement of the iron lung was made in 1932 by J. H. Emerson. He added a transparent airtight dome that could be fitted over the patient's head. It provided intermittent positive pressure at the head and mouth so the tank could be opened, enabling good and unhurried nursing care to the patient's immobile body.

During a poliomyelitis epidemic in England in 1938, the country had an inadequate supply of worthwhile ventilators. Lord Nuffield, owner of the Morris automobile factory in Oxford, promised to provide the Both cabinet tank type respirator, free of charge, to any hospital in the Empire that wanted one. This effort helped more widespread distribution and use.

Inherent Complications of the Iron Lungs. Good nursing care was nearly impossible in the first iron lungs. Simple procedures, e.g., taking the temperature or blood pressure, counting the pulse, giving a bed bath, or turning the patient to prevent bed sores, were nearly impossible before Emerson developed his transparent dome. Many pa-

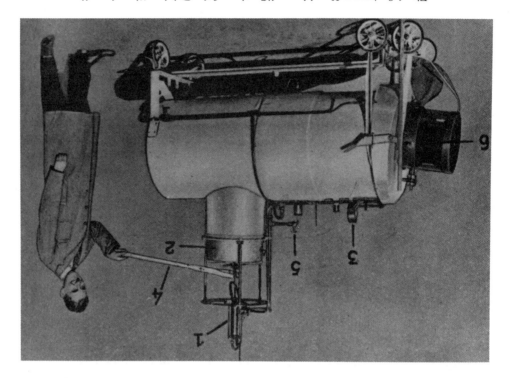

Fig. 1-8. August Krogh's modification of the Drinker "iron lung."

tients suffered from claustrophobia, disorientation, and loneliness from being encapsulated in the big tank. Visiting relatives, whom they might see approaching upside-down if they were privileged enough to have the necessary mirror, could not even hold their hands. Their necks were always sore from the necessarily tight collar, which in the best of cases felt like a shirt collar two sizes too small. Very often it caused open circular wounds and chronic headaches. It was so constricting that the patients could constantly hear their own pulses.

Perhaps the most important benefit of the iron lung was that it represented a stepping-off point for Emerson. Actually, three generations of the Emerson family have had an enormously beneficial influence on respiratory care advances. In 1909 Grandfather H. Emerson described the influence of artificial respiration on pulmonary edema. His still youthful son, John Haven Emerson, has provided the medical profession with an endless number of intelligently designed and usable pieces of equipment. Finally, George P. Emerson seems to be following the same line. He has been of great help to this author.

Cuirass Ventilators

Cuirass ventilators were also rigid, intermittent negative-pressure containers. However, they covered only the patient's chest or chest and abdomen, leaving the extremities and pelvis accessible. Two additional advantages over the iron lungs were their economy and portability.

According to Woollam, the first cuirasses were made by Ignez von Hauke of Austria in 1874, by Alexander Graham Bell in 1882, and by Rudolph Eisenmenger of Piski, Hungary in 1901 (Fig. 1-9). In 1927 the "Dr. Eisenmenger Biomotor," a motor-driven version, was patented in the United States. It was reported to be an "extraordinary success." A great number of cuirasses are de-

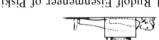

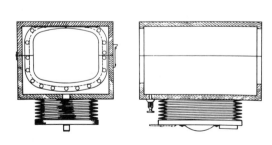

Fig. 1-9. In 1901 Rudolf Eisenmenger of Piski, Hungary patented a portable respirator which consisted of a "simple, two-part box" enclosing only the patient's chest. Courtesy of J. H. Emerson Company.

scribed in Woollam's excellent thesis, most of them developed in the United Kingdom, United States, France, or Sweden.

Eventually, Collier and Affeldt compared cuirasses with tank respirators. They found that if they took the tidal volume produced by the tank as 100 percent, the thoracoabdominal cuirass produced 61–63 percent but the thoracic cuirass only 47 percent. Bryce-Smith and Davis found that the cuirass required much more negative pressure to produce the same tidal volume as the tank. In 1948 in a preliminary report of 827 cases of poliomyelitis, Bergman reported with pride the results of use of the Swedish "Sahlin-Stille" cuirass. Fifteen percent of the patients survived, which "by far exceeds the general Swedish mortality. Those—indeed many—cases which we cannot save by the respirators are at least spared the torments of suffocation." He suggested, however, that "only 2 percent of all treated cases could be saved for a useful social life."

In 1955 Pask stated that:

It is very much to be hoped that further development will occur in this field, for the cuirass respirators must surely embarrass the circulation less than nearly all other types . . . IF it can be made comfortable enough for continuous use over long pe-

...riods, IF it can be made capable of producing really adequate ventilation in all patients, and IF it can be so modified that it be possible to nurse the patient in the prone position, then surely the future for this type of respirator must be very important.

Professor Pask's three "IFs" accurately summed up the problems of cuirass ventilation.

In 1953 Toker, and later Green and Coleman, described a completely new use for the cuirass when he successfully used a "Kifa" cuirass to ventilate patients during general anesthesia for bronchoscopy and laryngoscopy, a procedure which previously had presented a very difficult problem for the anesthetist. Wallace and his associates produced the longest single series of 248 such patients. They failed to adequately ventilate only 16 of these because of poor fit of the shell, obesity, or chronic lung disease. The present author has found that the Emerson wrap-around "raincoat" ventilator driven by a vacuum cleaner may be the best for these difficult cases because the rigid metallic supporting shell and the covering raincoat adapt better to patients with unusual shapes (Fig. 1-10).

A few users still advocate tank respirators in the acute stages of some respiratory disease and for some cases of chronic paralysis in special chronic hospital units. There are also a considerable number of patients living at home whose lives depend on the use of the cuirass respirator. Some have used it for over 25 years.

From an educational viewpoint, I must agree with Woollam that "it is unfortunate that a generation of anaesthetists is being trained who have little or no knowledge of the tank or cuirass."

Sauerbruch's Differential Pressure Chamber

Sauerbruch's differential pressure chamber appeared in 1904 when Ernst Ferdinand Sauerbruch, assistant to von Mikulicz in Breslau, Germany, published his dramatic experimental work, "The Pathology of Open Pneumothorax and the Basic Principle of My Method of Eliminating It." Unfortunately, this treatise represented a significant deviation from the sequential ventilator development pattern which had preceded its publication and delayed further progress by some 30 to 40 years. Sauerbruch transformed the operating room into a sort of enlarged pleural space (Fig. 1-11). He constructed a small airtight operating room where the patient's body and the surgeons were inside, and the patient's head outside. The hole around the patient's neck was airtight. By continuous suction, Sauerbruch created a subatmospheric pressure inside the operating room equal to the pleural pressure, and the patient's head and upper airways were exposed to atmospheric pressure. In this way he expanded the lungs during open thoracotomy and theorized that the patient could breathe spontaneously while receiving inhalation anesthesia. Sauerbruch's "pneumatic chamber," as this contraption was called, solved a theoretical problem from the physiological point of view. However, even the most technically perfect chamber broke down during clinical use for several reasons: the surgeon and his assistants had very little room for movement; the heat was almost unbearable; and it was extremely difficult to communicate satisfactorily with the anesthetist outside the chamber. For these and other reasons, the differential pressure method was abandoned and today is nothing more than a historical curio.

The use of differential pressure chambers was never popular in the United States except with one surgeon, Willy Meyer, at the German Hospital in New York. In 1909 he and his brother Julius constructed a chamber for positive and/or negative differential pressure (Fig. 1-12). It was comprised of an outer negative chamber, which served as the operating room, and a positive inner pressure chamber, in which the anesthetist remained. Thus the surgeon could operate under negative pressure around the thorax or under positive pressure around the patient's head. A combination could also be employed, and a change from one to the other was possible during the same operation.

BACK TO THE DIRECT APPROACH

Controlled breathing had long been practiced by physiologists who kept their curarized animals alive by this means. Conditions of controlled breathing were clearly described in Meltzer's work, ''Respiratory Changes of Intrathoracic Pressure,'' which he published in 1892. The tubes employed were introduced through a tracheotomy. Apparently no one noticed the difference when Auer and Meltzer introduced oral intubation in 1909. Today controlled ventilation has become an integral part of general anesthesia, and physicians and respiratory therapists find it difficult to believe that a mystique still enshrouded tracheal intubation as late as 1950.

During the last decade of the nineteenth century, knowledge of respiration and the support thereof was more than adequate for the purpose of open chest surgery. It included understanding basic physiological principles, tracheal intubation with cuffed tubes, oxygen compressed in tanks, ventilators, devices for producing continuous positive pressure or intermittent positive pressure with retard of expiration, and apparatus for the administration of general anesthesia. In 1899 Rudolph Matas of New Orleans wrote: ''The procedure that promises the most benefit is . . . rhythmic main-

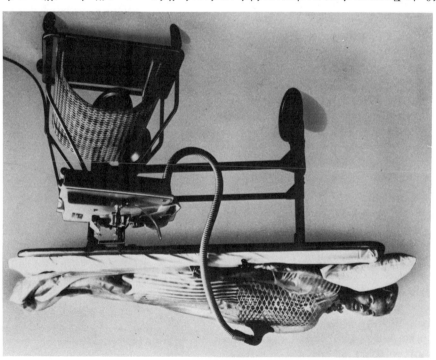

Fig. 1-10. An Emerson chest respirator which employed a light garment (''raincoat'') over the patient to effect the air seal and a shell over the chest and abdomen to hold the plastic garment away from the body. Intermittent negative pressure was developed inside the shell by a vacuum cleaner. Courtesy of J. H. Emerson Company.

tenance of artificial respiration by a tube in the glottis" (Fig. 1-13). On the European continent the simplest direct approach, combining artificial respiration with tracheal intubation, was presented by Franz Kuhn in Kassel, Germany in 1905. He was the first to pass a suction catheter through an endotracheal tube. In 1910 Läwen and Sievers, in Friedrich Trendelenburg's department in Leipzig, reported a piston ventilator which applied alternating positive and negative pressure, with supplemental oxygen through an endotracheal tube (Fig. 1-14).

The period from 1880 to 1910 was one of high hopes and a flurry of activity for thoracic surgeons. However, it failed because of a lack of antibiotics and blood transfusions. Mortality from sepsis and hemorrhage was high. Surgical techniques were often not sufficiently developed, bronchi and vessels being ligated en bloc. Billau's underwater drain was forgotten. The chest was closed air-tight, with sudden deaths resulting from bronchial leak and tension pneumothorax. For these reasons, and not because of failures to support ventilation, clinical activities decreased and experimental work increased.

For many decades the dangers of pneumothorax were overestimated because no apparent distinction was made between open and tension varieties. One of the mistakes involved the application of observa-

Fig. 1-11. Ernst Ferdinand Sauerbruck of Breslau, Germany developed a differential pressure chamber in 1904.

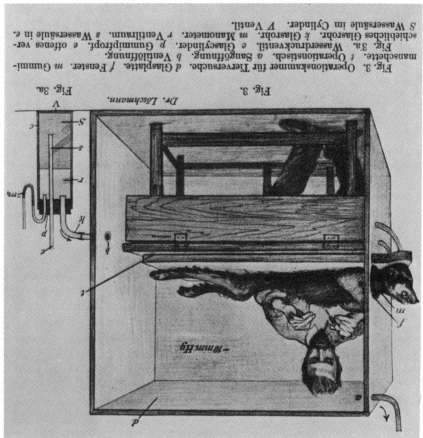

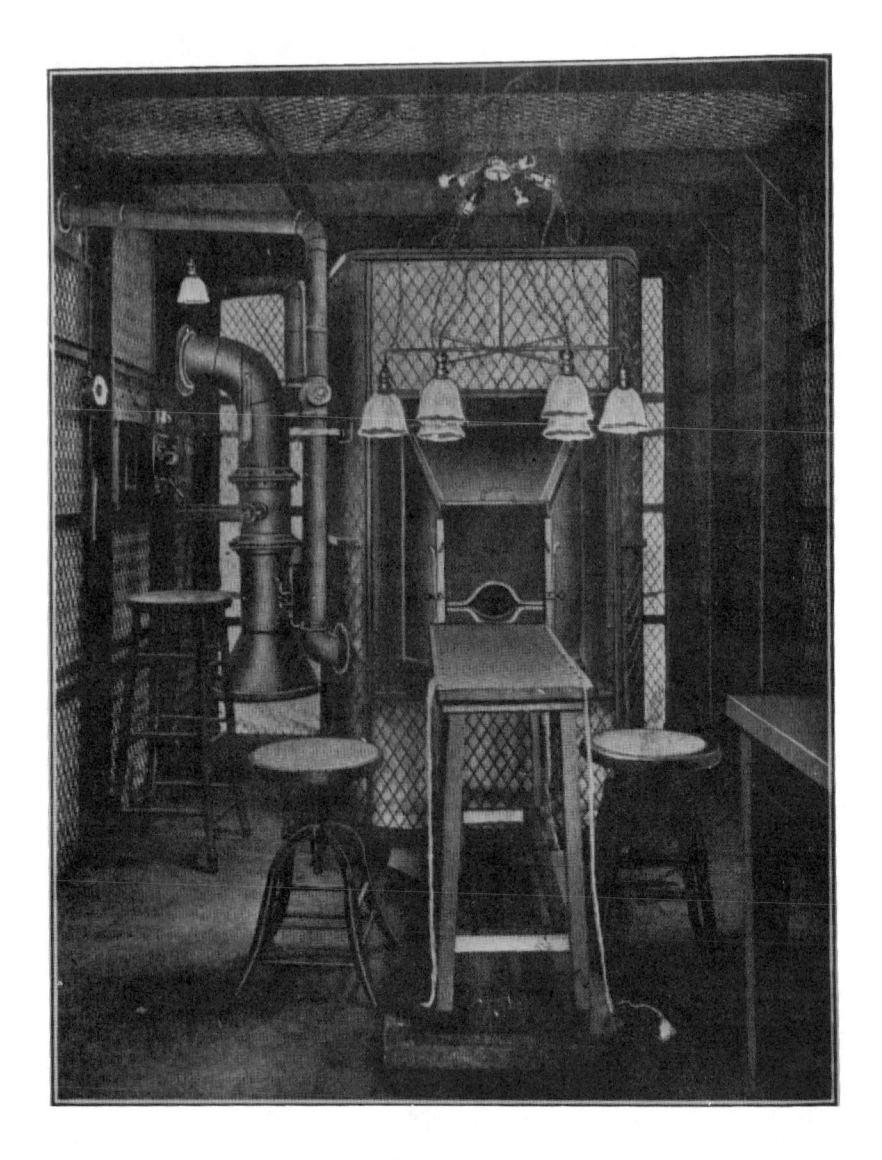

Fig. 1-12. In 1909 Dr. Willy Meyer of New York constructed a differential pressure chamber in which to perform thoracic surgical procedures.

tions made in animals directly to man. Not until the second decade of this century did the French surgeon Duval point out the fundamentally different nature of human and animal mediastina. In man the mediastinum is sufficiently firm to prevent spontaneous tearing if only one pleural space is opened. In contrast, because of the dog's delicate mediastinal septum, a unilateral open pneumothorax at once becomes bilateral.

Experimental Thoracic Surgery

From 1910 to 1930 significant advances occurred in experimental surgical and phys-

the end of the intratracheal catheter''), ex-actly the shape of the ones used today. He also developed the first modern laryngo-scope:

> The back of the tongue is touched with 10 percent cocaine; the patient is then anes-thetized, preferably by chloroform, in the usual manner and the catheter inserted into the trachea. This may be accom-plished by means of the Jackson direct lar-yngoscope so modified that it is deficient at the side in a manner permitting of the withdrawal of the instrument without the necessity of pushing the catheter through it—without detaching it from—the gas bag.

This laryngoscope was the first to use bat-teries in the handle. Janeway also appre-ciated the potentially adverse effect of pos-itive pressure on circulation. In many respects he was 20–30 years ahead of his time.

Unfortunately, as so often happens, these brilliant experimental surgeons evolved sat-isfactory solutions to the anesthetic and res-piratory problems they faced while they were young, enthusiastic, and idealistic, but they did not follow up their developments. Few interested assistants were available; anesthetic techniques were crude, poorly taught, and practiced by members of the house or nursing staff who were unenthu-siastic but could not avoid administering anesthesia for the next (not infrequently fatal) case. Perhaps the inventors did not try to persuade others of their ideas; or maybe as they grew older they saw that there was no money in research and much to be had in the treatment of patients. Their brilliant ideas languished and withered with nobody to follow up on them. Janeway left the field in 1914 to become a pioneer in radiother-apy. His respiratory machine was available at Presbyterian Hospital, but it was deemed too complicated to use and it never became popular (Fig. 1-15). Elsberg, one of the few surgeons who learned laryngoscopy for tra-

iological laboratories. Negative- and posi-tive-pressure cabinets never became pop-ular among American surgeons. Instead, they developed a variety of intralaryngeal tubes for direct introduction of air into the lungs from pumps especially devised for this purpose. In 1910, for example, the Phil-adelphia surgeon George Morris Dorrance and the New York surgeon C. A. Elsberg, as well as Läwen and Sievers from Tren-delenburg's department in Leipzig, all pub-lished outstanding works on these proce-dures. In 1913 Henry H. Janeway of New York described an ingenious machine for anesthesia and artificial respiration with a cuffed endotracheal tube (''a little rubber occluding bag with double wall, pulled over

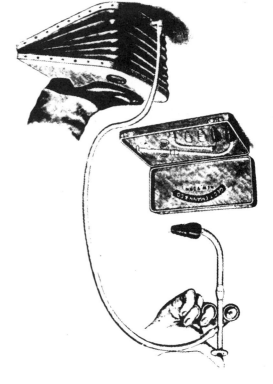

Fig. 1-13. In 1899 Rudolph Matas of New Or-leans described a procedure of artificial respi-ration achieved with endotracheal intubation and manual insufflation of air using the Fell-O'Dwyer Bellows.

cheal intubation and who developed the clinical usefulness of Meltzer's and Auer's insufflation methods, made a much better living as a neurosurgeon.

Small Portable Resuscitators

In 1907 the idea of using positive airway pressure during resuscitation was rediscovered by Heinrich Dräger of Lübeck, Germany. His famous "Pulmotor" was a small apparatus built into a suitcase. It consisted of two small concertina bags and a very stiff spring-and-toggle mechanism which activated a valve, giving a mixture of oxygen and air, sometimes with 5 percent carbon dioxide, at 3 kPa (20 mm Hg) pressure during inspiration. During expiration, a subatmospheric pressure of −3 kPa was applied, a dangerously low level that could easily cause airway collapse in certain patients.

The Pulmotor was designed for resuscitation in mines and gained great popularity over the next 40 years, particularly with fire departments and police rescue units. The general medical standard of resuscitation during the mid-1930s is illustrated by the fact that as a medical student I observed surgeons calling the fire department to bring their Pulmotor to treat patients in hospitals which had absolutely no means of resuscitation.

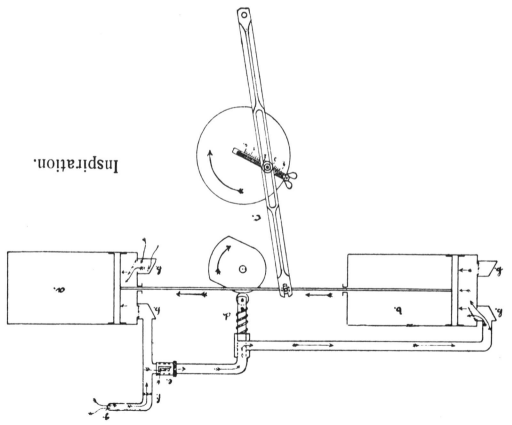

Inspiration.

Fig. 1-14. Lawen and Sievers of Leipzig, Germany developed a double-piston respirator in 1910. It provided mechanical inspiration and facilitated exhalation in intubated patients.

A great number of other smaller, hand-held resuscitators gained popularity during the many years before ventilators became commonly used. A few examples are the Kreiselman resuscitator (about 1940); Neff inflation valve (1945); Burn valve, especially designed for the Air Force (1946); Mushin and Hillard "Cardiff" valve (1953); Fink valve (1954); Digby-Leigh valve (1956); Frumin nonrebreathing valve; and Reed "Dewsbury" inflation valve (1959). Undoubtedly the most popular hand-operated resuscitator is the "Ambu-bag" designed in 1954 by Henning Ruben of Copenhagen. It is a simple, reliable instrument used for manual resuscitation in the emergency room and during transportation inside and outside the hospital—a resuscitator so good it has been copied dozens of times by other manufacturers. Today, rightfully so, it is found in most hospitals throughout the world.

Tracheal Intubation

Although Chevalier Jackson of Pittsburgh devoted his life to instructing anesthesiologists in "the technique of inserting intratracheal insufflation tubes," few paid any attention to the advantages of the technique. Positive-pressure methods which did not require intubation were preferred—tracheal intubation was still considered very difficult and very dangerous.

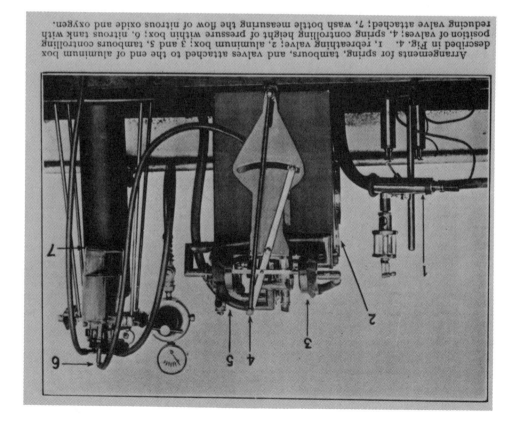

Arrangements for spring, tambours, and valves attached to the end of aluminum box described in Fig. 4. 1, rebreathing valve; 2, aluminum box; 3 and 5, tambours controlling position of valves; 4, spring controlling height of pressure within box; 6, nitrous tank with reducing valve attached; 7, wash bottle measuring the flow of nitrous oxide and oxygen.

Fig. 1-15. Janeway's anesthesia machine, which was constructed about 1910 at Columbia University.

Nevertheless, improvement in method-ology was achieved during the First World War by Ivan Whiteside Magill and E. S. Rowbotham of London while they served as anesthetists with the British Army plastic surgery unit in France. They modified, sim-plified, and publicized tracheal intubation. To them goes our gratitude for intubation as we know it today.

While studying in London in 1947, I had the privilege and great pleasure to listen to and learn from these two physicians. Magill was a technical master in anesthesia, charming and delightful to observe but somewhat less accomplished as a teacher. Rowbotham was a better teacher (and showman), who demonstrated his points in a direct, dry way. He was a chain-smoker and always smoked while giving anesthesia. While demonstrating that explosions only happened to those who did not know what they were doing, he enjoyed observing our reactions as he rested his lit cigarette on the ether vaporizer during ether anesthesia.

MODERN VENTILATORS

The evolution of present-day ventilators has been described in such a masterly fash-ion by Mushin, Rendell-Baker, Thompson, Mapleson, and Hillard that I refuse to even try to compete with them; instead, I prefer to quote them extensively, especially in the following pages.

Modern ventilators can, in fact, be traced back to Scandinavian initiatives taken in 1915 by Holger Mølgaard of Copenhagen, T. Thunberg of Lund, and especially by K. H. Giertz of Stockholm, in 1916. However, these three outstanding scientists all made the same unforgivable mistake! They pub-lished in Danish or Swedish, which in the scientific community was similar to writing in water. The data were hidden, lost, and forgotten almost as soon as it was written. Giertz, formerly one of Sauerbruch's as-sistants, showed experimentally that arti-ficial ventilation obtained through positive-pressure rhythmic insufflation was superior to every form of constant differential pres-sure breathing. He enlisted the help of the skilled ear, nose, and throat surgeon Paul Frenckner to evolve a series of endotra-cheal tubes. He also convinced the exper-imental engineer Emil Anderson of the AGA Company to develop an air-driven ventilator, the "Spiropulsator." Its essen-tial valve was the AGA flasher for auto-matic sea buoys, designed to send out pre-cisely timed flashes of burning acetylene. Clarence Crafoord used the Spiropulsator while working on the technical problems of pneumonectomy. The first commercial model of the Spiropulsator was offered in 1940; Mushin et al. write:

> Crafoord found the interest of his Amer-ican colleagues lukewarm, at best, when he demonstrated the "Spiropulsator" dur-ing operations on their patients. Among the exceptions were the experimental car-diac surgeons, Beck and Mautz of Cleve-land, who had already made their own sim-ilar version in 1939.

Unfortunately, Crafoord's demonstration in the USA ended with a loud BANG when the cyclopropane found it's way back to the source of the compressed air created by a vacuum cleaner with a sparking motor.

At the beginning of World War II, I was unable to import a Spiropulsator from Swe-den and was compelled, therefore, to com-mence the design and construction of my first piston ventilator in German-occupied Denmark (Fig. 1-16). Ole Lippmann of the medical instrument company of Simonsen and Weel had an excellent workshop in Co-penhagen with several highly skilled me-chanics. The mechanic who did most of my work was Arne Fin Schram, later the foun-der and owner of the competing instrument firm "Dameca." Because of the war, ma-terials were scarce. The piston and cylin-der, for example, had to be made from a discarded piece of dirty old sewer pipe from the streets of Copenhagen. The ventilator

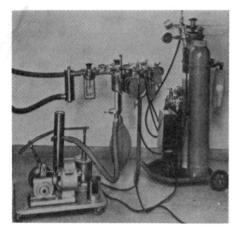

Fig. 1-16. In 1940 Ernst Trier Mörch designed his first piston ventilator.

rate was changed by a rheostat acting on an old electric brush-motor which sent out a continuous shower of sparks during the administration of nitrous oxide and ether. This, the first clinically proven volume ventilator, was used in a great number of thoracic operations performed by Erik Husfeldt, Tage Kjaer, and Jens Lyn Hansen between 1940 and 1949 in Denmark.

At a relatively early stage in my new career as anesthesiologist in Denmark, Henry Beecher from Harvard visited Copenhagen. After one of his lectures, he was asked about his technique for thoracic surgery anesthesia. He told the bewildered audience that he rarely used endotracheal tubes, never used curare or controlled respiration, and certainly never used a mechanical respirator. There I was, a young, unproved candidate for a new and important job, using all the commodities the "prophet" from Harvard had just condemned. My only defense was that most of my patients survived.

During 1946 and 1947 I was privileged to study anesthesia under Sir Robert Macintosh and William W. Mushin; I have never met better teachers. My first meeting with Sir Robert Macintosh was in the winter of 1945 when I applied for a position in his and Mushin's masterly teaching program. I

went to his office, and his secretary informed me that the professor was out skating on the meadows of Oxford. She asked me if I could skate, and when I answered affirmatively she gave me a pair of Sir Robert's skates. Thus we met while executing turns and pirouettes; both he and Mushin were elegant skaters.

Here again, I wish to quote from the masterpiece by Mushin et al:

> When Trier Mörch in a paper to the Royal Society of Medicine in London in 1947 enthusiastically advocated mechanical controlled respiration, he found in his audience some eager to try this new approach, one of them being Cecil Gray. By this time, surgeons in many European countries no longer needed to be convinced that the abolition of spontaneous respiration greatly eased their work within the chest and ensured excellent oxygenation and carbon dioxide elimination. The work of Ralph Waters of Madison on the carbon dioxide absorption and the use of cyclopropane was familiar to British anesthetists, and these methods were in widespread use by the time the war broke out. In 1941, Nosworthy described controlled respiration with cyclopropane for thoracic surgery. However, automatic apparatus for controlled respiration was at this time virtually unknown in the field. In Britain, the ready availability of skilled anesthetists, trained to meet the needs of the armed forces but back in civilian life, meant that increasingly, the surgeons left these problems to their colleagues.

The good reception of Mörch's advocacy of ventilators was in marked contrast to that accorded to Janeway and Jackson by an earlier generation of doctors. (This, however, was probably due as much to the advancements in blood transfusion, antibiotics, and surgical techniques as it was to timing and luck.)

A pharmacologist, Dennis E. Jackson of Cincinnati, Ohio, had repeatedly demonstrated the first commercially available anesthesia machine with a built-in ventilator and carbon dioxide absorption apparatus as early as 1927. Exasperated by their lack of acceptance, he wrote:

> 378 years ago Vesalius had demonstrated what artificial respiration may often accomplish. . . . It would appear, however, that the interval of time required for artificial respiration in the dog to evolute into artificial respiration in man may be almost as great as that required for an animal comparable to the dog to evolute into a man.

In 1944 K. B. Pinson of Manchester devised an automatic ventilator, "the pulmonary pump" (Fig. 1-17). He incorporated many refinements, but the apparatus consisted essentially of two piston pumps: One took over respiration, and the other employed suction to evacuate secretions or pus from the trachea and bronchial tree. Observing this very unusual and interesting ventilator in use was a pleasure. Dr. Pinson had come to the hospital the evening before surgery and assembled the pump in the operating room corridor. The next morning, however, it was discovered that the pump

was too large to fit through the door to the operating room. The case was postponed until the following day, the pump disassembled and then reassembled inside the operating room. Indeed, it worked very well!

During the Second World War, a motorcycle engineer, J. H. Blease of London, produced an anesthetic apparatus for a local physician. When the physician suddenly died, Mr. Blease found himself pressed into providing emergency anesthesia during the air raids on Merseyside. Put off by

> . . . the drudgery of manually controlled ventilation for thoracic surgery, in 1945 he built the first prototype of what was to become the "Pulmoflator." Though the reception of this prototype by some was skeptical, the convenience provided was especially appreciated when the introduction of curare during surgery necessitated artificial respiration throughout many other operations besides thoracic ones.

Blease's efforts were followed by designs of Esplen's "Aintree" ventilator in 1952 and the "Fazakerley" ventilator in 1956.

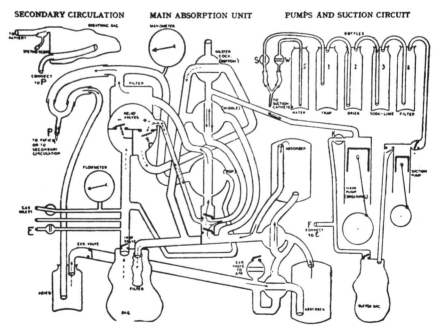

Fig. 1-17. A "simplified" illustration of "the pulmonary pump" devised in 1944 by K. B. Pinson of Machester.

ANESTHESIOLOGY PRINCIPLES IN RESPIRATORY CARE

One of the most revolutionary changes in respiratory care was attributable to the anesthesiologist Bjørn Ibsen of Copenhagen. In 1952 Scandinavia was struck by a poliomyelitis epidemic of unprecedented severity, and thousands of patients were hospitalized. From 24 July to 3 December the Hospital for Communicable Diseases in Copenhagen admitted 2722 polio patients, 315 of whom required respiratory support. Early in the epidemic, all patients were treated by the one tank and six cuirass respirators available. Uncuffed tracheostomy tubes were used to secure an open airway. Adequate humidification of inspired gas was not available. Effective chest physical therapy was hampered by body-enclosing respirators. Of the first 31 patients with respiratory paralysis admitted, 27 died within 3 days. When the 32nd patient, a 12-year-old girl was nearing a terminal state of respiratory insufficiency, Ibsen was consulted, and a tracheotomy was promptly performed, followed by insertion of a cuffed tracheostomy tube and initiation of manual artificial ventilation with a conventional Water's to-and-fro system. Improved oxygenation and correction of respiratory acidosis were followed by shock, but blood transfusions reestablished adequate circulation. Thus the patient had been improved by the measures usually carried out by the anesthetist in the operating theater.

The therapeutic principles demonstrated by Ibsen now became the accepted methods for management of respiratory paralysis throughout Northern Europe. Teams of "ventilators" consisting of nurse-anesthetists, interns, and medical students provided manual artificial ventilation and respiratory care in shifts during the epidemic. For several months the medical school in Copenhagen closed to allow its students to volunteer as "ventilators." At the peak of the epidemic, such teams were able to ventilate 75 patients simultaneously.

At first, professor H. C. A. Lassen was faced with a seemingly hopeless situation. About 500 patients were already in the hospital, and 50–60 new cases were coming in every day. However, with Ibsen's help, he quickly created an organization that worked extremely well. To give an impression of the magnitude of the task, Ibsen stated that within each 24-hour period the teams included 260 extra nurse auxillaries, 250 medical students, and 27 technicians just to handle the 250 large gas cylinders. A team of epidemiologists, ear-nose-throat specialists, and anesthesiologists worked with an excellent laboratory staffed by two full-time specialists and 15 technicians. Eventually, x-ray technicians and physiotherapists joined in as well. I cannot resist mentioning three of my now American friends who participated as anesthesiologists in this stupendous epoch: Henrik H. Bendixen (Columbia University, New York), Henning Pontoppidan (Massachusetts General Hospital, Boston), and Christian C. Rattenborg (University of Chicago).

The importance of care during transportation was demonstrated by many early tragic experiences when lay people alone accompanied the patients in the ambulance to the hospital. Aspiration often occurred, and on arrival at the hospital many patients were found to be moribund, some even dead.

Ibsen stressed that equipment for emergency respiration and suction must be available, even in the patient's home. He wanted help to come to the patient, not for the patient to go to the help. Thus teams went all over the country, by ambulance or by plane, to ensure safe patient transportation. When suctioning and ventilation, with either a bag and mask or a bag connected to an oral endotracheal or tracheostomy tube, were performed by trained personnel, a striking difference in results was noted in Copenhagen. Regional centers were soon established all over the country, and the overall mortality rate of patients with respiratory paralysis was reduced from 87 percent to less than 30 percent.

Most of the essential principles of positive-pressure mechanical ventilation and airway care were implemented during the 1952 Danish epidemic. Chest physical therapy with meticulous attention to postural drainage, manual assistance to coughing, and tracheobronchial aspiration of secretions were now universally applied. Inspired gas with partial rebreathing was humidified, albeit incompletely, in the to-and-fro system. More effective bypass humidifiers soon became available. Oxygen toxicity was avoided by using mixtures of nitrogen and oxygen. Orotracheal intubation preceded tracheotomy, thus eliminating the hazard of emergency tracheotomy without airway control. Large-bore, cuffed tracheostomy tubes were used to facilitate controlled ventilation and airway protection. Because blood gas and pH measurements were not available, adequacy of oxygenation was judged by clinical observation, measuring arterial oxygen saturation, or oximetry. Intermittent pulmonary hyperinflation, a forerunner of the "sighing" described in 1959 by Mead and Collier, were empirically applied to overcome the complaint of dyspnea commonly expressed by patients with ventilatory failure, despite what seemed to be adequate oxygenation and ventilation. As the patient's ability to breathe spontaneously improved, weaning was accomplished by gradual reduction in the number of assisted breaths, the forerunner of present-day intermittent mandatory ventilation (IMV). In many respects, and on an entirely empirical basis, the ventilation pattern provided by an "educated hand" proved to be physiologically superior to that provided by early mechanical ventilators. Toward the end of the epidemic, when a few Engström, Lundia, and Bang ventilators became available, they were often referred to as "mechanical students."

Similar experiences were reported in the United States. During a minor poliomyelitis epidemic in Kansas during 1951–1952, I treated a few patients with intermittent positive-pressure ventilation (IPPV) from my first American-made piston ventilator. Van Bergen of Minneapolis adopted Ibsen's methods of treatment during the polio epidemics in Minnesota and Western Canada in 1952 and developed his own ventilator. The New England region was struck by a severe epidemic of paralytic poliomyelitis in 1955. Anesthesiologists again assumed an important role in the care of patients with respiratory paralysis (Pontoppidan). At the Massachusetts General Hospital, an entire floor was converted to a poliomyelitis respiratory failure unit. At the height of that epidemic, 49 patients were mechanically ventilated at one time: Forty-six were in tank respirators and three were on the Jefferson ventilator, an early version of a volume-preset device capable of providing controlled ventilation. Once again, the superiority of IPPV was demonstrated, as it had been in 1899 by Matas, in 1905 by Kuhn, in 1910 by Läwen and Sievers, in 1916 by Giertz, in 1948 by Bower et al., and in 1952 by Ibsen. However, complications from inadequate humidification and tracheal trauma from tracheostomy tubes with high-pressure cuffs were still evident. Measurement of arterial oxygen saturation was the only clinically available method for assessing the adequacy of oxygenation at that time.

In 1960 one of my more memorable experiences was thrust on me when I suddenly became responsible for the care of Alon P. Winnie, now Chairman of the Department of Anesthesiology at the University of Illinois but then a surgical intern at Cook County Hospital in Chicago who was rotating through the anesthesia service. At 7 a.m. one morning he walked in complaining of a severe headache. Knowing that he was a popular party man, I presumed that he just had a hangover, so I gave him two aspirins and asked him to get going. An hour later he looked and was really sick, so I released him from work. I have never seen any case of bulbospinal poliomyelitis so violent and fulminant. By 4:00 p.m. I had performed a tracheostomy on him and connected him to a Mörch piston respirator placed under his bed.

(Winnie has an unusual sense of humor. One of his favorite fables was his admiration for my taking care of "the whole patient". On the evening of his admission he had a date with a beautiful young student nurse. Realizing that he would not be able to fulfill this obligation, I took her out dancing in the Pump Room at the Ambassador Hotel. Now this is Winnie's version)!

Ancillary Uses of Mechanical Ventilator

Finally, after several months of serious, paralytic poliomyelitis, Al Winnie was discharged from Cook County Hospital. In gratitude, Al threw a party in his 3rd floor apartment near the hospital for all the interns and residents who had cared for him. The main beverage streamed merrily from 2 large kegs of beer until at midnight the party was in grave danger when the pump failed, and beer would no longer leave the keg.

Unseen by the rest of the party, Trier Mörch sneaked out, returned to the hospital, found the very ventilator which had been breathing for Winnie only a few months earlier and dragged it across the street, and up the long, steep stairway. After a few on-the-spot modifications, Mörch adjusted the machine to run at low volume, high speed and high pressure to pump air into the kegs, and—mirabile dictu—the beer was again streaming down the throats of an appreciative crowd. Never did one mechanical ventilator save so many "patients" at one time!

Tracheobronchial Suction

Infection around the tracheostomy tube is always present. One of the many means to keep the infection to a minimum is careful, gentle aspiration with a sterile catheter (to be done as rarely as possible). It is difficult for our younger colleagues to realize how such care was carried out a score or more years ago.

In those days, before disposable plastic suction catheters were introduced, suction was performed with one red rubber urethral catheter of the type used on old prostatic men. In better hospitals the catheter was changed at *least* once daily! After use, it was "cleansed" by sucking saline (which also had been sterile in the early morning) through it; it was then stored in a container with some old cloudy alcohol, hoping that this procedure would resterilize it. When needed next time, it was taken from the solution and introduced into the trachea, which now also suffered the additional chemical irritation of the alcohol.

At Cook County Hospital we never had enough nurses; very often one nurse alone would look after 40 sick patients. To these dedicated but badly overworked nurses' irritation and consternation, I insisted on 10 red rubber catheters, preferably of the coudé type, for each patient daily. Each catheter was wrapped in a separate towel and sterilized. I was undoubtedly the first, at least in the Middle West, to use sterile catheters for each suctioning. I still have not completely accommodated to today's expense and waste of beautiful, sterile, disposable catheters.

Piped-In Artificial Ventilation

The recovery room at Cook County Hospital in Chicago had space for 50 patients in 2 large rooms. In a corner of each room was a Mörch Piston Respirator connected to a 25 mm (1 inch) pipe, which was mounted on all the walls. At each patient station was an outlet with a stopcock. Rhythmic pulses of compressed air could thus be available at each station without moving the respirator. From the stopcock a rubber hose could guide the air to a plastic cylinder surrounding a concertina shaped bag. The humidified air-oxygen mixture inside the concertina bag could then be directed to the patient at the desired volume and pressure. In this way 1,2, or 3 patients could be ventilated from the same respirator.

THE END OF POLIOMYELITIS ANTERIOR ACUTA

Introduction of the Salk and the Sabin poliomyelitis vaccines and their use in mass immunization campaigns in the United States practically eradicated poliomyelitis. The National Foundation for Infantile Paralysis shifted its attention to other fields, and the polio respirator centers it had supported closed about 1960. As a result, the use of mechanical ventilators declined sharply during the next few years. Those few patients requiring ventilator support were cared for on general hospital wards. Complications and mortality rates were high, in large measure because of inexperience of the personnel and mechanical failure of airway equipment or ventilators. For the most part, only a few patients with potentially reversible neuromuscular diseases or drug-induced coma, particularly from barbiturates, were treated successfully.

Eventually, an increase in the number of patients requiring mechanical ventilation prompted the reestablishment of respiratory units, now most often called intensive or critical care units.

INTERMITTENT POSITIVE-PRESSURE BREATHING

IPPB was described by Irwin Ziment of the University of California at Los Angeles. In 1937 Barach, Eckman, and Ginsburg and in 1945 Motley, Cournand, and Werkö, all of Columbia University in New York, were among the first to suggest that IPPB had therapeutic indications other than the maintenance of artificial respiration in completely apneic subjects. Barach and co-workers treated patients with pulmonary edema and other pulmonary diseases. Their studies found important application in the methods of oxygen delivery to pilots flying at high altitudes during World War II. Motley et al. treated a number of conditions, including respiratory insufficiency caused by barbiturates, carbon monoxide, or alcohol; paralysis caused by central nervous system pathology; acute asthmatic attacks; and postoperative thoracic surgery cases. They used the "Burns pneumatic balance resuscitator" developed for the Air Force.

Around that time, V. Ray Bennett developed the "Bennett clinical research model (Ben X-2) valve" which permitted intermittent delivery of oxygen under pressure during inspiration; subsequently the Bennett family of respirators was introduced into pulmonary medicine as a result of the studies of Motley and his colleagues. By 1950 IPPB had started its meteoric use as a major type of therapy for various disorders of the lung. Shortly thereafter, entry of Bird pressure-cycled respirators into the medical field led to a form of competition in which the operational characteristics of the rival instruments became the major consideration, overshadowing the questionable therapeutic value of IPPB.

Nevertheless, for many years the Bird equipment was very popular in the United States and abroad. Bird nebulizers were superior and were used extensively in the treatment of chronic obstructive pulmonary disease (COPD). Forrest Bird maintained an attractive school for inhalation therapy and provided a free IPPB clinic in Palm Springs, California at a time when very few such facilities existed.

Many other ventilators subsequently were introduced, some of which received enthusiastic commendations, although little evidence suggested that there was any one outstanding model or even that IPPB was clinically efficacious.

A major turning point in development occurred in 1954 when Engström introduced his excellent and highly sophisticated piston ventilator, which the following year was used by Björk and Engström for postoperative support of pulmonary resection patients. This therapy, which they pioneered, is still widely accepted for cardiac surgical patients, as well as for many other individuals who have undergone a variety of major operative procedures.

CRUSHING INJURIES OF THE CHEST

During the 1950s the treatment of severe crushed chest injuries was directed for the first time toward the maintenance of adequate ventilation. N. K. Jensen of Minneapolis used what was later described as positive end-expiratory pressure (PEEP) in 1952, and in 1953 tracheostomy was advocated by Carter and Guiseffi. In June 1954 an acute emergency led A. E. Avery, D. W. Benson and me to devise a new management technique for this problem.

A husky 51-year-old worker was directing a pack train in a Chicago steel mill. As the train approached, he stepped back, forgetting that he stood in front of a furnace. He was slowly crushed and rolled into an 8-inch "sausage." Upon admission to the hospital, he was moribund and in deep shock, with multiple bilateral fractures of all ribs, costochondral separations, bilateral tension hemopneumothoraces, fractures of the sternum, clavicles, and pelvis, crushing injuries of the liver and genitourinary tract, paralytic ileus, and acute gastric dilatation.

His chest wall was partially stabilized with soft tissue traction by the method of Hudson; long metal pins were passed under the pectoralis and serratus anterior muscles; spreader bows were attached, and traction was applied from an overhead frame. In spite of all efforts, he was slowly dying from shock, pulmonary edema, and respiratory acidosis. We then realized that his major problem was inadequate ventilation and that we had to breathe for him. An Ambu bag and later a Mörch piston ventilator were attached to his tracheostomy tube. The patient improved minute by minute from a semicomatose state with respiratory acidosis to a comfortable and alert state with respiratory alkalosis.

The two most important factors in this treatment were: First, NO active muscular movements of the ribs were allowed because this would displace the many fragments. This state was achieved by deliberate overventilation until apnea occurred. (Only if acidosis was present was it necessary to give sedatives or narcotics.) Second, NO negative pressure was applied in the chest in order to prevent paradoxical respirations.

We were amazed to observe how rapidly the numerous rib fragments moved back into place under the influence of IPPV. Because the force of air pressure on each fragment was proportional to the underlying pulmonary area, the lungs acted as splints. The patient was kept overventilated in respiratory alkalosis for 30 days. CO_2 and pH of the blood were checked twice daily. He was discharged from the hopsital 51 days after the injury and returned to work. Since that case in 1954, this therapy has been preferred for severe cases of crushed chest.

The Mörch piston ventilator (Fig. 1-18) used in this case was the first modern volume unit and became very popular during the mid-1950s. In was simple to use, having only two variants: rate and volume. The cylinder was an 8-inch (20 cm) diameter sleeve from a large diesel engine, and the piston rings were made of Teflon, which is nearly indestructible. Rate selection was controlled by a robust mechanism built originally for antiaircraft guns in the U.S. Navy. A stainless steel 12 mm (0.5 inch) ball in the exhalation valve was from a ball bearing.

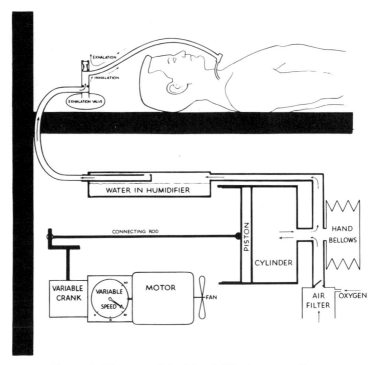

Fig. 1-18. Diagram of the Mörch III piston ventilator.

The cylinder assembly was the only part in contact with air going to the patient and could be sterilized easily by boiling, autoclaving, or treating with chemicals. The entire unit was so low it could be placed under the patient's bed; thus it did not take up any additional floor space, an important consideration because most hospital rooms were small. It was a very reliable machine which required almost no maintenance. The chief physician at the largest "respirator center" in Chicago tried all the ventilators. When I asked him why he used the Mörch so rarely, he answered, "Oh, we keep the Mörch in reserve for when the other machines fail."

SAGA OF THE UNCUFFED TRACHEAL TUBE

In Kansas City in 1952 I was treating a polio patient using a cuffed tracheostomy tube and the Mörch piston ventilator. One night the occlusive cuff ruptured. The nurse called me, and I was afraid we might lose the patient before I could get there (I lived 15 min from the hospital). However, she told me to take my time because she had simply increased the volume until the chest moved normally. This episode convinced me that we did not need a cuff at all. Any leak which was present depended on the ratio of the diameters of the trachea and the tracheal tube and on several other factors. We found empirically that the correct volume was about three times the tidal volume; thus if an adult patient needed 500 ml tidal volume but the leak around the tube was 1000 ml, the ventilator had to be set to deliver a 1500 ml tidal volume. Many patients could tell us the correct volume as well as when they had bronchial obstruction (often delineating which side the obstruction was on). In patients with polio who had normal or even decreased lung thorax compliance, the volume of air moving down the tracheal tube at a high velocity was greater than that lost even in the presence of a sizable leak.

This uncuffed system was described in 1956 by Mörch, Saxton and Gish. Possible advantages included the absence of tracheal pressure necrosis, a real risk if the cuff was overinflated; improved pulmonary toiletry as the leaking air blew particulate matter or secretions up into the pharynx, where the patient or nursing staff could remove them; the ability to talk—even if it was—only the time while—the machine was—blowing the air up—between the vocal cords. To be able to talk at all was a major improvement.

I treated a patient in Michigan who broke his neck diving in a gravel pit in 1960, and today he is still alive and talking—synchronously with the ventilator inflation. In most patients, however, it is desirable to use a cuff on the endotracheal or tracheostomy tube. Ideally, the cuff should be inflated until there is a "microscopic" annular space between its wall and the trachea; one should be able to hear a tiny leak, big enough to prevent pressure damage to the mucosa but so small it does not interfere with effective ventilation.

Motion of the tracheostomy tube transmitted from the rhythmic inflation and deflation of the connecting tubes can be decreased by positioning a swivel connector between the tracheal tube and the ventilator circuit. I invented the first such swivel adaptor and described it with Saxton in 1956.

THE ERA OF "ASSISTED" VENTILATION

In the United States, unlike Scandinavia, Britain, and some other countries of Europe, the value of controlled respiration during anesthesia—to say nothing of automatic ventilation—was strongly disputed as late as the 1950s. Though puzzled over the occurrence of both metabolic and respiratory acidosis, both surgeons and anesthesiologists doubted the value of automatically controlled ventilation. The dangers of explosion and the unsatisfactory pulmonary ventilation sometimes produced by stubborn anesthesiologists who did not learn to use the machines appropriately were thought to outweigh any possible advantages. Instead, they preferred:

> . . . respiration carefully assisted by the anesthetist, by squeezing the bag just as the patient inspires . . . feeling that this . . . gives the most effective type of ventilation. [One anesthesiologist commented that he] did not mean to imply that we have a closed mind about ways of improving the situation. [Maybe] it would be desirable for the surgeons to consider the possibility of other operating positions for these cases. We anesthetists, on our side, must find improved ways of *assisting respiration.*

As late as 1951, when I became head of the Department of Anesthesia at the University of Chicago, I was told by a surgeon on the staff "NO endotracheal tube, NO controlled respiration, NO curare, and—naturally—NO automatic breathing machines!" When I objected, it was hesitatingly conceded that only in extreme emergency situations would I be permitted to do whatever I deemed best for the patient. Shortly thereafter, an "emergency situation" occurred followed by others in slowly increasing numbers until we practiced the type of anesthesia I was used to. There were no objections (because the patients were doing better than previously).

Many anesthesiologists in the United States insisted that assisted ventilation was safer than controlled ventilation. They resisted the introduction of ventilators which, as a result, were quite rare in American operating rooms during the 1950s and early 1960s. The impetus for their adoption and increasing use came from cardiac surgeons involved in a concerted attack on the problems of open heart surgery.

CONTROLLED VENTILATION

Surgical pioneers (e.g., Beck and Blalock of Johns Hopkins; Brunn, Churchill, and Crafoord of Stockholm; Graham of St. Louis; and Nissen of Basel, Switzerland) and cardiac surgeons (including Albritten and Gibbon, the pioneer of pump oxygenators, of Philadelphia; and Dennis of New York), like Läwen, Sievers, and Mautz before them, showed that mechanical artificial ventilation enhanced the results of their work by providing more efficient carbon dioxide elimination and oxygenation.

One of the first commercially available anesthesia ventilators in the United States resulted from efforts in Philadelphia. Beck's technical assistant, Kenneth Wolfe, with the help of the engineer H. J. Rand, produced a simple and sturdy successor to the Mautz ventilator for everyday use in cardiac surgery in 1950. John Gibbon's brother, who was the president of an engineering company, and his engineer Chris Andreason improved it and produced the widely used "Jefferson ventilator." The benefits of automatic ventilation slowly became recognized by surgeons and anesthesiologists alike, and other anesthesia ventilators became commercially available, including the Mörch surgical ventilator (1955), the Stephenson "CRU" (1956), the Bennett ventilator (1957), and the Bird Mark 4 ventilator (1959).

The Mörch anesthesia ventilator incorporated several unique features: (1) It was the first ventilator in the United States to have a concertina-shaped bellows, an idea taken from the Blease and Oxford ventilators (Fig. 1-18). This feature enabled a reading of the tidal volume. (2) It was available as a separate unit or as a built-in component of several popular anesthesia machines. (3) It was the first ventilator in which all the parts in contact with the inspired gas could easily be cleaned or even sterilized. (4) It was the first ventilator that could be used either as a pressure-sensitive assistor or as a volume-controlled ventilator. (5) Most of the controls could be operated by foot.

The working principle was that of an air pressure amplifier based on two commercially available valves made by Johnson Control, Inc. (Milwaukee, WI). The first was an air-driven switch intended as a remote control for an electrical switch to enable its use in areas with flammable or explosive gases and liquids. This switch was activated by a large diaphragm in the ventilator and thus was sensitive to small variations in pressure. It regulated the air to a second three-way valve with larger openings for the air or oxygen that acted on the concertina breathing bag.

A bewildering array of ventilators for use in and out of the surgical suite have since been produced, some of which seem to have pursued sophistication as an end in itself. Often we have to decide whether to sacrifice reliability and simplicity for the sometimes dubious advantages that a highly sophisticated piece of apparatus may provide. Many of the newer ventilators are described elsewhere in this book.

EXPANDED FIELDS FOR SUPPORTIVE VENTILATION

Until the mid-1950s, ventilation had been applied only in 1909 by H. Emerson for the treatment of pulmonary edema in the field of resuscitation, for poliomyelitis, and in a few pioneering cases of anesthesia. By the late 1960s, however, mechanical ventilation was used widely in other areas, and new/rediscovered techniques appeared.

Idiopathic Respiratory Distress Syndrome

The idiopathic respiratory distress syndrome (IRDS) occurs primarily in premature infants. Infants so affected need resuscitation because each breath requires an extraordinary effort. With progression of the disease, they become tachypneic, often with alternating periods of apnea. If left untreated, they die. Yet careful support, from simple increases of inspired oxygen to fully controlled mechanical ventilation, is associated with a better than 80 percent survival.

Adult Respiratory Distress Syndrome

Adult RDS (ARDS) usually is caused by serious pulmonary injury or illness. Most of the patients have no history of previous pulmonary or cardiac illness. Symptoms and signs vary but usually include severe dyspnea, tachypnea, bloody sputum, cyanosis, and elevated minute ventilation. The lungs become "stiff" with patchy alveolar infiltrates and may require 40 to 60 cm H_2O inspiratory pressure (or more) to achieve adequate tidal volumes. Without adequate treatment, death may occur within 24–48 hours.

Pulmonary dysfunction of this type has been known since World War I and has been called "shock lung," "wet lung," "Da Nang lung," "posttraumatic pulmonary insufficiency," etc. It has been the focus of extensive research and treatment because of the high rates of associated morbidity and mortality, which still occur. Prolonged artificial ventilation is still a mainstay of support.

Positive End-Expiratory Pressure

More than four decades ago Barach and associates recognized that breathing with an elevated airway pressure was often therapeutic in the resolution of pulmonary edema associated with congestive heart failure. They increased airway pressure with a motor-driven blower and an expiratory valve, both connected to the patient's airway through a face mask. This technique—constant (or continuous) positive-pressure breathing (CPPB)—was used in 1952 by H. K. Jensen of Minneapolis to treat pulmonary contusion in spontaneously breathing patients with crush injuries of the chest.

In 1959 Frumin, Bergman, Holaday, et al. found that their patients' arterial oxygen tension was improved by adding positive end-expiratory pressure (PEEP). This observation was later confirmed by Ashbaugh et al. from Denver and McIntyre et al. from Toronto in the treatment of ARDS.

PEEP may prevent alveolar collapse by maintaining positive airway pressure throughout the respiratory cycle. A higher functional residual capacity and better overall ventilation/perfusion ratio results. Other potential benefits include a reduction in pulmonary blood flow and capillary stasis and congestion.

Intermittent Mandatory Ventilation

Weaning of patients from prolonged mechanical ventilation may present difficult problems. Several measurable variables have been used to predict whether ventilator support can be discontinued (Bendixen et al., 1965; Pontoppidan et al., 1970). Trial-and-error methods often were resorted to, with their inherent dangers of hypoventilation, hypoxia, undue stress, and anxiety.

Some of these problems were lessened when Kirby et al. introduced intermittent mandatory ventilation (IMV) as a treatment mode for neonates with IRDS in 1971; and Downs et al. from the University of Florida in Gainesville, proposed IMV as an aid to wean adult patients from mechanical ventilatory support.

IMV requires a system in which the patient may breathe spontaneously from a reservoir while the ventilator provides positive-pressure (mandatory) breaths of adjustable volume and timed intervals. As the patient's ability to breathe improves, the number of mandatory breaths is gradually reduced until completely spontaneous ventilation is achieved. Other variables (V_T, PEEP, F_{IO_2}, etc.) may be maintained constant during the period of rate adjustment.

One potential shortcoming of IMV is that the positive-pressure inflation may be out of phase with the patient's spontaneous ventilation. To avoid the possibility of poor coordination between patient and ventilator, synchronized IMV (SIMV),* also called intermittent demand ventilation (IDV) or intermittent assisted ventilation (IAV), has been popularized by several investigators, including Svein Harboe at the University of Oslo, Norway. Harboe used a new, improved model 900B of the Siemens-Elema servo ventilator which produced patient-triggered sighs during spontaneous breathing. The expired minute volume (EMV) was displayed continuously on the panel during spontaneous breathing as well as during controlled ventilation, with or without PEEP or CPAP.

IMV and IAV have many alleged advantages. For example, the patient starts quickly to train his own respiratory muscles, which may prevent the irregular breathing patterns frequently seen after prolonged disuse with controlled mechanical ventilation (Pontoppidan et al., 1970). In addition, regular "sighing" offered by IMV/IAV may prevent atelectasis (Bendixen et al., 1964).

FLUIDIC-CONTROLLED VENTILATORS

Fluidic-controlled ventilators have become popular in many countries because they are less sensitive to outside interferences, e.g., temperature fluctuation, vibration, and electricity. Also there are no moving mechanical parts. Fluidic systems utilize moving streams of liquid or gas for sensing, logic, amplification, and controls. Most elements operate either on wall attachment or beam deflection principles.

When a high-speed stream of air or other fluids emerge from a nozzle, air is entrained from all sides (the Bernoulli effect). When a wall is placed close to the jet on one side, less air enters from that side, causing pressure to fall even more here and the jet to be "sucked" over against the wall. This is called the surface or wall attachment effect. As is often the case, the basic phenomenon is by no means new. It was reported in 1800 by Thoman Young and is also called the "Coanda effect" after a Romanian aeronautic engineer, Dr. Henri Coanda, who designed, built, flew, and in 1910 destroyed the first jet-propelled aircraft in Paris.

Coanda's first, last, and only test flight took place at the Issy-les-Moulineaux airport, just outside the old walls around Paris. To start his test, Coanda took his flying machine to the end of the field farthest away from the Paris wall. At the start, the airplane emerged from a sheet of flame and a cloud of smoke, flying straight for the Paris wall. Coanda reported:

> . . . apparently I had given it too much fuel—when I looked over the side, I saw raw flames shooting out, and that should not be. Not with my wooden wings full of petrol. I ducked inside to adjust matters. A moment later, things felt very differently. I looked outside again to find myself many feet in the air. Straight ahead of me was the Paris wall. I didn't know what to do. I pulled on the control wheels, the machine went up on one wing and I was thrown out. The machine crashed right at the foot of the wall.

Fortunately, Coanda was not seriously hurt, but the plane was burnt and nobody was interested in his jet engine. To his dismay, Coanda noted that the mica deflector plates, intended to deflect the exhaust away from the fuselage, actually had pulled the flames toward it. Later, he invented a flying saucer as well as improved burners for central heating furnaces, and developed a revolutionary new agricultural insecticide spray, but he did nothing further related to fluidic controls.

Today's knowledge of fluidic systems is based mainly on the systematic and ingenious teamwork around 1959 of Billy M. Horton, Raymond W. Warren, and Ronald E. Bowles at the Army's Harry Diamond Laboratories in Washington, D.C. The first fluidic ventilator was designed for the Army in 1964 by Barila, Meyer, and Mosley and other anesthesiologists from the Walter Reed Army Institute for Research working with engineers from the Harry Diamond Laboratories.

Commercial versions of the U.S. Army's simple resuscitators and ventilators have since been designed and built by several companies, e.g., Bowles Fluidic Corporation, in cooperation with the Rectec Co. in Portland, Oregon (1967); Senko Medical (Japan), Mine Safety Appliance Co (U.S.), and French companies that made the ventilators called ''Airox R'' and ''VP 2000,'' which utilized pure fluidic components in 1969 for resuscitation and respiratory therapy. The first versatile complex, commercial fluidic ventilator, the ''Hamilton Standard PAD,'' appeared in 1970 and was very similar to the Corning Co.'s ventilator described in 1973 by R. K. Smith. This was followed by the ''Monaghan 225'' in 1973, the ''Ohio Medical 550'' in 1974, and the North American Dräger in 1975.

HIGH-FREQUENCY VENTILATION

In 1667 Robert Hook reported to the Royal Society in London:

> . . . I formerly tryed of keeping a Dog alive after his Thorax was all display'd by cutting away of the Ribbs and Diaphragme; and after the Pericardium of the Heart also was taken off.—the Dog being kept alive

by the Reciprocal blowing of the Lungs with Bellows, and they suffered to subside, for the space of an hour or more, after his Thorax and been so display'd and his Aspera arteria cut off just below the epiglottis, and bound on upon the nose of the Bellows.

The exact function of the lungs was at that time in some doubt, and Hooks reported that:

> Some eminent Physitians had affirm'd that the Motion of the Lungs was necessary to Life upon the account of promoting the Circulation of the Blood, and that it was conceiv'd, the Animal would immediately be suffocated as soon as the Lungs should cease to be be moved.

Hook did not believe this and to disprove it carried out another experiment which he describes as follows:

> I caused another pair of Bellows to be immediately joyn'd to the first, by a contrivance, I had prepar'd, and pricking all the outer-coat of the Lungs with the slendar point of a very sharp pen-knife, this second pair of Bellows was mov'd very quick, whereby the first pair was always kept full and always blowing into the Lungs; by which means the Lungs also were alwayes kept very full, and without any motion; there being a continual blast of Air forc'd into the Lungs by the first pair of Bellows, supplying it as fast, as it could find its way quite through the Coat of the Lungs by the small holes priked in it, as was said before. This being continues for a pretty while, the Dog lay still—and his Heart being very regularly. . . .

Hook foreshadowed future oxygenators when he reported that:

> . . . I shall shortly try, whether suffering the Blood to circulate through a vessel, so as it may be openly exposed to the fresh Air, will not suffice for the life of an Animal.

On 2 March 1955 J. H. Emerson of Arlington, Massachusetts applied for a United

States patent, later granted as No. 2,913,197: Apparatus For Vibrating Portions of a Patient's Airway.

> This invention pertains to an apparatus for treating a patient by vibrating a column of gas which is in communication with his airway at a rate which is greater than the patient's normal rate—from 100 to more than 1500 vibrations per minute—vibrating the column of gas doubtless causes the gas to diffuse more rapidly within the airway and therefore aids in the breathing function by circulating the gas more thoroughly to and from the walls of the lungs.

Modern era high-frequency ventilation (HFV) was introduced in 1967 and later widely publicized by Ulf Sjöstrand in Sweden as a means to maintain respiratory gas exchange without major changes in intrapleural pressure or thoracic volumes. For the experimenter, HFV offers a means of ventilation which does not interfere with accurate observation and measurement of cardiovascular responses to pharmacological and other interventions. To the clinician, HFV hopefully will minimize additional cardiovascular impairment in patients whose ventilatory and/or cardiovascular systems are severely compromised.

An impressive amount of research has been performed and published. It is still difficult to compare the experiences of different investigators because of the variability in techniques, waveforms at different frequencies [most often between 1 Hz (60/min) and 20 Herz (1200/min)], tidal volume, amplitude, energy source, and pressure.

THE FUTURE

Fifty years from now, future colleagues may review our current efforts and wonder at primitive and bewildering changes in concepts, theories, and practices of mechanical ventilation. Indeed, in this area no previous time has been as restlessly changing and as interesting as our own. Improvements will continue; for example, the era of servo and computerized equipment has just begun. Adaptation of the servo control method was attempted by Frumin and Lee in 1957 with their "Autoanestheton," in which end-expired carbon dioxide was sampled and the results used to adjust the ventilator through a feedback circuit. Similar concepts may be based on the oxygen tension, pH, or brain activity, as was reported during the 1940s by Albert Faulconer at the Mayo Clinic. More recently, the Siemens-Elema Servo 900 series of ventilators have been developed to compensate for changes in the patient's airway resistance or compliance.

Large numbers of ventilators, monitors, and other "gadgets" have been invented, and some are even useful! A good ventilator gives us a third hand, so that we can better observe and treat the patient. There will always be a need for well-educated, conscientious physicians, nurses, and respiratory therapists who understand the monitors and who use them well in our most important task: to safeguard those who sleep and those whose lives and very survival are in our hands.

ADDENDUM

I thank the editors for inviting me to write this chapter. I am old enough to be part of history, to have been in the midst of this wonderful and progressive century. Many of the personalities mentioned are or were my teachers, many my friends, and I thank y'all!

REFERENCES

Abel FL, Waldhausen JA: Effects of anesthesia and artificial ventilation on caval flow and cardiac output. J Appl Physiol 25:479, 1968

Abel FL, Waldhausen JA: Respiratory and cardiac effects on venous return. Am Heart J 78:266, 1969

Abrahams N, Fisk GC, Vonwiller JB, Grant GC: Evaluation of infant ventilators. Anaesth Intensive Care 3:6, 1975

Adams H, Ellis BN, Kaye G: A new respiratory pump. Aust J Exp Biol Med Sci 28:657, 1950

Adams AP, Eronomides AP, Finlay WEI, Sykes MK: The effects of variations in inspiratory flow waveform on cardio-respiratory function during controlled ventilation in normo-, hypo- and hypervolemic dogs. Br J Anaesth 42:818, 1970

Adamson TM, Collins LM, Delan M, et al: Mechanical ventilation in newborn infants with respiratory failure. Lancet 2:227, 1968

Adelman MH, Berman RA, Touroff ASW: A new method of automatic controlled respiration. J Thorac Surg 19:817, 1950

Adelman MH, Berman RA, Touroff ASW: Automatic controlled respiration. Anesthesiology 10:673, 1949

Adelman MH, Megibow SJ, Blum L: A method of automatic controlled respiration for anesthesia in the dogs. Surgery 28:1040, 1950

Agostoni E, Miserocchi G: Vertical gradient of transpulmonary pressure with active and artificial lung expansion. J Appl Physiol 29:705, 1970

Agostino R, Orzalesi M, Nodari S, et al: Continuous positive airway pressure (CPAP) by nasal cannula in the respiratory distress syndrome (RDS) of the newborn. Pediatr Res 7:50, 1973

Ahlgren EW and Stephen CR: Mechanical ventilation of the infant. Anesthesiology 27:692, 1966

Ahlström H, Jonson B, Svenningsen NW: Continuous positive airway pressure with a face chamber in early treatment of idiopathic respiratory distress syndrome. Acta Paediatr Scand 62:433, 1973

Allbritten FF, Haupt GJ, Amadeo JH: The change in pulmonary alveolar ventilation achieved by aiding the deflation phase of respiration during anesthesia for surgical operations. Ann Surg 140:569, 1954

Almeida JJ Cabral de: Novo método de respiração controlada mecânicamente. Rev Bras Anestesiol 1:117, 1951

Amaha K, Liu P, Weitzner SW, et al: Effects of constant chest compression on the mechanical and physiological performance of different ventilators. Anesthesiology 28:498, 1967

Ambiavagar M, Jones ES: Resuscitation of the moribund asthmatic; use of intermittent and positive pressure ventilation, broncheal lavage and intravenous infusion. Anaesthesia 22:375, 1967

Andersen EW, Ibsen B: The anaesthetic management of patients with poliomyelitis and respiratory paralysis. Br Med J 1:786, 1954

Andersen MN, Kuchinbak K: Depression of cardiac output with mechanical ventilators. J Thorac Surg 54:182, 1967

Andersen E, Crafoord C, Frenckner P: A new and practical method of producing rhythmic ventilation during positive pressure anesthesia. Acta Otolaryngol (Stockh) 28:95, 1939

Angrist SW: Fluid control devices. Sci Am 211:81, 1964

Ankeney JL, Hubay CA, Hackett PR, et al: The effect of positive and negative pressure respiration on unilateral pulmonary blood flow in the open chest. Surg Gynecol Obstet 98:5, 1954

Arp JL, Dillon RE, Humphries TJ, et al: A new approach to ventilatory support of infants with respiratory distress syndrome. Part I. The Arp infant respirator. Anesth Analg 48:251, 1969

Arp JL, Dillon RE, Humphries TJ, et al: A new approach to ventilatory support of infants with respiratory distress syndrome. Part II. The clinical applications of the Arp infant respirator. Anesth Analg 48:517, 1969

Arthur DS, Mathur AK, Nisbet HIA, et al: The effect of artificial ventilation on functional residual capacity and arterial oxygenation. II. Comparison of spontaneous respiration and artificial ventilation at similar arterial carbon dioxide tensions, tidal volumes and inspiratory gas flow rates. Can Anaesth Soc J 22:432, 1975

Ashbaugh DG: Effect of ventilatory methods and patterns on physiologic shunt. Surgery 68:99, 1970

Ashbaugh DG, Bigelow DB, Petty TI, et al: Acute respiratory distress in adults. Lancet 2:319, 1967

Ashbaugh DG, Petty TL: Positive end-expiratory pressure: physiology, indications and contraindications. J Thorac Cardiovasc Surg 65:165, 1973

Ashbaugh DG, Petty TL, Bigelow DB, et al: Continuous positive pressure breathing (CPPB) in adult respiratory distress syndrome. J Thorac Cardiovasc Surg 57:31, 1969

Asmussen E, Nielsen M: Efficacy of artificial respiration. J Appl Physiol 3:95, 1950

Astrup P, Goetzche H, Neukirk F: Lab investigation during treatment of patients with poliomyelitis and respiratory paralysis. Br Med J 1:780, 1954

Avery AE, Mörch ET, Benson DW: Critically crushed chests: a new method of treatment with continuous hyperventilation to produce alkalotic apnea and internal pneumatic stabilization. J Thorac Surg 32:291, 1956

Babinski M, Klain M, Smith RB: High frequency jet ventilation. American Society of Anesthesiology Annual Meeting, New Orleans, 1977 (abstract)

Baker AB: Artificial respiration, the history of an idea. Med Hist 15:344, 1971

Baker AB: Physiological responses to artificial ventilation. Thesis, University of Oxford, 1971

Bang C: A new respirator. Lancet 1:723, 1953

Barach AL: Principles and Practices of Inhalation Therapy. p. 52. Lippincott, Philadelphia, 1944

Barach AL, Barach B, Echman M, et al: An appraisal of intermittent positive breathing as a method of increasing altitude tolerance. CAM Reports No. 399, November 1944

Barach AL, Bickeman HA, Petty TL: Perspectives in pressure breathing. Resp Care 20:627, 1975

Barach AL, Eckman M, Ginsburg E, et al: Studies on positive pressure respiration. Aviat Med 17:290, 1946

Barach AL, Fen WO, Ferris EB, et al: The physiology of pressure breathing. J Aviat Med 18:73, 1947

Barach AL, Martin J, Eckman M: Positive pressure respiration and its application to the treatment of acute pulmonary edema. Ann Intern Med 12:754, 1938

Barach AL, Martin J, Eckman M: Positive pressure respiration and its application to the treatment of acute pulmonary edema. Proc Soc Clin Invest 16:664, 1937

Baratz RA, Ingraham RC: Renal hemodynamics and antidiuretic hormone release associated with volume regulation. Am J Physiol 198:565, 1960

Baratz RA, Philbin DM, Patternson RW: Plasma antidiuretic hormone and urinary output during continuous positive pressure breathing in dogs. Anesthesiology 34:510, 1971

Barker E, Singer R, Elkinton J, et al: The renal response in man to experimental respiratory alkalosis and acidosis. J Clin Invest 36:515, 1957

Barnes CH: Bristol Aircraft Since 1910, pp. 20, 70. Putnum, London, 1964

Barrie H: Simple method of applying continuous positive airway pressure in respiratory distress syndrome. Lancet 1:776, 1972

Bates DV, Macklem PT, Christie RV: Respiratory Function in Disease: An Introduction to the Integrated Study of the Lung. pp. 441–470. Saunders, Philadelphia, 1971

Baumeister J, Blood MJ, Marsh A, et al: The use of tracheotomy, intermittent positive pressure, and sedation treatment in children with poliomyelitis. J Kans Med Soc 53:281, 1952

Beaver RA: Pneumoflator for treatment of respiratory paralysis. Lancet 1:977, 1953

Beckman M, Norlander O: Pulmonary ventilation during thoracic surgery. Acta Chir Scand [Suppl] 245:27, 1959

Beecher HK: Principles of anesthesia for lobectomy and total pneumonectomy. Acta Med Scand [Suppl] 90:146, 1938

Beecher HK, Murphy AJ: Acidosis during thoracic surgery. J Thorac Surg 19:50, 1950

Behress CW: What is fluidics. Appliance manufacture, July 1968

Bendixen HH, Bullwinkel B, Hedley-Whyte J: Atelectasis and shunting during spontaneous ventilation in anesthesia patients. Anesthesiology 25:297, 1964

Bendixen HH, Egbett LD, Hedley-Whyte J, et al: Respiratory Care. Mosby, St. Louis, 1965

Bendixen HH, Hedley-Whyte J, Laver MB: Impaired oxygenation in surgical patients during general anesthesia with controlled ventilation: a concept of atelectasis. N Engl J Med 269:991, 1963

Bendixen HH, Kinney JM: History of intensive care. In Kinney J, Bendixen H, Powers S (eds): Manual of Surgical Intensive Care. Saunders, Philadelphia, 1977

Bendixen AH, Smith GM, Mead J: Pattern of ventilation in young adults. J Appl Physiol 19:195, 1964

Bergen FHV, Buckley JJ, Weastrehead DSP, et al: A new respirator. Anesthesiology 17:708, 1956

Bergman NA: Effects of different pressure breathing patterns on alveolar-arterial gradients in dogs. J Appl Physiol 18:1049, 1963

Bergman NA: Effects of varying respiratory waveforms on gas exchange. Anesthesiology 28:390, 1967

Bergman NA: Intrapulmonary gas trapping during mechanical ventilation at rapid frequencies. Anesthesiology 37:626, 1972

Bergman R: Eight hundred cases of poliomyelitis treated in the Sahlin respirator. Acta Paediatr Scand 36:470, 1948

Berneus B, Carlsten A: Effect of intermittent positive pressure ventilation on cardiac output in polio. Acta Med Scand 152:19, 1955

Berry PR, Pontoppidan H: Oxygen consumption and blood gas exchange during controlled and spontaneous ventilation in patients with respiratory failure. Anesthesiology 29:177, 1968

Binda RE, Cook DR, Fischer CG: Advantages of infant ventilators over adapted adult ventilators in pediatrics. Anesth Analg 55:769, 1976

Birnbaum GL, Thompson SA: The mechanism of asphyxial resuscitation. Surg Gynecol Obstet 75:79, 1942

Bjerager K, Sjöstrand U, Wattwil M: Long-term treatment of two patients with respiratory insufficiency with IPPV/PEEP and HFPPV/PEEP. Acta Anaesth Scand [Suppl] 64:55, 1977

Björk VO: Principles and indication for treatment of ventilatory insufficiency. Bull Soc Int Chir 15(3):249, 1956

Björk VO, Engström CG: Notre expérience de la respiration artificielle en chirurgie thoracique. Anesth Analg (Paris) 12:1955

Björk VO, Engström CG: The treatment of ventilatory insufficiency after pulmonary resection with tracheotomy and prolonged artificial respiration. J Thorac Cardiovasc Surg 30:356, 1955

Björk VO, Engström CG, Friberg O, et al: Ventilatory problems in thoracic anaesthesia: a volume-cycling device for controlled respiration. J Thorac Surg 31:117, 1956

Blaisdell FW, Lewis FR: Respiratory Distress Syndrome of Shock and Trauma. Saunders, Philadelphia, 1977

Blaisdell FW, Schlobohm RM: The respiratory distress syndrome: a review. Surgery 74:251, 1973

Bland RD, Kim MH, Light MJ, et al: High-frequency mechanical ventilation of low-birth weight infants with respiratory failure from hyaline membrane disease: 92% survival. Pediatr Res 11:531, 1977

Bland RD, Kim MH, Light MJ, et al: Mechanical ventilation at high respiratory frequencies in severe hyaline membrane disease—an alternative treatment? Crit Care Med 8:275, 1980

Bohm DJ, Miyasaka K, Marchak B, et al: Ventilation by high frequency oscillation. J Appl Physiol 48:710, 1980

Borg U, Eriksson I, Lyttkens L, et al: High-frequency positive-pressure ventilation (HFPPV) applied in bronchoscopy under general anaesthesia—an experimental study. Acta Anaesth Scand [Suppl] 64:69, 1977

Borg U, Lyttkens L, Nilsson LG, et al: Physiologic evaluation of the HFPPV pneumatic valve principle and PEEP—an experimental study. Acta Anaesth Scand [Suppl] 64:37, 1977

Boros SJ, Matalon SV, Ewald R, et al: The effect of independent variations in inspiratory-expiratory ratio and end-expiratory pressure during mechanical ventilation in hyaline membrane disease. J Pediatr 91:794, 1977

Bower AG, Bennett VR, Dillon JB, et al: Investigation of the care and treatment of poliomyelitis patients. Ann West Med Surg 4:561, 1950

Brauer L: Die ausschaltung der Pneumothorax folgen mit Hilfe des Überdruckverfahrens. Mitt Grenzgeb Med Chir 8:583, 1904

Braun E: Apparatus for resuscitating asphyxiated children. Boston Med Surg J 120:9, 1889

Braunwald E, Binion JT, Morgan WL, et al: Alteration in central blood volume and cardiac output induced by positive pressure breathing and counteracted by metaraminol. Circ Res 5:670, 1957

Breathing Machines and Their Use in Treatment: Report of the Respirators (Poliomyelitis) Committee. Medical Research Council, London, 22 November 1939

Breathing Mechanics for Medical Use. Proposed JSO Standard Specifications. International Standards Organization Technical Committee 121, Boston, 1972

Brecker GA: Venous Return. Grune & Stratton, New York, 1956

Breivik H, Grenvik A, Miller E, et al: Normalizing low atrial CO_2 tension during mechanical ventilation. Chest 63:525, 1973

Briscoe WA, Forster RE, Comroe JH: Alveolar ventilation at very low tidal volumes. J Appl Physiol 7:27, 1954

Brown EB Jr: Physiological effects of hyperventilation. Physiol Rev 33:445, 1953

Browne AGR, Pontoppidan H, Chiang H: Physiological criteria for weaning patients from prolonged artificial ventilation. American Society of Anesthesiologists Annual Meeting, 1972

Brundin T, Hendenstierna G, McCarthy G: Effect of intermittent positive pressure ventilation on cardiac systolic time intervals. Acta Anaesth Scand 20:278, 1976

Bryce-Smith R, Davis HS: Tidal exchange in respirators. Anesth Analg 33:73, 1954

Bryce-Smith R, Mitchell JV, Parkhouse J: The Nuffield Department of Anaesthesia. Oxford 1937–1962. University Press, Oxford.

Bull PR: A water driven respirator. Med J Aust 34:238, 1947

Bunnell J, Karlson K, Shannon D: High frequency positive pressure ventilation in dogs and rabbits. Am Rev Resp Dis 117:289, 1978

Burger EJ Jr, Macklem PT: Airway closure: demonstration of breathing 100 per cent oxygen at low lung volumes and by N_2 washout. J Appl Physiol 25:139, 1968

Burke JF, Pontoppidan H, Welch CE: High output respiratory failure: an important cause of death ascribed to peritonitis or ileus. Ann Surg 158:581, 1963

Burns HL: A pure fluid cycling valve for use in breathing equipment. Inhal Ther 14:11, 1969

Burns HL: Pneumatic balance resuscitator. Air Surg Bull 2:306, 1945

Burns HL: Specifications: RETEC Automatic Respirator Model A-30, RETEC Inc., Portland, Oregon, 1967

Burton CG, Gee GN, Hodgkin JE: Respiratory Care. Lippincott, Philadelphia, 1977

Bushman JA, Askill S: An adjustable annular fluid logic ventilator. Br J Anaesth 43:1197, 1971

Bushnell LS, Pontoppidan H, Hedley-Whyte, J et al: Efficiency of different types of ventilation in longterm respiratory care: mechanical versus spontaneous. Anesth Analg 45:696, 1966

Butler J, Smith BH: Pressure-volume relationships of the chest in the completely relaxed anaesthetized patient. Clin Sci 16:125, 1957

Butler WJ, et al: Ventilation by high frequency oscillation in humans. Anesth Analg 59:577, 1980

Campbell DI: A compact versatile, fluidic controlled ventilator. Anaesth Intensive Care 4:7, 1976

Campbell EJM, Nunn JF, Peckett BW: A comparison of artificial ventilation and spontaneous respiration with particular reference to ventilation-blood flow relationships. Br J Anaesth 30:166, 1958

Carden E: Positive-pressure ventilation during anaesthesia for bronchoscopy: a laboratory evaluation of two recent advances. Anesth Anal Curr Res 52:402, 1973

Carden E, Burns WW, McDevitt NB, et al: A comparison of venturi and side-arm ventilation in anaesthesia for bronchoscopy. Can Anaesth Soc J 20:569, 1973

Carden E, Chir B, Schwesinger WB: The use of nitrous oxide during ventilation with the open bronchoscope. Anesthesiology 39:551, 1973

Carden E, Crutchfield W: Anaesthesia for microsurgery of the larynx (a new method). Can Anaesth Soc J 20:378, 1973

Carden E, Ferguson GB: A new technique for micro-laryngeal surgery in infants. Laryngoscope 93:691, 1973

Carden E, Trapp WG, Oulton J: A new and simple method for ventilating patients undergoing bronchoscopy. Anesthesiology 33:454, 1970

Carlon GC, Fay C, Klain M, et al: High frequency positive pressure ventilation in management of patients with bronchopleural fistula. Anesthesiology 52:160, 1980

Carr DT, Essex HE: Certain effects of positive pressure respiration on the circulatory and respiratory system. Am Heart J 31:53, 1946

Cartwright RY, Hargrave PR: Pseudomonas in ventilators. Lancet 1:40, 1970

Chakrabarti MK, Sykes MK: Cardiorespiratory effects of high frequency positive pressure ventilation in the dog. Br J Anaesth 52:475, 1980

Cheney FW, Wayne EM: Effects of continuous positive pressure ventilation on gas exchange in acute pulmonary edema. J Appl Physiol 30:378, 1971

Civetta JM, Barnes JA, Smith LO: Optimal PEEP and intermittent mandatory ventilation in the treatment of acute pulmonary failure. Resp Care 20:551, 1975

Civetta JM, Brous R, Gabel JC: A simple and effective method of employing spontaneous positive pressure ventilation. J Thorac Cardiovasc Surg 63:312, 1972

Civetta JM, Hudson J, Kirby RR, et al: Mechanical ventilatory support. Crit Care Med 3:114, 1977

Clowes GHA, Cook WA, Vujovic V, et al: Pattern of circulatory responses to the use of respirators. Circulation [Suppl I] 31:157, 1965

Coanda H: Keynote address to the Third Fluid Amplification Symposium, 26 October 1965. Kindly provided by JM Kirshner, Harry Diamond Laboratories, Washington, D.C., 1965

Coleman E: Dissertation on Natural and Suspended Respiration. 2nd Ed. Cox, London, 1802

Collier CR, Affeldt JE: Ventilatory efficiency of the cuirass respirator in totally paralyzed chronic polio patients. J Appl Physiol 6:531, 1954

Comroe JH Jr, Dripps R: Artificial respiration. JAMA 130:381, 1946

Conway CM: Haemodynamic effects of pulmonary ventilation. Br J Anaesth 47:761, 1975

Conway CM, Payne JP: Hypoxemia associated with anaesthesia and controlled respiration. Lancet 1:12, 1964

Cooper JD, Grillo HC: The evaluation of tracheal injury due to ventilatory assistance through cuffed tubes: a pathologic study. Ann Surg 169:334, 1969

Corbet AJS, Ross JA, Beaudry PH, et al: Effect of positive-pressure breathing on a-ADO$_2$ in hyaline membrane disease. J Appl Physiol 38:33, 1975

Cournand A: Recent observations on the dynamics of the pulmonary circulation. Bull NY Acad Med 23:27, 1947

Cournand A, Motley HL, Werkö L: Mechanism underlying cardiac output change during intermittent positive pressure breathing. Fed Proc 6:92, 1947

Cournand A, Motley HL, Werkö L, et al: Physiological studies of effects of intermittent positive pressure breathing on cardiac output in man. Am J Physiol 152:162, 1948

Courtois MLH: Mémoire sur les asphyxie, avec la description d'un nouvel instrument propre à rappeler le méchanism de la respiration. J de Med Chir Pharm 82:361, 1790

Cox LA, Chapman EDW: A comprehensive volume cycled lung ventilator embodying feedback control. Med Biol Eng 12:160, 1974

Crafoord C: On the technique of pneumonectomy in man. Acta Chir Scand [Suppl 64] 81:1, 1938

Crafoord C: Pulmonary ventilation and anesthesia in major chest surgery. J Thorac Surg 9:237, 1940

Crafoord C: Thirty-five years experience with controlled ventilation in thoracic surgery. Int Anesthesiol Clin 10:1, 1972

Craig DB, McCarthy DS: Airway closure and lung volumes during breathing with maintained airway positive-pressures. Anesthesiology 36:540, 1972

Crampton Smith, A: Effect of mechanical ventilation on the circulation. Ann NY Acad Sci 121:733, 1965

Cross DA: A variation of the intermittent mandatory ventilation assembly. Anesthesiology 44:182, 1976

Cullen SC, Comroe JH Jr, Brown EB, et al: Problems in ventilation. Anesthesiology 15:416, 1954

Cullen W: A letter to Lord Cathcart, President of the Board of Police in Scotland concerning the recovery of persons drowned and seemingly dead. London, 1776. Quoted in: Herholdt JD, Rafn CG: An Attempt at an Historical Survey of Life-Saving Measures for Drowning Persons and Information of the Best Means by Which They Can Again Be Brought Back to Life. H Tikiob, Copenhagen, 1796.

Cumarasamy N, Nussli R, Vischer D, et al: Artificial ventilation in hyaline membrane disease: the use of positive end-expiratory pressure and continuous positive airway pressure. Pediatrics 51:629, 1973

Cutler EC: The origin of thoracic surgery. N Engl J Med 208:1233, 1933

Daily WJR, Meyer HPP, Sunshine P, et al: Mechanical ventilation of the newborn infants, III, IV, V. Anesthesiology 34:119, 1971

Daily WJR, Smith PC: Mechanical ventilation of the newborn infant. Curr Probl Pediatr 1:1–37, 1971

Daily WJR, Sunshine P, Smith PC: Mechanical ventilation of the newborn infant: five year experience. Anesthesiology 34:132, 1971

Dalziel J: On Sleep and an Apparatus for Promoting Artificial Respiration. British Association for Advancement of Science Report No. 2, p. 127, 1838

Dameron JT, Greene DG: Use of the Burns valve as a simple respirator for intrathoracic surgery in the dog. J Thorac Surg 20:706, 1950

D'Avignon P, Sundell L, Werneman H: Treatment in cuirass and/or positive pressure respirator: primary lethality, invalidity, and physical fitness of respirator patients after one year. Acta Med Scand 154:316, 1956

Dehan FH: La respiration mecaniquement controlée en chirurgie thoracique. Acta Chir Belg 49:938, 1950

deLemos R, Mclaughlin GW: Technique of Ventilation in the Newborn: the Use of IMV. Physiologie Appliquèe de la Ventilation Assistée Chez le Nouveau-née. Report of Colloquium. Pont-a-Moussou, France, 27–28 September 1973, pp. 173–178

deLemos RA, Armstrong RG, Kirby RR, et al: A new pediatric volume ventilator evaluation in 90 newborn infants (abstract). American Thoracic Society, 1971

deLemos RA, McLaughlin GW, Robison EJ, et al: Continuous positive airway pressure as an adjunct to mechanical ventilation in the newborn with respiratory distress syndrome. Anesth Analg 52:328, 1973

deLemos RA, Wolsdorf J, Nachman R, et al: Lung injury from oxygen in lambs; the role of artificial ventilation. Anesthesiology 30:609, 1969

Dennis C, Karlson KE, Eder WB, et al: A simple, efficient respirator and anesthesia bag for open chest surgery. Surg Forum 583, 1950

Desautels D: Ventilator classification: a new look at an old subject. Curr Rev Resp Ther 1:82, 1979

Desautels D, Bartlett JL: Methods of administering intermittent mandatory ventilation (IMV). Resp Care 19:187, 1974

Dickinson DG, Wilson JL, Graham BG: Studies in respiratory insufficiency. I. Carbon dioxide and oxygen studies in early respiratory paralysis in poliomyelitis. Am J Dis Child 3:265, 1953

Dobkin AB: Ventilators and Inhalation Therapy. Little, Brown, Boston, 1972

Doctor NH: A device for mechanical ventilation suitable for newborn and infants during anaesthesia. Br J Anaesth 36:259, 1964

Donald I: Augmented respiration; emergency positive-pressure patient-cycled respirator. Lancet 1:895, 1954

Dorrange GM: On the treatment of traumatic injuries of the lungs and pleura: with the presentation of a new intratracheal tube for use in artificial respiration. Surg Gynecol Obstet 11:160, 1910

Downes JJ: CPAP and PEEP: a perspective. Anesthesiology 44:1, 1976

Downes JJ: Mechanical ventilation of the newborn. Anesthesiology 34:116, 1971

Downes JJ, Nicodemus HF, Pierce WS, et al: Acute respiratory failure in infants following cardiovascular surgery. J Thorac Cardiovasc Surg 59:21, 1970

Downs JB, Block AJ, Vennum KB: Intermittent mandatory ventilation in the treatment of patients with chronic obstructive pulmonary disease. Anesth Analg 53:437, 1974

Downs JB, Douglas ME, Sanfelippo PM, et al: Ventilatory pattern, intrapleural pressure and cardiac output. Anesth Analg 56:88, 1977

Downs JB, Klein EF, Desautels D, et al: Intermittent mandatory ventilation—a new approach to weaning patients from mechanical ventilators. Chest 64:331, 1973

Downs JB, Klein EF, Modell JH: The effect of incremental PEEP on PaO_2 in patients with respiratory failure. Anesth Analg 52:210, 1973

Downs JB, Mitchell LA: Intermittent mandatory ventilation following cardiopulmonary bypass. Crit Care Med 2:39, 1974

Downs JB, Perkins HM, Modell JH: Intermittent mandatory ventilation: an evaluation. Arch Surg 109:519, 1974

Downs JB, Perkins HM, Sutton WW: Successful weaning after five years of mechanical ventilation. Anesthesiology 40:602, 1974

Drinker CK: Development of the school of public health (at Harvard University). Harvard Med Alumni Bull 10:9, 1935

Drinker CK: Pulmonary Edema and Inflammation. Harvard University Press, Cambridge, 1945

Drinker P, McKhann CF: The use of a new apparatus for the prolonged administration of artificial respiration in a fatal case of poliomyelitis. JAMA 92:1658, 1929

Drinker P, Shaw LA: An apparatus for the prolonged administration of artificial respiration. J Clin Invest 7:229, 1927

Drury DR, Henry JP, Goodman J: Effects of continuous pressure breathing on kidney function. J Clin Invest 26:945, 1947

Duffin J: Fluidics and pneumatics principles and applications in anaesthesia. Can Anaesth Soc J 24:126, 1977

Dunn PM: Continuous positive airway pressure (CPAP) using the Gregory box. Proc R Soc Med 67:245, 1974

E & J resuscitator: report from Council of Physical Therapy. JAMA 121:1219, 1943

Egan DF: Fundamentals of Oxygen Therapy. Mosby, St. Louis, 1977

Eger EI II, Hamilton WK: Positive negative pressure ventilation with a modified Ayre's T-piece. Anesthesiology 19:611, 1958

Elam JO, Brown ES, Janney CD: Ventilator. Anesthesiology 17:504, 1956

Elam JO, Kerr JH, Janney CD: Performance of ventilators—effect of changes in lung-thorax compliance. Anesthesiology 19:56, 1958

El-Naggar M: "Weaning." Middle East J Anaesthesiol 3:401, 1972

Elsberg CA: Clinical experiences with intratracheal insufficiency (Meltzer) with remarks upon the value of the method for thoracic surgery. Ann Surg 52:23, 1910

Elsberg CA: The value of continuous intratracheal insufflation of air (Meltzer) in thoracic surgery: with description of an apparatus. Med Rec 77:493, 1910

Emerson H: Artificial respiration in the treatment of edema of the lungs. Arch Intern Med 3:368, 1909

Emerson JH: Respiratory problems in poliomyelitis. Presented at the National Foundation for Infantile Paralysis Conference, Ann Arbor, MI, March 1952, p 11

Emerson JH: The Evolution of "Iron Lung." J.H. Emerson Co., Cambridge, MA, 1978

Emerson resuscitator: report from Council of Physical Therapy. JAMA 119:414, 1942

Enghoff E: Konstgjord Andning, pp. 19–66. Almqvist & Wiksell, Uppsala, 1956

Enghoff H: Bemerkungen zur Frage des Schädlischen Raumes. Uppsala Läkarföreningens Forhandlinge 44:191, 1938

Enghoff H: Der Barospirator: Untersuchungen über seine Wirkungsweise mit besonderer Berüchsichtigung die Pneumographischen Methodik. Scand Arch Physiol 51:1, 1927

Engström CG: Respirator enligt nyt princip. Svensk Läkartidn 50:545, 1953

Engström CG: The clinical application of prolonged controlled ventilation. Acta Anaesth Scand [Suppl] 13:25, 1963

Engström CG: Treatment of severe cases of respiratory paralysis by the Engström universal respirator. Br Med J 2:666, 1954

Engström CG, Herzog P: Ventilation nomogram for practical use with the Engström respirator. Acta Anaesth Scand 6:49, 1959

Engström CG, Herzog P, Norlander OD, et al: Ventilation nomogram for the newborn and small children to be used with the Engström respirator. Acta Anaesth Scand 6:175, 1962

Engström CG, Norlander OD: A new method for analysis of respiratory work by measurement of actual power as a function of gas flow, pressure and time. Acta Anaesth Scand 6:49, 1962

Epstein RA: The sensitivities and response times of ventilatory assistors. Anesthesiology 34:321, 1971

Eriksson I: The role of the conducting airways in N_2-washout during high frequency mechanical ventilation. Anesthesiology (Suppl) 55:354, 1981

Eriksson I, Heijman L, Sjöstrand U: High-frequency positive-pressure ventilation (HFPPV) in bronchoscopy during anaesthesia. Opusc Med 19:14, 1972

Eriksson I, Jonzon A, Sedin G, et al: The influence of the ventilatory pattern on ventilation, circulation and oxygen transport during continuous positive-pressure ventilation—an experimental study. Acta Anaesth Scand [Suppl] 64:149, 1977

Eriksson I, Lyttkens L, Nilsson LG, et al: The importance of frequency and relative insufflation time in ventilation during bronchoscopy under general anaesthesia. Svenska Läkarsällskabets Handlingar Opusc Med 21:142, 1976

Eriksson I, Nilsson LG, Nordström S, et al: High-frequency positive pressure ventilation (HFPPV) during transthoracic resection of tracheal stenosis and during perioperative bronchoscopic examination. Acta Anaesth Scand 19:113, 1975

Eriksson I, Sjöstrand U: A clinical evaluation of high-frequency positive-pressure ventilation (HFPPV) in laryngoscopy and under general anaesthesia. Acta Anaesth Scand [Suppl] 64:101, 1977

Eriksson I, Sjöstrand U: Effects of high frequency positive-pressure ventilation (HFPPV) and general anaesthesia on intrapulmonary gas distribution in patients undergoing diagnostic bronchoscopy. Anesth Analg 59:585, 1980

Eriksson I, Sjöstrand U: Experimental and clinical evaluation of high-frequency positive-pressure ventilation (HFPPV) and the pneumatic valve principle in bronchoscopy under general anesthesia. Acta Anaesth Scand [Suppl] 64:83, 1977

Eriksson I, Sjöstrand U: High frequency positive-pressure ventilation (HFPPV) during laryngoscopy. Opusc Med 19:278, 1974

Erlanson P, Lindholm T, Lindquist B, et al: Artificial respiration in severe renal failure with pulmonary insufficiency. Acta Med Scand 166:81, 1960

Esplen JR: A new apparatus for intermittent pulmonary inflation. Br J Anaesth 24:303, 1952

Esplen JR: Differential pressure respiration in thoracic operations. Br J Anaesth 23:214, 1951

Esplen JR: The Fazakerley respirator. Br J Anaesth 28:176, 1956

Fairley HB: Respiratory insufficiency. Int Anesthesiol Clin 1:351, 1963

Fairley HB, Britt BA: The adequacy of the air-mix control in ventilators operated from an oxygen source. Can Med Assoc J 90:1394, 1964

Fairley HB, Hunter DD: Mechanical ventilators: an assessment of two new machines for use in the operating room. Can Anaesth Soc J 10:364, 1963

Fairley HB, Hunter DD: The performance of respirators used in the treatment of respiratory insufficiency. Can Med Assoc J 90:1397, 1964

Fairley HB, Schlobohm RM, Singer MM, et al: The appropriateness of intensive respiratory care. Crit Care Med 1:115, 1973

Falke KJ, Pontoppidan H, Kumar A, et al: Ventilation with end-expiratory pressure in acute lung disease. J Clin Invest 51:2315, 1972

Falor WH, Kelly TR, Reynolds CW: Mechanical elimination of respiratory acidosis during open thoracic procedures. Surg Forum 5:536, 1954

Fanaroff AA, Klaus MH: Evaluation and care of the newborn infant. In Lough MD, et al. (ed): Pediatric Respiratory Therapy. p. 30. Year Book, Chicago, 1974

Faridy EE, Perman HS, Riley RL: Effect of ventilation on surface forces in excised dogs' lungs. J Appl Physiol 21:1453, 1966

Feeley TW, Hedley-Whyte J: Current concepts: weaning from continuous ventilatory supplemental oxygen. N Engl J Med 292:903, 1975

Feeley TW, Saumaurez R, Klick JM, et al: Positive end-expiratory pressure in weaning patients from continuous ventilation: a prospective randomized trial. Lancet 2:725, 1975

Fell GE: Artificial respiration. Surg Gynecol Obstet 10:572, 1910

Fell GE: Forced respiration in opium poisoning. Buffalo Med Surg J 28:145, 1887

Fenn WO, Chadwick E: Effect of pressure breathing on blood flow through the finger. Am J Physiol 151:270, 1947

Fenn WO, Otis AB, Rahn H, et al: Displacement of blood from the lungs by pressure breathing. Am J Physiol 151:258, 1947

Ferris BG, Mead J, Whittenberger JL, et al: Pulmonary function in convalescent poliomyelitis patients. III. Compliance of the lungs and thorax. N Engl J Med 247:390, 1952

Flaum A: Experience in the use of a new respirator (Sahlin type) in the treatment of respiratory paralysis in poliomyelitis. Acta Med Scand [Suppl] 78:849, 1936

Fleming WH, Bowen JC: A comparative evaluation of pressure-limited and volume-limited respirators for prolonged post-operative ventilatory support in combat casualties. Ann Surg 176:49, 1972

Fleming WH, Bowen JC: Early complications of long-term respiratory support. J Thorac Cardiovasc Surg 64:729, 1972

Fletcher PR, Epstein MAF, Epstein RA: Alveolar pressure during high frequency ventilation (HFV). Fed Proc 39:576, 1980

Fletcher PR, Epstein MAF, Epstein RA: A new ventilator for physiologic studies during high frequency ventilation. Resp Physiol 47:21, 1982

Fletcher PR, Epstein RA: A high frequency ventilator for physiologic studies. Anesthesiology 53:399, 1980

Fletcher PR, Epstein RA: Experimental studies in high-frequency ventilation. Anesthesiology 53:401, 1980

Fletcher PR, Epstein RA: Measurement of alveolar pressure during HFV. Anesthesiology (Suppl) 55:358, 1981

Folkow B, Pappenheimer JR: Components of the respiratory dead space and their variation with pressure breathing and with bronchoactive drugs. J Appl Physiol 8:102, 1955

Fothergill J: A case published in the last volume of Medical Essays of recovery of a man dead in appearance, by distending the lungs with air. Lettsam JC (ed): The Works of John Fothergill, M.D. C Dilly, London, 1784

France EM: Some eighteenth century authorities on resuscitation of the apparently drowned. Anaesthesia 30:530, 1975

Frank I, Noack W, Lunkenheimer PP, et al: Light- and electronmicroscopic investigations of pulmonary tissue after high-frequency positive-pressure ventilation (HFPPV). Anaesthesist 24:171, 1975

Fredberg JJ: Augmented diffusion in the airways can support pulmonary gas exchange. J Appl Physiol 49:232, 1980

Fredberg JJ, Mean J: Impedance of intrathoracic airway models during low frequency period flow. J Appl Physiol 47:347, 1979

French-Brevet d'Invention (patent) P.V. No. 956.441, No. 1 386.37. entitled: Appareils distributeurs à membranés, granted 14 December 1964

Frenkner P: Bronchial and tracheal catheterization. Acta Otolaryngol Scand [Suppl] 20:97, 1934

Frost GT, Dupuis YG, Bain JA: A modification of the Bird Mark VIII ventilator to deliver continuous positive pressure breathing and intermittent mandatory ventilation. Can Anaesth Soc J 22:719, 1975

Frumin MJ: Clinical use of a physiological respirator producing N_2O amnesia-analgesia. Anesthesiology 18:290, 1957

Frumin MJ, Bergman NA, Holaday DA, et al: Alveolar arterial O_2 differences during artificial respiration in man. J Appl Physiol 14:694, 1959

Frumin MJ, Lee ASJ: A physiologically oriented artificial respirator which produces N_2O-O_2 anesthesia in man. J Lab Clin Med 49:617, 1957

Frumin MJ, Lee ASJ, Papper EM: Intermittent positive-pressure respirator. Anesthesiology 21:220, 1960

Frumin MJ, Lee ASJ, Papper EM: New valve for nonrebreathing systems. Anesthesiology 20:383, 1959

Gagge AP, Allen SC, Marborger JP: Pressure breathing. Aviat Med 16:2, 1945

Gallagher TJ, Civetta JM, Kirby RR, et al: High level PEEP, cost vs value. Annual Meeting of American Society of Anesthesiologists, 1976 (abstract)

Galloon S: The Toronto ventilating laryngoscope. Br J Anaesth 45:912, 1973

Galloon S, Rosen N: Changes in airway resistance and alveolar trapping with positive-negative ventilation. Anaesthesia 20:429, 1965

Gammanpila S, Bevan DR, Bhudu R: Effect of positive and negative expiratory pressure on renal function. Br J Anaesth 49:199, 1977

Garzon AA, Seitzer B, Karlson KE: Physiopathology of crushed chest injuries. Ann Surg 168:128, 1968

Gauer OH, Henry JP, Sieker HO, et al: Effect of negative pressure breathing on urine flow. J Clin Invest 33:287, 1954

Gett PM, Sherwood-Jones JG, Shepherd GF: Pulmonary oedema associated with sodium retention during ventilator treatment. Br J Anaesth 43:460, 1971

Gibbon JH, Haupt GJ: The need for adequate pulmonary ventilation during surgical operation. Surg Clin North Am 35:1553, 1955

Gibbon JH, Stayman JW, Allbritten FF: Controlled respiration in thoracic and upper abdominal operations. Minnesota Med 33:1031, 1950

Giertz KH: Studier över tryckdifferensandning enligt Sauerbruch och över konstgjord andning (rytmisk luftinblåsning vid intrathoracala operationer). Ups Läkareför Forh (Suppl) 22:1, 1916

Gillick JS: The inflation-catheter technique for ventilation during bronchoscopy. Anesthesiology 40:503, 1974; Can Anaesth Soc J 23:534, 1976

Gioia FR, Harris AP, Hamburger C, et al: Peripheral circulatory changes with high frequency ventilation. Anesthesiology (Suppl) 55:357, 1981

Gioia FR, Rinehart G, Parke SD, et al: Pulmonary blood flow during high frequency ventilation. Anesthesiology (Suppl) 55:356, 1981

Giordano J, Harken A: Effect of continuous positive pressure ventilation on cardiac output. Am Surg 41:221, 1975

Gold MI: Impedance in anoxia. Anesthesiology 30:663, 1969

Goldstein DH, Slutsky AS, Ingram RH, et al: CO_2 elimination by high frequency ventilation (4–10 Hz) in normal subjects. Am Rev Resp Dis 123:251, 1981

Goodwyn E: Dissertatio Medica Inauguralis de Morbo Morteque Submersorum Investigandis. Edinburgh 1786

Goodwyn E: La Connexion de la Vie Avec la Respiration. Paris, An VI, 1798

Goodwyn E: The connexion of life with respiration; or an experimental inquiry into the effects of submersion, strangulation, and several kinds of noxious airs, on living animals; with an account of the nature of disease they produce; its distinction from death itself; and the most effectual means of cure. Printed by T. Spilsbury, Snow-hill. For J. Johnson, in St. Paul's Church-yard, 1788

Gordh T: Postural circulatory and respiratory changes during ether and intravenous anesthesia: experimental analysis of significance of postural changes during anesthesia with special regard to value of head down posture in resuscitation. Acta Chir Scand (Suppl 102) 92:1, 1945

Gordh T, Linderholm H, Norlander O: Pulmonary function in relation to anesthesia and surgery evaluated by analysis of oxygen tension of arterial blood. Acta Anaesth Scand 2:15, 1958

Gordon AS, Frye CW, Langston HT: The cardiorespiratory dynamics of controlled respiration in the open and closed chest. J Thorac Surg 32:431, 1956

Gotoh F, Meyer J, Takagi Y: Cerebral effects of hyperventilation in man. Arch Neurol 12:419, 1965

Green NW: The positive pressure method of artificial respiration. Surg Gynecol Obstet 2:512, 1906

Green NW, Janeway HH: Artificial respiration and intrathoracic oesophageal surgery. Ann Surg 52:58, 1910

Greenfield LJ, Ebert PA, Benson DW: Effect of positive pressure ventilation on surface tension properties of lung extracts. Anesthesiology 25:312, 1964

Greer JR, Donald I: A volume controlled patient-cycled respirator for adults. Br J Anaesth 30:3236, 1958

Gregory GA: Respiratory care of newborn infants. Pediatr Clin North Am 19:311, 1971

Gregory GA, Kitterman JA, Phibbs RH, et al: Treatment of the idiopathic respiratory distress syndrome with continuous positive airway pressure. N Engl J Med 184:1333, 1971

Grenard S, et al: Advanced Study in Respiratory Therapy. Glenn Educational Medical Services, Monsey, NY, 1971

Grenvik A: Acute respiratory failure; with special reference to current management of life threatening failure in an intensive care unit. In: Current Therapy. Saunders, Philadelphia 1983

Grenvik A: Respiratory, circulation and metabolic effects of respiratory treatment: a clinical study in post-operative thoracic surgical patients. Acta Anaesth Scand [Suppl] 19:1, 1966

Gunkler WA, Mahoney EB: A respirator for use in intrathoracic surgery in the dog. Surgery 26:821, 1949

Gwathmey JT: Anesthesia. Appleton, New York, 1914

Haddad C, Richards CC: Mechanical ventilation of infants: significance and elimination of ventilator compression volume. Anesthesiology 29:365, 1968

Haggard HW: Devils, Drugs and Doctors. Pocket Books, New York, 1959

Haglund G, Waldinger A: En ny övertrycksrespirator. Nord Med 53:804, 1955

Hardy MJ: The de Havelland Mosquito. p. 20. Arco, New York.

Harris AP, Gioia F, Hamburger C, et al: Peripheral circulatory changes with high frequency ventilation. Anesthesiology (Suppl) 555:357, 1981

Harrison VC, Heese H de V, and Klein M: The effects of intermittent positive pressure ventilation on lung function in hyaline membrane disease. Br J Anaesth 41:908, 1969

Hedenstierna G, McCarthy G, Bergström M: Airway closure during mechanical ventilation. Anesthesiology 44:114, 1976

Hedley-Whyte J, Laver MB: O_2 solubility in blood and temperature correcting factors for Po_2. J Appl Physiol 19:901, 1964

Hedley-Whyte J, Pontoppidan H, Morris MJ: The response of patients with respiratory failure and cardiopulmonary disease to different levels of constant volume ventilation. J Clin Invest 45:1543, 1966

Heese H de V, Harrison VC, Klein M, et al: Intermittent positive pressure ventilation in hyaline membrane disease. J Pediatr 76:183, 1970

Heifetz M, DeMyttenaere S, Rosenberg B: Intermittent positive pressure inflation during microscopic endolaryngeal surgery. Anaesthesist 26:11, 1977

Heijman K, Heijman L, Jonzon A, et al: High-frequency positive-pressure ventilation during anaesthesia and routine surgery in man. Acta Anaesth Scand 16:176, 1972

Heijman K, Sjöstrand U: Treatment of the respiratory distress syndrome—a preliminary report. Opusc Med 19:235, 1974

Heijman K, Sjöstrand U: Treatment of the respiratory distress syndrome by HFPPV and PEEP and by CPAP. In Stembera ZK, et al. (eds): Perinatal Medicine. p. 336. Thieme, Stuttgart, 1974

Heijman L, Nilsson LG, Sjöstrand U: High-frequency positive-pressure ventilation (HFPPV) in neonates and infants during NLA and routine plastic surgery, and in postoperative management. Acta Anaesth Scand [Suppl] 64:111, 1977

Heijman L, Sjöstrand H: Some anaesthetic techniques in operations for cleft lip and palate. Abstracts of the Society of Anaesthiae Sueciae, Karlskoga-Kristineham 1974

Heironimus T: Mechanical Artificial Ventilation. Charles C Thomas, Springfield, IL, 1970

Hellsten H: Lundia respiratorn. Svensk Lakartidn 50:1512, 1953

Herholdt JD, Rafn CG: An attempt at an historical survey of life-saving measures for drowning persons and information on the best means by which they can again be brought back to life. Printed at Tikiob Booksellers with M. Seest, Copenhagen, 1796. Re-edited by Henning Poulsen; English translation by DW Hannah and A Rousing, 1960. Scan Soc Anaest.

Herzog P: Advice and practical instruction for use of the Engström respirator. Opusc Med Stockh 9:280, 1964

Herzog P, Norlander OP: Distribution of alveolar volumes with different types of positive pressure gas-flow patterns. Opusc Med 13:3, 1968

Hewitt PB, Chamberlain JH, Seed RF: The effect of carbon dioxide on cardiac output on patients undergoing mechanical ventilation following open heart surgery. Br J Anaesth 45:1035, 1973

Hewlett AM: Artificial ventilation. In Gray TC, Utting JE, Nunn JF (eds): General Anesthesia. Vol I. pp. 573–590. Butterworth, London, 1980

Hill DW: Recent developments in the design of electronically controlled ventilators. Anaesthesia 15:234, 1966

Hill DW, Moore V: The action of adiabatic effects on the compliance of an artificial thorax. Br J Anaesth 37:19, 1965

Hill JD, Main FB, Osborn JJ, et al: Correct use of respirator on cardiac patients after operation. Arch Surg 91:775, 1965

Hirsch H: Uber künstliche Atmung durch Ventilation der Trachea. Thesis, University of Giessen, Germany, 1905

Hjalmarson O: Mechanics of breathing in newborn infants with pulmonary disease. Thesis, University of Gothenburg, Sweden, 1974

Holaday DA, Rattenberg CC: Automatic lung ventilators. Anesthesiology 23:493, 1962

Holmdahl M: The effect on inadequate gaseous interchange in the postoperative period upon the circulation. Acta Chir Scand 113:402, 1957

Hubay CA, Brecher GA, Clement FL: Etiological factors affecting pulmonary arterial flow with continuous respiration. Surgery 38:215, 1955

Hubay CA, Waltz RC, Brecher GA, et al: Circulatory dynamics of venous return during positive-negative pressure respiration. Anesthesiology 15:445, 1954

Hudson LD: The use of positive end-expiratory pressure in the adult respiratory distress syndrome. In Fontoni A (ed): Atti del 2° Corso Naziole di Aggiornamento in Rianimazione, Napoli, p. 472. 1974

Humphreys GH, Moore RL, Barkley H: Studies of the jugular, carotid and pulmonary pressures of anesthetized dogs during positive inflation of the lungs. J Thorac Surg 8:553, 1939

Humphreys GH, Moore RL, Maier HC, et al: Studies of the cardiac output of anaesthetised dogs during continuous and intermittent inflation of the lungs. J Thorac Surg 7:438, 1938

Hunsinger DC: Respiratory Technology: a Procedure Manual. Prentice-Hall, Reston, VA, 1973

Hunter AR: The classification of respirators. Anaesthesia 16:231, 1961

Hunter J: Observation on certain parts of the animal oeconomy. Philos Trans R Soc Lond 66:1776

Hunter J: Proposals for the recovery of people apparently drowned. Philos Trans R Soc Lond 66:412, 1776

Ibsen B: From anaesthesia to anaesthesiology. Acta Anaesth Scand [Suppl] 61:65, 1975

Ibsen B: The anaesthetist and positive pressure breathing. In Lassen HCA (ed): Management of Life-Threatening Poliomyelitis. p. 14. Livingstone, Edinburgh, 1956

Ibsen B: The anesthetist's viewpoint on the treatment of respiratory complications in poliomyelitis during the epidemic in Copenhagen in 1952. Proc R Soc Med 47:72, 1954

Ibsen B: Treatment of respiratory complications in poliomyelitis. Dan Med Bull 1:9, 1954

Ingestedt S, Jonson B, Nordström L, et al: A servo-controlled ventilator measuring expiratory minute volume, airway flow and pressure. Acta Anaesth Scand [Suppl] 47:9, 1972

Inkster JS, Lunn JN: A device for mechanical ventilation suitable for newborn and infants during anesthesia. Br J Anaesth 38:381, 1964

Inkster JS, Pearson DT: Some infant ventilator systems: a description of their characteristics and functions. Br J Anaesth 39:667, 1967

Jackson C: The Life of Chevalier Jackson, An Autobiography. Macmillan, New York, 1938

Jackson C: The technique of insertion of intratracheal insufflation tubes. Surg Gynecol Obstet 17:507, 1913

Jackson DE: A universal artificial respiration and closed anesthesia machine. J Lab Clin Med 12:998, 1927

Jackson DE: The use of artificial respiration in man, report of a case. Cincinnati J Med 11:515, 1930

Jacobs HJ: The burns pneumatic balance resuscitator. J Aviat Med 18:436, 1947

James NR: An automatic machine for controlled respiration. Med J Aust 6:325, 1950

Janeway HH: An apparatus for intratracheal insufflation. Ann Surg 56:328, 1912

Janeway HH: Intratracheal anaesthesia by nitrous oxide and oxygen under conditions of differential pressure. Ann Surg 58:927, 1913

Janeway HH, Green NW: Experimental intrathoracic esophagus surgery. JAMA 53:1975, 1909

Jansson L, Jonson B: A theoretical study on flow patterns of ventilators. Scand J Res Dis 53:237, 1972

Jardine AD, Harrison MJ, Healy TEJ: Automatic flow interruption bronchoscope: a laboratory study. Br J Anaesth 47:385, 1975

Jensen HK: Recovery of pulmonary function after crushing injuries of the chest. J Dis Chest 22:319, 1952

Johansson H: Studies on inspiratory gas flow patterns during artificial ventilation. Linkoping Univ Med Diss 18:24, 1974

Johansson L, Silander T: Twenty-one years of thoracic injuries: a clinical study of 313 cases. Acta Chir Scand [Suppl] 245:91, 1959

Johnston RP, Donovan DJ, MacDonnell KF: PEEP during assisted ventilation. Anesthesiology 40:308, 1974

Jonzon A: High-frequency positive-pressure ventilation and carotid sinus nerve stimulation. Acta Univ Upsaliensis 138:1972

Jonzon A: Phrenic and vagal nerve activities during spontaneous respiration and positive-pressure ventilation. Acta Anaesth Scand [Suppl] 64:29, 1977

Jonzon A, Öberg PÅ, Sedin G, et al: High frequency low tidal volume positive pressure ventilation. Acta Physiol Scand 80:21A, 1970

Jonzon A, Öberg A, Sedin G, et al: High-frequency positive-pressure ventilation by endotracheal insufflation. Acta Anaesth Scand [Suppl] 43:1971

Jonzon A, Sedin G, and Sjöstrand U: High-frequency positive-pressure ventilation (HFPPV) applied for small lung ventilation and compared with spontaneous breathing and continuous positive airway pressure (CPAP). Acta Anaesth Scand [Suppl] 53:23, 1973

Joyce JW, Woodward KE, Barila T: A fluid amplifier-controlled respirator. Proceedings of the Conference on Engineering in Medicine and Biology. Vol. 7. p. 20. Abstract 145. Institute of Electrical and Electronic Engineers, New York, 1965

Junger T, Laurent B: The polio epidemic in Stockholm 1953. XI. Biochemical laboratory investigation. Acta Med Scand [Suppl] 316:71–79, 1956

Kadosch M, Paulin C, Gilbert J, et al: Appareil de respiration artificielle basé sur le principe des commutateur fluides, sans pièce mobile. J Fr Med Chir Thorac 20:5, 1966

Kattwinkel J, Fleming D, Cha CC, et al: A device for administration of continuous positive airway pressure by the nasal route. Paediatrics 52:131, 1973

Keats AS: A simple and versatile mechanical ventilator for infants. Anesthesiology 29:591, 1968

Keiskamp DHG: Automatic ventilation in paediatric anaesthesia using a modified Ayre's T-piece with negative pressure during expiratory phase. Anaesthesia 18:46, 1963

Keith A: The mechanism underlying the various methods of artificial respiration. Lancet 1:745, 825, 895, 1909

Kellcher WH, Kinnier Wilson AB, Ritchie RW, et al: Notes on curiass respirator. Br Med J 2:413, 1952

Kelman GR, Nunn JF: Computer Produced Physiological Tables for Calculations Involving the Relationships Between the Blood Oxygen Tension and Content. Butterworth, London, 1968

Kelman GR, Prys-Roberts C: Circulatory influences of artificial ventilation during nitrous oxide anaesthesia in man. I: Introduction and methods. Br J Anaesth 39:523, 1967

Kenney LJ, Schosser RJ: Severe crushing injury of the chest; management with the Mörch respirator. J Michigan Med Soc 57:225, 1958

Kety SS, Schmidt CF: The effects of altered arterial tensions of carbon dioxide and oxygen on cerebral blood flow and cerebral oxygen consumption in normal young men. J Clin Invest 27:484, 1948

Khambatta HJ, Sullivan SF: Effects of respiratory alkalosis on oxygen consumption and oxygenation. Anesthesiology 38:53, 1973

Kilburn KH: Shock, seizures, and coma with alkalosis during mechanical ventilation. Ann Intern Med 65:977, 1966

Kilburn KH, Sieker HO: Hemodynamic effects of continuous positive and negative pressure breathing in normal man. Circ Res 8:660, 1960

Kirby RR: High levels of positive end-expiratory pressure (PEEP) in acute respiratory insufficiency. Chest 67:156, 1975

Kirby RR: Intermittent mandatory ventilation in the neonate. Crit Care Med 5:18, 1977

Kirby RR: Is intermittent mandatory ventilation a satisfactory alternative to assisted and controlled ventilation. American Society of Anesthesiology Refresher Course Lecture, 1975

Kirby RR, Desautels D, Smith RA: Mechanical ventilation. In Burton GG, Hodgkin JE (eds) Respiratory Care: A guide to clinical practice. pp. 556–647. Lippincott, Philadelphia 1984

Kirby RR, Downs JB, Civetta JM, et al: High level positive end-expiratory pressure (PEEP) in acute respiratory insufficiency. Chest 67:156, 1975

Kirby RR, Graybar GB (eds): Intermittent mandatory ventilation: Int Anesthesiol Clin 18:No. 2, 1980

Kirby RR, Perry JC, Calderwood HW, et al: Cardiorespiratory effects of high positive end-expiratory pressure. Anesthesiology 43:533, 1975

Kirby RR, Robison EJ, Schulz J, et al: A new pediatric volume ventilator. Anesth Analg 50:533, 1971

Kirby R, Robison E, Schulz J, et al: Continuous flow ventilation as an alternative to assisted or controlled ventilation in infants. Anesth Analg 51:871, 1972

Kirschner JM: Fluid Amplifiers. McGraw-Hill, New York, 1966

Kirschner JM: Fluidics. I. Basic Principles. TR-1498, Harry Diamond Laboratory (U.S. Army), Washington, DC, 1968

Kirschner JM, Horton BM: A brief history of fluidics (from the viewpoint of the Harry Diamond Laboratories). Presented at the 7th National Fluidics Symposium, Tokyo, 1972

Kite C: On submersion of Animals; its Effects on the Vital Organs; and the Most Probable Method of Removing Them. Mem Med Soc London 1792, III, pp 215–308

Klain M, Smith RB: Fluidic technology. Anaesthesia 31:750, 1976

Klain M, Smith RB: High frequency percutaneous transtracheal jet ventilation. Crit Care Med 5:280, 1977

Klein RL, Safar P, Grenvik A: Respiratory care in blunt chest injury: retrospective review of 43 cases. In: Abstracts of Scientific Papers, Annual Meeting of ASA, New York, pp. 145–146, 17–21 October 1970

Kolton M, Cattran C, Bryan AC, et al: High frequency oscillation and mean lung volume. Anesthesiology (Suppl) 55(3A):353, 1981

Komesaroff D, McKie B: The "bronchoflator": a new technique for bronchoscopy under general anaesthesia. Br J Anaesth 44:1057, 1972

Kotheimer TG, Dickie KJ, DeGroot WJ: Mechanical determinants of inspiratory oxygen concentration in a pressure-cycled ventilator. Am Rev Respir Dis 103:679, 1971

Kreiselman J: New resuscitation apparatus. Anesthesiology 4:608, 1943

Kristensen HS, Lunding M: Two early Danish respirators designed for prolonged ventilation. Acta Anaesth Scand [Suppl] 67:96, 1978

Krogh A: En respirator efter Philip Drinker's princip. Hosp Tidende 75:629, 1932

Kuhn F: Perorale intubation mit Überdrucknarkose. Dtsch Z Chir 76:148; 78:467, 1905, 1907

Kumar A, Falke KJ, Geffin G, et al: Continuous positive-pressure ventilation in acute respiratory failure—effects on hemodynamics and lung function. N Engl J Med 283:1430, 1970

Kumar A, Pontoppidan H, Baratz RA, et al: Inappropriate response to increased plasma ADH during mechanical ventilation in acute respiratory failure. Anesthesiology 40:215, 1974

Kumar A, Pontoppidan H, Falke KJ, et al: Pulmonary barotrauma during mechanical ventilation. Crit Care Med 1:181, 1973

Kuwabara S, McCaughey TJ: Artificial ventilation in infants and young children using a new ventilator with the T-piece. Can Anaesth Soc J 13:576, 1966

Lassen HCA: A preliminary report of the 1952 epidemic of poliomyelitis in Copenhagen. Lancet 1:37, 1953

Lassen HCA: The Management of Respiratory and Bulbar Paralysis in Poliomyelitis. Monograph Series No. 26, pp. 157–211. World Health Organization, Geneva. 1955

Laver MB: Prevention of post-operative respiratory complications. In Saidman LJ, Moya F (eds): Complications of Anesthesia. pp. 31–39. Charles C Thomas, Springfield, IL, 1970

Laver MB, Morgan J, Bendixen HH, et al: Lung volume compliance and arterial oxygen tension during controlled ventilation. J Appl Physiol 19:725, 1964

Läwen and Sievers: Zur Praktischen Anwendung der instrumentellen künstlichen Respiration am Menschen. Münch Med Wochenschr 57:2221, 1910

Lawler PGP, Nunn JF: Intermittent mandatory ventilation. Anaesthesia 32:138, 1977

Lecky JH, Quinsky AJ: Postoperative respiratory management. Chest 62:503, 1972

Lee CJ, Lyons JH, Konisberg S, et al: Effects of spontaneous and positive pressure breathing of ambient air and pure oxygen at one atmosphere pressure on pulmonary surface characteristics. J Thorac Cardiovasc Surg 53:759, 1967

Lee ST: A ventilating bronchoscope for inhalation anesthesia and augmented ventilation. Anesth Analg 52:89, 1973

Lee ST: A ventilating laryngoscope for inhalation anaesthesia and augmented ventilation during laryngoscopic procedures. Br J Anaesth 44:874, 1972

Lehr J: Circulating currents during high frequency ventilation. Fed Proc 39:576, 1980

Lenaghan R, Silva YJ, Walt AJ: Hemodynamic alterations associated with expansion rupture of the lung. Arch Surg 99:339, 1969

Lenfent C, Howell BJ: Cardiovascular adjustments in dogs during continuous pressure breathing. J Appl Physiol 15:425, 1960

Leroy J: Recherches sur l'asphyxie. J Physiol (Paris) 8:97, 1828

Leroy J: Seconde mémoire sur l'asphyxie. J Physiol (Paris) 8:97, 1828

Levine M, Gilbert R, Auchincloss JH Jr: A comparison of the effects of sighs, large tidal volumes, and positive end-expiratory pressure in assisted ventilation. Scand J Respir Dis 53:101, 1972

Little DM Jr: The methodology of controlled respiration. Ann NY Acad Sci 66:939, 1957

Llewellyn MA, Swyer PR: Assisted and controlled ventilation in the newborn period: effect on oxygenation. Br J Anaesth 43:926, 1971

Llewellyn MA, Swyer PR: Positive expiratory pressure during mechanical ventilation in the newborn. Proceedings Society of Pediatric Research, p. 224, 1970

Loredo MA, Avila JD, Gonzales CG: Apparatus for effortless inhalation anesthesia. Curr Res Anesth Analg 28:352, 1949

Lough MD, Doershuk CF, Stern RC: Pediatric Respiratory Therapy. Year Book, Chicago, 1974

Lucas BGB: A portable resuscitator. Br J Med 1:541, 1949

Luedke J, Kosmatka A: A new method of weaning from respiratory support. Resp Care 18:561, 1973

Lunkenheimer PP, Frank I, Ising H, et al: Intrapulmonaler Gaswechsel unter simulierter Apnoe durch transtrachealen, periodischen intrathorakalen Druckwechsel. Anaesthesist 22:232, 1973

Lunkenheimer PP, Rafflenbeul W, Keller H, et al: Application of transtracheal pressure-oscillations as a modification of "diffusion respiration." Br J Anaesth 44:627, 1972

Lunn JN, Mapleson WW, Chilcoat RT: Effects of changes of frequency and tidal volume of controlled ventilation: measurements at constant arterial P_{CO_2} in dogs. Br J Anaesth 47:2, 1975

Lutch JS, Murray JF: Continuous positive pressure ventilation—effects on systemic oxygen transport and tissue oxygenation. Ann Intern Med 76:193, 1972

Lyager S: Influence of flow pattern on the distribution of respiratory air during intermittent positive pressure ventilation. Acta Anaesth Scand 12:191, 1968

Lyager S: Ventilation/perfusion ratio during intermittent positive pressure ventilation—importance of no-flow interval during the insufflation. Acta Anaesth Scand 14:211, 1970

Lyons J, Moore F: Posttraumatic alkalosis—incidence and pathophysiology of alkalosis in surgery. Surgery 60:93, 1966

Maloney JV, Affeldt JE, Sarnoff SJ, et al: Electrophrenic respiration. 9. Comparison of effects of positive pressure breathing on the circulation during haemorrhage and barbiturate poisoning. Surg Gynecol Obstet 92:672, 1951

Maloney JV, Derrick WS, Whittenberger JL: A device producing regulated assisted respiration. Surg Forum 588, 1950

Maloney JV, Derrick WS, Whittenberger JL: Device producing regulated assisted respiration: prevention of hypoventilation and mediastinal motion during intrathoracic surgery. Anesthesiology 13:23, 1952

Maloney JW, Elam JO, Handford SW, et al: Importance of negative pressure phase in mechanical respirator. JAMA 152:212, 1953

Maloney JV, Elam JO, Handford SW, et al: Imsponse to intermittent positive and alternating positive-negative pressure respirations. J Appl Physiol 6:453, 1954

Maloney JV, Whittenberger JL: The direct effects of pressure breathing on the pulmonary circulation. Ann NY Acad Sci 66:931, 1957

Mannino FL, Feldman BH, Heldt GP, et al: Early mechanical ventilation in RDS with a prolonged inspiration. Pediatr Res 10:464, 1976

Mapleson WW: Physical aspects of automatic ventilators: basic principles. In Mushin WW, Rendell-Baker L, Thompson PW (eds): Automatic Ventilation of the Lungs. pp. 42–79. Blackwell, Oxford, 1959

Mapleson WW: The effect of changes of lung characteristics on the functioning of automatic ventilation. Anaesthia 17:300, 1962

Mapleson WW: Volume-pressure characteristic of the ''one gallon'' reservoir bag. Br J Anaesth 26:11, 1954

Marcotte RJ, et al: Differential intrabronchial pressure and mediastinal emphysema. J Thorac Surg 9:346, 1940

Margand PMS, Chodoff P: Intermittent mandatory ventilation; an alternative weaning technique: a case report. Anesth Analg 54:41, 1975

Markland E, Boucher RF: A Guide to Fluidics. p. 2. Macdonald, London, 1971

Martin AM Sr, Simmons RL, Heisterkamp CA III: Respiratory insufficiency in combat casualties. I. Pathologic changes in the lungs of patients dying of wounds. Ann Surg 170:30, 1969

Masud KZ, Byoan M, Hoffman R, et al: Hemodynamic effects of IMV and HFV in patients with acute respiratory failure. Anesthesiology (Suppl) 55:355, 1981

Matas R: Artificial respiration by direct intralaryngeal intubation with a modified O'Dwyer tube and a new graduated air-pump in its application to medical and surgical practice. Am Med 3:97, 1902

Matas R: Intralaryngeal insufflation for the relief of acute surgical pneumothorax: its history and methods with a description of the latest devices for this purpose. JAMA 34:1468, 1900

Matas R: On the management of acute traumatic pneumothorax. Ann Surg 29:409, 1899

Matilla MAK: The role of the physical characteristics of the respirator in artificial ventilation of the newborn. Acta Anaesth Scand [Suppl] 56:1, 1974

Mattila MAK, Suntarinen T: Clinical and experimental evaluation of the Loosco baby respirator. Acta Anaesth Scand 15:229, 1971

Mautz FR: A mechanism for artificial pulmonary ventilation in the operating room. J Thorac Surg 10:544, 1941

Mautz FR: Mechanical respirator as adjunct to closed system anesthesia. Proc Soc Exp Biol 42:190, 1939

Mautz FR: Surgery: thoracic, physical consideration. In Glasser O (ed): Medical Physics. pp. 1514–1519. Year Book, Chicago, 1944

Mautz FR, Beck CS, Chase HF: Augmented and controlled breathing in transpleural operation. J Thorac Surg 17:283, 1948

Mead J: The distribution of gas flow in the lungs. In: Ciba Foundation Symposium: Circulatory and Respiratory Mass Transport. pp. 204–209. Churchill, London, 1969

Mead J, Collier C: Relationship of volume of lungs to respiratory mechanisms in anesthetized dogs. J Appl Physiol 14:669, 1959

Mead J, Whittenberger JL: Lung inflation and hemodynamics. In: Fenn WO, Rahn H (eds): Handbook of Physiology, Section 3: Respiration. Vol I. p. 477. American Physiological Society, Washington, DC, 1964

Meier A, Baum M: The influence of the internal compliance of a respirator on the alveolar gas distribution. Acta Anaesth Scand [Suppl] 63:1, 1976

Meltzer SJ: Der gegenwärtige Stand der intratrachealen Insufflation. Berl Klin Wochenschr 51:677, 743, 1914

Meltzer SJ: History and analysis of the methods of resuscitation. Med Rec 92:190, 1939

Meltzer SJ, Auer J: Continuous respiration without respiratory movements. J Exp Med 11:622, 1909

Merlis JK, Degelman J: Improved artificial respirator for animal experimentation. Science 114:692, 1951

Meyer JA, Joyce JW: The fluid amplifier and its application in medical devices. Anesth Analg 47:710, 1968

Meyer W: Anesthesia in differential pressure chambers, cabinets and other apparatus for thoracic surgery. In Keen WW (ed): Surgery, Its Principles and Practice. p. 953. Saunders, Philadelphia, 1913

Meyer W: Pneumonectomy with the aid of differential air pressure. JAMA 53:1978, 1909

Minkowski A, Monset-Couchard M, Amiel-Tison: Symposium on artificial ventilation. Biol Neonate 16:1, 1970

Modell JH: Intermittent mandatory ventilation in the treatment of patients with chronic pulmonary disease. Anesth Analg 54:119, 1975

Modell JH: Ventilation/perfusion changes during mechanical ventilation. Dis Chest 55:447, 1969

Mölgaard H: Fysiologisk Lungekirurgi. pp. 1–370. Gyldendal, Copenhagen, 1915

Monckcom W, Patterson RW: Ventilation-perfusion inequalities resulting from hypocapnic changes in lung mechanics. J Thorac Cardiovasc Surg 63:577, 1972

Moore FD, Lyon JH, Peirce EC, et al: Post-Traumatic Pulmonary Insufficiency: Pathophysiology of Respiratory Failure and Principles of Respiratory Care after Surgical Operations, Trauma, Hemorrhage, Burns and Shock. pp. 12–125. Saunders, Philadelphia, 1969

Moore RL, Humphreys GH, Wreggit WR: Studies on the volume output of blood from the heart in anesthetized dogs before thoracotomy and after thoracotomy and intermittent or continuous inflation of the lungs. J Thorac Surg 5:195, 1935

Morales ES, Krumperman LW: The effects of instrumentation on gas flows during bronchoscopy using the Sanders ventilating attachment. Anesthesiology 38:197, 1973

Mörch ET: Anaesthesi. Munksgaard, Copenhagen, p. 405, 1949

Mörch ET: Anaesthesien under intrapleurale operationer. Nord Med 36:2234, 1947

Mörch ET: Controlled respiration by means of special automatic machines as used in Sweden and Denmark. Proc R Soc Med 40:39, 1947

Mörch ET: Et nyt obstetrisk analgesi-apparat. Ugeskr Laeger 110:856, 1948

Mörch ET, Avery E, Benson DW: Hyperventilation in the treatment of crushing injuries of the chest—problems in pulmonary physiology and pathology. Surg Forum 6:270, 1955

Mörch ET, Benson DW: Automatic artificial respiration during anesthesia. In: Proceedings: Third Congress of the Scandinavian Society of Anaesthesiologists, Copenhagen, pp. 30–46, 1954

Mörch ET, Engel R, Light GA: Effects of pressure breathing on the peripheral circulation: motion picture observations in the bat wing and rabbit ear chamber. Arch Surg 79:493, 1959

Mörch ET, Saxton GA: Tracheostomy tube connectors. Anesthesiology 17:366, 1956

Mörch ET, Saxton GA, Gish G: Artificial respiration via the uncuffed tracheostomy tube. JAMA 160:864, 1956

Morgan BC, Crawford EW, Guntheroth WG: The hemodynamic effects of changes in blood volume during intermittent positive pressure breathing. Anesthesiology 30:297, 1965

Morgan BC, Crawford EW, Hornbein TF, et al: Hemodynamic effects of changes in arterial carbon dioxide tension during intermittent positive pressure ventilation. Anesthesiology 28:866, 1967

Morgan BC, Crawford EW, Winterscherd LC, et al: Circulatory effects of intermittent positive pressure ventilation. Northwest Med 67:149, 1968

Morgan BC, Martin WE, Hornbein TF, et al: Hemodynamic effects of intermittent pressure respiration. Anesthesiology 27:584, 1966

Morgan WL, Binion JT, Sarnoff SJ: The circulatory depression induced by high level of positive pressure breathing counteracted by metaraminol. J Appl Physiol 10:26, 1957

Morton JHV: Respiratory patterns during surgical anaesthesia. Anaesthesia 5:112, 1950

Motley HL: Physiological and clinical studies on man with the pneumatic balance resuscitation "Burns model. Memorandum Report TSEAL-3-660-49. O, AAF Hedgs. ATSC, Engineering Div, Aero Med Lab Wright Field, 23 August 1945

Motley HL, Cournand A, Eckman M, et al: Physiology studies on man with pneumatic balance resuscitator "Burns model." J Aviat Med 17:431, 1946

Motley HL, Cournand A, Werkö L, et al: Intermittent positive pressure breathing. JAMA 137:370, 1948

Motley HL, Cournand A, Werkö L, et al: Observation on the clinical use of intermittent positive pressure. J Aviat Med 18:417, 1947

Motley HL, Cournand A, Werkö L, et al: Physiological and clinical studies of intermittent pressure respirators and manual methods for producing artificial respiration in man. Report No. TSEEA-697-79-F. Army Air Forces, Engineering Division. Memorandum, 6 September 1946

Motley HL, Cournand A, Werkö L, et al: Physiological studies on man with pneumatic balance resuscitator "Burns model." J Aviat Med 17:431, 1946

Motley HL, Lang LP, Gordon B: Use of intermittent positive pressure breathing combined with nebulization in pulmonary disease. Am J Med 5:853, 1948

Mousel LH, Stubbs D, Kreiselman L: Anesthetic complications and their management. Anesthesiology 7:69, 1946

Moylan FMB, Walker AM, Kramer SS, et al: The relationship of bronchopulmonary dysplasia to the occurrence of alveolar rupture during positive pressure ventilation. Crit Care Med 6:140, 1978

Munson ES, Eger EI II: Continuous ventilation in the newborn. Anesthesiology 24:871, 1963

Murdaugh HV, Seiker HO, Manfredi F: Effect of altered intrathoracic pressure on renal hemodynamics, electrolyte excretion and water clearance. J Clin Invest 38:834, 1959

Murphy FT: A suggestion for a practical apparatus for use in intrathoracic operations. Boston Med Surg J 152:428, 1905

Musgrove AH: Controlled respiration in thoracic surgery: a new mechanical respirator. Anaesthesia 7:77, 1952

Mushin WW, Faux N: Use of the Both respirator to reduce postoperative morbidity. Lancet 2:685, 1944

Mushin WW, Mapleson WW, Lynn JN: Problem of automatic ventilation in infants and children. Br J Anaesth 34:514, 1962

Mushin WW, Rendell-Baker L: Modern automatic respirators. Br J Anaesth 26:131, 1954

Mushin WW, Rendell-Baker L: Principles of Thoracic Anaesthesia. Blackwell, Oxford, 1953

Mushin WW, Rendell-Baker L: The Principles of Thoracic Anaesthesia Past and Present. p. 172. Charles C Thomas, Springfield, IL, 1953

Mushin WW, Rendell-Baker L, Thompson PW: Automatic Ventilation of the Lungs. Blackwell, Oxford 1959, 1980; and FA Davis, Philadelphia, 1969

MacDonell K, Lefemine AA, Moon HS, et al: Comparative hemodynamic consequences of inflation hold, PEEP, and interrupted PEEP. Ann Thorac Surg 19:552, 1975

Macintosh RR: New use of Both respirator. Lancet 2:745, 1940

MacNaughton FI: Catheter inflation ventilation in tracheal stenosis. Br J Anaesth 47:1225, 1975

Macrae J, McKendrick GDW, Claremont JM, et al: Positive-pressure respiration: management of patients treated with Clevedon respirator. Lancet 2:21, 1954

Macrae J, McKendrick GDW, Claremont JM, et al: The Clevedon positive-pressure respirator. Lancet 2:971, 1953

McIntyre RW, Laws AK, Ramachandran PR: Positive expiratory pressure plateau: improved gas exchange during mechanical ventilation. Can Anaesth Soc J 16:477, 1969

McLaughlin GW, Kirby GG, Kemmerer WT, et al: Indirect measurement of blood pressure in infants using doppler ultrasound. J Pediatr 79:300, 1971

McLellan L: Resuscitation apparatus. Anaesthesia 36:307, 1981

McMahon SM, Halpin GM: Modification of intrapulmonary blood shunt by end-expiratory pressure application in patients with acute respiratory failure. Chest 59:27S, 1971

McPherson SP: Respiratory Therapy Equipment. Mosby, St. Louis, 1977

McPherson SP, Glasgow GD, William AA, et al: A circuit that combines ventilator weaning methods using continuous flow ventilation (CFV). Resp Care 20:261, 1975

Naess K: A simple apparatus for artificial respiration, built of a vacuum window wiper. Acta Physiol Scand 22:376, 1951

Nash G, Blennerhassett JB, Pontoppidan H: Pulmonary lesions associated with oxygen therapy and artificial ventilation. N Engl J Med 276:368, 1967

Nash G, Bowen JA, Langlinais PC: "Respirator lung": a misnomer. Arch Pathol 91:234, 1971

National Fluid Power Association: Recommended Standard Graphic Symbols for Fluidic Devices and Circuits. NFPA/T3.7.2-1968. National Fluid Power Association, Thiensville, WI, 1968

National Fluid Power Association: What You Should Know About Fluidics. National Fluid Power Association, Thiensville, WI, 1972

Nause FP: Crushed chest, treatment using a mechanical respirator. Wis Med J 59:697, 1960

Neff W, Phillips W, Gunn G: Anesthesia for pneumonectomy in man. Anesthesiology 3:314, 1942

Nennhaus HP, Javis H, Julian OC: Alveolar and pleural rupture: hazards of positive pressure respiration. Arch Surg 94:136, 1967

Nicotra MB, Stevens PM, Viroslav J, et al: Physiologic evaluation of positive end-expiratory pressure ventilation. Chest 64:10, 1973

Nightingale DA, Richards CC, Glass A: An evaluation of rebreathing on a modified T-piece system during continuous ventilation for anaesthesia in children. Br J Anaesth 37:762, 1965

Nilsson E: On treatment of barbiturate poisoning. Acta Med Scand [Suppl] 253:1, 1951

Nilsson LG, Lyttkens L, Sjöstrand U, et al: Positive end-expiratory pressure (PEEP)—an experimental study on dogs. Opusc Med 21:117, 1976

Nisbet HIA, Dobbinson TL, Steward DJ, et al: The effect of artificial ventilation on FRC and arterial oxygenation. Can Anaesth Soc J 21:215, 1974

Nissen R: Historical development of pulmonary surgery. Am J Surg 89:9, 1955

Nordenström B: Contrast examination of the cardiovascular system during increased intrabronchial pressure. Acta Radiol Scand [Suppl] 200:1, 1960

Nordström L: Haemodynamic effects of intermittent positive-pressure ventilation with and without an end-inspiratory pause. Acta Anaesth Scand [Suppl] 47:29, 1972

Nordström L: On automatic ventilation. Acta Anaes Scand [Suppl] 47:1, 1972

Nordström S, Eriksson I, Nilsson LG, et al: High frequency positive pressure ventilation (HFPPV) during transthoracic resection of tracheal stenosis and during preoperative bronchoscopic examination. Acta Anaesth Scand 19:113, 1975

Norlander O: Anaesthesiologische Gesichtspunkte der Handhabung Thoracchirurgischer Fälle während und nach der Operation. Thoraxchirurgie 6:162, 1958

Norlander O: Functional analysis of force and power of mechanical ventilation. Acta Anaesth Scand 8:57, 1964

Norlander O: Management of respirator and anesthesia patients: monitoring and developments. Med Prog Technol 3:15, 1974

Norlander O, Björk VO, Crafoord C, et al: Controlled ventilation in medical practice. Anaesthesia 16:285, 1961

Norlander O, Herzog P: An Engström respirator designed for high frequency ventilation. Opusc Med 18:74, 1973

Norlander O, Holmdahl MH, Matell G, et al: Clinical experience with a new modular Engstöm care system (ECS 2000) ventilator. In Arias A, Llaurado R, Nalda MA, Lunn JN (eds): Recent Progress in Anaesthesiology and Resuscitation. pp. 516–518. Excerpta Medica, Amsterdam, 1975

Norlander O: The use of respirators in anesthesia and surgery. Acta Anaesth Scand [Suppl] 30:1, 1968

Norlander O, Pitzela S, Edling N, et al: Anaesthesiological experience from intracardiac surgery with the Crafoord-Senning-heart-lung machine. Acta Anaesth Scand 2:181, 1958

Northrup WP: Apparatus for artificial forcible respiration. Med Surg Rep Presbyterian Hosp (NY) 1:127, 1896

Northway WR Jr, Rosal RC, Porter DY: Pulmonary disease following respiratory therapy of hyaline membrane disease: bronchopleural dysplasia. N Engl J Med 276:357, 1967

Nosworthy MD: Anaesthesia in chest surgery. Proc R Soc Med 34:479, 1941

Nunn JF: Physiological aspects of artificial ventilation. Br J Anaesth 29:540, 1957

Nunn JF, Bergman NA, Coleman AJ: Factors influencing the arterial oxygen tension during anaesthesia with artificial ventilation. Br J Anaesth 37:898, 1965

Nystrom G, Blalock A: Contribution to the technique of pulmonary embolectomy. Thorac Surg 5:169, 1936

Obdrzalek J, Kay JC, Noble WH: The effects of continuous positive pressure ventilation on pulmonary oedema, gas exchange and lung mechanics. Can Anaesth Soc J 22:399, 1975

O'Donoline W Jr, Baker JP, Beil GM, et al: The management of acute respiratory failure in a respiratory intensive care unit. Chest 58:603, 1970

O'Dwyer J: Fifty cases of croup in private practice treated by intubation of the larynx, with a description of the method and of the dangers incident thereto. Med Res 32:557, 1887

O'Dwyer J: Intubation of the larynx. NY Med J 42:145, 1885

Okmian L: Artificial ventilation by respirator for newborn and small infants during anaesthesia. Acta Anaesthesiol Scand [Suppl] 20:1, 1966

Opie LH, Smith AC, Spalding JMK: Conscious appreciation of the effects produced by independent changes of ventilator volume and of end-tidal Pco_2 in paralyzed patients. J Physiol (Lond) 149:494, 1959

Opie LH, Spalding JMK, Smith AC: Intrathoracic pressure during intermittent positive pressure respiration. Lancet 1:911, 1961

Orth OS, Wilhelm RL, Waters RM: The question of pulmonary drainage with artificial respiration. J Thorac Surg 14:220, 1945

Orton RH: Controlled respiration. Med J Aust 2:255, 1947

Oulton JL, Donald DM: A ventilating laryngoscope. Anesthesiology 35:540, 1971

Parham FW: On the management of acute traumatic pneumothorax. Ann Surg 29:409, 1899

Parham FW: Thoracic resection for tumor growing from the bony wall of the chest. Transactions of the Southern Society of Anesthetists 11:223, 1898

Parson EF, Travis K, Shore N, et al: Effect of positive pressure breathing on distribution of pulmonary blood flow and ventilation. Am Rev Resp Dis 103:356, 1971

Patterson JR, Russell GK, Pierson DJ et al: Evaluation of a fluidic ventilator: a new approach to mechanical ventilation. Chest 66:706, 1974

Peck CH: Intratracheal insufflation anesthesia (Meltzer-Auer): observation on a series of 216 anaesthesiae with the Elsberg apparatus. Ann Surg 56:192, 1912

Pedersen B: Respirator treatment of neonates. Acta Anaesth Scand 16:38, 1972

Perea EJ, Criado A, Moreno M, et al: Mechanical ventilators as vehicles of infection. Acta Anaesth Scand 19:180, 1975

Peslin RL: Étude sur modèles de la distribution aérienne au cours de la ventilation instrumental. Bull Physiol Pathol Resp 2:253, 1966

Peslin RL: The physical properties of ventilators in the inspiratory phase. Anesthesiology 30:315, 1969

Peters RM: The Mechanical Basis of Respiration. J Churchill, London, 1969

Peters RM, Hutchin P: Adequacy of available respirations to their tasks. Ann Thorac Surg 3:414, 1967

Petrén K, Sjövall E: Eine studie über die tödliche akute Form der Poliomyelitis. Acta Med Scand 64:260, 1926

Petty TL: IMV vs IMC. Chest 67:630, 1975

Petty TL: Intensive and Rehabilitative Respiratory Care. Lea & Febiger, Philadelphia, 1974

Petty TL, Ashbaugh DG: The adult respiratory distress syndrome. Chest 60:233, 1971

Petty TL, Bigelow DB, Broughton JO: A new volume cycled ventilator. Resp Ther 2:33, 1972

Petty TL, Nett LM, Ashbaugh D: Improvement in oxygenation in the adult respiratory distress syndrome by positive end-expiratory pressure (PEEP). Resp Care 16:173, 1971

Phillein DM, Baratz RA, Patterson RW: The effect of carbon dioxide on plasma antidiuretic hormone levels during intermittent positive pressure breathing. Anesthesiology 33:345, 1970

Pierce HF: An artificial respiration and ether apparatus for use with compressed air. J Lab Clin Med 9:197, 1923

Pilcher J: Prolonged orotracheal intubation without tracheostomy for respiratory failure. B J Dis Chest 61:95, 1967

Pinson KB: Mechanically controlled respiration in thoracic surgery. Anaesthesia 4:79, 1949

Pinson KB, Bryce AG: Constant suction in thoracic surgery: description of an anaesthetic apparatus. Br J Anaesth 19:53, 1944

Plum F, Lukas DS: An evaluation of the cuirass respirator in acute poliomyelitis with respiratory insufficiency. Am J Med Sci 221:417, 1951

Plum F, Wolff HG: Observations on acute poliomyelitis with respiratory insufficiency. JAMA 146:442, 1951

Plut HG Jr, Miller WF: New volume ventilator. Inhal Ther 13:91, 1968

Poisvert M, Cara M: Un nouveau concept en ventilation artificielle: la cellule logique. Ann Anesthesiol Fr 8:411, 1967

Poisvert M, Galinski R, Hurtland JP, et al: A propos de l'utilisation clinique d'un respirateur a cellules logiques. Ann Anesthesiol Fr 8:445, 1967

Poling HE, Wolfson B, Siker ES: A technique of ventilation during laryngoscopy and bronchoscopy. Br J Anaesth 47:382, 1975

Pontoppidan H: Mechanical aid to lung expansion in non-intubated surgical patients. Am Rev Respir Dis 122:109, 1980

Pontoppidan H: Pathophysiology of postoperative pulmonary complications. In: Anesthesiology and Intensive Care Medicine. Springer, Berlin, 1979

Pontoppidan H: Pneumonia treated by extracorporeal membrane oxygenation. N Engl J Med 292:1174, 1975

Pontoppidan H, Berry PR: Regulation of the inspired oxygen concentration during artificial ventilation. JAMA 201:11, 1967

Pontoppidan H, Geffin B, Lowenstein E: Acute respiratory failure in the adult. N Engl J Med 287:690, 743, 799, 1972

Pontoppidan H, Hedley-Whyte J, Bendixen HH, et al: Ventilation and oxygen requirements during prolonged artificial ventilation in patients with respiratory failure. N Engl J Med 273:401, 1965

Pontoppidan H, Laver MB, Geffin B: Acute respiratory failure in the surgical patients. Adv Surg 4:163, 1970

Pontoppidan H, Rie MA: Pathogenesis and therapy of acute lung injury. In Prakash O (ed): Applied Physiology in Clinical Respiratory Care. Ch. 5. Martinus Nijhoff, The Hague, 1982

Pontoppidan H, Wilson RS, Rie MA, et al: Respiratory intensive care. Anesthesiology 47:96, 1977

Poulsen H, Skall-Jensen J, Staffeldt I, et al: Pulmonary ventilation and respiratory gas exchange during manual artificial respiration and expired-air resuscitation on apnoeic normal adults. Acta Anaesth Scand 3:129, 1959

Powers SR Jr, Mannal R, Neclerio M, et al: Physiologic consequences of positive end-expiratory pressure (PEEP) ventilation. Ann Surg 128:265, 1972

Price HL, Conner EH, Dripps RD: Some respiratory and circulatory effects of mechanical respirators. J Appl Physiol 6:517, 1954

Price HL, Conner EH, Elder JD, et al: Effect of sodium thiopental on circulation response to positive pressure inflation of lung. J Appl Physiol 4:629, 1952

Prys-Roberts C, Kelman GR, Greenbaum R, et al: Circulatory influences of artificial ventilation during nitrous oxide anesthesia in man. II. Results: the relative influences of mean intrathoracic pressure and arterial carbon dioxide tension. Br J Anaesth 39:533, 1967

Pyle P, Darlow M, Firman JE: A treated ultra-high-efficiency for mechanical ventilators. Lancet 1:136, 1969

Qvist J, Pontoppidan H, Wilson RS, et al: Hemodynamic response to mechanical ventilation with PEEP: The effect of hyperventilation. Anesthesiology 42:45, 1975

Radford EP: Ventilation standards for use in artificial respiration. J Appl Physiol 7:451, 1955

Ramanathan S, Sinha K, Arismendy J, et al: Bronchofiberscopic high frequency ventilation. Anesthesiology (Suppl)55(3A):352, 1981

Randall HT, McPherson RC, Haller JA, et al: Treatment of flail chest injuries with a piston respirator. Am J Surg 104:22, 1962

Reba I: Applications of the Coanda effect. Sci Am 214:84, 1966

Rees GJ, Owen-Thomas JB: A technique of pulmonary ventilation with a nasotracheal tube. Br J Anaesth 38:901, 1966

Reicher J: Pulmonary suck and blow as respiratory analeptic. Arch Surg 53:77, 1946

Reynolds EOR: Methods of mechanical ventilation for hyaline membrane disease. Proc R Soc Med 67:10, 1974

Reynolds EOR: Pressure waveform and ventilator settings for mechanical ventilation in severe hyaline membrane disease. Int Anesthesiol Clin 12:259, 1974

Reynolds EOR, Taghizadeh A: Improved prognosis of infants mechanically ventilated for hyaline membrane disease. Arch Dis Child 49:505, 1974

Reynolds JA: A method of recording pulmonary ventilation. J Sci Instrum Series 2:1, 1968

Reynolds RN: A pulmonary ventilator for infants. Anesthesiology 25:712, 1964

Richardson B: Artificial respiration. In Druitt R (ed): The Surgeons Vade Mecum. 10th Ed. Churchill, London, 1870

Robinson S: A classical cone with a rubber drum over the base of dog's face. Ann Surg 47:184, 1908

Robinson S: Experimental surgery of the lungs. I. Thirty animal operations under positive pressure. Ann Surg 47:184, 1908

Robinson S, Leland GA: Survey of the lungs under positive and negative pressure. Surg Gynecol Obstet 9:255, 1909

Rochford J, Welch RF, Winks DW: An electronic time-cycled respirator. Br J Anaesth 30:23, 1958

Rogers EJ: Physics vs physiology in infant ventilation. Resp Ther 2:1, 1972

Roos A, Thomas LJ, Nagel EL, et al: Pulmonary vascular resistance as determined by lung inflation and vascular pressure. J Appl Physiol 16:77, 1961

Rossing TH, Slutsky AS, Lehr JL, et al: Tidal volume and frequency dependence of carbon dioxide elimination by high frequency ventilation. N Engl J Med 305:1375, 1981

Rotherman EB Jr, Safar P, Robin ED: CNS disorder during mechanical ventilation in chronic pulmonary disease. JAMA 189:993, 1964

Ruben H: A new nonrebreathing valve. Anesthesiology 16:643, 1955

Russell WR, Schuster E: Respiration pump for poliomyelitis. Lancet 2:707, 1953

Russell WR, Schuster E, Smith AC, et al: Radcliffe respiration pump. Lancet 1:539, 1956

Safar P: Long term resuscitation in intensive care units. Anesthesiology 25:216, 1964

Safar P: Respiratory Therapy. Davis, Philadelphia, 1965

Safar P, Berman B, Diamond E, et al: Cuffed tracheostomy tube vs. tank respirator for prolonged artificial ventilation. Arch Phys Med 43:487, 1962

Safar P, Davis G: Modified Mörch piston respirator. Anesthesiology 25:81, 1964

Safar P, Grenvik A: Critical care medicine: organizing and staffing intensive care units. Chest 59:535, 1971

Safar P, Grenvik A: Multidisciplinary intensive care. Mod Med 39:92, 1971

Safar P, Kunkel HG: Prolonged artificial ventilation. Clin Anesth Resp Ther 1:93, 1965

Safar P, Nemoto EM, Severinghaus JW: Pathogenesis of central nervous system disorder during artificial hyperventilation in compensated hypercarbia in dogs. Crit Care Med 1:15, 1973

Sahlin B: En ny respiratortyp. Hygeij Revy 20:129, 1931

Sahlin B: Zehn Fälle von Atemlähmung mit dem Barospirator Behandelt. Acta Med Scand 79:75, 1932

Sahn SA, Lakshmenarayan S, Petty TL: Weaning from mechanical ventilation. JAMA 235:2208, 1976

Saklad M: Inhalation Therapy and Resuscitation. Blackwell, Oxford, 1953

Saklad M, Wickliff D: Functional characteristics of artificial ventilators. Anesthesiology 28:718, 1967

Sanders RD: Two ventilating attachments for bronchoscopes. Del Med J 39:170, 1967

Sandison JW, McCormick PW, Sykes MK: Intermittent positive pressure respiration after open heart surgery. Br J Anaesth 35:100, 1963

Sarnoff SJ, Maloney JK, Whittenberg JL: Electrophrenic respiration. V. Effect on the circulation of electrophrenic respiration and positive pressure breathing during the respiratory paralysis of high spinal anesthesia. Ann Surg 132:921, 1950

Sauerbruch EF: Ueber die physiologischen und physikalischen Grundlagen bei intrathoracalen Eingriffen in meiner pneumatischen Operations—Kammer. Arch Klin Chir 73:977, 1904

Sauerbruch EF: Master Surgeon. Cromwell, New York, 1953

Sauerbruch EF: Zur Pathologie des öffennen Pneumothorax und die Grundlagen meines Verfahrens zu seiner Ausshaltung. Mitt Grenzgeb Med Chir 8:399, 1904

Scales JT, Kinnier Wilson AB, Holmes Sellors T, et al: Cuirass respirators: their design and construction. Lancet 1:671, 1953

Schmid ER, Knopp TJ, Rehder K: Intrapulmonary gas transport and perfusion during high frequency oscillation. J Appl Physiol 51:1507, 1981

Schwerma H, Ivy AC: Safety of modern alternating positive and negative pressure resuscitation. JAMA 129:1256, 1945

Scott DB, Stephen GW, Davie IT: Haemodynamic effects of a negative (subatmospheric) pressure expiratory phase during artificial ventilation. Br J Anaesth 44:171, 1972

Scullin G: The jet propelled genius and his mighty blow. Time Magazine 36:41, 1950

Secher O, Wandall HH, Clemmesen T, et al: The Mölgaard positive-pressure anaesthetic apparatus. Acta Chir Scand [Suppl] 283:8, 1961

Sedin G, Heijman K, Heijman L, et al: High-frequency positive-pressure ventilation during anaesthesia in man. Opusc Med 18:82, 1973

Selmeyer JP, Liberatore JM: Respiratory distress syndrome and continuous positive airway pressure. Lancet 2:1422, 1972

Severinghaus J, Swenson E, Finley T, et al: Unilateral hypoventilation produced in dogs by occluding one pulmonary artery. J Appl Physiol 16:53, 1961

Shaw LA, Drinker P: An apparatus for the prolonged administration of artificial respiration. J Clin Invest 8:33, 1929

Shinnick JP, Johnston RF, Oslick T: Bronchoscopy during mechanical ventilation using the fiberscope. Chest 65:613, 1974

Singer MM: Intermittent mechanical ventilation in the treatment of patients with chronic obstructive pulmonary disease. Anesth Analg 53:441, 1974

Sjöberg A, Engström CG, Svanborg N: Diagnostiska och kliniska ron vid behandling av bulbospinal polio-myelit (med film och demonstration av ny respirator). Nord Med 47:536, 1952

Sjöstrand U: Anesthésie générale et bronchoscopie. Ann Anesth Fr 17(8):871, 1976

Sjöstrand U: Pneumatic systems facilitating treatment of respiratory insufficiency with alternative use of IPPV/PEEP, HFPPV/PEEP, CPPB or CPAP. Acta Anaesth Scand [Suppl] 64:123, 1977

Sjöstrand U: Review of the physiological rationale for and development of high-frequency positive-pressure ventilation—HFPPV. Acta Anaesth Scand [Suppl] 64:165, 1977

Sjöstrand U: Summary of experimental and clinical features of high-frequency positive-pressure ventilation—HFPPV. Acta Anaesth Scand [Suppl] 64:165, 1977

Sjöstrand U (ed.): Experimental and clinical evaluation of high-frequency positive-pressure ventilation (HFPPV). Acta Anaesth Scand [Suppl] 64:1, 1977

Sjöstrand U, Eriksson I, Heijman L, et al: High-frequency positive-pressure ventilation (HFPPV) in bronchoscopy under general anaesthesia: preliminary communication. Opusc Med 21:113, 1976

Sjöstrand U, Jonzon A, Sedin G: Ventilazione a pressione positiva con alta frequenza: studio sperimentale ed espereinza clinica. In Fantoni A (ed): Atti del 3° Corso Nazionale di Aggiornamento in Rianimazione. p. 13. Piccin Editore, Padua, 1973

Sjöstrand U, Jonzon A, Sedin G, et al: High-frequency positive-pressure ventilation. Opusc Med 18:74, 1973

Skillman JJ, Malhorta JV, Pallotta JA, et al: Detriments of weaning from continuous ventilation. Surg Forum 22:198, 1971

Sladen A, Laver MB, Potoppidan H: Pulmonary complications and water retention in prolonged mechanical ventilation. N Engl J Med 279:448, 1968

Sliom CM: Infant ventilator systems. Br J Anaesth 40:306, 1968

Slocum HC, Hayes GW, Laezman BL: Ventilator techniques of anesthesia for neurosurgery. Anesthesiology 22:143, 1961 (abstract)

Slutsky AS, Brown R, Lehr J, et al: High-frequency ventilation: a promising new approach to mechanical ventilation. Med Istrum 15:229, 1981

Slutsky AS, Drazen J, Ingram RH, et al: Effective pulmonary ventilation with small volume oscillation at high frequency. Science 209:609, 1980

Smith C: Continuous ventilation employing a modified Ayre's technique. Anesth Analg 44:842, 1965

Smith RA: Respiratory Care. In Miller RD (ed): Anesthesia. Churchill Livingstone, New York, p. 1379, 1981

Smith RB, Babinski M, Petruscak J: A method for ventilating patients during laryngoscopy. Laryngoscope 84:553, 1974

Smith RB, Lindholm CE, Klain M: Jet ventilation for fiberoptic bronchoscopy under general anaesthesia. Acta Anaesth Scand 20:111, 1976

Smith RB, MacMillan BB, Petruscak J, et al: Transtracheal ventilation for laryngoscopy. Ann Otol 82:347, 1973

Smith RE: Modified Both respirators. Lancet 1:679, 1953

Smith RK: Respiratory care application for fluidics. Resp Ther 3:29, 1973

Smith-Clarke GT: Mechanical breathing machines. Proc Inst Mech Eng 171:52, 1957

Smith-Clarke GT, Galpine JF: Positive-negative pressure respirator. Lancet 1:1299, 1955

Soper RL: The pneumatic balance valve and its applications: a preliminary report. Br Med J 4733:717, 1951

Spalding JMK: Pressure and duration of inspiration during artificial respiration by intermittent positive pressure. Lancet 1:1099, 1955

Spalding JMK, Crampton Smith A: Clinical Practice and Physiology of Artificial Respiration. Davis, Philadelphia, 1963

Spalding JMK, Crampton Smith A: Clinical Practice of Artificial Respiration with Some Physiological Observations. Blackwell, Oxford, 1963

Spearman CB: Control of inspiratory oxygen concentration and addition of PEEP or CPAP with the Bourns pediatric ventilator. Resp Care 18:405, 1973

Speidel BD, Dunn PM: Effect of continuous positive airway pressure on breathing pattern of infants with respiratory-distress syndrome. Lancet 1:302, 1975

Spenser FC: Use of a mechanical respirator in the management of respiratory insufficiency following trauma or operation for cardiac or pulmonary disease. J Thorac Cardiovasc Surg 38:758, 1959

Speranza V, Beckman M, Norlander O: Il trattamento del insufficienza ventilatoria con la ventilazione artificiale a mezzo del respiratore di Engström. Chir Gen 9:417, 1957

Speranza V, Beckman M, Norlander O: L'insufficienza ventilatoria in chirurgia. Chir Gen 7:498, 1959

Spoerel WE, Greenway RE: Technique of ventilation during endolaryngeal surgery under general anesthesia. Can Anaesth Soc J 20:369, 1973

Spoerel WE, Narayanan PS, Singh NP: Transtracheal ventilation. Br J Anaesth 43:932, 1971

Stahlman MT, Malan AT, Shepard FM, et al: Negative pressure assisted ventilation in infants with hyaline membrane disease. J Pediatr 76:174, 1970

Stange G, Gebert E, Van de Loo C: Intubationslose Narkose bei direkter Laryngoscopie. Laryngol Rhinol 53:339, 1974

Steen SN, Lee ASJ: Prevention of inadvertent excess pressure in closed system. Anesth Analg 39:264, 1960

Steigman AJ, Rumph PH: The positive pressure respirator dome. Am J Nurs 52:311, 1952

Steinbereithner K, Baum M, Meier A: The influence of a respirator internal compliance on "pendelluft." Excerpta Med Int Congr Series 387:163, 1976

Sterling GM: The mechanism of bronchoconstriction due to hypocapnia in man. Clin Sci 34:377, 1968

Steuart W: Demonstration of apparatus for inducing artificial respiration for long periods. Med J South Afr 13:147, 1918

Stone JG, Sullivan SF: Failure of shallow ventilation to produce pulmonary shunting in the anesthetized dog. Anesthesiology 32:338, 1970

Straub H, Meyer JA: An evaluation of a fluid amplifier, face mask respirator. In: Proceedings of the Third Fluid Amplification Symposium. Vol. 3. p. 309. 1965

Styles J, Robinson JS, Jones JG: Continuous ventilation and oedema. Br J Anaesth 42:522, 1970

Sugarman HJ, Olofsson KB, Pollack TW, et al: Continuous positive pressure end-expiratory pressure ventilation (PEEP) for the treatment of diffuse interstitial pulmonary edema. J Trauma 12:263, 1972

Sugerman JH, Rogers RM, Miller LD: Positive end-expiratory pressure (PEEP): indications and physiological considerations. Chest 62:86, 1972

Suter PM, Fairley HB, Isenberg MD: Optimum end-expiratory airway pressure in patients with acute respiratory failure. N Engl J Med 292:284, 1975

Suwa K, Bendixen HH: Change in Paco$_2$ in the mechanical dead space during artificial ventilation. J Appl Physiol 24:556, 1968

Suwa K, Geffin B, Pontoppidan H, et al: A monogram for deadspace requirement during prolonged artificial ventilation. Anesthesiology 29:1206, 1968

Swensson A: Artificial respiration in general surgery. Acta Chir Scand 113:417, 1957

Swensson A: Artificial respiration in severe abdominal disease. Arch Dis Child 37:149, 1962

Swyer PR: Methods of artificial ventilation in the newborn (IPPV). Biol Neonate 16:3, 1970

Sykes MK, Adams AP, Finlay WEI, et al: The effects of variations in end-expiratory inflation pressure on cardiorespiratory function in normo- hypo- and hypervolemic dogs. Br J Anaesth 42:669, 1970

Sykes MK, Lumley J: The effect of varying inspiratory:expiratory ratios on gas exchange during anaesthesia for open-heart surgery. Br J Anaesth 41:374, 1969

Sykes MK, McNicol MW, Campbell EJM: Respiratory Failure. Davis, Philadelphia, 1969

Sykes MK, Young WE, Robinson BE: Oxygenation during anesthesia with controlled ventilation. Br J Anaesth 37:314, 1965

Taylor G, Gerbode F: Observations on the circulatory effects of short duration positive pressure pulmonary inflation. Surgery 30:56, 1951

Thatcher VS: History of Anesthesia. Lippincott, Philadelphia, 1953

Thompson SA: The effect of pulmonary inflation and deflation upon the circulation. J Thorac Surg 17:323, 1948

Thompson SA, Lange K, Rocky EE: The use of fluorescein to demonstrate the effect of artificial respiration upon the circulation. J Thorac Surg 16:710, 1947

Thompson SA, Quimby EH, Smith BC: The effect of pulmonary resuscitative procedures upon the circulation as demonstrated by the use of radio-active sodium. Surg Gynecol Obstet 83:387, 1946

Thompson SA, Rockey EE: The effect of mechanical artificial respiration upon maintenance of circulation. Surg Gynecol Obstet 84:1059, 1947

Thunberg T: Andning utan andningsrörelser. Hygiejnisk Revy, Uppsala Sweden 13:147, 1924.

Thunberg T: Der Barospirator: Ein neuer apparat für künstliche Atmung nach einem neuen Prinzip. Skan Arch Physiol 48:80, 1926

Tiegel M: Ein einfacher apparat zur Überdrucknarkose. Zbl Chir 22:679, 1908

Todd HM, Toutant SM, Shapiro HM, et al: Intracranial pressure effects of low and high frequency ventilation. Anesthesiology 53:196, 1980

Tossack W: Medical Essays and Observations. Vol. V. Part 2. p. 605. Society of Gentlemen of Edinburgh, Edinburgh, 1744

Trier-Mörch E: *see* Mörch ET

Trimble C, Smith DE, Rosenthal MH, et al: Pathophysiological role of hypocarbia in post-traumatic pulmonary insufficiency. Am J Surg 122:633, 1971

Trippenbach T: Effects of vagal blockade in artificially ventilated rabbits. Acta Physiol Pol 24:491, 1973

Tuffier T, Hallion L: Opérations intrathoracique avec respiration artificielle per insufflation. C R Soc Biol 48:951, 1896

Ueda H, Neclerio M, Leather RP, et al: Effect of positive end-expiratory pressure ventilation on renal function. Surg Forum 23:209, 1972

Ulf B, Eriksson J, Lyttkens L, et al: High frequency positive-pressure ventilation (HFPPV) applied in bronchoscopy under general anesthesia. Acta Anaesth Scand [Suppl] 64:69, 1977

Urban BJ, Weitzner SW: The Amsterdam infant ventilator and the Ayre's T-piece in mechanical ventilation. Anesthesiology 40:423, 1974

Uzawa T, Ashbaugh DG: Continuous positive pressure breathing in acute hemorrhagic pulmonary edema. J Appl Physiol 26:427, 1969

Van Bergen FH, Buckley JJ, Weatherhead DSP, et al: A new respirator. Anesthesiology 17:708, 1956

Vandam LD: Ten years ago: re-evaluation of critically crushed chests. Surv Anesthesiol 1:523, 1966

Van Vliet PKJ, Fisk GC, Gupta JM: Artificial ventilation in respiratory failure in the newborn. Med J Aust 2:648, 1971

Vesalius A: de Humani Corporis Fabrica Libra Septem. Basel, 1555

Vidyasagar D, Chernick V: Continuous positive transpulmonary pressure in hyaline membrane disease. Pediatrics 48:296, 1971

Vidyasagar D, Pildes RS: Use of the Amsterdam infant ventilator for continuous positive pressure breathing. Crit Care Med 2:89, 1974

Vilee CA, Vilee DB, Zuckerman J: Respiratory Distress Syndrome. Academic Press, New York, 1973

Visscher MB: The physiology of respiration and respirators with particular reference to poliomyelitis. In: National Foundation for Infantile Paralysis Round Table Conference. p. 156. Minneapolis, October 1947

Volgyesi G, Misbet HIA: A new position ventilator for use in respiratory studies. Can Anaesth Soc J 19:662, 1972

Volhardt F: Ueber Künstliche Atmung durch Ventilation der Trachea und eine einfache Vorrichtung zur rhytmischen, künstlichen Atmung. Münch Med Wochenschr 55:209, 1908

Volpitto PP, Woodburg RA, Abreu BE: Influence of different forms of mechanical artificial respiration on the pulmonary and systemic blood pressure. JAMA 126:1066, 1944

Waltz RC, Hubay CA, Ankeney JL, et al: Experimental study of pulmonary histopathology following positive and negative pressure respiration. Surg Gynecol Obstet 99:5, 1954

Watrous WG, Davis FE, Anderson BM: Manually assisted and controlled respiration: a review. Anesthesiology 12:33, 1951

Watson WE: Observation on physiological dead space during intermittent positive pressure respiration. Br J Anaesth 34:504, 1962

Watson WE: Some observations on dynamic lung compliance during intermittent positive pressure respiration. Br J Anaesth 34:153, 1962

Watson WE, Smith AC, Spalding JMK: Transmural central venous pressure during intermittent positive pressure breathing. Br J Anaesth 34:274, 1962

Weenig CS, Pietak S, Hickey RF, et al: Relationship of pre-operative closing volume to functional residual capacity and alveolar-arterial oxygen difference during anesthesia with controlled ventilation. Anesthesiology 41:3, 1974

Weil H, Shubin H: The new practice of critical care medicine. Chest 59:473, 1971

Weil H, Williams TB, Burk RH: Laboratory and clinical evaluation of a new volume ventilator. Chest 67:14, 1975

Weitzner SW, Urban BJ: A new ventilator utilizing fluid logic. JAMA 207:1126, 1969

Weitzner SW, Urban BJ: Fluid amplifiers: a new approach to the construction of ventilators. In: Proceedings of the 4th World Congress on Anesthesiology. pp. 1068–1074. Excerpta Medica, Amsterdam, 1968

Werkö L: The influence of positive pressure breathing on the circulation in man. Acta Med Scand [Suppl] 193:1, 1947

Werl H, Williams TB, Buck RH: Laboratory and clinical evaluation of a new volume ventilator. Chest 67:14, 1975

West JB: Ventilation/Blood Flow and Gas Exchange. Blackwell, Oxford, 1970

Whittenberger JL: Artificial respiration. Physiol Rev 35:611, 1955

Whittenberger JL (ed): Artificial Respiration. Harper & Row, New York, 1962

Whittenberger JL: Medical progress: resuscitation and other uses of artificial respiration: part I. N Engl J Med 251:775, 1954

Whittenberger JL: Medical progress: resuscitation and other uses of artificial respiration: part II. N Engl J Med 251:816, 1954

Whittenberger JL: Respiratory problems in poliomyelitis. In: National Foundation for Infantile Paralysis Conference. p. 10. Ann Arbor, Michigan, March 1952

Whittenberger JL, McGregor M, Berglund E, et al: Influence of state of inflation of the lung on pulmonary vascular resistance. J Appl Physiol 5:878, 1960

Whittenberger JL, Sarnoff EJ: Physiological principles in the treatment of respiratory failure. Med Clin North Am 34:1335, 1950

Wiggers CJ: The dynamics of lung inflation. In: Physiology in Health and Disease. 5th Ed. Lea and Febiger, New York p. 422 1949

Williams MH Jr, Shin CS: Ventilatory failure: etiology and clinical forms. Am J Med 48:477 1970

Williams TM: An automatic breathing attachment to Boyle's apparatus. Br J Anaesth 24:222, 1952

Wilson JL: The Use of the Respirator in Poliomyelitis. National Foundation of Infantile Paralysis, New York, 1942

Wilson RF, Gibson D, Percivel AT, et al: Severe alkalosis in critically ill surgical patients. Arch Surg 105:197, 1972

Wilson RS, Pontoppidan H: Respiratory care. Mod Med 39:100, 1971

Woillez EJ: Du spirophore, appareil de sauvetage pur le traitment de l'asphyxie et principalement de l'asphyxie des noyes et des nourveaunes. Bull Acad Méd Paris 5:611, 1876; also Dict Encyclopedique Sci Méd Paris Series 13:609, 1876

Woollam CHM: The development of apparatus for intermittent negative pressure respiration. Anaesthesia 31:537, 666, 1976

Woollam H, Smith TC, Stephan G, et al: Effects of extremes of respiratory and metabolic alkalosis on cerebral blood flow in man. J Appl Physiol 24:60, 1968

Wood DW, Downes JJ, Lecks HI: The management of respiratory failure in childhood status asthmaticus: experience with 30 episodes and evolution of a technique. J Allerg 42:261, 1968

Wyche MQ, Teichner RL, Kallo ST, et al: Effects of continuous positive pressure breathing on functional residual capacity and arterial oxygenation during intra-abdominal operations: studies in man during nitrous oxide and d-tubocurarine anesthesia. Anesthesiology 38:68, 1973

Yakaitis RW, Cooke JE, Redding JS: Re-evaluation of relationship of hyperkalemia and P_{CO_2} to cardiac arrhythmias during mechanical ventilation. Anesth Analg 50:368 1971

Young J, Crocker D: Principles and Practice of Respiratory Therapy. Year Book, Chicago, 1976

Zapol WM, Snider MT, Schneider RC: Extracorporeal membrane oxygenation for acute respiratory failure. Anesthesiology 46:27, 1977

Ziment I: Intermittent positive pressure breathing. In Burton GG, Gee GN, Hodgkin JE (eds): Respiratory Care. pp. 546–582. Lippincott, Philadelphia, 1977

2

Physical Principles and Functional Designs of Ventilators

Charles B. Spearman
Howard G. Sanders, Jr.

> If anything can go wrong it will, and that which goes wrong will be whatever can do the most damage.
> Murphy's Law (paraphrased)

PHYSICAL PRINCIPLES OF VENTILATORS

The physical characteristics of mechanical ventilators are important to the clinician because they establish the framework within which most mechanical ventilatory support is provided. Physiological parameters—e.g., minute ventilation, distribution of inspired air, alveolar gas exchange, distribution of pulmonary blood flow, venous return and cardiac output, oxygen consumption, and work of breathing—can all be affected by the physical characteristics and available modes of the ventilator. A basic understanding of the physical aspects of ventilators is essential to their proper clinical application. Most ventilators in common use today have similar operational characteristics. The classification which follows is intended to provide a basic overview to prepare the reader for later chapters on clinical use of ventilatory support

and individual ventilator descriptions. Specific ventilators are mentioned only as examples of the principles discussed. Terminology for the variety of ventilatory support modes is also introduced in this chapter.

Positive Versus Negative Pressure Ventilation

Normally, movement of air into the lungs is provided by contraction of the respiratory muscles, producing a "negative" or subatmospheric intrapleural and intraalveolar pressure. A pressure gradient is thereby established between the upper airway (atmospheric) and alveoli (subatmospheric), and air flows into the lungs. During expiration, which is usually passive, the natural recoil of the lung tissue causes an increase in alveolar pressure so that the pressure gradient is reversed (positive intraalveolar pressure to atmospheric upper airway pressure), and air flows out of the lungs.

Mechanical support of air movement into the lungs can be provided either by applying a subatmospheric pressure around the chest or by generating a positive pressure above atmospheric pressure to the upper airway. The necessary pressure gradient develops because the alveoli are at atmospheric pressure just before inspiration. As intraalveolar pressure rises during positive-pressure ventilation, intrapleural pressure also rises to levels potentially above atmospheric pressure. When gas flow into the upper airway ceases, the lungs usually deflate passively. Upper airway pressure is equal to atmospheric pressure and the higher intraalveolar pressure causes the air to flow out of the lungs. Intrapleural pressure also falls during this time and returns to a subatmospheric level if alveolar pressure is allowed to return to atmospheric pressure.

Mechanical ventilatory support by "negative-pressure" ventilation can be provided by three basic types of ventilators[60,63,70,88]: those which completely surround the patient's entire body, often referred to as "tank ventilators" or "iron lungs"; those which fit only around the chest; and those which fit around the abdomen.[53] The chest and abdominal units are called cuirass ventilators, the chest unit being the most common. The abdominal unit pulls the abdominal wall forward and the diaphragm downward during inspiration.[53] Although negative-pressure ventilators are still utilized to provide support for patients with various neuromuscular disorders, they are seldom employed in the critically ill patient with respiratory failure. The remainder of this chapter is devoted to positive-pressure ventilation systems.

Ventilator Power and Control Systems

The power source required to operate mechanical ventilators is provided by either compressed gases, electricity, or both. The control system refers to the decision-making or logic component which starts and stops inspiration and expiration. Ventilators may be controlled by electronic, pneumatic, or fluidic means, or by combinations of the three.

Pneumatic Ventilators. Pneumatic ventilators require some source of compressed gas in order to provide a positive-pressure breath. The gas may be compressed air and/or oxygen and is usually pressurized to 50 psig. Internally, this pressure is regulated by mechanisms that include reducing valves (e.g., Bennett PR-2) or a highly resistant needle valve or venturi mechanism (e.g., Bird Mark 7).[60,63] All controls are influenced by gas pressure and are therefore considered pneumatic in nature.

Some pneumatic ventilators utilize more refined fluidic controls.[60,63,84] These components have no moving parts and depend solely on gas flow and pressure to function. A ventilator which requires a compressed gas source to operate and utilizes fluidic logic for its decision-making is referred to as pneumatically powered and fluidically controlled. The Monaghan 225/SIMV volume ventilator is an example of such a unit.

Electronic Ventilators. Ventilators which require only an electrical source to provide mechanical ventilation are referred to as electronically powered and controlled. Compressed oxygen is required only to provide a fraction of inspired oxygen (F_{IO_2}) greater than that of room air but is not required as a driving or controlling force. These ventilators continue to provide positive-pressure ventilation with room air even when oxygen failure occurs. The primary logic systems for controlling inspiration and expiration are provided by electrical components. Examples of electronically powered and controlled ventilators include the Emerson 3-PV and Bennett MA-1. The Emerson uses an electrical motor to drive a piston in a cylinder, and this piston provides the positive inspiratory pressure. In the MA-1, an electrical compressor provides the compressed air necessary to drive a bellows system during inspiration.

Combined Power Ventilators. Certain ventilators utilize both pneumatic and electrical power sources. Compressed air and oxygen are often required to provide a variable F_{IO_2} and the driving force during mechanical inspiration. Most often the electrical power is utilized for timing, phasing, and monitoring. Because these ventilators cannot provide mechanical inspiration with only one of the two sources, they are considered to be *both* pneumatically and electronically powered.

Some pediatric ventilators provide a continuous flow of gas into their delivery circuit while utilizing either electronic or a combination of electronic and fluidic components for controlling inspiratory and expiratory phasing. The BEAR CUB BP 2001 is an example of a pneumatically and electrically powered, electronically controlled infant ventilator. The Sechrist IV-100B is pneumatically and electrically powered and is controlled by a combination of electronic and fluidic components.

The Servo 900 series ventilators by Siemens are units which also require pneumatic and electrical power sources. The pneumatic source is part of the driving system, whereas the logic functions are primarily electronic. Therefore these ventilators are classified as being pneumatically and electrically powered and electronically controlled.

Drive Mechanisms

Each mechanical ventilator must have a system which provides the *force* with which the positive-pressure gas flow is generated. The mechanism providing this force is considered the driving system. A knowledge of driving systems is important because each general type suggests certain performance characteristics. The general categories presented here are simplified but cover the most commonly used drive mechanisms.

Single and Double Circuit Systems. Driving systems can be broadly subdivided into *single-circuit* and *double-circuit* types. If the gases within the driving mechanism go directly to the patient, the device is considered a single-circuit device. If gas from the driving mechanism is used to compress another system, e.g., a bag or bellows, which in turn delivers gas to the patient, the unit is considered a double-circuit device.

A common example of a single-circuit ventilator system is shown in Figure 2-1. Here the drive system is a piston within a cylinder. When the piston moves forward (to the right), it expels gas from the cylinder directly into the tubing system connected to the patient. Other sources can also be used to provide a single-circuit drive mechanism, including pneumatic systems and spring-driven bellows. Examples of single-circuit ventilators using a piston include the Emerson 3-PV and 3-MV models. Pneumatically driven single-circuit units are represented by the Bird Mark series and Bennett PR series ventilators. The Siemens Servo 900 series are examples of single-circuit, spring-loaded bellows ventilators.

Figure 2-2 shows a double-circuit system. In this example, a piston is again utilized to provide the driving power. However, gases from the piston are not sent directly to the patient. Instead, these gases pressurize a chamber and compress a bag which contains gas the patient is to receive. The piston is considered the driving circuit, and the bag and connecting tubing comprise the patient circuit. A collapsible bellows or concertina bag can be utilized instead of the bag as part of the patient circuit, and other driving sources can be used in place of the piston. Engström 150 and 300 series ventilators are piston-driven, double-circuit ventilators which produce unique pressure and flow patterns partly because of their double-circuit design.[63] Bennett MA-1 and Monaghan

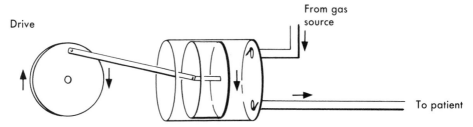

Fig. 2-1. Single-circuit drive mechanism. In this example, gas passes directly from the cylinder to the patient circuit. The drive mechanism is a rotary-driven piston. (Reprinted with permission from Spearman CB, Sheldon RL (eds): Egan's Fundamentals of Respiratory Therapy. 4th Ed. Mosby, St. Louis, 1982).

225/SIMV ventilators are double-circuit ventilators using a collapsible bellows.

Piston-Driven Ventilators. A piston moving back and forth through a cylinder has provided a convenient method for providing positive-pressure ventilation for several decades.[63] Pistons are coupled to one of two basic components which provide the to-and-fro movement: a rotary drive or a linear drive mechanism.

Rotary-Driven Piston. A rotary-driven piston is one that is connected to the edge of a wheel which is, in turn, powered by an electrical motor. As the piston moves back, one-way valves allow fresh gas to fill the cylinder. On the forward stroke these gases are then pushed into the patient's circuit, causing inspiration (single-circuit, as shown in Figure 2-1).

The flow pattern from a rotary-driven, single-circuit piston is unique and is shown in Figure 2-3. As the rotary wheel turns, the piston is moved through the cylinder in an accelerating, then decelerating fashion, producing a similar pattern of air flow. This flow profile occurs because at the beginning of inspiration the movement of the piston's connecting rod is mostly upward rather than forward. Subsequently, the motion is transferred to a more forward direction as the wheel continues to rotate, and gas flow out of the cylinder accelerates. When the wheel is one-quarter through its rotation, the piston has moved one-half of its total forward

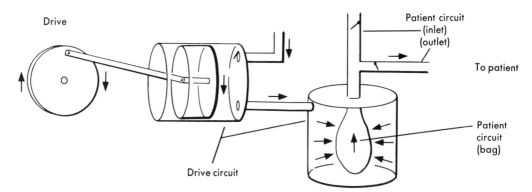

Fig. 2-2. Double-circuit drive mechanism using a rotary-driven piston. Gas passes from the cylinder to a rigid cannister and compresses a bag. Gas contained within the bag is then delivered into the patient circuit. The two gas sources are separate. A collapsible bellows may be substituted for the bag in the patient circuit. (Reprinted with permission from Spearman CB, Sheldon RL (eds): Egan's Fundamentals of Respiratory Therapy. 4th Ed. Mosby, St. Louis, 1982).

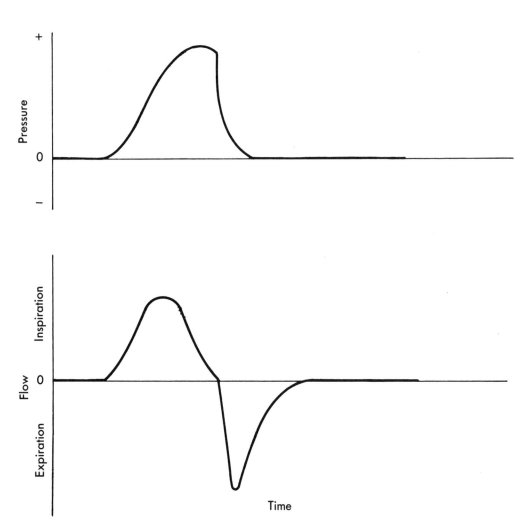

Fig. 2-3. Pressure (sigmoidal) and flow (sinusoidal) waveforms associated with a rotary-drive piston mechanism (Fig. 2-1). (Reprinted with permission from Spearman CB, Sheldon RL (eds): Egan's Fundamentals of Respiratory Therapy. 4th Ed. Mosby, St. Louis, 1982.)

distance and peak flow is reached. The remainder of inspiration occurs with the forward motion of the piston being transferred progressively in a downward direction, causing a deceleration of inspiratory flow. This accelerating then decelerating inspiratory flow pattern is often termed sinusoidal, or like a sine-wave, although it is more precisely one-half of a sine-wave. During the remainder of the cycle, the wheel continues its rotation and pulls the piston backward through the cylinder, which is refilled with fresh gas for the next breath. The patient is not affected by this refilling because of the one-way valve system which interrupts the ventilator-airway communication during exhalation. The patient's exhalation occurs independently of the piston stroke, and the wave-form produced for expiratory flow (Fig. 2-3) is primarily a function of the lung-chest wall compliance, airway resistance, and tubing circuit resistance (not shown).

The Emerson models 3-PV and 3-MV ventilators are examples of rotary-driven piston devices. Because these ventilators utilize a rather powerful electrical motor to turn the rotary wheel, relatively high pressures can be generated at the airway with very little influence on the inspiratory flow pattern. This sine-wave flow pattern is similar to that produced during typical spontaneous breathing and may have some theoretical advantages over other flow patterns.[18]

Linear-Driven Piston. Piston ventilators may also utilize a driving system which moves the piston at a constant rate of speed throughout the inspiratory phase. Thus the movement is said to be linear. These devices can be powered in several ways, two of which are depicted in Figure 2-4. A rotating gear connected to the piston's rod by cogs or teeth can produce a constant piston movement and therefore a constant flow. High-tension springs can also be used to drive the piston at a relatively constant rate. This constant flow is often described as a square-wave and is discussed later in this chapter.

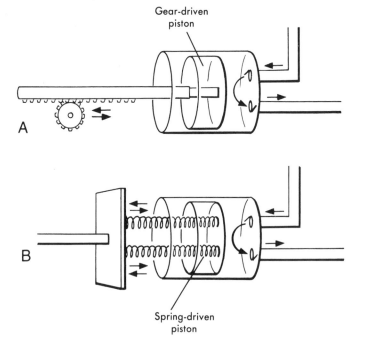

Fig. 2-4. Single-circuit gear (A) and spring (B) piston drive mechanisms. (Reprinted with permission from Spearman CB, Sheldon RL (eds): Egan's Fundamentals of Respiratory Therapy. 4th Ed. Mosby, St. Louis, 1982.)

The Bourns LS 104–150 Infant Ventilator utilizes a gear system to provide a linear-driven piston, and the no longer manufactured Searle VVA unit utilized a relatively high spring tension drive system with its piston-like component.[60,63]

Pneumatically Driven Ventilators. Numerous ventilators utilize compressed gases as the primary driving force during inspiration. Various methods are used to control the amount and pattern of both pressure and flow in pneumatically driven ventilators, and three are presented here.

High-Pressure Drive with High Internal Resistance. The simplest form of a pneumatic drive system can be constructed from a high-pressure source gas (3–50 psig oxygen or compressed air), incorporating an adjustable resistance to control pressure and flow rate. These driving forces equal 200 to over 3500 cm H_2O and represent 2–35 times the typical maximum pressure developed at the airway. To avoid sudden pressurization in the patient with these high-pressure systems, a highly resistant valve is used. This "needle valve" adjusts the size of an orifice at the outlet of the high-pressure source and therefore controls the flow rate.

The flow pattern produced by this type of system is generally constant or square-wave in nature because the driving force is relatively high. It can exist in either a single- or double-circuit configuration (Fig. 2-5). In a single-circuit device, the driving source passes through its high internal resistor directly into the patient. In a double-circuit system, the driving source compresses a bag or bellows containing gases for the patient. An example of a single-circuit ventilator with a high-pressure pneumatic drive

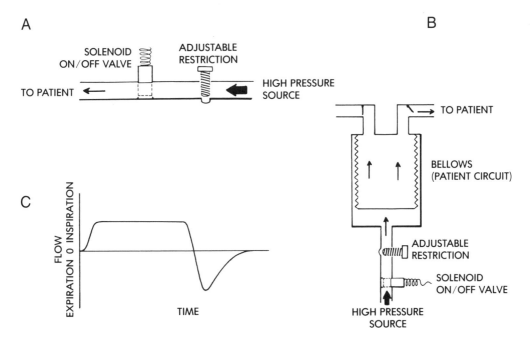

Fig. 2-5. High-pressure pneumatic drive systems with high internal flow resistance. (A) Single-circuit system. (B) Double-circuit system. Adjustable restrictions control flow from high-pressure source gas. Electrical solenoids open (solid line drawings) and close (dashed line drawings), creating inspiration and expiration, respectively. (C) Constant inspiratory flow pattern typical of these systems.

system is the Bird Mark 7 on its "100 percent" setting, as the venturi mechanism is bypassed. The Monaghan 225/SIMV ventilator is a double-circuit unit that uses a high-pressure drive system.[60]

Low-Pressure Drive System. Another pneumatic drive system is one which regulates the pressure to a relatively low level, e.g., 60 cm H_2O pressure or less. A number of mechanisms may incorporate this principle, two of which are described here.

Some ventilators utilize a venturi or injector as their driving force. Generally, a high-pressure source of compressed air and/or oxygen is used to drive the jet of the venturi. The pressure applied to the small orifice of the jet establishes a high forward velocity, and air is entrained by this gas.[75] The amount of pressure that can be generated by the venturi is proportional to, but much less than, the pressure applied to the jet, assuming that the entrainment area is left open and without valves.

Pressure-reducing valves are also used in ventilators with a low driving pressure.[60] In these systems, adjustment of the spring tension within the reducing valve establishes the desired driving pressure.

The flow pattern created by low-pressure drive systems of the venturi or reducing valve types is quite similar. Both systems are susceptible to back pressure caused by increased airway resistance, decreased lung-thorax compliance, etc., such that flow decreases as pressure in the patient system increases. As an example, a ventilator using a low-pressure drive is set to produce 20 cm H_2O driving pressure. At the beginning of inspiration, if the pressure in the patient's airway is 0 cm H_2O, the gradient between the ventilator and the patient is 20 cm H_2O (20 cm H_2O drive − 0 cm H_2O patient) and flow begins at its highest level. As pressure increases in the patient's airway through inspiration, this pressure gradient progressively decreases until finally the airway pressure equals the driving pressure. Concomitantly, flow also de-

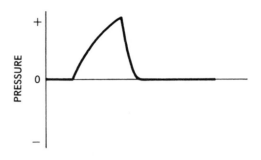
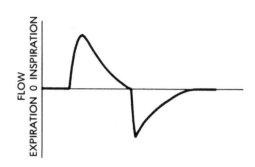
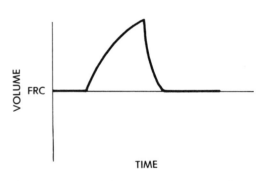

Fig. 2-6. Pressure, flow, and volume waveforms of a ventilator with a low-pressure drive system. Note that flow during inspiration reaches its peak early and then tapers, whereas pressure continues to rise.

creases progressively until it finally reaches 0. Figure 2-6 shows theoretical airway pressure and flow patterns produced by a ventilator with a low-pressure drive mechanism. Examples of devices using a low-pressure venturi drive mechanism include the Hand-E-Vent from Ohio Medical Prod-

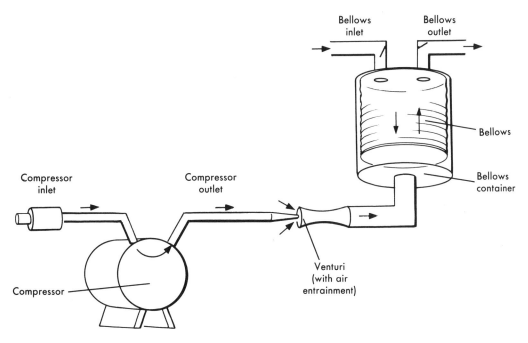

Fig. 2-7. Double-circuit compressor-bellows drive mechanism using a venturi. The pressure decrement occurring through the venturi tube increases output from the compressor while additional ambient air is entrained. (Reprinted with permission from Spearman CB, Sheldon RL (eds): Egan's Fundamentals of Respiratory Therapy. 4th Ed. Mosby, St. Louis, 1982.)

ucts and Bird Asthmastik from Bird Corp. The Bennett PR-1 and PR-2 ventilators are examples of low-pressure drive units which utilize an adjustable reducing valve.[60]

Compressor-Driven Bellows. Compressors are commonly used to provide the driving force for double-circuit ventilators. A bellows is usually used for patient gases, and the compressor pressurizes the bellows container to drive it upward, emptying part or all of its contents into the patient circuit (Fig. 2-7). Some compressors or blowers can produce moderate pressures of 100 cm H_2O or more at flow rates exceeding 100 L/ minute and apply their output directly to the bellows container. An example of such a ventilator is the CCV-2, SIMV unit by Ohio Medical Products.

Other models use compressors which produce pressures of several pounds per square inch gauge (psig) (e.g., 6–12 psig), but at flow rates less than 50 L/minute. In these systems, a venturi is used to reduce the maximum pressure and increase the flow from the compressor. Figure 2-7 diagrams such a system and shows the compressor being used to drive the jet of a venturi while the output of the venturi drives the bellows. The MA-1 and MA-2 + 2 ventilators from Puritan-Bennett are examples of ventilators using this type of driving system.

Generally, these driving mechanisms produce a relatively square flow pattern until the pressure in the patient circuit increases to within a few centimeters of water pressure of the maximum driving force, at which time some decrease or tapering of flow occurs.

Initiation of Inspiration

Various mechanisms are available for initiating inspiration in modern mechanical ventilators. The way in which a ventilator is cycled on or "triggered" is a convenient way to categorize the modes of ventilatory support which are available. These modes vary from complete automatic cycling by the ventilator, through a combination of patient- and ventilator-triggered breaths, to a combination of ventilator breaths and spontaneous breathing.

Initiation of the inspiratory phase is often referred to as "cycling," although this term is also applied to the termination of inspiration and the initiation and termination of expiration as well.[63] We indicate which phase change we are referring to with this term for the remainder of this chapter. The term "triggering" is also synonymous with starting inspiration.

Control Mode (Time-Cycled or Triggered). Control mode or controlled ventilation is provided when the positive-pressure breaths automatically start by some timing mechanism, regardless, or in the absence, of any patient effort. In this mode the patient receives a pressurized breath at time intervals determined by the setting of the timing mechanism only. Patients receiving control mode ventilation (CMV) may be totally dependent on the ventilator for support as they are often apneic from either disease processes or drugs, e.g., neuromuscular blocking agents and sedatives.

A variety of systems are available in modern ventilators to establish a control rate.[60,63] The most common are described here.

Single Rate Control. Some ventilators have an electrical timer system which divides each minute into a set number of breaths. Actually, these timers establish the number of times per minute inspiration *should* begin, whereas some other mechanism (described later in this chapter) causes inspiration to end.

The controls can be calibrated in breaths per minute (BPM) or in time increments between breaths. In both cases the timer itself is doing the same thing: starting the inspiratory phase at regular intervals. For example, if the timer initiates a mechanical breath every 5 seconds, the control can be calibrated to read "12 BPM" or "5 seconds" of total ventilatory cycle time. The Puritan-Bennett MA-1 and the BEAR-2 ventilators use single rate control knobs which are calibrated in BPM, whereas the Emerson 3-MV uses a single control calibrated in seconds of total time.

Inspiratory and Expiratory Timers. Other ventilators divide the phases of breathing with separate timers. In this case, inspiration is started by one timer and expiration by another. Any change in either of the timers can affect the resulting mechanical rate. As an example, if inspiration lasts 2 seconds and expiration 3 seconds, the total ventilatory cycle time is 5 seconds and the set control rate 12 BPM (60 divided by 5 seconds total). The Emerson 3-PV ventilator uses electrical timers whereas the Babybird uses pneumatic timers for establishing a control rate.

Independent Expiratory Timer. Another approach to setting an automatic rate for the control mode is the use of an electronic or pneumatic *expiratory* timer. The inspiratory phase begins when this expiratory time ends. The length of inspiration is subject to several factors, e.g., flow rate and tidal volume or pressure setting; therefore the rate can be altered not only by the setting of the expiratory timer but also by variables that occur during inspiration. An example of such an electronically controlled system is the Ohio CCV-2, SIMV ventilator, which establishes a control rate based on an expiratory time setting plus tidal volume and flow settings for the inspiratory time. The Bird Mark 7 has a pneumatic timer for the expiratory phase, whereas inspiratory time is controlled by flow and pressure settings. Because the patient's lung condition can influence the flow pattern during the breath and change inspiratory time accordingly, only a maximum expiratory time can be "guaranteed" rather than an actual respiratory rate.

Assist Mode (Patient-Cycled or Triggered). When a ventilator senses a slight inspiratory effort by the patient and responds by triggering a pressurized breath, assist mode or assisted ventilation is provided. Assist mode ventilation (AMV) implies that the patient's efforts are responsible for the ventilator providing a positive-pressure breath. The number of ventilator breaths occurring per minute is determined solely by the patient's efforts and is quite variable, depending on a variety of factors.

Assist mechanisms can function various ways. Most respond to a change in *pressure* within the patient's tubing circuit. In some ventilators a flexible diaphragm is displaced by the drop in pressure as the patient begins to make an inspiratory effort. If, for example, the diaphragm is moved enough for two electrical contacts to touch, inspiration can be triggered. If the amount of effort required by the patient to trigger inspiration is adjustable, the ventilator is said to have a *sensitivity* or *patient effort* control. If the amount of pressure drop necessary is decreased, the system becomes *more* sensitive, requiring *less* patient effort.

Pressure transducers are also used in some ventilators to provide an assist mode. Here, more sophisticated electronic logic systems are needed to compare a signal on a reference control (e.g., sensitivity) to the signal produced by the pressure transducer in order to trigger an assist breath.

A flow-sensing device can also be used to detect an inspiratory effort. Generally, a slight drop in pressure creates a change in flow. If monitored electronically, the change in flow can also cycle the ventilator on in response to the patient's breathing effort.

Assist mode and sensitivity adjustments are provided by a diaphragm and electrical contact system on the Puritan-Bennett MA-1, whereas a pressure transducer system is used for the Siemens Servo 900B ventilator.[60] A thermistor bead is used with the BEAR-1 to detect the change in flow caused by an inspiratory patient effort.[60]

Assist-Control Mode. An automatic rate mechanism may be combined with an assist mechanism to provide an assist-control mode. In this case the control rate is thought of as the "back-up" system and provides the minimum allowable breaths per minute. Should the patient desire to breathe at a rate faster than the control rate, the assist mechanism is triggered. This mode of ventilatory support is very common to modern ventilators, and some cannot be used as strict "controllers" or "assistors" only. Assist-control mode is a convenient way to allow patients to establish their own ventilatory rate while maintaining a minimum rate in case of respiratory depression or apnea.

Figure 2-8 illustrates the difference between control mode and assist mode in terms of the pressure waveform for each. Pressure is shown on the vertical axis, and time is on the horizontal axis. Note that for control mode the time intervals between the beginning of one positive-pressure breath and the beginning of the next are quite regular. During assist mode ventilation, a characteristic drop in pressure occurs at the beginning of each breath, indicating that the patient's inspiratory effort triggered or started each breath. The time intervals for the assisted breaths are not as regular as for controlled ones.

Intermittent Mandatory Ventilation. When spontaneous breathing is *combined* with a controlled mechanical rate from a ventilator, the pattern of ventilation is referred to as intermittent mandatory ventilation (IMV).[50,83,86] The control rate set on the ventilator is provided at preset time intervals, whereas between these breaths the patient inhales from a source of fresh gas at the desired rate and tidal volume. The spontaneous breathing component of IMV infers that the size and number of breaths received are related solely to the patient's ability to

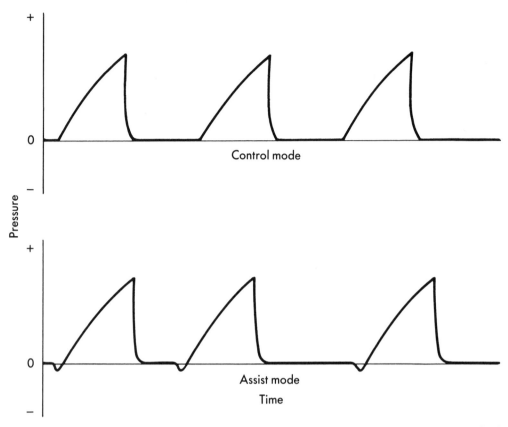

Fig. 2-8. Pressure-time waveforms for control mode and assist mode IPPV. In this example the slight "negative" pressure generated by the patient's voluntary inspiratory effort triggers the ventilator during assist mode breathing. (Reprinted with permission from Spearman CB, Sheldon RL (eds): Egan's Fundamentals of Respiratory Therapy. 4th Ed. Mosby, St. Louis, 1982.)

inhale spontaneously. The mandatory breaths are those given by the ventilator at regular intervals in a fashion similar to the control mode. Indeed, the primary difference between control mode and IMV is that when a patient attempts to breathe spontaneously between mechanical ventilator breaths in a control mode no fresh gas is available.

IMV allows the patient to participate in the ventilation process to varying degrees and may allow them to maintain some of the physiological advantages of spontaneous breathing.[12,50,79] IMV has been used for over a decade in all age groups as both a primary mode of ventilatory support and a means for weaning patients from the ventilator,[20,50,51,54] although not all patients are candidates for IMV.[24,57]

Most ventilators can be modified easily to supply a source of fresh gas for spontaneous breathing, and many have such a system built in.[19,61,63,85]

Synchronized Intermittent Mandatory Ventilation. When the mechanical breaths during IMV are provided by an "assist" mechanism, the technique is referred to as synchronized IMV (SIMV). That is, the mechanical breaths are *synchronized* with the patient's efforts in the same manner as on an assist mode.

In order to accomplish this synchronization, some patient efforts are "ignored" by the ventilator (spontaneous breaths), whereas others trigger a pressurized, mechanical breath (SIMV breath). Special timing circuits are necessary for this coordination, and ventilators with this mode utilize different logic or counting patterns.[60] Should the patient not make a sufficient effort to trigger an assist breath within a predetermined time period, most ventilators with SIMV automatically cycle. Therefore they tend to function in an assist-control fashion for the mandatory breaths.

No study to date has shown clear physiological advantages of SIMV compared to IMV for critically ill patients. One study of these modes could not demonstrate significant differences between them when comparing hemodynamic parameters, blood gas values, and pulmonary barotrauma.[42] Other terms for SIMV are intermittent assisted ventilation (IAV) and intermittent demand ventilation (IDV).[40,60,78]

Figure 2-9 shows pressure waveforms comparing IMV and SIMV.

Mandatory Minute Volume. Recently another mode combining spontaneous and mechanical ventilation has been introduced.[44,65] In this system a constant flow of gas equal to the minimum allowable *minute volume* is fed into either a constant-pressure reservoir or a collecting bellows. The patient breathes as much as desired from the constant-pressure reservoir, and excess flow is collected in the bellows. Once the collecting bellows contains a preset amount of this ''excess'' flow, a mechanism triggers the ventilator and the bellows content is delivered as a pressurized tidal volume to the patient. If the patient breathes less of the constant flow, the collecting bellows is filled sooner and a pressurized breath is delivered more often. Should the patient's spontaneous breathing equal the constant flow, the collecting bellows does not fill and no mandatory breaths are given. If the patient breathes more than the set minute volume, a valving system allows additional gas to enter. This unique system can deliver any amount of the preset minute volume as pressurized, mandatory breaths, automatically compensating for changes in the level of spontaneous breathing.[65] In contrast, the mechanical rate for IMV must be manually adjusted as the patient's requirements change.

The clinical efficacy of this mode of ventilatory support is not well documented as yet. The Engström Erica is an example of a ventilator capable of providing a modification of the mandatory minute volume (MMV) method just described.

Ventilation at High Rates. During the past decade reports of systems using ventilatory frequencies of 60 to over 900/minute have appeared in the medical literature.[6,11,13,29,30,49,59,80,81] Although conventional ventilators have been used at high rates, most high-frequency systems are uniquely designed to provide high-rate ventilation in combination with or independent of conventional ventilators.[6,11,13,80,81]

High-frequency ventilation (HFV) is a generic term often used to refer to all high-frequency ventilator systems. However, at least three subcategories of HFV have been defined, based primarily on their frequency range, tidal volumes, and operational characteristics.[81]

High-frequency positive-pressure ventilation (HFPPV)[81] describes ventilation provided by a special pneumatic valve at rates of 60 to 110/minute. The tidal volume with each cycle is less than normal, although total minute ventilation may be considerably greater.

High-frequency jet ventilation (HFJV) is used most commonly at 100 to 200 BPM, although some systems can produce much higher rates. In these systems, a high-pressure jet pulses gas down the airway at volumes one to three times the predicted anatomical dead space. The jet, which may be constructed from a 14- to 18-gauge needle or catheter, can be used with or without entrainment of other gas.[13]

High-frequency oscillation (HFO) systems produce very high rates. A piston

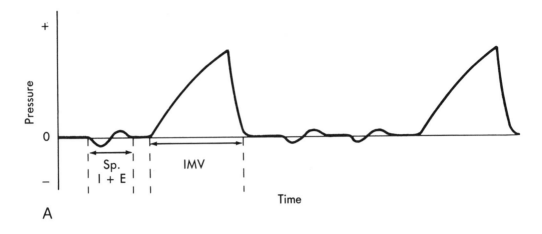

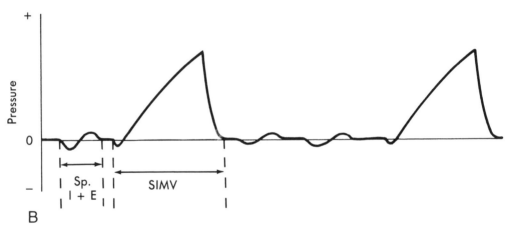

Fig. 2-9. Difference between IMV and SIMV illustrated by pressure waveforms wherein spontaneous inspiration and expiration (Sp. I + E) are shown combined with ventilator (IMV and SIMV) breaths. (A) Regularity between IMV breaths is similar to control-mode. (B) Patient-triggered SIMV breaths are similar to assist-mode breaths. (Reprinted with permission from Spearman CB, Sheldon RL (eds): Egan's Fundamentals of Respiratory Therapy. 4th Ed. Mosby, St. Louis, 1982.)

which moves rapidly back and forth is most commonly used to move air into and out of the airway.[11] An additional flow of gas continuously flushes the system. Volumes delivered by HFO systems are very difficult to measure but are assumed to be equal to or smaller than anatomical dead space. Though mostly experimental, some clinical experience has been gained in adults and neonates using HFO.[11,59]

How HFV with very small volumes produces adequate ventilation is not well understood.[30,49] At lower rates and larger volumes, ventilation probably occurs mostly by bulk flow in a manner similar to that of conventional ventilation, whereas very high rates and smaller volumes may increase the radial and axial diffusion and mixing of gases in the airways.[11,29,30,49,59,81]

Physical Principles During Mechanical Inspiration

During conventional mechanical ventilation, certain characteristics of inspiration have been used to classify ventilators. One system, reported by Mushin et al., utilizes positive pressure.[63] Although few ventilators fit precisely into these categories under all conditions, they are described here for completeness, together with certain clinical implications.

Pressure Generators. *Constant-Pressure Generators.* When a ventilator applies a relatively constant pressure to the airway throughout inspiration, it is termed a constant-pressure generator. Generally, the mechanisms employed are similar to the low-pressure drive systems previously discussed. Figure 2-10 illustrates theoretical pressure, flow, and volume waveforms for an ideal pressure generator. In each of the examples illustrated, the amount and pattern of applied *pressure* is the same. However, the *flow* pattern and *volume* delivery vary in response to changes in lung or airway characteristics.

Flow is at its highest level at the beginning of inspiration in a pressure generator because the difference in pressure between the ventilator and the patient's lung is greatest at this time. As pressure in the patient's airway increases, the gradient decreases and flow is reduced. If the ventilator and alveolar pressures equilibrate before inspiration ends, flow tapers to zero and the volume delivered is held constant until inspiration is terminated. The tidal volume delivered is a function of the pressure applied, the patient's compliance, and airway resistance (Fig. 2-10A).

Figure 2-10B illustrates the effects of decreased lung compliance on flow and volume for the same pressure generator as in Figure 2-10A. Note that flow tapers to zero quickly, and the lung volume is decreased as ventilator and alveolar pressures equilibrate earlier in the cycle.

Figure 2-10C illustrates the effects of increased airway resistance. Here the flow pattern shows a more gradual taper than in Figure 2-10A, although in the example zero flow is reached before end-inspiration. The flow tapers more slowly because the resistance to flow in the airways impedes the equilibration of alveolar pressure and ventilator pressure. The lung volumes achieved at end-inspiration in Figure 2-10A and 2-10C are the same, indicating that the lung-thorax compliance was the same for both. However, the increased airway resistance in Figure 2-10C caused that volume to be reached later in the breath.

Constant-pressure generators and the low-pressure driving systems (discussed earlier in the chapter) are similar, particularly in the general flow and volume changes which occur with changing patient conditions. A true constant-pressure generator, however, produces the same pressure pattern breath after breath, even when patient conditions vary. A low-pressure drive system may produce the same peak airway pressure each breath (e.g., Puritan-Bennett PR-2), although the pressure pattern or waveform produced can vary substantially. Few pure pressure generators are used in clinical medicine today, although occasionally pediatric ventilators are used so that they produce such a pattern.[9,28,41,60,71,76]

Non-Constant-Pressure Generators. Theoretically, a non-constant-pressure generator produces a constant *pattern* of pressure from one breath to the next, but the pressure itself is not constant *during* the breath. As an example, the pressure may increase throughout inspiration (non-constant pressure), but each breath resembles the last in terms of the pressure pattern.[63] Some ventilators approach these operational characteristics, but none can consistently reproduce the same pattern of pressure rise regardless of changing patient conditions; thus none are pure non-constant-pressure generators.

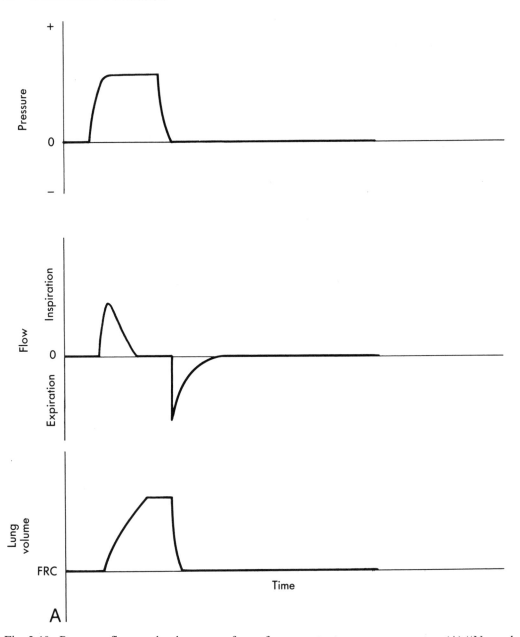

Fig. 2-10. Pressure, flow, and volume waveforms for a constant-pressure generator. (A) "Normal conditions. (B) Decreased lung compliance. (C) Increase in airway resistance. A decrease in volume delivery occurs in (B), whereas in *C* a slowly tapering inspiratory flow is present. (Reprinted with permission from Spearman CB, Sheldon RL (eds): Egan's Fundamentals of Respiratory Therapy. 4th Ed. Mosby, St. Louis, 1982.) (Figure continues.)

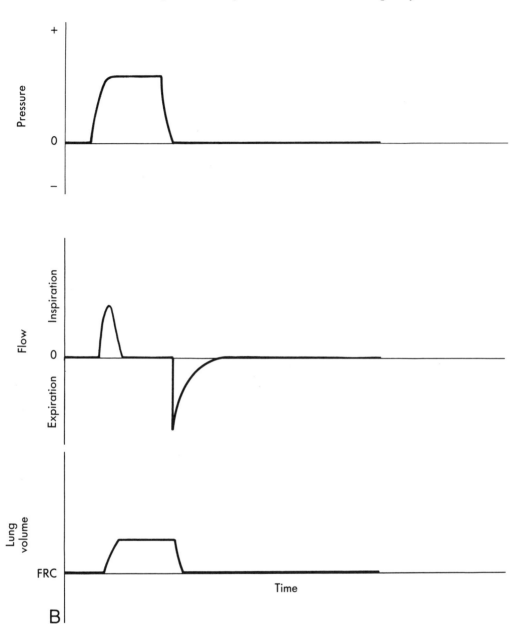

Fig. 2-10 (Continued). (B).

Flow Generators. *Constant-Flow Generators.* When a very high pressure is generated within a ventilator, the potential is present for the ventilator to produce a *flow pattern* that is reproducible regardless of changing patient conditions. Such a ventilator is called a *flow generator.*[63] If the ac-

tual *flow rate* is the same *during* the breath and the flow *pattern* is the same breath to breath, the ventilator is a constant-flow generator.

Ventilators using high-pressure driving systems with high internal resistance (Fig. 2-5) are constant-flow generators. The driv-

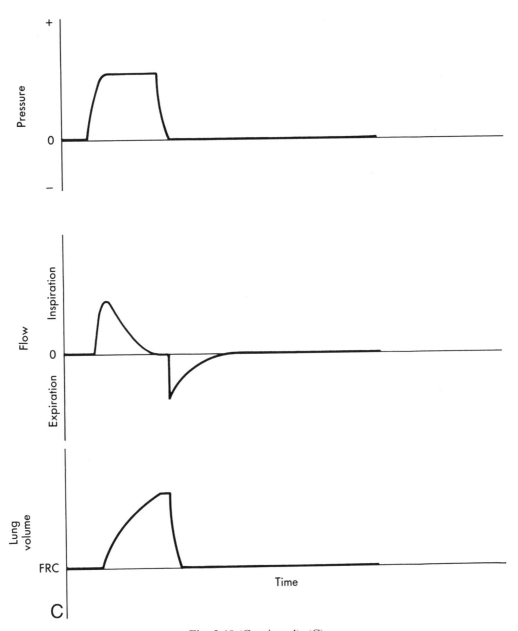

Fig. 2-10 (Continued). (C).

ing force is so high that resistance and compliance changes in the ventilator circuit and patient's lungs do not decrease the pressure gradient sufficiently to alter the flow rate during each breath. Figure 2-11 illustrates this point. In Figures 2-11A and 2-11B, inspiratory time is held constant. Note that the flow pattern remains the same, whereas the pressure increases when decreased lung compliance is encountered (Fig. 2-11B). The constant flow pattern during inspiration is commonly referred to as a square-wave.

Some ventilators function as constant-flow generators only when inspiratory pres-

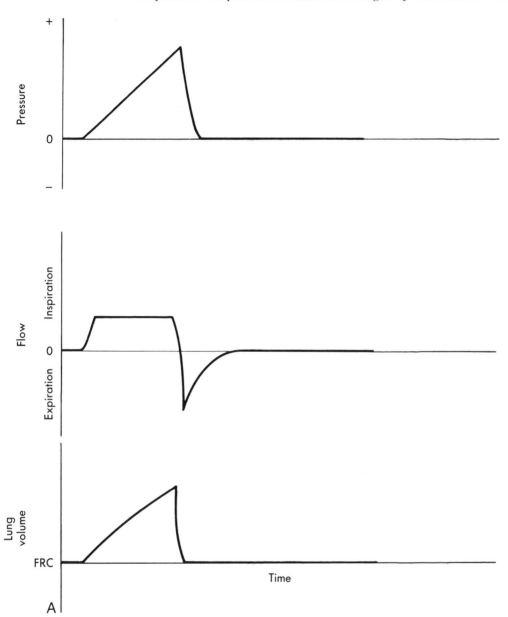

Fig. 2-11. Pressure, flow, and volume waveforms for a constant-flow generator under "normal" conditions (A) and with decreased compliance (B). Note that in (B) inspiratory flow remains unchanged whereas inspiratory pressure and expiratory flow increase. Lung volume remains relatively unchanged for the purpose of illustration. (Reprinted with permission from Spearman CB, Sheldon RL (eds): Egan's Fundamentals of Respiratory Therapy. 4th Ed. Mosby, St. Louis, 1982.) (Figure continues.)

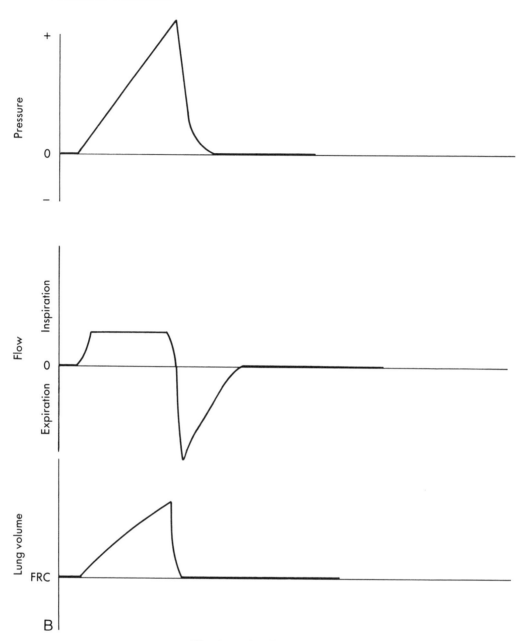

Fig. 2-11 (Continued). (B).

sures are relatively low. When high airway pressure is necessary and that pressure approaches the available driving pressure, flow decreases. The Siemens Servo 900 B and Puritan-Bennett MA-1 ventilators have driving pressures equal to or greater than 100 cm H_2O and normally produce a rela-

tively constant flow at typical airway pressures.[60] They are not pure constant-flow generators, as airway pressures close to their driving pressures can be encountered in some clinical situations. The Bourns LS 104–150 piston ventilator and the Monaghan 225/SIMV ventilator are closer to pure constant-flow generators because their driving systems have high force potential.

Non-Constant-Flow Generators. Non-constant-flow ventilators are exemplified by rotary-driven piston ventilators, producing a sine-wave flow pattern. Because the motor driving the piston can produce a high force, the flow *pattern* produced remains the same in spite of varying patient conditions. Figure 2-12 shows pressure and flow patterns typical of such a ventilator. "Normal" conditions are represented by Figure 2-12A, whereas Figures 2-12B and 2-12C illustrate increased airway resistance and decreased compliance, respectively. Although the *pressure* pattern produced is different for each example, the inspiratory *flow* pattern is the same in all three figures. The Emerson 3-PV and 3-MV ventilators are examples of non-constant-flow generators.

Ending the Inspiratory Phase

Various terms have been used to indicate the changeover from inspiration to expiration during mechanical ventilation, the most common being "cycle" and "limit." Neither is fully descriptive, however, because cycle is also used to indicate the changeover from expiration to inspiration, and limit is used to indicate the maximum value for components of the respiratory cycle other than inspiratory time. In this chapter we use the term *cycle* for both the initiation and termination of inspiration, and we distinguish which changeover is occurring. When the term *limit* is used, it refers to a maximal setting or value.

Terminal cycling of the inspiratory phase can be accomplished by *pressure, volume, time, flow,* or a combination of these.

Pressure-Cycled Ventilators. When the inspiratory phase ends because a preset pressure is reached, pressure cycling is occurring. Other factors (e.g., length of inspiration, volume delivered, and flow rate

produced) are usually variable during pressure-cycled ventilation. Worsening lung compliance or airway resistance generally causes the set pressure to be reached sooner, resulting in a shorter inspiration and a smaller delivered volume. If the ventilator is one which has a low-pressure drive system or uses a venturi, the flow rate pattern may also be affected by the changing lung and airway conditions.

Pressure-cycled ventilators are most commonly used to administer intermittent positive-pressure breathing (IPPB) therapy on a short-term basis, although they are occasionally used for continuous mechanical ventilation as well.[86]

Several mechanisms are used to provide pressure cycling. The Bird Mark series ventilators balance magnetic attraction against gas pressure.[60] The positive-pressure buildup during inspiration is exerted against a diaphragm to which a metal plate is attached. When sufficient pressure is developed, the metal plate is moved out of the magnetic force area. This sudden shift in diaphragm position closes a pneumatic switch which ends inspiration. The amount of pressure required to cause these events to occur can be increased by moving the magnet closer to the metal plate, causing its attraction for this plate to increase.

Fluidic components, e.g., Schmitt triggers, can also be used to sense pressure within a ventilator circuit and cause a changeover to expiration to occur.[61,63,84] This mechanism is present in the Monaghan 225/SIMV ventilator, although in this unit pressure cycling is generally a secondary or safety cycling mechanism.

Volume-Cycled Ventilators. In contrast to pressure-cycled ventilators, volume-cycled ventilators end inspiration when a preset volume has been delivered from the ventilator. In this case, applied pressure becomes the greater variable. Inspiratory time and flow may or may not vary with different patient characteristics, depending

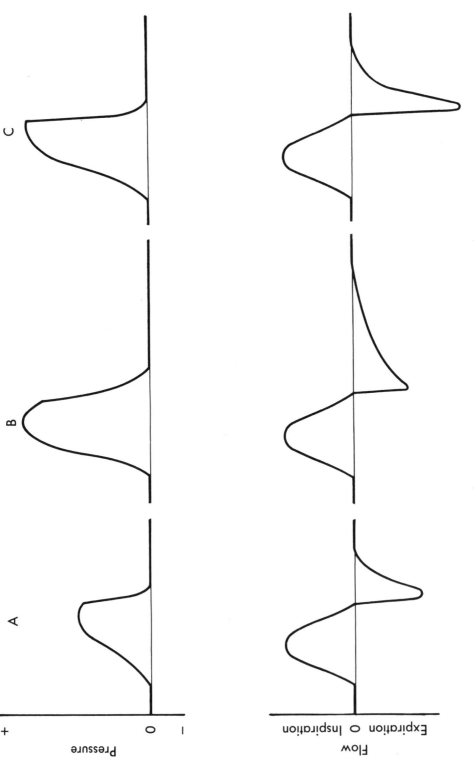

Fig. 2-12. Non-constant-flow generator (sine-wave type) pressure and flow waveforms. (A) "Normal" conditions. (B) Increased pressure and slow expiratory flow caused by increased airway resistance. (C) Increased pressure and expiratory flow caused by a decrease in lung compliance. Note that all inspiratory flow patterns remain the same. (Reprinted with permission from Spearman CB, Sheldon RL (eds): Egan's Fundamentals of Respiratory Therapy. 4th Ed. Mosby, St. Louis, 1982.)

mostly on whether the ventilator is a flow generator.

Contrary to popular belief, volume-cycled ventilators do not always deliver precise volumes to patients requiring different pressures to ventilate because some of the volume distends the delivery tubing and/or is compressed within the circuitry.[35,56,72,88] This characteristic of volume-cycled ventilator performance is discussed later in the chapter.

One method of detecting that a volume has been delivered is to monitor the position of the bellows during inspiration. As an example, an electronic switch on the top of a bellows can be tripped when the bellows is emptied, cycling the ventilator into the expiratory phase. The amount of volume in the bellows is determined by how much gas enters during refill. The Ohio CCV-2/SIMV volume ventilator functions in this manner.[60]

A moving bellows can also be monitored electrically by connecting it to a potentiometer. At the beginning of inspiration, the bellows is full. As it is pushed upward during the breath, the potentiometer signals the ventilator's logic system continuously. When that signal matches another signal set as a reference control, inspiration is terminated. This is the basic mechanism of the volume control system for the Puritan-Bennett MA-1 and MA-2 ventilators.[60]

A flow sensor may also be employed. Volume cycling occurs when the desired volume has passed through the flow sensor, and an on-off valve stops flow. In the BEAR-1 ventilator, a vortex shedding flow sensor is used for this purpose.[60]

Other methods are employed less commonly for volume cycling.[60,63]

Time-Cycled Ventilators. Time-cycled ventilators end inspiration when a preset time has ended. Depending on the individual ventilator's characteristics, pressure, volume, and flow may be variables as lung compliance and airway resistance change. Some time-cycled ventilators are also flow generators and produce a consistent flow pattern and inspiratory time. Under these circumstances, the ventilator produces the same volume at each breath as well. Pressure generators can also be time-cycled, in which case flow and volume are variable with changing patient conditions.

Timing mechanisms can be either pneumatic or electronic. Some ventilators use a gas chamber with an adjustable flow into it to time inspiration. The greater the flow in, the shorter the breath lasts and vice versa. The Baby Bird utilizes a pneumatic timing circuit, whereas the Sechrist IV-100B has quartz oscillators as the major component of its electronic timing system.

Flow-Cycled Ventilators. If a ventilator has a flow pattern which changes during inspiration, inspiration can be terminated when a specific flow level is reached. Puritan-Bennett PR-1 and PR-2 ventilators are sometimes considered to be flow-cycled, although the level of flow causing end-inspiration is not readily adjustable. Instead, these ventilators utilize a gravity-dependent valve which closes and stops inspiration when a critically low level of flow passes through it. This flow-cycling mechanism is activated because the pressure set on the ventilator is nearly equalized on both sides of the Bennett valve. Therefore these units may be considered to be pressure-cycled as well.

Combined Cycling. Many of the ventilators used in critical care units have more than one cycling mechanism available. As an example, a volume-cycled ventilator may use a pressure-cycling feature as a safety backup system. If inspiratory pressure reaches a preselected level before completion of the preselected tidal volume delivery, the pressure-cycling mechanism overrides the volume-cycling one and ends inspiration. This system is employed in the Bennett MA-1 and MA-2 + 2 ventilators.

The BEAR-1 ventilator has a time-cycling mechanism as a secondary backup to its volume-cycling control. The I:E ratio system can end inspiration if it is prolonged beyond one-half of the total ventilatory cycle time as set by the rate control.[60]

Inspiratory Limits. As the term "limit" is used here, it infers that some parameter, e.g., pressure or volume, can be set for a maximum allowable value; however, inspiration is not ended or cycled off when that value is reached. As an example, a pressure relief valve can be used to limit pressure during inspiration by allowing the excess gases to vent when the preselected pressure is reached. The pressure is "held" at that level until the breath is volume- or time-cycled off. The Bourns LS 104–150 infant piston ventilator is volume-cycled, yet it has a pressure relief or "pop-off" valve which can limit the pressure during inspiration. Pressure limiting occurs in a similar fashion with Babybird and Babybird-2 ventilators, whereas time is used as the cycling mechanism.

Some ventilators are primarily time-cycled but are intended to be used as "volume ventilators." The Servo 900B and 900C ventilators are examples of units that are primarily time-cycled but "attempt" to deliver a consistent volume each breath. If the driving force in these ventilators is inadequate to maintain the necessary flow, volume delivery decreases but inspiratory *time* does not vary. Because this circumstance rarely occurs, these ventilators usually are considered to be volume-limited. Regardless of the cycling mechanism used, most ventilators with either tidal volume or minute volume controls available are considered "volume ventilators."

Inspiratory Hold

After the active portion of inspiration ends, some ventilators utilize a "static" period before the beginning of expiration. Two forms of inspiratory holds are commonly used: volume holds and pressure holds.

This feature is also variously termed inflation hold and end-inspiratory pause.

A volume hold occurs after a volume-cycling mechanism has stopped inspiratory flow; the exhalation valve is maintained in a closed position, "holding" the delivered volume in the patient system for a given period of time. During this period, pressure in the patient circuit tends to equilibrate with pressure in the patient's alveoli, and a further internal distribution of gases can occur. Figure 2-13 illustrates a typical waveform during a volume hold.

Generally, a timer is used to establish how long the volume hold period lasts. Therefore this particular part of inspiration is time-cycled off. On some ventilators the timer is calibrated in seconds, whereas in others cycling is based on a percentage of the total time set by the rate control (e.g., Siemens Servo 900B).

Volume hold maneuvers have been used to improve the distribution of inspired gases,[18,55] to decrease the V_D/V_T ratio,[31,55] and for monitoring changes in static compliance and airway resistance.[7,8]

A pressure hold is accomplished by using a pressure limit system, e.g., a relief valve described above under Inspiratory Limits. Once the pressure is reached, it is "held" at that level until inspiration ends. Given enough time, lung pressure equilibrates with this pressure limit. This mechanism varies from the volume hold, in which tidal volume delivery before the hold period and bulk flow from the ventilator is stopped. Gas from the set tidal volume redistributes throughout the ventilator circuit and the patient's airways during the hold period, and a characteristic drop in pressure occurs. With a pressure hold, gas actively flows from the ventilator during the hold period. At first, when the pressure relief valve begins to vent, the flow is divided between the relief valve and the patient because lung pressure is still less than circuit pressure due to airway resistance. As the lung pressure equalizes with the applied pressure,

A

B

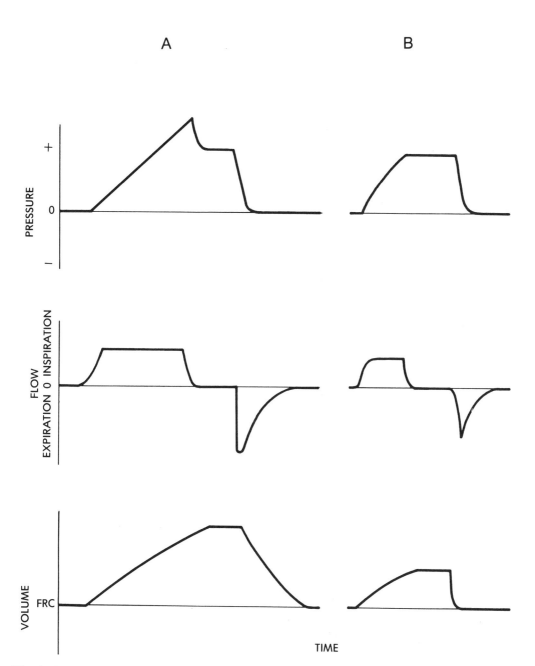

Fig. 2-13. Pressure, flow, and volume waveforms during mechanical ventilation with inspiratory hold. (A) Volume hold. (B) Pressure hold. See text for description.

more flow vents out the relief valve; finally all the flow vents, and pressures are equal throughout the system and the patient.

A basic clinical difference between these types of inspiratory hold may be noted when patient conditions change. As an example, if compliance changes, the pressure varies in a volume hold whereas the volume remains the same. In a pressure hold system, the pressure remains the same whereas the volume varies.

Expiratory Phase Maneuvers

Under normal conditions expiration is a passive event caused by lung recoil. Expiratory flow is determined by the pressure gradient from the lung to the atmosphere and the resistances to that flow caused by the airways, ventilator tubing, and valving system. Alteration of the expiratory phase has important clinical implications. Three types of expiratory maneuver are described here.

Expiratory Resistance or Retard. Patients with chronic obstructive pulmonary disease (COPD) have been observed to use "pursed lip breathing."[2,3,62] By so doing, they increase expiratory airway resistance, presumably moving the equal pressure point toward the proximal airway and thereby decreasing air trapping. It is thought that air trapping is relieved by this maneuver, either by its effect on the internal pressure of the flaccid airways or by slowing the respiratory rate.[2,62] Provision of resistance to expiratory air flow during continuous ventilatory support (by decreasing the orifice size through which the patient exhales) mimics this effect. After termination of inspiration, pressure within the airway drops to baseline levels less rapidly when retardation is used than during a typical ventilator breath (Fig. 2-14).

Retardation of expiratory flow can be accomplished by regulating the diameter of the outlet or exhalation valve of the ventilator tubing circuit with an adjustable orifice device or by placing endotracheal tube connectors at the exhalation valve outlet. Some ventilators have an adjustable resistance system, e.g., the Puritan-Bennett MA-1 or the Siemens Servo 900B. The MA-1 control is not calibrated, whereas the Servo 900B adjusts the *maximum* expiratory flow allowed and is calibrated in liters per minute.

All ventilator circuits impose *some* additional resistance to expiratory gas flow compared to normal spontaneous breathing. The amount of resistance is determined primarily by the diameter of the tubing and its connectors, valves, and outlets as well as the length of the tubing. Any continuous flow through the circuit (as occurs with some IMV apparatus) can add additional expiratory resistance as both the continuous flow and the patient's expiratory flow must pass through the same exhalation valve orifice. Excessive intrathoracic pressure can develop during a cough or forced exhalation when the circuit's expiratory resistance is high unless a sensitive pressure relief valve opens abruptly. IPPV with added expiratory resistance increases the mean airway and intrathoracic pressures compared to IPPV alone and can *cause* air trapping if the I:E ratio and/or respiratory rate is increased.

Negative End-Expiratory Pressure. Negative end-expiratory pressure (NEEP) applies a subatmospheric pressure to the airway during the expiratory phase. This "negative" pressure is seen at end-expiration (Fig. 2-15). NEEP has been suggested to reduce the mean airway and intrathoracic pressures during positive-pressure mechanical ventilation, thereby augmenting venous return to the right heart.[63] Excessive NEEP can promote airway collapse in both normal and emphysematous patients, and these side effects tend to negate its purported benefits.

Subatmospheric pressure at the airway during exhalation can be generated by entraining air through the exhalation valve

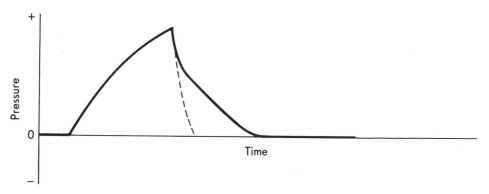

Fig. 2-14. Pressure waveform typical of increased expiratory resistance (retard). Dotted line shows expiratory pattern of system without increased resistance for comparison. (Reprinted with permission from Spearman CB, Sheldon RL (eds): Egan's Fundamentals of Respiratory Therapy. 4th Ed. Mosby, St. Louis, 1982.)

from the expiratory side of the ventilator circuit. Typically, a venturi or similar device is employed.[60] An increase in flow to the jet of the venturi device is associated with increased entrainment of gas out of the circuit and lowering of airway pressure. Systems for applying NEEP are available for or present in the Bird Mark 8, the Puritan-Bennett MA-1, and the Engström 300 series ventilators.

Positive End-Expiratory Pressure. PEEP maintains a positive airway pressure during expiration. It can be utilized during both mechanical ventilation and sponta-

neous breathing. When combined with assist or control modes, it is sometimes called mechanical ventilation with PEEP (MV/ PEEP), IPPV/PEEP or continuous positive-pressure ventilation (CPPV).[1,23,38] When spontaneous breathing utilizes positive expiratory pressure, various terms are used.[23] Continuous positive-pressure breathing (CPPB) and continuous positive airway pressure (CPAP) describe breathing in which the positive pressures during inspiration and expiration are similar.[3,23,38] (Inspiratory and expiratory pressures fluctuate about the same amount as during sponta-

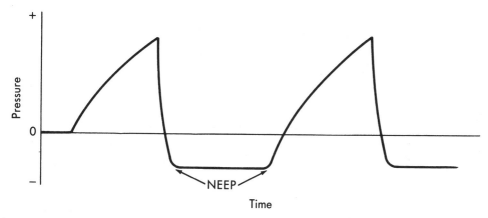

Fig. 2-15. Pressure waveform typical of IPPV with NEEP. (Reprinted with permission from Spearman CB, Sheldon RL (eds): Egan's Fundamentals of Respiratory Therapy. 4th Ed. Mosby, St. Louis, 1982.)

neous breathing without a positive-pressure baseline.) When PEEP is applied following a spontaneous peak inspiratory pressure at or below atmospheric pressure, the terms spontaneous PEEP (sPEEP) and expiratory positive airway pressure (EPAP) have been used.[23,34,37,77,87] Mechanical ventilation also can be combined with these spontaneous breathing modes resulting in IMV/CPAP or IMV/sPEEP.[50,86] Pressure waveforms depicting these techniques are illustrated in Fig. 2-16.

Expiratory positive pressure can be applied by a variety of devices, some of which are presented here.[39,48,88]

Underwater Column. A simple method directs the exhaled gases under water (Fig. 2-17). After bubbling through the water, the gases are vented to the atmosphere. The PEEP level is adjusted by changing the height of the water above the port of gas entry. Raising the water height increases the pressure at and below which further exhalation of gas does not occur. Hence the exhaled volume decreases, and this gas is "trapped" within the patient circuit and lungs.

If the entry and exit ports on the water column are not restrictive, the PEEP device will have little flow resistance. Therefore, although a positive pressure is present at end-expiration, little or no expiratory flow resistance (or retard) is encountered. If the entry or exit ports are small in diameter, resistance to flow is present and the pressure after a mechanical inspiration takes longer to return to the baseline PEEP level. This flow dependency of airway pressure causes the mean airway pressure to be higher than if the same PEEP level is applied with a resistance-free water column.

Water-Weighted Diaphragm. The J. H. Emerson Co. produces a water column PEEP device which does not require the exhaled gases to bubble through the water (Fig. 2-18). Instead, the water is separated from the patient's airway by a flexible dia-

phragm. The diaphragm seat is on the exhalation port which connects to the patient circuit by a large-bore tube. Airway pressure below the diaphragm must be greater than the hydrostatic force exerted by the water column for gas to move the diaphragm off the seat and vent to the atmosphere. When gas and water forces are equal, the diaphragm seals the exhalation port and further exhalation is prevented. The height of the water column regulates the PEEP level.

This device is relatively free of resistance under moderate flow rate conditions. The Emerson 3-PV and 3-MV ventilators apply positive pressure *above* the water level in the valve during mechanical inspiration, forcing the diaphragm to remain seated. Thus the unit functions as a combination exhalation/PEEP valve.

Venturi PEEP Valve. Some ventilators incorporate a venturi tube to apply PEEP.[60] One method applies the output pressure of the venturi tube against a one-way valve through which the patient's exhaled air must pass (Fig. 2-19). A high-pressure gas source drives the jet of the venturi. More pressure applied to the jet results in more pressure exerted against the one-way valve; therefore more pressure is required to open the valve during exhalation. When the pressure on the patient side of the one-way valve exceeds the opposing venturi pressure, exhaled air moves through the valve and venturi tube and out through open ports to the atmosphere.

The flow dependence of this type of venturi PEEP valve is primarily a function of the one-way valve resistance and the venturi tube which is often the narrowest portion of the system. If the one-way valve has a low resistance and the passages for gas flow are relatively wide, the flow-dependent resistance will be low. Two infant ventilators, the Bourns LS 104–150 and BP 200, utilize this type of venturi PEEP device.

Spring-Loaded Disk Valve. A spring-loaded valve used for pressure limiting can

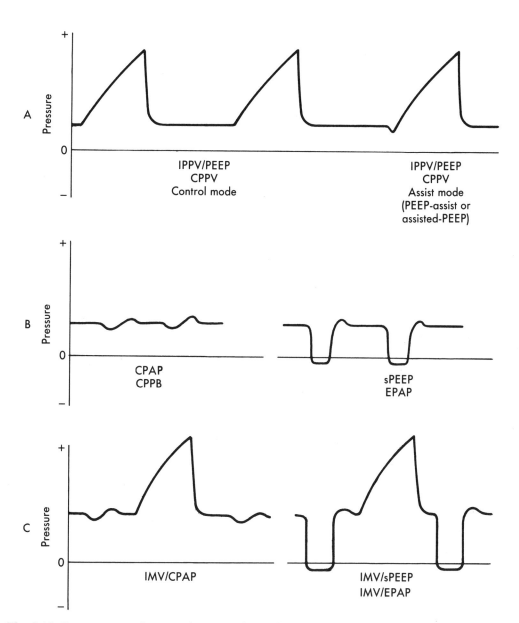

Fig. 2-16. Pressure waveforms and commonly used terminology for various techniques of ventilatory support. PEEP or CPAP is present in each illustration. (Reprinted with permission from Spearman CB, Sheldon RL (eds): Egan's Fundamentals of Respiratory Therapy. 4th Ed. Mosby, St. Louis, 1982.)

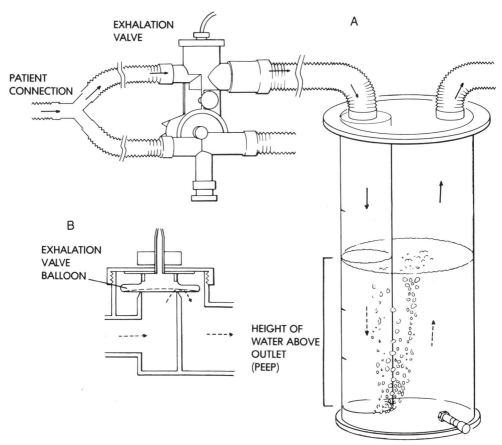

Fig. 2-17. Water column PEEP device. (A) Typical ventilator circuit. (B) Detail of the exhalation valve balloon. Flexible balloon moves off the seat (dotted lines), allowing exhaled gas to pass on to the water column.

also be used to create PEEP (Fig. 2-20). An adjustable spring provides tension (force) against a disk which rests on the exhalation port, sealing it from the atmosphere. Expiratory gas pressure opposes the spring tension on the disk. When gas pressure is greater than the spring tension, the disk moves away from its port and the gas vents to the atmosphere. When the gas pressure equals the force of the spring, the disk seals the port and prevents further egress. The PEEP level is raised by compressing the spring, which increases its force on the disk.[48]

Some spring-loaded valves also cause significant expiratory resistance, whereas oth-

ers offer little resistance to flow.[48,88] The final effect is related primarily to the length of the spring and its movement and the area of the opening for gas flow.[65,88]

Pressurized Exhalation Balloon Valve. Fig. 2-21 shows examples of an exhalation balloon valve PEEP system with different methods of applying pressure within the balloon. In Figure 2-21A, a small venturi applies its output pressure to the balloon. As gas flow to the venturi jet is increased, balloon pressure also increases. In Figure 2-21B, an adjustable reducing valve applies pressure to the balloon. Greater pressure from the reducing valve results in greater pressure within the balloon. In Figure 2-

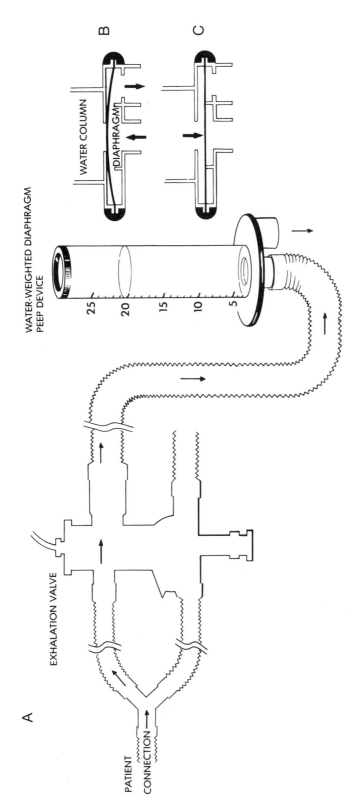

Fig. 2-18. Water-weighted diaphragm PEEP device. (A) Typical ventilator circuit. (B) Detail of diaphragm mechanism. When airway pressure is higher than that of the water column, the diaphragm is displaced upward and exhaled gas passes out of the circuit. When pressures equalize, the diaphragm "seats" and expiratory flow ceases.

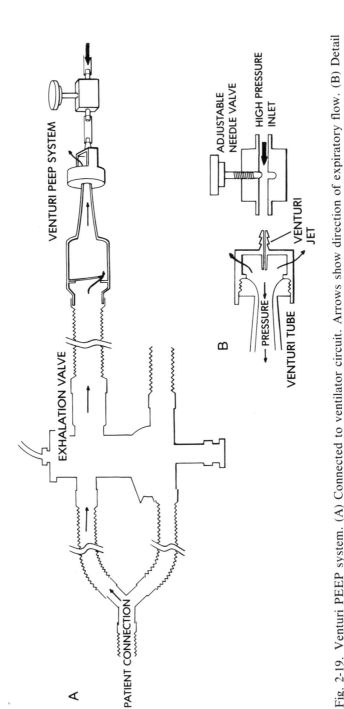

Fig. 2-19. Venturi PEEP system. (A) Connected to ventilator circuit. Arrows show direction of expiratory flow. (B) Detail of adjustable needle valve and venturi.

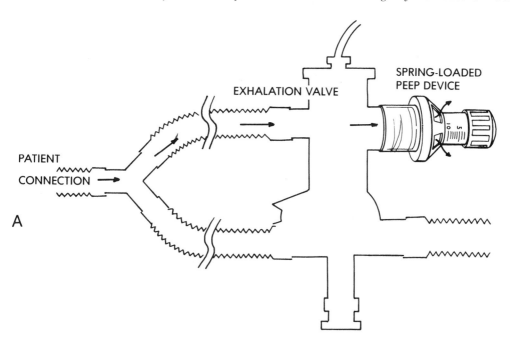

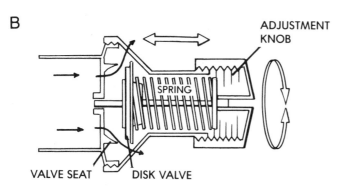

Fig. 2-20. Spring-loaded disk valve. (A) Typical ventilator circuit. Arrows show direction of expiratory flow. (B) Detail of spring-loaded valve. See text for description.

21C, a system with adjustable flow against a fixed restriction pressurizes the balloon. As flow is increased, a pressure increase results as the resistance of the fixed orifice is increased.

In all three examples the pressure in the balloon opposes pressure in the patient circuit. Because the area of the balloon applying pressure against the gas outlet is greater than the area below the valve, the pressure within the balloon is less than that within the patient circuit.[48] Pressure in the patient circuit, acting against a smaller area, must exceed the lower pressure in the balloon, which acts on a larger area in order for gas to flow to the atmosphere. These systems

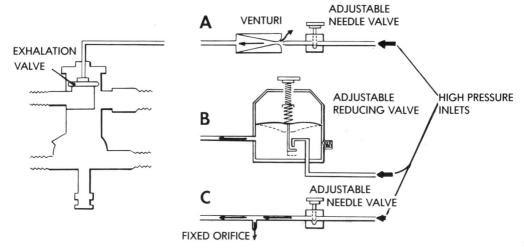

Fig. 2-21. "Trapped" pressure in exhalation valve balloon can be used to generate PEEP in the patient circuit. (A), (B), (C) Three ways gas pressure within the balloon is controlled. See text for descriptions.

can have flow resistance if the opening area for gas flow is small or if the balloon cannot easily deflate.

Systems such as these are the basis of the PEEP mechanisms in several ventilators.[60,63] Venturi pressure applied to an exhalation balloon is used in the BEAR-2 and Puritan-Bennett MA-2 ventilators. The Puritan-Bennett MA-1 has an optional PEEP attachment which utilizes a reducing valve to apply PEEP.[60] Flow adjustment against a fixed leak to regulate pressure within the exhalation balloon is the mechanism used by the Monaghan 225/SIMV ventilator.[60]

Magnetic PEEP Valve. Some devices utilize opposing magnetic and gas pressure forces to create PEEP[48] (Fig. 2-22). A valve with a metal component rests in the expiratory gas flow path. A variable position magnet can be moved closer to the valve to increase the attractive force. When force generated by the airway pressure is greater than that of magnetic attraction, the valve moves off its seat and expiration occurs. When the forces are equal, the valve shuts and PEEP is generated. Thus stronger magnetic attraction is associated with higher PEEP.

These devices may require a greater pressure to open the valve than to hold it open. Initially, the valve is close to the magnet but moves away slightly once opening occurs. The change in distance is reflected by a lower pressure. Flow dependency for these valves occurs primarily because of the limited opening area through which expiratory gases pass.

Fixed or Adjustable Orifice. These systems produce PEEP through resistance to a continuous gas flow. An increase in flow or decrease of the orifice size raises the PEEP level. Such devices are totally flow-dependent. Without gas flow, pressure is zero. A prototype system of this type was described by Barach and Molomut in 1942.[4] Continuous flow passed into a reservoir bag and "metered" mask. The expiratory port size was variable so that back pressure (PEEP) could be adjusted. The CPAP system of Gregory et al. for infants also used an adjustable orifice and continuous flow to provide positive expiratory pressure.[38] The Babybird ventilator utilizes flow against an

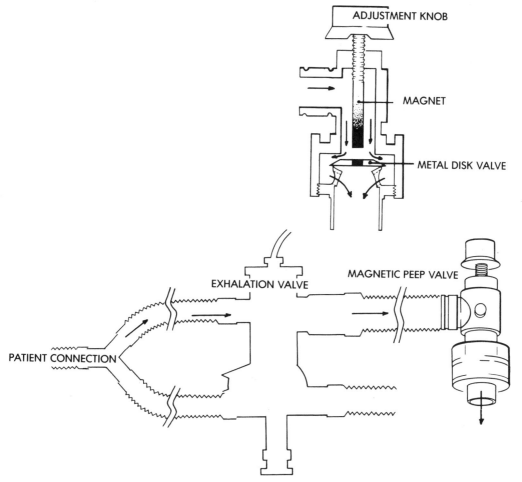

Fig. 2-22. Magnetic PEEP valve. (A) Connected to ventilator circuit. Arrows show direction of expiratory flow. (B) Detail of magnetic valve. See text for description.

adjustable outlet orifice to raise baseline pressure.[51,60] Because these systems are flow-dependent, under certain conditions they generate a combination of expiratory resistance (retard) and PEEP.

General Characteristics of Ventilation Methods

In our discussion thus far, several methods of ventilatory support have been suggested. This section discusses some general technical and clinical differences for the most common types of positive-pressure ventilation: pressure-cycled, volume-cycled, time-cycled with a volume limit, and time-cycled with a pressure limit.

Pressure-Cycled Ventilation. As previously mentioned, pressure-cycled ventilators terminate the inspiratory phase when a preset pressure is reached, regardless of the volume delivered. Therefore such ventilators are susceptible to changes in compliance and air flow resistance.[22,25,70] As lung compliance decreases or flow resistance increases, they reach their set pressures prematurely and the delivered volume decreases. Under these circumstances, overall hypoventilation may result during control mode ventilation. During assist mode ventilation, the patient may respond to the lower tidal volumes by increasing his/her respiratory rate, which increases the I:E ratio and elevates the mean airway pressure.

Raising the peak pressure can restore the tidal volume within the individual ventilator's limitations. However, as compliance and/or resistance to air flow improve, delivered volumes may now increase excessively, leading to hyperventilation and respiratory alkalosis. This potential variation in ventilation makes monitoring of these variables imperative when pressure-cycled ventilation is provided to critically ill patients.

Many patients can be successfully ventilated with pressure-cycled ventilators when adequate supervision and monitoring by a knowledgeable clinician are provided. Patients with normal lungs who receive ventilatory support for short periods postoperatively, patients with relatively stable COPD, and patients weaning from controlled ventilation can be adequately supported by pressure-cycled ventilators with proper management.

Pressure-cycled ventilators can sometimes provide better leak compensation than volume-cycled ventilators.[70] If the leak is not great enough to prevent cycling, these units can provide sufficient volume and flow to "ventilate" both the leak and the patient. In contrast, similar leakage in a volume-preset ventilator decreases the amount of gas received by the patient.[70] Naturally, any such leak should be eliminated, but occasionally this is not possible. Should the leak be large enough to prevent pressure-cycling, a time-cycling mechanism may be needed to terminate inspiration (e.g., Bennett PR-2). Some ventilators, e.g., the Bird Mark 14, the Bird ventilator, and the Ben-

nett PR-2, have special controls which provide additional flow to compensate for the leak.

Generally, pressure-cycled ventilators have peak flows of 80–100 L/minute and peak pressures of 50–60 cm H_2O, and are therefore somewhat limited in their capabilities. Pneumatic oxygen controllers or blenders can be adapted to provide control of delivered oxygen. PEEP and CPAP systems generally can be applied only with special adaptations.[48]

Ventilators using low-pressure drive systems (venturis or reducing valves described earlier in the chapter) produce a flow pattern which responds to back pressure within the patient system.[21] The decreasing flow rate tends to decrease turbulence, and we have observed repeatedly that specific volumes can be delivered with such ventilators at a lower peak airway pressure in postoperative patients than when the same volume is delivered as a square-wave flow pattern from a volume ventilator.

Most pressure-cycled ventilators, e.g., the Bird Mark series and Bennett PR series, are pneumatically powered and are therefore useful as back-up devices to electrically powered volume-cycled or time-cycled ventilators in intensive care units. They are also used for ground and air transport systems, primarily because of their small size and light weight. Such uses require that respiratory therapists, physicians, and nurses be thoroughly familiar with their function and clinical application.

Volume-Cycled Ventilation. Volume-cycled ventilators are the primary types used in critical care units today. Many patients receiving ventilatory support undergo frequent and often rapid changes in lung compliance or airway resistance. Most clinicians believe that volume-cycled ventilators are capable of maintaining more constant ventilation under these circumstances when compared to pressure-cycled ventilators.[5,22,25,46,58,70,73] As compliance or resistance worsens, the driving pressure needed to deliver the volume increases automatically. If the pressure reaches a predetermined safety limit, inspiration is terminated by a secondary pressure cycling mechanism or the excess (nondelivered) volume vents to the ambient level through a relief valve, preventing any additional increase of pressure. Modern volume-cycled ventilators are usually capable of high airway pressures (100–150 cm H_2O).[60,63]

Volume-cycled ventilators do not deliver constant tidal volumes under all conditions. The inspiratory positive pressure acts on the patient circuit and the ventilator's internal pneumatic system. Gas is compressed by this pressure whereas flexible tubing and other components expand. Hence part of the preset volume (compressible volume) is lost to the patient because it never reaches the airway.

The volume not received by the patient depends on the pressure generated and the compliance of the system. If the components in which compression occurs are fairly stiff or rigid, the amount of gas compressed is approximately 1 ml/cm H_2O for each liter of available space. If a ventilator has a rigid delivery system of 4 L, 4 ml of gas/cm H_2O pressure would be compressed during inspiration. This factor, called the *compressibility factor,* is 4 ml/cm H_2O in this example. If the system is somewhat distensible under pressure, the factor is greater (4.5 or 5 ml/cm H_2O). This value is sometimes termed the *compliance factor* but is generally interchangeable with the compressibility factor.

The significance of the compressed volume during "volume" ventilation depends on a variety of factors, including the preset tidal volume compared to the compressibility factor and the extent of compliance and resistance changes (Fig. 2-23). If the compressibility factor is large and small tidal volumes are selected, the ventilator tends to function more like a pressure ventilator in terms of volume delivery. As an example, if the factor is 5 ml/cm H_2O and

the tidal volume is 300 ml, this entire amount could be compressed within the system if 60 cm H_2O inflation pressure was applied. The patient would not be ventilated. If end-inspiratory pressure was only 20 cm H_2O, the compressed volume would be one-third the set volume ($5 \times 20 = 100$ ml compressed), whereas a 40 cm H_2O pressure would cause 200 ml of the set volume to be lost, with a resultant substantial reduction of the patient's ventilation. These large decreases in patient-delivered tidal volume are similar to the changes in volume which might be experienced when a pressure-cycled ventilator is used under similar conditions.

The volume in which gas may be compressed is limited primarily to external tubing circuits in some ventilators, whereas others have significant *internal* volume as well.[49,66,88] This fact presents the clinician with a practical problem in volume measurement. Gas collected at a ventilator's exhalation valve is a mixture of that which entered the patient's airway and that compressed primarily in the *external* tubing circuit. (Generally the gas compressed in an internal compartment—bellows or piston cylinder—does not vent through the exhalation valve. Instead, it simply reexpands as that compartment refills immediately after end-inspiration and remains inside the ventilator.)

A simplified ventilator with both internal and external spaces for compressible volumes is illustrated in Fig. 2-24. The set tidal volume, provided by the excursion of the bellows, is 800 ml. Because this bellows begins the inspiratory phase in its full position and empties only part of its volume during the breath, a significant amount of space is available to compress gas within the bellows at end-inspiration. This end-inspiratory internal volume is 2 L, providing a compressibility factor of about 2 ml/cm H_2O. The tubing circuit is the external source of compressible volume and in Figure 2-24 contains 3 L, yielding a compress-

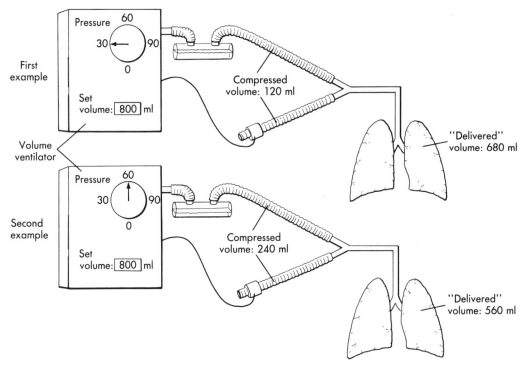

Fig. 2-23. Comparison of tidal volume delivery to a patient when different end-inspiratory pressures occur during volume-cycled ventilation. The first example with a 30 cm H_2O peak pressure results in 680 ml received out of a preset volume of 800 ml. In the second example, a 60 cm H_2O peak pressure results in only 560 ml received. (Reprinted with permission from Spearman CB, Sheldon RL (eds): Egan's Fundamentals of Respiratory Therapy. 4th Ed. Mosby, St. Louis, 1982.)

ibility factor of 3 ml/cm H_2O. Thus a total of 5 ml/cm H_2O is compressed during inspiration and is not delivered to the patient. However, only the 3 ml/cm H_2O compressed in the external circuit is collected with the patient's exhaled gas because the internal system returns to atmospheric pressure as the bellows refills. The one-way valve near the bellows outlet closes, and the "trapped" gases in the bellows simply reexpand.

If end-inspiratory pressure is 40 cm H_2O, 80 ml is compressed internally (2 × 40), 120 ml is compressed externally (3 × 40), and the patient receives the remaining 600 ml. Only the 120 ml and 600 ml volumes are collected in the spirometer at the exhalation valve, whereas the 80 ml volume remains in the bellows. The spirometer reading is 720 ml, which differs from the set volume of 800 ml. To calculate what portion of the

exhaled gas was received by the patient, 3 ml/cm H_2O is subtracted from the *collected* volume recorded by the spirometer. To determine what the patient received compared to the *set* volume of 800 ml, the *total compressibility factor* of 5 ml/cm H_2O is used (800 ml set − 200 ml compressed both internally and externally = 600 ml). Using the *total* factor with the *spirometer* reading *underestimates* the volume received by the patient.

Time-Cycled Ventilation. Pure time-cycled ventilators end the inspiratory phase once a preset time has passed and manifest relative disregard for airway pressure or volume. However, most time-cycled ventilators are commonly used so that they are also pressure- or volume-limited.

Time-cycled, volume-limited ventilation. When a time-cycled ventilator is a constant- or non-constant-flow generator, the volume

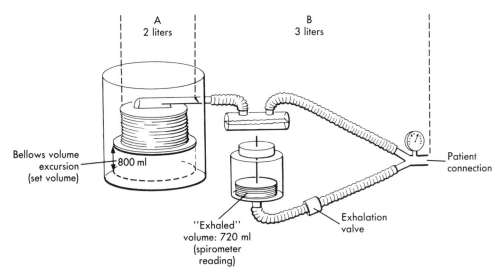

Fig. 2-24. Internal compressed volume (A) and tubing circuit compressed volume (B) reduce the tidal volume received by a patient during volume-cycled ventilation. Gases compressed internally are not measured on a spirometer. See text for further description of this example. (Reprinted with permission from Spearman CB, Sheldon RL (eds): Egan's Fundamentals of Respiratory Therapy. 4th Ed. Mosby, St. Louis, 1982.)

is also controlled. With a constant-flow generator, the relationship is expressed as:

Volume (liters)   (1)

$$= \frac{\text{inspiratory time (seconds)} \times \text{flow rate (LPM)}}{60}$$

To use such a ventilator when the desired tidal volume and inspiratory time are known, the necessary flow rate can be found through rearrangement of Eq. 1:

Flow rate (LPM) needed   (2)

$$= \frac{\text{desired volume (liters)}}{\text{inspiratory time (seconds)}} \times 60$$

Non-constant-flow generators which are time-cycled produce the same flow *pattern* during the same interval each breath; therefore a consistent tidal volume results. The most common ventilators of this type are the piston-driven, time-cycled ventilators, e.g., the Emerson 3-PV and 3-MV units. In these devices the piston stroke establishes the volume, and the rotary drive and inspiratory time setting generate the flow pattern

and flow rate, respectively, for that volume. In both examples, inspiration ends after passage of a preselected time interval, even though tidal volume remains constant from one breath to the next. Such ventilators are referred to as time-cycled and volume-limited, and have limitations of volume delivery similar to those described for volume-cycled ventilators. Flow and pressure waveforms for time-cycled, volume-limited ventilators are similar to those shown in Figures 2-11 and 2-12.

Time-Cycled, Pressure-Limited Ventilation. When a pressure relief valve is used to limit the maximum pressure during a time-cycled breath, both flow and volume delivery can vary with changes in the patient's airway resistance and compliance. This pattern is commonly employed with pediatric ventilators.[28,41,60] In the Babybird-2 and Bear Cub BP-200 pediatric ventilators, a flow of gas enters the patient's circuit at all times. Periodically, an expiratory valve is closed and the continuous flow is diverted, under pressure, into the patient's airway. If the pressure limit is reached before inspiratory time is over, some or all of the flow begins to vent through the relief valve, and pressure holds constant for the remainder of the breath.

The volume received by the patient is related primarily to two factors so long as lung pressure equilibrates with the ventilator pressure limit during inspiration: (1) applied pressure; and (2) the patient's lung-thorax compliance. If a peak pressure 30 cm H_2O above PEEP is applied during inspiration and equilibrates with alveolar pressure, then 30 times the patient's compliance equals the volume received. As an example, if the patient's compliance is 1.5 ml/cm H_2O, a 30 cm H_2O pressure results in a tidal volume of 45 ml ($1.5 \times 30 = 45$). Should this compliance value change to 2 ml/cm H_2O, the patient's volume would increase to 60 ml for the same 30 cm H_2O pressure. If the applied pressure does not equilibrate in the alveoli—because of excessive airway resistance, inadequate inspiratory time, or both—the volume may be quite variable.

Examples of time-cycled, pressure-limited ventilation under changing patient conditions are shown in Fig. 2-25. In all three examples, sufficient time is allowed for equilibration of the applied pressure within the lung. Note that the inspiratory time and pressure limit are the same in each example. The periods of zero flow and flattening of the volume curved indicate that pressure in the lung equals the pressure limit applied. Relatively normal conditions are illustrated in Figure 2-25A, whereas a decreased volume delivery results from reduced compliance in Figure 2-25B. The same volume delivery as in Figure 2-25A requires more time in Figure 2-25C because of an increase in airway resistance.

Other variables can also change the volume received during time-cycled, pressure-limited ventilation. If the patient is actively inspiring while the ventilator is in its inspiratory phase, the volume delivered can be greater than if the patient is apneic. An active exhalation during the breath reduces the volume delivery.

Flow and volume waveforms are not easily monitored in pediatric continuous-flow, time-cycled, pressure-limited ventilation; therefore changes in resistance and compliance are not easily detected. Analysis of the pressure waveform (which is more easily obtained) has been recommended but thus far has been done only in the laboratory using a lung simulator.[76]

FUNCTIONAL DESIGNS OF OTHER VENTILATOR FEATURES AND SYSTEMS

Air-Oxygen Blending Systems

Most modern ventilators used in critical care can be connected to an oxygen blending system or have one as an integral component part. In general, these systems can be categorized into two types: (1) those requiring both pressurized oxygen and air; and (2) those requiring only pressurized oxygen.

Pressurized Oxygen and Air Blenders. Pressurized oxygen and air blenders generally require inputs from 40–50 psig oxygen and air sources. These gas pressures are then either reduced and matched at a lower pressure (e.g., 10–12 psig), or the higher of the two pressures is reduced to match the lower pressure (Fig. 2-26). Air and oxygen at equal pressures are then connected to a *proportioning* valve with a single outlet for the blended gases. Because the pressures entering the proportioning valve are equal and the outlet pressure is the same as well, the pressure gradient across this valve is the same for each gas. The *amount* of each gas which passes through the valve is *proportional* to the orifice size for each gas. The valve is constructed so that one side is opened *proportionately* as the other side closes during rotation of the selection knob. When the opening for air is equal to the opening for oxygen (and the pressure gradient across the valve is equal for each gas),

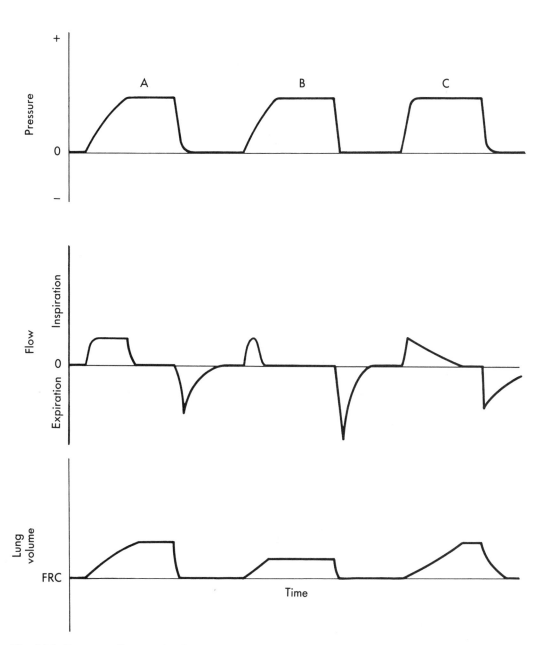

Fig. 2-25. Pressure, flow, and volume waveforms for time-cycled, pressure-limited ventilation during different patient conditions. (A) Normal. (B) Reduced compliance. (C) Increased airway resistance. See text for descriptions. (Reprinted with permission from Spearman CB, Sheldon RL (eds): Egan's Fundamentals of Respiratory Therapy. 4th Ed. Mosby, St. Louis, 1982.)

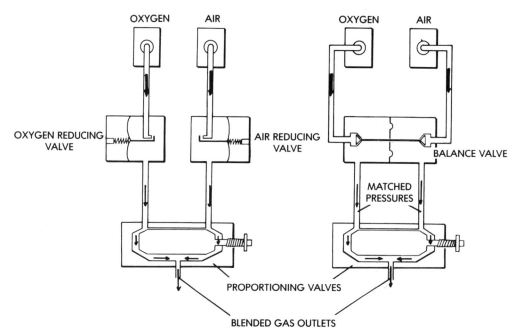

Fig. 2-26. Oxygen blending systems requiring pressurized oxygen and air sources. (A) Separate reducing valves set for identical pressures are used to lower oxygen and air pressures proximal to the proportioning valve. (B) Both gases are connected to a balance valve, which reduces the higher gas pressure to match the lower pressure proximal to the proportional valve.

the mixture will contain approximately 60 percent oxygen (half the gas is air containing 20.9 percent oxygen and the other half contains 100 percent oxygen). If total occlusion of both sides is possible, concentrations of oxygen from 20.9% to 100 percent will be available.

The BEAR-2 and BEAR-CUB ventilators utilize the system in which compressed air and oxygen are reduced and matched (Fig. 2-26A), whereas the Bird oxygen blender and Puritan-Bennett AO-1 mixer are examples of higher-pressure types which match the higher input pressure to the lower input pressure (Fig. 2-26B).[60]

Pressurized Oxygen Only Blending Systems. Some ventilators require only pressurized oxygen. In these systems oxygen pressure is reduced to nearly atmospheric level. The reduced pressure oxygen and a source of filtered room air for blending then refill the delivery system (Fig. 2-27). A proportioning valve is used to blend air and oxygen. However, the pressure gradient across the valve is from nearly atmospheric pressure for the air and oxygen inlets to a few centimeters of H_2O below atmospheric pressure within the delivery system during its refilling phase. Oxygen blending systems such as these are used in the Puritan-Bennett MA-1 and MA-2 ventilators and the Ohio CCV-2, SIMV ventilator.[60]

Venturi systems utilizing entrainment of room air to mix with 100 percent oxygen have been used; however, these systems are susceptible to back pressure, which causes a decrease in air entrainment and an increase in oxygen concentration.[60,75] If a venturi system is used to premix oxygen and air in a reservoir system and the venturi itself is not exposed to inspiratory positive pressure, reasonably accurate blending can occur. Very early models of the Puritan-Bennett MA-1 utilized such a system, as did the previously produced Ohio 560.[60]

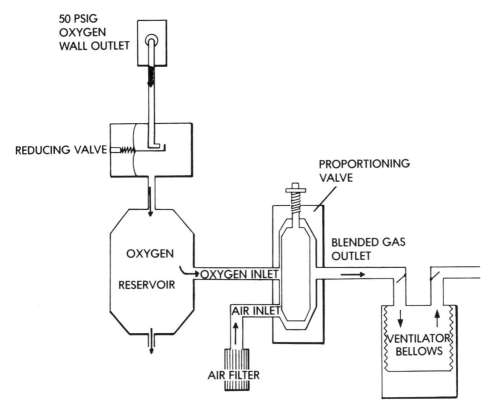

Fig. 2-27. Pressurized oxygen blending system. Oxygen is reduced to near atmospheric pressure in the reservoir. Air and oxygen inlets to the proportioning valve are both at atmospheric pressure. Gas is "pulled" across the valve as the bellows fall during refill.

Various alarms are available for the blenders. Some monitor only pressures within the systems, whereas others utilize oxygen analyzers to measure oxygen concentration. Some blending systems partially or totally stop supplying gas when one input source fails, whereas others switch entirely over to the remaining gas source regardless of the concentration set on the proportioning valve. Clinicians must be thoroughly familiar with the oxygen system being used so that they can anticipate and respond appropriately in cases of failure.

Humidification Systems

Normally, when the upper airway is intact, inspired air is warmed to near body temperature and is nearly saturated with water vapor by the time it reaches the level of the carina.[47,74] When endotracheal or tracheostomy tubes are used to provide mechanical ventilation, the natural warming and moisturizing functions of the nose, mouth, and trachea are bypassed. Nevertheless, the alveolar air is saturated with water vapor at body temperature even when dry air is inspired. The water deficit of inspired air and the heat needed to warm this air must come from the mucosal surfaces below the artificial airway. Adverse effects of such breathing on mucociliary clearance are well known.[5,65,73,79,86,88]

To avoid this "added burden" on the respiratory tract, heated humidification systems should be utilized whenever artificial airways are used. In general, they are capable of providing saturated gas over a wide range of temperatures in their simulation of the upper airway functions of heat and moisture control.

The assumption that one must provide gases at 100 percent relative humidity and body temperature (so-called "body humidity") when patients are intubated may be invalid. Some controversy exists concerning the optimal range for humidity and temperature for such patients. Research on anesthetized animals and patients presents conflicting data for lung tissue and surfactant changes, mucous flow, and pulmonary complications at various levels of temperature and humidity.[14,15,26,27,90] When all heat and humidity requirements are supplied externally, natural heat and water vapor losses from the airway are stopped. The clinical significance of this situation is not well understood at present. However, at 50–70 percent body humidity mucociliary clearance of secretions is impaired. This function improves when temperatures of 32–42°C with 33 mg/L of water vapor are used. Because body humidity equals about 44mg/L at 37°C, 33 mg/L provides 75 percent body humidity.

Delivered gas for intubated patients should be kept at 80–100 percent relative humidity at temperatures of 32–37°C (90–99°F), and temperature must be monitored closely. Our own clinical experience agrees with that of others for the general use of these guidelines.[88]

Heated Humidifiers. Humidification systems have been evaluated extensively.[52,60,69] Three basic types of heated humidifiers produce water vapor with little or no aerosol: pass-over or blow-by, bubbler or cascade, and wick. Because the bubbler and wick types are the most commonly used, they are described here.

Bubbler and Cascade Humidifiers. In bubbler and cascade humidifiers, gas must pass under and be dispersed through water as relatively small bubbles (Fig. 2-28). This process creates a large surface area for exposure of the gas to the heated water, and evaporation is enhanced. Temperature control is generated by heated rods immersed in the water or a heated plate at the bottom of the humidifier jar. Those using heating rods generally require more agitation of the water for even heating than do the units having a heated plate.

The most commonly used bubbler-style humidifier is the Puritan-Bennett Cascade model. It is produced specifically to provide a relatively low resistance at intermittent high ventilator flow rates. Other examples of bubble humidifiers are the Ohio Heated Humidifier and Chemetron's MICH humidifier system.

Wick-Type Heated Humidifiers. Some humidifiers incorporate a water-absorbing material referred to as a wick. These units are actually "blow-by" humidifiers because gas flowing through them passes over the water next to the saturated wick, which usually rests against a heated plate (Fig. 2-29).

Several manufacturers produce wick-type heated humidification systems.[60,69] Examples include the Bird Humidifier Model 3000, several models of the Conchatherm/Conchapak systems from Respiratory Care Inc., and the MR500 heated humidifier from Fisher and Paykel Medical, Inc.

Performance Limitations. Most heated humidifiers saturate the gas passing through them if enough heat is applied to the water.[52] In order to deliver the gas near body temperature at the end of a tubing circuit 4–6 feet long, it must be heated to a higher temperature before leaving the humidifier. Fig. 2-30 illustrates this point. In the example, a high-efficiency humidifier is heated so that its output temperature is 50°C. Saturated air at 50°C contains 84 mg/L water vapor. The room air surrounding the tubing is 22°C, and cooling of the warmed gas occurs as it moves through the tubing to the patient connection. In this example, the temperature at the patient Y connection is 37°C. Because the gas was sat-

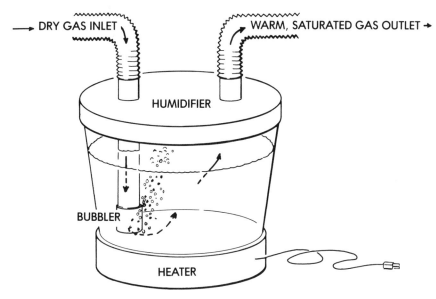

→ DRY GAS INLET

WARM, SATURATED GAS OUTLET →

HUMIDIFIER

BUBBLER

HEATER

Fig. 2-28. Heated bubbler humidifier. Large-bore tubing, low-resistance bubbling device with high surface area contact between gas and water and heated water provide an efficient ventilator humidification system.

urated (100 percent relative humidity) at the humidifier outlet, the temperature drop along the circuit path causes condensation of water vapor to occur, and the absolute humidity decreases from 84 mg/L to 44 mg/L. Nearly one-half of the original vapor produced condenses in the tubing circuit as the temperature decreases from 50°C to 37°C. Relative humidity, however, remains at 100 percent (saturated), so the patient is assured of an adequate moisture content of the inspired gas.

The amount of condensation can be reduced significantly by heating the delivery tubing between the humidifier and the patient connection.[64,93] Generally, the humidifier outlet temperature can be within 1–2°C of that at the patient connection, so very little condensation occurs.

"Servo-controlling" the humidifier can improve temperature control.[60] When this technique is employed, a probe monitors gas temperature near the patient connection, and water temperature within the humidifier is regulated to maintain the desired gas temperature. These systems tend to compensate for changes in ambient temperature, air currents around the tubing, and bedding insulating the tubing, etc. to ensure a relatively constant gas temperature. If a servo-control is not used, the gas temperature varies with environmental changes, whereas the water temperature remains relatively constant. Examples of servo-controlled humidifiers include the Puritan-Bennett Cascade II and the Dual Servo MR500.

Thermal mass within a humidifier influences its ability to react quickly to changing gas flow rates or ventilator cycling frequency. As an example, a unit containing 800–1000 ml of water responds to an increased ventilator rate by delivering more heat into the gas. This causes the air temperature breathed by the patient to increase until the "extra" heat in the water is dissipated. In some wick humidifiers, the volume of water and hence the thermal mass are very small. These units respond quickly to changing conditions, allowing some wick units to have a shorter "warm-up" time than some bubblers.[52]

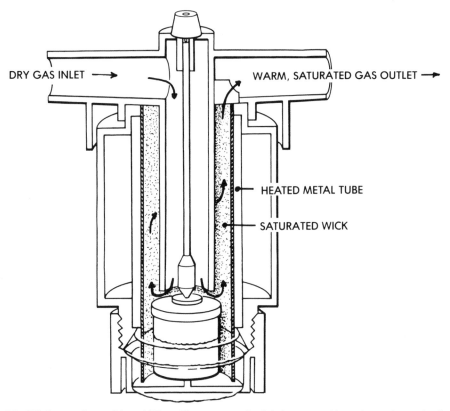

DRY GAS INLET →

WARM, SATURATED GAS OUTLET →

HEATED METAL TUBE

SATURATED WICK

Fig. 2-29. Wick-type heated humidifier. The saturated wick is warmed by a heated metal tube, and gas passing over the wick gains heat and water vapor.

Heat and Moisture Exchangers. Heat and moisture exchangers have been called "artificial noses" because they allegedly mimic the heating and humidifying functions of the nose.[5,73,89] They are placed so that they become part of the respiratory dead space or rebreathed volume. During exhalation, saturated gas from the patient condenses some water vapor and gives up some heat to the device. During the subsequent inspiration, the condensed water evaporates and heat is gained from the exchanger, raising the humidity and temperature of the inspired gas toward body levels. A newer design uses a porous material chemically treated to make it hygroscopic and is said to retain more water vapor during the expiratory phase.[32]

Heat and moisture exchangers may provide adequate humidity levels while intubated patients breathe room air or anesthetic gases in semiclosed anesthesia circuits; however, their use in critically ill patients who require mechanical ventilatory support for extended periods needs further study.[32,89,91,92] Generally, they provide no more than 50–80 percent body humidity when dry gases are breathed, and this level may be inadequate for patients with abnormal clearance of secretions. Condensing units which can provide 80 percent body humidity may prove to be useful for patients receiving mechanical ventilation whose airways are relatively normal.

Advantages of heat and moisture exchangers include the elimination of condensate in the tubing circuit, reduced compressible volume caused by the absence of a humidifier and water traps, and the avoidance of overheating which can occur with

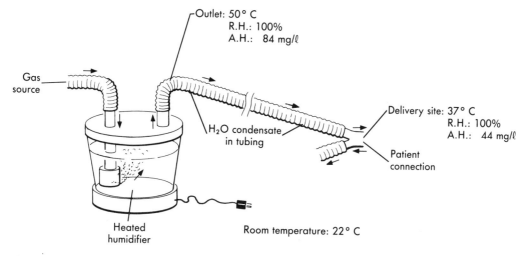

Fig. 2-30. Temperature and humidity changes in the tubing circuit with a heated humidifier. Hot gases saturated with water vapor cool during passage to the patient connection. Condensation occurs, decreasing the absolute humidity (A.H.), whereas the relative humidity (R.H.) stays at 100 percent. Note that in this example almost one-half of the original water vapor condenses in the tubing circuit. (Reprinted with permission from Spearman CB, Sheldon RL (eds): Egan's Fundamentals of Respiratory Therapy. 4th Ed. Mosby, St. Louis, 1982.)

heated humidifiers. Examples of currently available devices are the Servo Humidifier from Siemens-Elema and the Breathaid from Terumo Corp.

Delivery Circuits

Ventilator tubing circuits are varied in their configuration, but most have common features. We first describe a typical system for a volume-cycled ventilator, then compare two general methods for modifying the circuit to improve IMV.

Volume-Cycled Ventilator Circuit. Most ventilators utilize a tubing circuit with the primary components shown in Fig. 2-31. The inspiratory side has connecting tubing, a heated humidifier, support manifold, and sometimes a nebulizer and temperature probe. The expiratory limb is comprised of connecting tubing and a gas-powered exhalation valve. A Y connector connects the inspiratory and expiratory sides to each other and to the patient. Tubing between the

Y and the patient is considered *mechanical dead space* because its contents will be rebreathed. Some circuits also have a port for monitoring pressure at the Y as well as bacteria filters, water traps to collect condensate, adaptors for in-line oxygen monitoring, and adjustable relief valves.

During mechanical inspiration the exhalation valve is pressurized at a level equal to or greater than that received by the patient. Because the area under the valve (in the circuit) is smaller than the area within the valve, a surface area differential force is established and the valve is held closed.[48] Some ventilators use a predetermined pressure to charge the exhalation valve each breath.[60] During expiration, the valve is depressurized to baseline level (i.e., zero or PEEP), the valve "collapses," and the patient's exhaled gases and those compressed in the tubing circuit vent to the atmosphere.

Other ventilators, e.g., the Servo 900B and Bourns BP-200 models, do not utilize pneumatically powered exhalation valves. Instead, electronically controlled systems

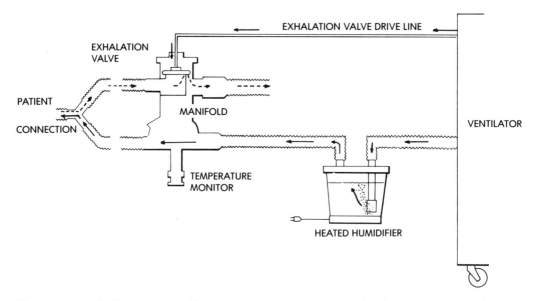

Fig. 2-31. "Typical" volume ventilator circuit. Solid arrows depict inspiratory flow; dashed arrows show expiratory flow.

are used and the tubing circuit requires only inspiratory and expiratory large-bore tubes without an expiratory drive line.

IMV Circuits. Since IMV was first popularized for adult ventilation, several modifications to the typical circuit have been suggested.[14–16,20,21,89,90] Two representative modifications are presented here. Both systems are designed to add a source of fresh gases for spontaneous breathing.

Continuous Flow-Through System with Reservoir Bag. The continuous flow-through system with a reservoir bag is illustrated in Fig. 2-32. A 3- to 5-L bag is connected to the inspiratory side of the ventilator circuit proximal to the heated humidifier. Continuous gas flow from an oxygen blender enters the bag until it is full, then passes through a one-way valve into the main portion of the patient circuit. Spontaneous breaths are taken from this continuous flow and, if necessary, from the bag.

When the ventilator cycles (mandatory mechanical breath), the one-way valve between the circuit and the bag is closed, preventing the continuous flow from entering the circuit. The valve also prevents the ventilator from "ventilating" the bag instead of the patient. When exhalation begins, the continuous flow moves through the circuit again. During spontaneous breathing, this configuration functions much like a continuous-flow CPAP system.[45,82,83] The spontaneous work of breathing is influenced by the flow through the circuit. Once inspiratory flow exceeds the continuous flow, additional gas must come from the reservoir bag. If the humidifier is a bubbler or cascade type, the water provides resistance to the patient's breathing. Inspiratory work is least when the continuous flow is higher than the patient's peak inspiratory flow rate (40–60 L/minute for most patients). Such high flow rates can raise the patient's baseline airway pressure by 2–5 cm H_2O, reflecting the circuit's resistance to gas flow. This pressure is sometimes called "inadvertent PEEP" and may be undesirable in some patients.

Another problem is that this high flow must be vented along with the patient's exhaled gas, producing an increase of expi-

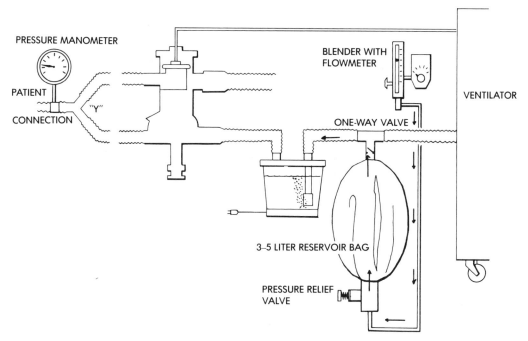

Fig. 2-32. Continuous-flow-through reservoir bag IMV system. Continuous gas flow from the blender fills the bag and flows through the circuit to allow spontaneous breathing. The pressure relief valve on the bag is used to vent excess flow during a mechanical breath. See text for description.

ratory resistance or retard. This effect is increased after a mechanical breath from the ventilator. When the ventilator cycles on, the continuous flow is "collected" within the reservoir bag until inspiration ends. As the exhalation valve opens at end-inspiration, the patient's exhaled gases, the continuous flow, and any gases collected in the reservoir bag must all pass through the same exhalation valve, resulting in a substantial increase of expiratory resistance. Some of this resistance can be reduced by a reservoir bag relief valve set for a pressure higher than PEEP but less than the peak pressure during a mechanical breath. In this way the relief valve is closed between mechanical breaths, and flow passes through the circuit as usual. When mechanical inspiration causes the one-way valve to close, the incoming continuous flow causes pressure in the bag to increase until the pressure relief valve opens, venting the extra flow to the atmosphere.

Another problem identified for continuous-flow systems can occur when the ventilator's flow rate is less than the continuous-flow rate.[68] In this case, the one-way valve between the reservoir bag and the circuit remains open, and the tidal volume from the ventilator is increased by the continuous flow. This sequence occurs only if the reservoir bag itself is relatively noncompliant. In our experience, if it can stretch, the pressure in the bag remains lower than that within the circuit, and the one-way valve remains closed during mechanical inspiration.

Lower continuous-flow rates can increase the spontaneous inspiration work, especially if the patient must "pull" gases from the bag through the humidifier's water. If the ventilator pressure manometer is connected to the circuit proximal to the humidifier, it reflects the additional pressure necessary to bubble gas through the water and is several centimeters of H_2O greater than the patient's airway pressure. If a relatively low-resistance humidifier (wick type) is used, the inspiratory work is decreased and the internal pressure manometer reading will be more accurate. A manometer connected at the patient Y best reflects the pressure at the proximal upper airway, regardless of the continuous-flow setting or the type of humidifer used.

A final problem inherent in continuous-flow systems involves the collection of exhaled gases for volume and gas concentration measurements. The continuous flow mixes with the exhaled gases, making such measurements extremely difficult. A pressure differential pneumotachometer placed between the circuit Y and the patient's airway "sees" only inspired and expired gas, and the continuous flow is not measured.[60,66,67] Systems which shunt the continuous flow proximal to a flow sensor so that only inspired and expired gases are monitored have been described.[60,61,94] An additional exhalation valve to isolate the patient's flow so that exhaled gas volumes and concentrations can be monitored has also been used.[43,94]

Because both ventilator-supplied and continuous-flow gas passes through the circuit's heated humidifier, no additional humidification system is needed. Also, only one PEEP device is required because all gas leaves the circuit through a single exhalation valve (unless a special monitoring system is applied). The primary advantage of continuous-flow systems seems to be the relatively low and adjustable work of breathing.[33]

Parallel Flow or "H" IMV System. Another method to provide gas for spontaneous breathing uses the system in Fig. 2-33. A T connector attaches the spontaneous breathing circuit to the inspiratory limb of the ventilator circuit. A one-way valve separates the two circuits so that it is closed by the mandatory mechanical breath and opened by a spontaneous effort. Blended gas from either a heated entrainment nebulizer or heated humidifier feed the T and bypass the one-way valve through an open-end length of reservoir tubing. This system has the shape of an H when it is connected, and the continuous flow is parallel to, rather than through, the main circuit.

During a spontaneous effort the patient creates a slight drop in pressure (usually 1–2 cm H_2O) which opens the one-way valve in the H system and inhales from the continuous flow of blended gases. During expiration the patient's exhaled air flows down the expiratory limb of the ventilator circuit, and the continuous flow goes through the reservoir tube. Thus the exhaled gas is separate from the continuous flow, and monitoring of gas volume and composition is accomplished more easily than with the continuous-flow-through system. Expiratory resistance is also less with this system.

Work of breathing is somewhat adjusted by using a low-resistance one-way valve. A spring-loaded valve with an adjustable spring tension can also be used such that increasing the spring tension increases the effort required to open the valve during a spontaneous inspiration.

This system requires an additional heated humidification system. If PEEP is applied to the ventilator circuit, the patient must lower the PEEP to zero plus whatever additional pressure decrement is needed to open the valve, similar to sPEEP and EPAP breathing modes.[34,37,48,77,87] To decrease the spontaneous work of breathing when PEEP is applied to the ventilator circuit, a similar level of pressure must be applied to the continuous-flow circuit.[10] So long as pressure in the parallel circuit is less than PEEP in the ventilator circuit, the continuous flow remains separated from the patient's exhaled air.

If an entrainment nebulizer is used to control the humidification and oxygen concen-

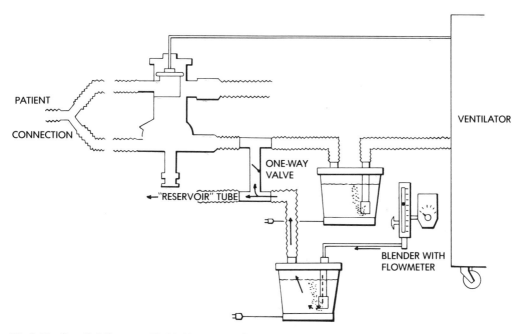

Fig 2-33. Parallel flow, or H, IMV system. Gas from the blender passes through a separate humidifier, past a one-way valve, and out the reservoir tube. See text for description.

tration in the parallel circuit, PEEP on this side of the one-way valve causes an increase in oxygen concentration and a decrease in total flow from the nebulizer (back pressure effect). A high flow oxygen blender and heated humidifier is more suitable as PEEP does not affect oxygen concentrations or gas flow with this apparatus.

Flow through the parallel circuit must exceed the peak inspiratory flow created by the patient to avoid inhalation of room air from the open reservoir (assuming no PEEP device is present). Alternatively, the reservoir volume can be increased to allow lower flow rates. If the volume of the reservoir is larger than the patient's spontaneous tidal volume, flow rates need only exceed the patient's spontaneous minute volume.

Other Systems. IMV is commonly available in modern ventilators, some of which use a continuous-flow system (e.g., 3-MV Emerson), whereas others employ a demand flow system. Demand systems produce flow in response to the patient's efforts, usually up to 100 L/minute or more. They may use a pneumatic valve (Puritan-Bennett MA-1 or BEAR-2) or sophisticated electronic systems (Servo 900C and Puritan-Bennett 7200 microprocessor).

Demand systems do not interfere with monitoring, and PEEP is generally automatically or manually compensated so that a demand-CPAP breathing pattern is available. Pneumatic demand valves often are not adjustable for work of breathing, whereas electronic systems can be.

Properly adjusted continuous-flow systems seem to provide the least change in airway pressure and the least work during spontaneous breathing, although some PEEP devices used with continuous flow can influence inspiratory and expiratory work and breathing resistance.[16,17,33,45]

REFERENCES

1. Ashbaugh DG, Petty TL: Positive end-expiratory pressure: physiology, indications

and contraindications. J Thorac Cardiovasc Surg 65:165, 1973

2. Barach AL: Physiotherapy of advanced disease states, In Petty TL (ed): Chronic Obstructive Pulmonary Disease. Marcel Dekker, New York, 1978

3. Barach AL, Bickerman HA, Petty TL: Perspectives in pressure breathing. Respir Care 20:627, 1975

4. Barach AL, Molomut N: Oxygen mask metered for positive pressure. Ann Intern Med 17:820, 1942

5. Bendixen HH, Egbert LD, Hedley-White J, et al: Respiratory Care. Mosby, St. Louis, 1965

6. Bland RD, Kim MH, Light MJ, et al: High frequency ventilation in severe hyaline membrane disease: an alternative treatment? Crit Care Med 8:275, 1980

7. Bone RC: Diagnosis of causes for acute respiratory distress by pressure-volume curves. Chest 70:740, 1976

8. Bone RC: Monitoring respiratory function in the patient with adult respiratory distress syndrome. Semin Respir Med 2:140, 1981

9. Boros SJ: Variations in inspiratory:expiratory ratio and airway pressure wave form during mechanical ventilation: the significance of mean airway pressure. J Pediatr 94:114, 1979

10. Brach BB, Yin F, Timms R, et al: Reduced inspiratory effort during intermittent mandatory ventilation with PEEP. Crit Care Med 4:142, 1976

11. Butler WJ, Bohn DJ, Bryan AC, et al: Ventilation by high frequency oscillation in humans. Anesth Analg 59:577, 1980

12. Bynum LJ, Wilson JE, Pierce AK: Comparison of spontaneous and positive pressure breathing in supine normal subjects. J Appl Physiol 40:341, 1976

13. Carlon GC, Meadownik S, Cole R, et al: Technical aspects and clinical implications of high frequency jet ventilation with a solenoid valve. Crit Care Med 9:47, 1981

14. Chalon J, Chandrakant P, Ali M, et al: Humidity and anesthetized patients. Anesthesiology 50:195, 1979

15. Chalon J, Loew DAY, Malebranche J: Effects of dry anesthetic gases on tracheobronchial ciliated epithelium. Anesthesiology 36:338, 1972

16. Culpepper J, Snyder J, Pennock B, et al: Effect of PEEP valve resistance on airway pressure and inspiratory work. Crit Care Med 11:220, 1983 (abstract)

17. Culpepper J, Snyder J, Pinsky M, et al: Resistance in the inspiratory limb of continuous pressure airway pressure systems. Crit Care Med 11:220, 1983 (abstract)

18. Damman JF, McAslan TC, Maffeo FJ: Optimal flow pattern for mechanical ventilation of the lungs. Crit Care Med 6:29, 1978

19. Desautels DA, Bartlett JL: Methods of administering intermittent mandatory ventilation (IMV). Respir Care 19:187, 1974

20. Downs JB, Klein EF, Desautels D, et al: Intermittent mandatory ventilation: a new approach to weaning patients from mechanical ventilation. Chest 64:331, 1973

21. Edwards WL, Sappenfield RS: Pressure-cycled ventilators and flow rate control. Anesth Analg 47:77, 1968

22. Elam JO, Kerr JH, Janney CD: Performance of ventilators: effects of changes in lung-thorax compliance. Anesthesiology 19:56, 1958

23. Eross B, Powner D, Grenvik A: Common ventilatory modes: terminology. Int Anesthesiol Clin 18:11, 1980

24. Fairley HB: Critique of intermittent mandatory ventilation. Int Anesthesiol Clin 18:191, 1980

25. Fleming WH, Bowen JC: A comparative evaluation of pressure-limited and volume-limited respirators for prolonged postoperative ventilatory support in combat casualties. Ann Surg 176:49, 1972

26. Forbes AR: Humidification and mucus flow in the intubated trachea. Br J Anaesth 45:874, 1973

27. Forbes AR: Temperature, humidity and mucus flow in the intubated trachea. Br J Anaesth 46:29, 1974

28. Fox WW, Shutack JG: Positive pressure ventilation: pressure and time-cycled ventilators. In Goldsmith JP, Karotkin EH (eds): Assisted Ventilation of the Neonate. Saunders, Philadelphia, 1981

29. Fredberg JJ: Augmented diffusion in the airways can support pulmonary gas exchange. J Appl Physiol 49:232, 1980

30. Froese AB, Bryan AC: High frequency ventilation. Am Rev Respir Dis 123:249, 1981 (editorial)

31. Fulheihan SF, Wilson R, Pontoppidan H: Effect of mechanical ventilation with end-inspiratory pause on gas exchange. Anesth Analg 55:122, 1976

32. Gedeon A, Mebius C: The hygroscopic condenser humidifier: a new device for general use in anesthesia and intensive care. Anaesthesia 34:1043, 1979

33. Gibney RTN, Wilson RS, Pontoppidan H: Comparison of work of breathing on high gas flow and demand valve continuous positive airway pressure systems. Chest 82:692, 1982

34. Gillick JS: Spontaneous positive end-expiratory pressure (sPEEP). Anesth Analg 56:627, 1977

35. Graybar G: The most advanced respiratory life support system. Chest 75:106, 1979 (Letter to Editor)

36. Graybar GB, Smith RA: Apparatus and techniques for intermittent mandatory ventilation. Int Anesthesiol Clin 18:53, 1980

37. Greenbaum DM, Millen EJ, Eross B, et al: Continuous positive airway pressure without tracheal intubation in spontaneously breathing patients. Chest 69:615, 1976

38. Gregory GA, Kitterman JA, Phibbs RH, et al: Treatment of the idiopathic respiratory distress syndrome with continuous positive airway pressure. N Engl J Med 284:1333, 1971

39. Hall JR, Rendleman DC, Downs JB: PEEP devices: Flow-dependent increases in airway pressures. Crit Care Med 6:100, 1978 (abstract)

40. Harboe S: Weaning from mechanical ventilation by means of intermittent assisted ventilation, I.A.V.: case reports. Acta Anaesth Scand 21:252, 1977

41. Harris TR: Physiologic principles. In Goldsmith JP, Karotkin EH (eds): Assisted Ventilation of the Neonate. Saunders, Philadelphia, 1981

42. Hasten RW, Downs JB, Hesman TJ: A comparison of synchronized and nonsynchronized intermittent mandatory ventilation. Respir Care 25:554, 1980

43. Henry WC, West GA, Wilson RS: An evaluation of a gas collection valve for use in metabolic measurements in high flow CPAP systems. Respir Care 27:282, 1982

44. Higgs BD, Bevan JC: Use of mandatory minute volume ventilation in the perioperative management of a patient with myasthenia. Br J Anaesth 51:1181, 1979

45. Holt TB, Hall MW, Bass JB, et al: Comparison of changes in airway pressure during continuous positive airway pressure (CPAP) between demand valve and continuous flow devices. Respir Care 27:1200, 1982

46. Hunter AR: The classification of respirators. Anaesthesia 16:231, 1961

47. Inglestent S: Studies on the conditioning of air in the respiratory tract. Acta Otolaryngol [Suppl] (Stockh) 131:1, 1956

48. Kacmarek RM, Dimas S, Reynolds J, et al: Technical aspects of positive end-expiratory pressure (PEEP): parts I, II, and III. Respir Care 27:1478, 1490, 1505, 1982

49. Kirby RR: High frequency positive pressure ventilation (HFPPV): what role in ventilatory insufficiency? Anesthesiology 52:109, 1980 (editorial)

50. Kirby RR, Graybar GB (eds): Intermittent mandatory ventilation. Int Anesthesiol Clin 18:1, 1980

51. Kirby RR, Robison EJ, Schulz J, et al: A new pediatric volume ventilator. Anesth Analg 50:533, 1971

52. Klein EF, Shah DA, Modell JH, et al: Performance characteristics of conventional and prototype humidifiers and nebulizers. Chest 64:690, 1973

53. Kristensen HS, Neukirch F: Very long term artificial ventilation (28 years). In Rattenborg CC, Via-Reque E (eds): Clinical Use of Mechanical Ventilation. Year Book, Chicago, 1981

54. Lawler PGP, Nunn JF: Intermittent mandatory ventilation. Anaesthesia 32:138, 1977

55. Lindahl S: Influence of an end-inspiratory pause on pulmonary ventilation, gas distribution, and lung perfusion during artificial ventilation. Crit Care Med 7:540, 1979

56. Lohand L, Charabarti MK: The internal compliance of ventilators. Anaesthesia 26:414, 1971

57. Luce JM, Pierson DJ, Hudson LD: Critical reviews: intermittent mandatory ventilation. Chest 79:678, 1981

58. Mapleson WW: The effects of changes of lung characteristics on the functioning of automatic ventilators. Anaesthesia 17:300, 1962

59. Marchak BE, Thompson WK, Duffty P, et al: Treatment of RDS by high frequency os-

cillatory ventilation: a preliminary report. J Pediatr 99:287, 1981
60. McPherson SP: Respiratory Therapy Equipment. 2nd Ed Mosby, St. Louis, 1981
61. McPherson SP, Glasgow GD, William AA, et al: Methods of administering intermittent mandatory ventilation (IMV). Respir Care 19:187, 1974
62. Mueller RE, Petty TL, Filley GF: Ventilation and arterial blood gas changes induced by pursed-lip breathing. J Appl Physiol 28:784, 1970
63. Mushin WW, Rendell-Baker L, Thompson PW, et al: Automatic Ventilation of the Lungs. 3rd Ed Blackwell, Oxford, 1980
64. Nelson D, McDonald JS: Heated humidification, temperature control, and "rainout" in neonatal ventilation. Respir Ther 7:41, 1977
65. Nunn JF: Applied Respiratory Physiology. Butterworth, London, 1977
66. Osborn JJ: A flow meter for respiratory monitoring. Crit Care Med 6:349, 1978
67. Osborn JJ: Monitoring respiratory function. Crit Care Med 2:217, 1974
68. Perel A, Pachys F, Olshwang D, et al: Mechanical inspiratory peak flow as a determinant of tidal volume during IMV and PEEP. Anesthesiology 48:290, 1978
69. Poulton TJ, Downs JB: Humidification of rapidly flowing gas. Crit Care Med 9:59, 1981
70. Rattenborg CC, Via-Reque E (eds): Clinical Use of Mechanical Ventilation. Year Book, Chicago, 1981
71. Reynolds EOR: Pressure wave form and ventilator settings for mechanical ventilation in severe hyaline membrane disease. Int Anesthesiol Clin 12:59, 1974
72. Robbins L, Crocker D, Smith RM: Tidal volume losses of volume-limited ventilators. Anesth Analg 46:294, 1967
73. Safar P (ed): Respiratory Therapy. Davis, Philadelphia, 1965
74. Sara C: The management of patients with a tracheostomy. Med J Aust 1:99, 1965
75. Scacci R: Air entrainment masks: jet mixing is how they work; the bernoulli and venturi principles are how they don't work. Respir Care 24:298, 1979
76. Schachter NE, Lehnert BE, Specht W: Pressure-time relationships of pressure-limited neonatal ventilators. Crit Care Med 11:177, 1983
77. Schmidt GB, Deepak SP, Bennett T, et al: EPAP without intubation. Crit Care Med 5:297, 1977
78. Shapiro BA, Harrison RA, Walton JR, et al: Intermittent demand ventilation (IDV): A new technique for supporting ventilation in critically ill patients. Respir Care 21:521, 1976
79. Shapiro BA, Harrison RA, Trout CA: Clinical Application of Respiratory Care (2nd Ed) Chicago, Year Book Medical Publishers, 1979
80. Sjöstrand U: High frequency positive pressure ventilation (HFPPV): A review. Crit Care Med 8:345, 1980
81. Sjostrand U, Eriksson IA: High rates and low volumes in mechanical ventilation—not just a matter of ventilatory frequency. Anesth Analg 59:567, 1980
82. Smith RA, Kirby RR, Gooding JM, et al: Continuous positive airway pressure (CPAP) by face mask. Crit Care Med 8:483, 1980
83. Smith RA: Respiratory care, In: Miller RD (ed): Anesthesia. New York, Churchill Livingstone, Inc. 1981
84. Smith RK: Resiratory care applications for fluidics. Resp Ther 3:29, 1973
85. Spearman CB: Control of inspired oxygen concentration and addition of PEEP or CPAP with the Bourns pediatric ventilator. Respir Care 18:405, 1973
86. Spearman CB, Sheldon RL, Egan DF: Egan's Fundamentals of Respiratory Therapy. (4th Ed), St. Louis, The CV Mosby Co, 1982
87. Sturgeon CL, Douglas ME, Downs JB, et al: PEEP and CPAP cardiopulmonary effects during spontaneous ventilation. Anesth Analg 56:633, 1977
88. Sykes MK, McNicol MW, Campbell EJM: Respiratory Failure. Oxford, England, Blackwell Scientific Publications, 1976
89. Toremalm NG: A heat and moisture exchanger for post-tracheostomy care. An experimental study. Acta Otolaryngol 52:461, 1960
90. Tsuda T, Noguchi H, Takumi Y, et al: Optimum humidification of air administered to a tracheostomy in dogs. Br J Anaesth 49:965, 1977

91. Walker AKY, Bethune DW: A comparative study of condenser humidifiers. Anaesthesia 31:1086, 1976

92. Weeks DB: Humidification of anesthetic gases with an inexpensive condenser-humidifier in the semiclosed circle. Anesthesiology 41:601, 1974

93. Weigl J: Proximal airway conditions—some theoretical considerations. Resp Ther 6:21, 1976

94. Weled BJ, Winfrey D, Downs JB: Measuring exhaled volume with continuous positive airway pressure and intermittent mandatory ventilation: techniques and rationale. Chest 76:166, 1979

3

Ventilator Performance Evaluation

David A. Desautels

> Science is a fascinating subject. One gets such a wholesale return of conjecture from such a trifling investment of facts.
>
> Mark Twain

People responsible for the purchase of mechanical ventilators must be rational, objective, calculating, and ever-aware of the sky-rocketing costs of health care. Only diligent control by all persons concerned can limit such expenditures. Consumers (patients), patient's families, respiratory therapists, nurses, and physicians must be the driving force behind ventilator pricing. The days when therapists should want to be the first in their locale with the newest gimmick should be a thing of the past. Decisions regarding what components of a ventilator are essential should be made unemotionally, without bias, and with special regard to the type of patient to be ventilated and the quality of support services to be provided. The most expensive and elaborate ventilator is not essential in a chronic care unit where complications are minimal, yet a quality product must be available to the consumer. Ventilators must meet their specifications and remain within those specifications with reasonable use without premature breakdowns.

One of the purposes of this chapter is to aid those who purchase ventilators to evaluate them by objective criteria. Such a purchase should be approached like that of an expensive automobile. Economic virtues, recommendations, flexibility, and need should be investigated. The possibility that the device in question might someday be used for a friend, loved one, or oneself should be considered. Personal inspection of ventilators that are already owned, on trial, or anticipated for purchase is essential. Such inspection should not be limited only to those ventilators with which one is familiar.

PERFORMANCE EVALUATION FORMS

A program that allows an objective and comprehensive evaluation of any ventilator should include forms based on classification and specifications by which similarities, differences, and the results of bench testing

VENTILATOR CLASSIFICATION ANALYSIS   MODEL_____
(Check if available)

I. Ventilator power variables			b. Pressure cycled	
A. Pressure differential			c. Volume cycled	
1. Subambient pressure			d. Flow cycled	
2. Positive pressure			e. Mixed cycled	
B. Power source			2. Limits	
1. Electrical			a. Pressure	
a. Mechanical			b. Volume	
b. Electronic			c. Mixed	
2. Gas			C. Expiratory phase	
a. Pneumatic			1. Classic methods generators	
b. Fluidic			a. Constant pressure	
3. Mixed power			b. Nonconstant pressure	
C. Gas transmission			c. Constant flow	
1. Direct			d. Nonconstant flow	
2. Indirect			2. Modified method	
D. Internal mechanism			a. Distending pressure	
1. Eccentric wheel piston			b. Subambient pressure	
2. Direct drive piston			c. Flow taper	
3. Solenoid/gate valve			D. Change from expiratory to inspiratory	
4. Venturi (injector)			1. Classic methods	
5. Compressor			a. Time cycled	
6. Bellows/bag			b. Pressure cycled	
7. High pressure gas			c. Volume cycled	
8. Spring			d. Mixed cycled	
9. Weight			2. Traditional	
II. Ventilator phase variables			a. Control	
A. Inspiratory phase			b. Assist	
1. Normal generators			c. Assist/control	
a. Constant pressure			d. Intermittent mandatory ventilation	
b. Nonconstant pressure			e. Synchronized intermittent mandatory ventilation	
c. Constant flow			III. High frequency ventilation	
d. Nonconstant flow			A. High frequency positive pressure ventilation	
2. Modified: inspiratory hold			B. High frequency oscillation	
B. Change from inspiratory to expiratory			C. High frequency jet ventilation	
1. Classic methods				
a. Time cycled				

Fig. 3-1. Form to evaluate a ventilator by its classification.

VENTILATOR SPECIFICATIONS - I   Model _____

Manufacturer _____   Cost _____

	Capability		Alarm/Monitor				
	Minimum	Maximum	Low	High	Type	Delay	Comment
Inspiration							
Rate (breath/min)							
Volume (ml)							
Flow rate (L/min)							
Pressure limit (cm H_2O)							
Time (sec)							
Effort (sensitivity) (cm H_2O)							
Hold (sec)							
Oxygen (%)							
Demand flow (L/min)							
Safety pressure limit (cm H_2O)							
Expiration							
Volume (ml)							
Time (sec)							
Positive end-expiratory pressure and continuous positive airway pressure (cm H_2O)							
Retard (L/min)							
Ratio of inspiration to expiration							
Ratio							
Inverse							
Sigh							
Rate (breath/hour)							
Volume (ml)							
Pressure limit (cm H_2O)							
Multiples							
Humidity							
Temperature (°C)							
Volume (ml)							

Fig. 3-2. Form to evaluate a ventilator by its specifications.

VENTILATOR SPECIFICATIONS - II   Model_____

Manufacturer_____Cost _____

(Check if available or fill in correct number)

OPTIONALS		WAVEFORM	
Power switch		Constant	
Lamp test		Decelerating	
Delay selector		Accelerating	
Pressure gauge		POWER	
Alarm reset		Electric	
Alarm volume		Gas	
Single breath trigger		V	
Sigh breath trigger		Psi	
Oxygen pressure gauge		Apneic period (sec)	
Air pressure gauge		Humidifier volume (ml)	
Elapse timer		CURRENT LEAKAGE (UV)	
Minute volume counter		ELECTRIC CONSUMPTION (watt)	
MODE SELECTOR		GAS CONSUMPTION (L/min)	
Control		MINUTE VOLUME	
Assist		Rate x tidal volume	
Assist/Control		Flow x inspiration time x expiration time	
Intermittent mandatory ventilation		Flow x inspiration time x I:E ratio	
Synchronized intermittent mandatory ventilaton		PHYSICAL DIMENSIONS	
Continuous positive airway pressure		Size	
Compressible volume (ml/cm H_2O)		Weight	
Resistance (cm H_2O/L/sec)			

Fig. 3-3. Form to evaluate a ventilator by its specifications (does not require testing at minimum and maximum settings).

and subjective evaluations can be recorded. Even a picture of the front panel and a schematic diagram of the various ventilators may be useful. The forms should be comprehensive yet succinct. Too much detail makes forms cumbersome and discourages thoroughness.

Various performance evaluation forms are presented in this chapter to assist in obtaining the most comprehensive and objective analysis possible (Figs. 3-1 through 3-6). Such forms help a prospective purchaser or user to compare ventilators objectively. Although some forms may seem irrelevant (e.g., the classification form), all are important for good decision-making.

As additional ventilators are evaluated for purchase, the forms may be accumulated so that eventually a complete file of objective, unsolicited information is available with which to make solid decisions, to keep ventilators within their specifications, to pass inspections, and to become oriented to new products.

VENTILATOR CLASSIFICATION

The *New World Dictionary* defines a ventilator as "a thing that ventilates; especially any opening or device used to bring in fresh air and drive out foul air." The American

VENTILATOR CONTROLS ORIENTATION
(Check if available)

I. Minute volume delivery		C. Environment controls	
A. Flow and time controls		1. Oxygen concentration	
1. Flow rate		2. Humidification: heater	
2. Time		3. Nebulizer	
a. Rate		D. Sigh controls	
b. Inspiratory time		1. Rate	
c. Expiratory time		2. Volume	
d. Inspiratory:expiratory ratio		3. Pressure	
B. Volume and time controls		4. Multiple sigh	
1. Volume		III. Expiratory modification controls	
a. Minute volume		A. Flow	
b. Tidal volume		1. Retard	
2. Time		2. Expiratory flow gradient	
a. Rate		B. Pressure	
b. Inspiratory time		1. Subambient pressure	
c. Expiratory time		2. Distending pressure	
d. Inspiratory:expiratory ratio		IV. Alarms	
II. Delivery modification controls		A. Minute volume	
A. Initiation		1. Power failure	
1. Manual trigger		2. High pressure	
2. Sensitivity		3. Low pressure	
a. Pressure sensitivity		4. High volume	
b. Volume sensitivity		5. Low volume	
B. Inspiratory modification controls		6. Long expiration	
1. Inspiratory hold		7. Short expiration	
2. Flow pattern		B. Supplemental alarms	
a. Biphasic flow		1. Oxygen concentration	
b. Flow taper		2. Distending pressure	

Fig. 3-4. Form for orientation to ventilator control knobs.

College of Chest Physicians describes a ventilator as "a device designed to augment or replace the patient's spontaneous ventilation." A ventilator is differentiated from a respirator, which is defined by the *New World Dictionary* as "1. a contrivance such as gauze worn over the mouth, or mouth and nose to prevent the inhalation of harmful substances, to warm the air breathed, etc. 2. An apparatus for giving artificial respiration. 3. A gas mask." The proper term "ventilator" is used throughout this chapter.

Proper classification cannot be summed up by a simple phrase such as "volume ventilator." Although such a description may have been meaningful during the 1960s when intermittent positive-pressure breathing was in vogue, it has little use at present. The sophistication in ventilators of the 1980s dictates an elaborate method of classification (Fig. 3-1).

Subjective Checklist for Ventilator Evaluation

(1 = poor, 2 = fair, 3 = average, 4 = good, 5 = excellent)

	Weight	1	2	3	4	5	Total
Ease of operation							
Durability							
Flexibility							
Cost							
Monitor/Alarms							
Dependability							
Simplicity							
Esthetics							

Fig. 3-5. Form for the subjective evaluation of ventilators.

Power Variables

See also Chapter 2.

Ventilators are first characterized according to power variables, which are subdivided into pressure differential, power source, mechanism of transmission, and internal mechanisms.[13-15] Pressure differential has been limited since the early 1960s primarily to positive-pressure ventilation; however, many iron lungs and chest cuirasses, which belong in the subambient pressure category, are still available. The power source is divided into electrical and gas components, each with further subdivisions: electronic or mechanical and fluidic or pneumatic, respectively. Many ventilators use several power sources. Examples include the Emerson ventilator, which has some electronic components but is basically a mechanical device, and the Puritan-Bennett MA-1 ventilator, which has some mechanical components but is primarily electronic. Similar overlap also occurs with fluidic and pneumatic ventilators.

The mechanism of transmission describes how gas is delivered to the patient. If the power source is the medium by which gas is transmitted, direct transmission is involved; if not, the gas is indirectly transmitted. Examples of direct-transmission ventilators include the Emerson 3-PV and Babybird, whereas the Puritan-Bennett MA-1 and the Bear-1 represent indirect-transmission types.

A ventilator also can be categorized according to the internal mechanism by which it operates. Here, the emphasis is on the mechanical components which are responsible for ventilator function. Many are similar from one ventilator to another, whereas others are unique. Some ventilators operate by more than one basic mechanism. Primary mechanisms include eccentric wheel pistons, direct-drive pistons, solenoid/gate valves, venturis, compressors, bellows/bags, high-pressure gas, springs, and weights. The drive mechanisms are directly responsible for the type of flow developed. As an example, an eccentric wheel piston develops a sinusoidal flow curve, whereas a solenoid gate valve produces a square-wave flow pattern.

Phase Variables

See also Chapter 2.

Mushin et al.'s classic description in the first edition of *Automatic Ventilation of the Lungs*[13] still remains the prototype of classification systems, even though relatively

Checklist for Inspection by the Joint Commission for the Accreditation of Hospitals

REQUIREMENTS FOR EACH VENTILATOR	A	B	C	D	E
Policy and procedure					
Assembly and operation instructions					
Objectives of use					
Orientation documents					
Continuing education documents					
Entry level knowledge documentation					
Quality assurance program					
Preventative maintenance program					
Specifications on file					
Component calibration records					
Pressure monitoring available					
Oxygen monitoring available					
Temperature monitoring available					
PIN index and diameter index safety system					
Infection control measures					
Cleaning and sterilizing procedures					
Adverse reaction criteria					
Equipment change requirements					
Instructions for discharged patients					
GENERAL REQUIREMENTS					
Samples of forms					
Records of equipment changes					
Prescription record on patient's chart					
Record of new piping installation testing					
Documentation of goals and objectives on patient's chart					
Efficacy of treatment on patient's chart					
Drugs and reagents in date					
Drug refrigerator documented at 40°C					
Documentation of long term oxygen use					

Fig. 3-6. Checklist with which to prepare ventilators for inspection by the Joint Commission on Hospital Accreditation.

few ventilators were available at that time and the field has undergone explosive growth. They divided the ventilatory cycle into four primary components: the inspiratory phase, the change from inspiratory to expiratory phase, the expiratory phase, and the change from expiratory to inspiratory phase. To begin inspiration, a positive-pressure ventilator must have an internal pressure different from (higher than) that of the lung; i.e., there must be a pressure differential. Factors of importance include the volume of gas to be delivered, the rate at which the gas must flow, the airway pressure required to move gas, and the alveolar pressure that results once gas has been delivered.[3,6,11-16,18-20,22]

Inspiratory Phase. The inspiratory phase (perhaps the most frequently misunderstood category) is dependent on either pressure or flow generators.[11,13-15]

Constant-Pressure Generator. A constant-pressure ventilator develops a low pressure and maintains a low-pressure gradient. Pure constant-pressure generators equilibrate with the patient's alveolar pressure within several time constants. A time constant (tau, T) is the time required for completion of 63 percent of an exponentially changing function when the total time for the function change is unlimited. The percent of the equilibrium value obtained in each time constant is related to the reciprocal of the natural log e:

$$\frac{1}{2.718} = 0.3679;\ 1.0 - 0.3679$$

$$= \underline{0.63}\ \text{(one time constant)}$$

$$(0.3679)^2 = 0.1354;\ 1.0 - 0.1354$$

$$= \underline{0.865}\ \text{(two time constants)}$$

$$(0.3679)^3 = 0.4971;\ 1.0 - 0.04971$$

$$= \underline{0.95}\ \text{(three time constants)}$$

In the ventilator/patient system the rate of change of pressure and volume depends on the product of total resistance and total compliance. If this value is 50 ml/cm H_2O/L/sec, the time constant is 0.5 seconds. This in turn means that in 0.5 seconds 63 percent of the equilibrium pressure and volume will be delivered, in 1.0 second 86.5 percent, in 1.5 seconds 95 percent, etc. Hence the ventilator inspiratory phase progresses toward equilibrium at an exponential rate so that, in the first time constant 63 percent of equilibrium is attained, in the second 86.5 percent, in the third 95 percent, and so forth.

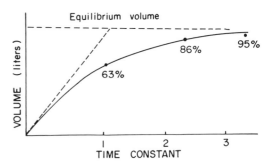

Fig. 3-7. Dynamic volume curve during mechanical ventilation with a constant-pressure generator.

A theoretical pure constant-pressure generator is represented by an inverted bellows connected to a lung. If a weight which generates exactly the pressure required for proper lung excursion is placed on the bellows, it is pushed down and gas flows into the lung until pressure is balanced between the bellows and the lung. However, perfect equilibrium is never attained, only approximated. After a specific (constant) period of time, even though equilibrium may be only 99.996 percent complete, the expiratory phase begins.

Examples of dynamic curves for constant-pressure generators demonstrate the exponential function of these ventilators. Volume (V) delivered to the lung relative to the volume attained at equilibrium may be determined at any time constant (Fig. 3-7). The volume to be delivered at equilibrium is equal to the product of system compliance and generated pressure.

$$V\ \text{(liters)} = PC$$

$$= (\text{cm } H_2O)\ (\text{L/cm } H_2O)\quad (1)$$

If 0.8 L (800 ml) is the equilibrium volume, in one time constant 63 percent of that volume, or 0.504 L (504 ml), is delivered.

Flow ($\dot{V}$) (Fig. 3-8) is determined relative to the initial flow capability of the constant-pressure generator, which is equal to pressure divided by the system's resistance:

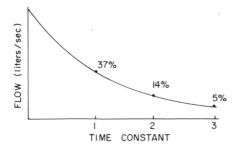

Fig. 3-8. Dynamic flow curve during mechanical ventilation with a constant-pressure generator.

$$\dot{V} = \frac{P}{R \text{ (patient + ventilation)}} \qquad (2)$$

$$= \frac{\text{cm } H_2O}{\text{cm } H_2O/L/\text{second}}$$

$$= L/\text{second}$$

Therefore if the pressure generated is 20 cm H_2O and the resistance of the system (patient and ventilator) is 30 cm $H_2O/L/\text{second}$, the initial flow into the lung is 0.67 L/second. In the first time constant flow is diminished to 37 percent of the initial value (1 − 0.63), in two time constants to 13.5 percent (1 − 0.865), etc.

Alveolar pressure (PA) (Fig. 3-9), relative to the pressure attained at equilibrium, may also be determined at any time constant. The alveolar pressure at equilibrium should equal that of the constant-pressure gener-

ator. This value is equal to the volume at equilibrium divided by the compliance of the system:

$$P_A = \frac{V}{C \text{ (patient + ventilator)}} \qquad (3)$$

$$= \frac{L}{L/\text{cm } H_2O}$$

$$= \text{cm } H_2O$$

As with volume, if the equilibrium pressure is 20 cm H_2O, in the first time constant PA is 63 percent or 12.6 cm H_2O, and in two time constants 86.5 percent or 17.3 cm H_2O of the equilibrium pressure.

As gas flows, "mouth" or oral pressure (PM) (Fig. 3-10) exceeds alveolar pressure by the ratio of the patient's resistance to the system's total resistance:

$$P_M = \frac{R \text{ (patient)}}{R \text{ (patient + ventilator)}} \times P \qquad (4)$$

$$= \frac{\text{cm } H_2O/L/\text{second (patient)}}{\text{cm } H_2O/L/\text{second} \atop \text{(patient + ventilator)}}$$

$$\times \text{ cm } H_2O$$

$$= \text{cm } H_2O$$

In this case, the instantaneous pressure must first be determined. The time constants are then applied to the difference between instantaneous pressure and equilibrium pressure. As an example, if the ratio

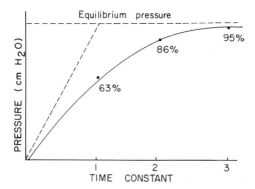

Fig. 3-9. Dynamic alveolar pressure curve during mechanical ventilation with a constant-pressure generator.

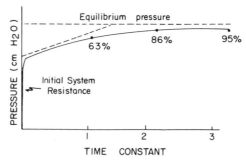

Fig. 3-10. Dynamic oral pressure curve during mechanical ventilation with a constant-pressure generator.

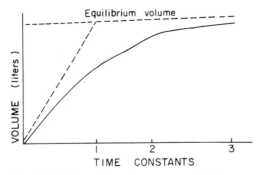

Fig. 3-11. Dynamic volume curve during mechanical ventilation with a non-constant-pressure generator.

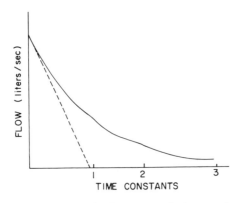

Fig. 3-12. Dynamic flow curve during mechanical ventilation with a non-constant-pressure generator.

affected by the patient's compliance and resistance. Equilibrium with the patient is developed within specific time constants, as with a constant-pressure generator, but each time constant is determined trigonometrically rather than arithmetically.

Dynamic curves for non-constant-pressure generators (Figs. 3-11 through 3-14) follow the same principles as those for constant-pressure generators except that with non-constant pressure, the curves may not be exponential and may vary at each time constant.

Constant-Flow Generator. The constant-flow generator theoretically is not influenced by changes in patient compliance and resistance because the ventilator pressure source is at least 10 times greater than that required for normal lung expansion. The pressure gradient is so large that time

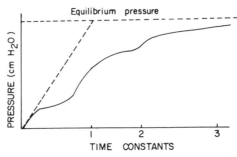

Fig. 3-13. Dynamic alveolar pressure curve during mechanical ventilation with a non-constant-pressure generator.

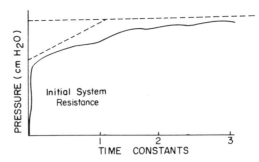

Fig. 3-14. Dynamic oral pressure curve during mechanical ventilation with a non-constant-pressure generator.

of the patient's resistance to the total resistance is 75 percent, 75 percent of the generated pressure is registered instantaneously on the pressure gauge before any gas flow occurs. If this value is 15 cm H_2O (75 percent of 20 cm H_2O), the first time constant relation of 63 percent is applied to the difference between equilibrium pressure and instantaneous pressure (20 − 15). Thus in the first time constant the oral pressure is 18.15 cm H_2O (15 + 3.15).

Non-Constant-Pressure Generator. In the non-constant-pressure ventilator, pressure, instead of remaining constant, is allowed to vary. It is the same at any designated point during each inspiration but is

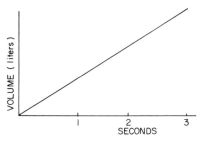

Fig. 3-15. Dynamic volume curve during mechanical ventilation with a constant-flow generator.

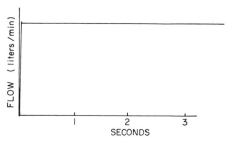

Fig. 3-16. Dynamic flow curve during mechanical ventilation with a constant-flow generator.

constants are measured in minutes rather than seconds, and inspiratory time is measured in seconds rather than time-constant increments. Most constant-flow generators have a high internal resistance as a safety feature. The necessity of this feature can be readily understood if a pure constant-flow generator, represented by a cylinder of gas at 2200 psig, is examined. If this gas source is connected to a patient's airway and a solenoid valve is placed between the cylinder and the patient, a pure constant-flow generator results. When the solenoid valve is opened for a fraction of a second, the patient's resistance and compliance have little effect on gas flow. However, in the absence of an internal reducing regulator, the patient is exposed to a high risk of injury.

Constant flow through a ventilator can be mistaken for that induced by a constant-flow generator, but there is a distinction, e.g., in the Babybird. A constant-flow generator applies only to the inspiratory phase, whereas constant flow through a ventilator applies to both inspiratory and expiratory phases.

The volume (Fig. 3-15) of gas flowing to the lung is determined by the elapsed time of gas flow:

$$V = \dot{V} \times t \qquad (5)$$

$$= L/second \times seconds = L$$

Because the internal resistance of the system is so great, most constant-flow generators have a time constant greater than 6

minutes, making such a value of little practical or clinical significance. Therefore elapsed time is determined in seconds. If the constant flow is 1.0 L/second, in 1 second 1 L is delivered, in spite of resistance and compliance factors of the patient, because of the high pressure differential.

Gas flow (Fig. 3-16) into the lung, as implied, proceeds at a constant rate. It is equal to the generating pressure (P_G) divided by the resistance of the system:

$$\dot{V} = P_G/R \qquad (6)$$

$$= \frac{cm\ H_2O}{cm\ H_2O/L/second}$$

$$= L/second$$

If $P_G = 4000$ cm H_2O and $R = 8000$ cm $H_2O/L/sec$, $\dot{V} = 0.5$ L/sec.

Alveolar pressure (Fig. 3-17) is calculated as the ratio of the ventilator flow to the compliance of the system:

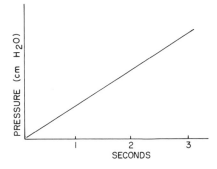

Fig. 3-17. Dynamic alveolar pressure curve during mechanical ventilation with a constant-flow generator.

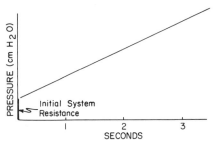

Fig. 3-18. Dynamic oral pressure curve during mechanical ventilation with a constant-flow generator.

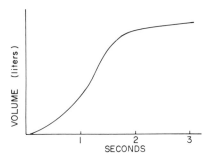

Fig. 3-19. Dynamic volume curve during mechanical ventilation with a non-constant-flow generator.

$$P_A = \dot{V}/C \qquad (7)$$

$$= \frac{L/second}{L/cm\ H_2O}$$

$$= cm\ H_2O/second$$

Note that this value varies as a function of time. If the flow is 0.5 L/sec and the compliance of the system is 0.05 L/cm H_2O, the alveolar pressure increases at 10 cm H_2O/sec.

Mouth, or oral, pressure (Fig. 3-18) exceeds alveolar pressure during gas flow; therefore a differential pressure equal to the product of the resistance of the patient and the flow of the system must be added to the alveolar pressure:

$$P_M = P_A + (R\ patient \times \dot{V}) \qquad (8)$$

$$= cm\ H_2O + (cm\ H_2O/L/second)$$

$$\times (L/second)$$

$$= cm\ H_2O$$

If the alveolar pressure in the first second is 10 cm H_2O and the differential pressure is 2.5 cm H_2O (resistance of patient = 5 cm H_2O/L/second and flow = 0.5 L/second), the oral pressure in the first second is 12.5 cm H_2O.

The reader should be aware that "pure" constant-flow generators and constant-pressure generators are theoretical constructs in the clinical setting. To the extent that a ventilator's functional characteristics approach one or the other of these cate-gories more closely, it is classified accordingly.

Non-Constant-Flow Generator. Ventilators of the non-constant-flow type generate sinusoidal flow curves. The pressure gradient, similar to that of constant-flow generators, is so large that flow is not influenced by the patient's compliance or resistance, and the flow curve never varies. Examples of dynamic function curves during mechanical ventilation with a non-constant-flow generator are shown in Figures 3-19 through 3-22.

Inspiratory Hold. An inspiratory plateau, or hold, is now incorporated into many ventilators. Several mechanisms are available. In some cases the ventilator holds pressure in the lung for a set period,

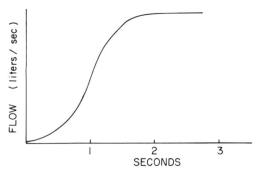

Fig. 3-20. Dynamic flow curve during mechanical ventilation with a non-constant-flow generator.

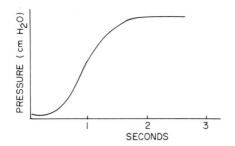

Fig. 3-21. Dynamic alveolar pressure curve during mechanical ventilation with a non-constant-flow generator.

whereas in others volume is maintained at a constant level. Finally, additional gas flow may be provided after the normal tidal volume delivery.

Inspiratory to Expiratory Phase. Elam et al.[6] classified ventilators as volume-limited and pressure-variable or pressure-limited and volume-variable, a system which was generally accepted until Mapleson[12] introduced the concepts of time, pressure, volume, and flow cycling. This method of classification has survived to the present despite the proposal of other systems, e.g., that of Hunter,[10,17] which classed ventilators as pressure-set and volume-set. An important distinction must be made between "cycling" and "limiting." Cycling refers to termination, whereas limiting implies re-

striction. Thus "pressure-cycled" is completely different from "pressure-limited." If a ventilator is pressure-cycled, it cycles to the expiratory phase once the designated pressure is reached. In contrast, a pressure-limited ventilator reaches and holds its designated pressure without cycling to the expiratory phase. Ventilators may be pressure- or volume-limited, but they cannot be time-limited; if time is limited and that time elapses, an exhalation must result. Such a ventilator is actually time-cycled.

Expiratory Phase. The same classification used for the inspiratory phase can also be applied to the expiratory phase. However, such a classification is limited in that expiration is most dependent on the functional characteristics of exhalation valves, which are widely variable. A more practical approach is to consider what therapeutic regimens are employed during expiration (distending or subambient pressure and retardation or modification of expiratory flow).

Expiratory to Inspiratory Phase. Mapleson[12] classified this phase similarly to the inspiratory to expiratory phase, i.e., that phases are cycled by time, pressure, volume, the patient, or a combination thereof. More useful, perhaps, is the system of Holaday and Rattenborg,[8] which describes assistors, controllers, and assistor-controllers to which may be added intermittent mandatory ventilation (IMV) and synchronized IMV (SIMV).

Assisted (patient-triggered) ventilation is regulated by the patient's spontaneous breathing effort, which initiates a positive-pressure breath response from the ventilator. Controlled ventilation is machine-initiated (time-cycled on) at a designated rate. With assistor-controllers, the assist mode is dominant unless the patient fails to trigger the ventilator within a specified period of time; in the latter event, the control mode dominates. Intermittent mandatory ventilation is a combination of *controlled* and *spontaneous* ventilation, whereas SIMV

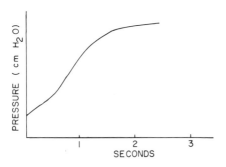

Fig. 3-22. Dynamic oral pressure curve during mechanical ventilation with a non-constant-flow generator.

represents a combination of *assisted* and spontaneous ventilation.

SPECIFICATIONS

Controls

Specifications pertain to ventilator controls without regard to ventilator classification. The majority of necessary information with which to evaluate specifications is shown in Figures 3-1 through 3-4. This information is not listed by priority, nor is all of it necessary to evaluate a ventilator satisfactorily.

The range (minimum to maximum) of each control is indicated in the manufacturer's manual or is measured by specific monitors or gauges. However, the specifications listed in the manual should not be considered constant for any ventilator: A ventilator that has been in use for even a brief time requires calibration to ensure specific levels of performance. Although some controls are not applicable to every ventilator, each control that is available should be evaluated to make comparison easier. If the range of a control is not given in the proper unit of measure, the necessary conversion should be made. As an example, the pressure limit may be stated in millimeters of mercury, but centimeters of H_2O, through common usage, is more appropriate for most ventilators. Though often not listed in the manufacturer's specifications, the inspiratory time is very helpful in comparisons. Should specifications for certain parameters not be available from the manufacturer, the following suggestions may help in assessing the requisite values.

Rate. Values can be determined best by counting the number of breaths per minute as the machine cycles at the lowest and the highest settings.

Volume. A respirometer may be used with volume at minimum and maximum values. It is advisable to make several measurements at the minimum setting, which tends to fluctuate most. If only minute volume is indicated, this value must be divided by the number of breaths counted. Alternatively, tidal volume (V_T) can be calculated from the inspiratory time[21]:

$$V_T = \dot{V} \times \text{inspiratory time} \qquad (9)$$

$$= \frac{\text{L/minute} \times \text{inspiratory time (seconds)}}{60 \text{ seconds/minute}}$$

(i.e., 30 L/minute for 1 second)

$$= \frac{30 \text{ L/minute}}{60 \text{ sec/minute}} \times 1 \text{ second}$$

$$= 0.5 \text{ L}$$

Flow Rate. To measure flow rate exactly requires expensive flowmeters or a pneumotachograph. A rough approximation can be made from tidal volume and inspiratory time:

$$\text{Flow} = \frac{V_T}{\text{inspiratory time}} \qquad (10)$$

$$= \frac{\text{L} \times 60 \text{ seconds/minute}}{\text{seconds}}$$

(i.e., 0.5 L for 1 second)

$$= 30 \text{ L/minute}$$

Pressure Limit. The pressure limit value should be measured at the minimum and maximum settings. The maximum deflection of the pressure gauge should not be assumed to be the pressure limit. Generally, the needle oscillates and moves back toward the true reading because of a damping effect.

Inspiratory and Expiratory Times. Inspiratory and expiratory times are difficult to determine exactly without expensive measuring devices. However, an approximate value can be determined easily:

Inspiratory time

$$= \frac{V_T \, (L)}{L/\text{minute}} \qquad (11)$$

$$= \frac{L \times \text{minute}/60 \text{ second}}{L/\text{minute}}$$

(i.e., 30 L/minute and 0.5 L)

$= 1$ second

Additionally, the inspiratory and expiratory times can be determined if the rate and the ratio of inspiration to expiration (I : E) are known. Calculation at a rate of 16 breaths/minute with an I : E ratio of 1 : 2 follow:

Respiratory cycle time

$$= \frac{60 \text{ seconds/minute}}{16 \text{ breaths/minute}}$$

$= 3.75$ seconds/breath

Fractional units of respiratory cycle

$$= \frac{\text{respiratory cycle time}}{I + E}$$

$$= \frac{3.75 \text{ seconds/breath}}{1 + 2} = \frac{3.75}{3}$$

$= 1.25$

Inspiratory time $= 1$ fractional unit

$= 1.25$ second

Expiratory time $= 2$ fractional units

$= 2.50$ seconds

Inspiratory Effort. The inspiratory effort can be measured by placing a T in line and measuring the deflection of a pressure gauge during inhalation with the airway occluded.

Inspiratory Hold. Similar to the measurement of inspiratory effort, a T may be placed in line in order to observe the level and duration of an inspiratory "plateau."

Oxygen Concentration. An oxygen analyzer should be placed in line to read the minimum and maximum oxygen concentrations.

Demand Flow. A flow rater or pneumotachograph is necessary during inspiration with continuous positive airway pressure to determine the maximum flow rate of the system. Efforts to obtain flow greater than the capacity of the system do not increase flow further.

Positive End-Expiratory Pressure/ Continuous Positive Airway Pressure. To measure PEEP and CPAP, a T is connected to the pressure gauge and the plateau pressure during expiration is observed. This measurement should *always* be made at the Y connector (patient/ventilator interface).

Retard. Retard is measured in liters per minute of flow. This requires a flow rater or pneumotachograph which is placed in the expiratory system to measure the flow of gas from the patient.

I : E Ratio. An accurate assessment of the I : E ratio requires pressure to be transduced onto a graphic recorder at a known speed. Once the graph is recorded, measurement of the time of each phase from the chart speed is a simple matter.

Other Factors. Each control also may have an alarm/monitor, the range of which should be listed. A minimum requirement is a method to monitor and sound an alarm if the minute volume is not delivered. Thus alarms for power failure, high and low pressures, high and low volumes, and long or short expiratory times may be necessary. Additional alarms to detect the failure to maintain oxygen concentration and PEEP are desirable. The type of alarm (audible, visual, or both) should be characterized. The alarm delay, or that period of time which elapses before the alarm is activated, should be recorded. Alarm systems for ventilators have undergone rapid development during the last few years, almost to the point that some ventilators are overloaded with them and basic functions tend to be overlooked.

One item of major importance in evaluating ventilator performance is the magnitude of peak flow at designated pressures. Pressure relief ("pop off") valves with known pressure limits are helpful for measuring the ability of the ventilator to work against significant "back pressure." If the valves are placed at the patient wye and the ventilator cycled, an in-line flow rater indicates the flow capabilities against the generated back pressure. Often a ventilator that functions well during a demonstration under ideal conditions fails in a clinical setting when significant back pressure is present.

A specification sheet should be a composite reflection of the major categories and components of most ventilators and should serve as a guide that can be adjusted as necessary to serve you best for ventilator comparison.

Schematic Diagram

A detailed schematic diagram of the internal mechanisms of a ventilator should be included in a ventilator performance evaluation. Such a diagram may be obtained from the ventilator manufacturer.

Front Panel

In order to clarify the functions available on a ventilator, one should obtain a diagram of the front panel and controls of the ventilator. Such diagrams are available from the manufacturer or may be found in this and other texts.[4,5,7,13-15,25]

Subjective Evaluation

The subjective evaluation has no rules; the ventilator should be graded according to one's feelings about anything from color, to control panel layout, to operation, etc.

However, the prospective purchaser should be fair and not make decisions based only on past experience or because a salesman may present the product poorly.

TEST BENCH EVALUATION

A test bench evaluation should be included in the ventilator performance evaluation program. Although a great deal can be learned from publications, manufacturers' information, and ventilator trials, until the ventilator actually has been tested under varied conditions a complete understanding of its advantages, disadvantages, and best application cannot be obtained. An operational test bench includes a lung analog to simulate physiological variables (e.g., compliance, resistance, and air leaks) and instruments to measure ventilator variables (e.g., flow, time, pressure, and volume). The measuring instruments need not be expensive and elaborate; simple tools are often better than expensive devices. Measurement of resistance can be expensive or—with a water-filled U tube, flowmeter, some tubing, and a flow rater—inexpensive.

Lung analogs have long presented a perplexing problem to physiologists. Considering the multitude of complex factors that influence the human lung, it is hardly surprising that our ability to mimic the lung and its function is less than satisfactory. From beer barrels to expensive wedge-type lung analogs, experts have tried to simulate natural lung functions during mechanical ventilation, although mechanical ventilation is anything but natural. Publication of the American National Standards for Breathing Machines for Medical Use, ANSI standards Z79.7, in January of 1976[2] brought some order out of the previously existing chaos relating to specific compliance and resistance testing. Without these standards, physicians and respiratory therapists would be faced with an extremely difficult job of product evaluation and comparison.

Once this test bench has been established, it may also be used for teaching and for testing new techniques. Flow, pressure, and volume curves can be demonstrated under a wide range of ventilator settings, and elaborate lung analogs can be useful in demonstrating how volume remains static or changes as a patient's compliance and resistance are altered; how gas can be trapped at some settings when the ventilator's flow taper is not functioning properly; what happens during an inspiratory plateau; how PEEP and CPAP work; and a multitude of other concepts that require observation for complete understanding.

PURPOSES OF AN EVALUATION PROGRAM

Ventilator Operation

How a ventilator is adjusted depends on the needs of the patient. If a patient requires a respiratory rate of 30 breaths/minute, the ventilator should provide that rate. A patient should never be made to breathe inappropriately because the ventilator cannot provide the proper rate. A variety of ventilatory modes should be available to meet ordinary and unusual requirements.

Additional mechanisms can modify or initiate mechanical breathing, including sensitivity control, which determines the spontaneous effort required to initiate a breath, and manual buttons which generate an inflation only when they are pushed.

Once the mode has been selected, a frequency must be chosen. Some ventilators use inspiratory and expiratory time controls rather than rate controls per se. The expiratory and inspiratory times determine the rate, the minute volume, or both. The expiratory time is extended to allow more spontaneous respiration with IMV and SIMV. Miscellaneous controls to modify

frequency include sigh rate, multiple sigh breaths, I:E ratio, and safety time-limit controls. An inspiratory hold modifies frequency by prolonging the inspiratory time through maintenance of either pressure or volume in the lung at the end of the inspiratory phase.

Although most critical care ventilators are generally referred to as "volume ventilators" (even though they often are not volume-cycled), pressure ultimately limits their capabilities. The pressure limit is determined by the operator; however, the pressure limit does not cycle the ventilator into the expiratory phase. The pressure setting on some ventilators, especially those that are constant-pressure generators, is the endpoint of ventilator function. If that pressure is attained and is in equilibrium with the alveoli within six time constants, the ventilator is classified as a constant-pressure generator, e.g., the Gill 1 ventilator or the Siemens 900B ventilator (when minute volume is high and the working pressure control is set at a low level).

Gas flow in a ventilator system occurs because of a pressure gradient. Hence pressure and flow are intrinsically related and interdependent. The settings for flow and inspiratory time generate a specific tidal volume into the circuit in time-cycled ventilators. Just as inspiratory flow can be modified, so also can the expiratory flow. An expiratory flow gradient may be used to eliminate inadvertent PEEP or an expiratory retard valve employed to decrease flow rate and prevent air trapping. Some recently introduced ventilators use an inspiratory flow taper to alter the square-wave flow pattern of many time-cycled ventilators.

Distending pressure controls maintain positive pressure during either expiration (PEEP) or throughout the entire respiratory cycle when the patient breathes spontaneously (CPAP). A threshold resistor which holds pressure, releases it for exhalation, and quickly reapplies the hold is preferable (Emerson). A flow resistor (restricted orifice), which of necessity increases or decreases pressure as flow increases or decreases, respectively, is sometimes employed (Babybird). The latter exerts an expiratory flow retard pattern as well as PEEP/CPAP, whereas a threshold resistor has minimal flow retardation. Consequently, the distending pressure is constant despite changes in flow in the latter.

Ventilator Malfunction

Extreme caution must be used in dealing with ventilators that have malfunctioned. Initially, the extent of the malfunction must be assessed. If it is clear that the malfunction is easily correctable and does not jeopardize the patient's well-being, the therapist can proceed with corrective action. However, if any doubt exists regarding the origin or extent of the malfunction or the means to correct it, the ventilator must be disconnected from the patient immediately and alternative manual or mechanical ventilation provided. A troubleshooting algorithm is useful and is usually available in the instruction manual which comes with the ventilator. If a significant problem is documented which is intrinsic to the ventilator, it should be detailed sufficiently for publication or forwarded to an organization such as the Emergency Care Research Institute (ECRI) which publishes hazard bulletins and investigates problems of more than passing interest to medical consumers.

Ventilator Comparison

To gain a perspective on available ventilators, one should first thoroughly evaluate those ventilators immediately at hand. To understand a ventilator's capabilities and limitations, the investigator should employ it under many clinical and laboratory settings. One difficulty with this approach is that familiarity may mask objectivity.

Use of forms similar to those presented earlier in this chapter is helpful in cataloging information and maintaining a neutral outlook. The forms which in all likelihood are of greatest use pertain to classification specifications. Probable clinical applications must be considered, particularly when flow rates and pressure-limit capabilities are important determinants of function. Specification forms help to remove some subjective aspects of decision-making; if they are properly used and weighed appropriately for each criterion for each ventilator, many dilemmas of decision-making are obviated.

If possible, once a particular "make and model" of ventilator is chosen, several "samples" should be tested. Surprising differences in performance in apparently identical machines may be detected. Ventilators, like automobiles, require periodic calibration and "tune-ups." In fact, the Joint Commission on Accreditation of Hospitals requires that ventilators be calibrated to manufacturers' specifications at intervals designated by the manufacturer (usually annually, but quarterly is preferable).

When comparing ventilators, one should initially compare the base or stripped models before considering optional accessories. If options are necessary to make products comparable, the additional cost must be considered in the final evaluation.

Often ventilators are modified by the user in order to achieve some perceived advantage in performance. Such changes must be well thought out. Should the integrity of the ventilator be affected in a way not approved by the manufacturer, the user becomes liable for any mishaps and the ventilator warranty is invalidated. After major alterations, animal studies are appropriate before the ventilator is applied clinically.

Ventilator Purchase

Ventilators to be considered for purchase should be submitted to an in-hospital trial and performance evaluation. New or trial equipment must be introduced cautiously to clinical use. Although manufacturers have utilized engineering prototypes, animal experiments, and clinical trials in the development of their product, the ventilator is new to the prospective buyer and staff. A proper orientation must be given to all personnel required to operate the device before it is used for patient care. Untrained persons should not use the ventilator under any circumstances. When in-service education is provided, the personnel signatures, date of training, and lecturer must be documented and filed.

Should a given hospital or teaching institution be involved with clinical trials or research protocols for ventilator development, such protocols normally must be approved by the Institutional Review Board. If the ventilator is a prototype developed after 28 May 1976, its use falls under the Food and Drug Administration (FDA) regulations concerning all new class-three medical devices.[23,24]

A thorough cost analysis helps and should be established when ventilator purchases are considered. In addition to depreciation, each of the following must be taken into account to arrive at a true estimate of dollar outlay:

1. Ventilator
2. Circuit
3. Sterilization
4. Repair
5. Preventive maintenance
6. Quality assurance
7. Additional monitoring
8. Replacement
9. Operation
10. Interest on money borrowed to purchase the ventilator

Justification for the purchase of very expensive ventilators may be difficult when one deals with health care administrators who are striving to reduce costs. Once a ventilator is chosen, data should be presented (if possible) to show that it can provide the best medical care for the fewest dollars. Later the decision to purchase should be evaluated objectively to determine if prepurchase considerations have actually been verified.

Joint Commission on Hospital Accreditation Inspection

A performance verification program should be instituted to comply with Joint Commission on Hospital Accreditation (JCAH) standards[1] and should include the records of repair, preventive maintenance, and quality control for each ventilator in use, as well as documentation of employment, orientation, and continuing education of persons using the ventilators.

A checklist to help with JCAH inspections is provided here (Fig. 3-6). This checklist, which is compiled from several JCAH documents and other support materials, should be used for each ventilator. Also, policies and procedures related to each type of ventilator in the department as well as for orientation and in-service and continuing education must be written.[9] Records of attendance at continuing education programs should be kept in the personnel files, together with an outline of the lecture, signatures of the lecturer, and persons attending. A separate schedule of lectures should also be maintained.

Many quality assurance programs can be built around each ventilator. These should contain criteria for evaluation, a detailed survey or collection of data, results, follow-up, and indications for corrective actions that may be taken. Each ventilator must have a repair and preventive maintenance record that contains the instructions, specifications, and manufacturer's suggested maintenance schedule. This requirement applies also to all ventilator components as well as to gases used.

For proper documentation, all ventilator therapy must be recorded on the patient's chart, including the diagnosis; goals and objectives of care; prescriptions; type, frequency, and duration of any treatment; type, dose, and diluent of medication; oxygen concentration; patient's vital signs at regular intervals; and results of therapy. All of these data must be accompanied by the initials of the responsible person.

Additional policies and procedures that must be available pertain to documents to substantiate the competence of any therapist on staff, tests on all newly installed gas piping systems, routine checks on existing systems, and compliance of ventilator systems with PIN index or DISS safety systems. Policies of infection control, which must address requirements and methods for ventilator equipment changes, cleaning, and sterilization, must also be maintained. Further documentation must substantiate the actions to be taken in the event of complications—how the complication is identified and how it should be corrected.

REFERENCES

1. Accreditation Manual for Hospitals, Joint Commission of Accreditation of Hospitals, 1984
2. American National Standards Institute, Inc: American National Standard for Breathing Machines for Medical Use. ANSI 279.7–1976, 26 January 1976
3. Baker AB, Babington PCB, Colliss JE, et al: Effects of varying inspiratory flow waveform and time in intermittent positive pressure ventilation. Br J Anaesth 49:1207, 1977
4. Burton GB, Gee GN, Hodgkin JE: Respiratory Care. 1st Ed. Lippincott, Philadelphia, 1977
5. Egan D: Fundamentals of Respiratory Therapy. 2nd Ed. Mosby, St. Louis, 1973
6. Elam JO, Kerr JH, Janney CD: Performance of ventilators: effects of changes in lung-thorax compliance. Anesthesiology 19:56, 1958
7. Heironimus TW, Bogeaut RA: Mechanical Artificial Ventilation. 3rd Ed. Charles C Thomas, Springfield, IL, 1977
8. Holaday DA, Rattenborg CC: Automatic lung ventilators. Anesthesiology 23:493, 1962
9. Hunsinger DL, Maurizi JJ, Lisnerski KS, et al: Respiratory Technology. 2nd Ed. Reston Publishing Co., Reston, VA, 1976
10. Hunter AR: The classification of respirators. Anaesthesia 16:231, 1961
11. Jansson L, Jonson B: A theoretical study on flow patterns of ventilators. Scand J Respir Dis 52:237, 1972
12. Mapleson WW: The effect of changes of lung characteristics on the functioning of automatic ventilators. Anaesthesia 17:300, 1962
13. Mushin WW, Rendell-Baker L, Thompson PW, et al: Automatic Ventilation of the Lungs. 1st Ed. Blackwell, London, 1959
14. Mushin WW, Rendell-Baker L, Thompson PW, et al: Automatic Ventilation of the Lungs. 2nd Ed. Davis, Philadelphia, 1969
15. Mushin WW, Rendell-Baker L, Thompson PW, et al: Automatic Ventilation of the Lungs. 3rd Ed. Blackwell, London, 1980
16. Nunn JF: Applied Respiratory Physiology. Butterworth, Boston, 1977
17. Perry D: A simplified diagram for understanding the operation of volume-preset ventilators. Respir Care 22:42, 1977
18. Peslin RL: The physical properties of ventilators in the inspiratory phases. Anesthesiology 30:3, 1969
19. Robbins LS, Crocker D, Smith RM: Tidal volume losses of volume-limited ventilators. Anesth Analg 46:428, 1967
20. Simbruner G, Gregory GA: Performance of neonatal ventilators: the effects of changes in resistance and compliance. Crit Care Med 9:509, 1981
21. Slonim NB, Hamilton LH: Respiratory Physiology. 2nd Ed. Mosby, St. Louis, 1971
22. Sullivan M, Saklad M, Demers R: Relationships between ventilator waveform and tidal-volume distribution. Respir Care 22:386, 1977
23. United States Department of Health & Human Services: Investigational Device

Exemption Regulation. Food & Drug Administration, Washington, DC, July 1980

24. United States Department of Health and Human Services: Guidelines for the Arrangement and Content of a Premarket Approval Application. Washington, DC, November 1980

25. Young JA, Crocker O: Inhalation Therapy. 2nd Ed. Year Book, Chicago, 1976

4

Monitoring Respiratory and Hemodynamic Function in the Patient with Respiratory Failure

Roger C. Bone

> When you can measure what you are
> speaking about, and express it in numbers,
> you know something about it; but when you
> can not measure it, when you can not ex-
> press it in numbers, your knowledge is of a
> meager and unsatisfactory kind: it may be
> the beginning of knowledge, but you have
> scarcely, in your thoughts, advanced to the
> stage of science.
> Lord Kelvin
> Popular Lectures and Addresses
> (1891–1894)

Care of a critically ill patient requires that data be gathered, stored, and analyzed in a logical fashion. Monitoring of a patient with respiratory failure can be defined as repeated or continuous observations made to detect change in a patient's condition. Monitoring is a fatiguing, repetitive task that machines do well and people do poorly. Monitoring decisions involve cost-benefit considerations, including the risks of invasive monitoring and economic costs.[7,8] Invasive monitoring requires meticulous manual skills for placement of sensors, costly equipment, and sterile procedures. Patient discomfort and potential complications of invasive procedures limit these procedures

to the few in whom benefits are likely. Improvement in patient outcome or decision-making ability results from increased information. The spectrum from noninvasive to highly invasive monitoring is shown in Table 4-1.

Respiratory emergencies are commonplace in the care of critical care patients. Zwillich et al. found 400 complications in a prospective analysis of 354 consecutive mechanically ventilated patients with a variety of causes of respiratory failure.[45] Respiratory monitoring may increase our ability to detect complications of mechanical ventilation[6] and should complement the clinician's clinical acumen through data ac-

Table 4-1. Monitoring Procedures

Noninvasive procedures
  Physical examination
  Electrical sensing with surface electrodes, e.g., ECG and EEG
  Impedance phlebography
  Arterial tonometry
  Gas sampling using skin surface probes
  Radiological examination
  Bedside mass spectrometry
  Expired gas analysis
Invasive procedures
  Intravenous injection and blood sampling from capillaries and peripheral veins
  Cutaneous needle electrodes for ECG and EEG
  Rectal probe for temperature
  Bladder catheter for renal function
  Tissue oxygen probe
  Intraarterial and venous gas tension and pH analysis
Highly invasive
  Arterial and central venous catheter
  Intracardiac probes
  Transcardiac probes for pulmonary artery catheter for pressures and flows
  Subarachnoid probes for pressure
  Intracranial probes for CSF pressures and flows

quisition by objective measurements. If used as an adjunct to clinical care rather than a substitute, such monitoring should improve patient care. Certain monitoring techniques might also help to define resolution or progression of lung disease and the results of therapeutic maneuvers during the course of respiratory failure.[6] Although monitoring of hemodynamic indices is often utilized in the patient with respiratory failure, few measurements of respiratory function are routinely performed. Measurement of hemodynamic parameters is essential for proper management of critically ill patients, and access to certain measurements of "respiratory function" in acute respiratory failure may also improve decision-making capabilities.

Arterial blood gas tensions are an essential index of lung function and are available routinely in most hospitals. However, exclusive reliance on blood gas measurements as an index of respiratory function is unwise because they are obtained intermittently and a variable time lapses before the results are available. In addition, arterial blood gas values offer an incomplete definition of pathological physiology. For example, most respiratory complications in the patient with respiratory failure cause the arterial oxygen tension (Pa_{O_2}) to decrease. Thus changes in Pa_{O_2} alone do not usually help to make a diagnosis. However, the Pa_{O_2} value is essential in ascertaining the severity of disease and guiding treatment once the diagnosis is made.

When monitoring a patient with respiratory failure, the overall importance of clinical and metabolic measurements is obvious. Daily weights, intake and output, and blood chemistries are important measurements that are usually available. Intermittent measurements are usually satisfactory because changes occur at a gradual rate. Rapidly changing respiratory measurements, e.g., gas flow rate and pressure, might, if frequently monitored, provide clues dictating immediate therapeutic intervention. Information obtained from measurements at a patient's airway cannot substitute for blood gas measurements or chest roentgenograms, but it can have special advantages. The measurements are noninva-

Table 4-2. Symbols

‾ Dash above any symbol indicates a mean value
· Dot above any symbol indicates a time derivative
Primary symbols
  V = gas volume
  V̇ = gas volume/unit time
  P = gas pressure
  F = fractional concentration in dry gas phase
  (f) = respiratory frequency (breaths/unit time)
  Q̇ = volume of blood/unit time
  C = concentration of gas in blood phase
  S = percent saturation of hemoglobin with O_2 or CO_2
Examples
  V_A = volume of alveolar gas; V_T = tidal volume
  $\dot{V}_E$ = minute volume; $\dot{V}_{O_2}$ = O_2 consumption
  $P_{A_{O_2}}$ = alveolar O_2 pressure; $P\bar{c}_{O_2}$ = mean capillary O_2 pressure
  $F_{I_{O_2}}$ = fractional concentration of inspired O_2
  $\dot{Q}_S$ = shunt blood flow; $\dot{Q}_t$ = cardiac output
  R = $\dot{V}_{CO_2}/\dot{V}_{O_2}$
  Ca_{O_2} = ml O_2/100 ml arterial blood
  $S\bar{v}_{O_2}$ = saturation of Hb with O_2 in mixed venous blood

sive, and with appropriate equipment the information can be provided continuously and without significant time delay.

Techniques that are available to all well-equipped and well-staffed intensive care units (ICUs) with access to a pulmonary function laboratory and which are then generally applicable are considered first, followed by a consideration of computerized monitoring. This format should allow the clinician to judge the applicability of more sophisticated techniques to a particular clinical setting. Symbols used in this chapter are defined in Table 4-2.

DIAGNOSTIC STUDIES

The simplest and most valuable patient monitoring is intelligent observation by experienced personnel. In the evaluation of pulmonary competence over short or long time intervals, physical examination and radiological examination continue to be of prime importance. As more sophisticated diagnostic studies become available, there is a tendency for clinical specialists to neglect these fundamental techniques. The time has not yet arrived when it is safe to do so, and it probably never will. Newer techniques should supplement, not supplant, the basic methods.

Measurements that are appropriate for the patient with respiratory failure and which directly or indirectly provide information about respiratory function in most ICU settings are listed in Table 4-3. Not all of these measurements are necessary in every patient treated for respiratory failure. Selection of tests should be made based on the likelihood of their providing information valuable for clinical decision-making. Selected variables, their units, formulas, and normal values are presented in Table 4-4.

Physical Examination

Heart Rate and Blood Pressure. Tachycardia is an abnormality often suggesting

Table 4-3. Bedside Measurements

Physical examination

Body weight

Urine output, plasma and urine osmolality, specific gravity, osmolar and free water clearance

Radiological examination

Electrocardiogram (ECG)

Hematocrit and hemoglobin

Arterial blood gases

Intraarterial monitoring

Tidal volume (V_T), expired minute volume ($\dot{V}_E$), and inspiratory force

Physiological dead space (V_D) or the ratio of dead space ventilation to total ventilation (V_D/V_T)

Bedside measurements of lung mechanics

Hemodynamic monitoring

Physiological shunt oxygen delivery

Inspired and expired gas measurements

blood volume or flow deficits. Usually the increase in heart rate is proportional to the degree of cardiac impairment and/or hypovolemia; however, an increased heart rate is not specific and may result from anxiety, stress, fever, etc. Bradycardia in the face of low cardiac output is ominous and suggests inadequate coronary blood flow.

The blood pressure is usually measured with a sphygmomanometer or an arterial catheter. The sphygmomanometer is not applicable for situations where continuous monitoring is required. Measurements from the arterial catheter are continuous but, as with other invasive techniques, can be associated with complications. An arterial tonometer is now being developed which uses a force transducer to measure intraluminal arterial blood pressure externally. The principle of the tonometric method is based on the relationship of arterial pressure to the displacement of a force-sensing transducer located over a superficial artery. Advantages of the method include atraumatic, nonocclusive, and continuous monitoring of arterial blood pressure. Present-day tonometer sensors are relatively sophisticated devices using well-defined algorithms which detect lateral and vertical

Table 4-4. Selected Variables: Their Units, Formulas, and Normal Values

Abbreviation	Variable Name	Formula	Normal Values	Unit
MAP	Mean arterial pressure	MAP = diastolic + $\frac{1}{3}$ pulse pressure	85–95	mm Hg
CVP	Central venous pressure	Direct measurement	0–10	cm H_2O
Hgb	Hemoglobin concentration	Direct measurement	12–15	g/dl
MPAP	Mean pulmonary arterial pressure	Direct measurement	10–18	mm Hg
WP	Pulmonary arterial wedge pressure	Direct measurement	2–12	mm Hg
CI	Cardiac index	Cardiac output/B.S.A.	2.5–3.5	L/min/M^2
LVSW	Left ventrical stroke work	LVSW = S1 × MAP × 0.0144	44–68	kgM/M^2
LCW	Left cardiac work	LCW = C1 × MAP × 0.0144	3–3.5	kgM/M^2
SVR	Systemic vascular resistance	SVR = 80 (MAP − CVP)/CI	1200–1800	dynes·sec/cm^5·M^2
PVR	Pulmonary vascular resistance	PVR = 80 (MPAP − WP)/CI	150–250	dynes·sec/cm^5·M^2
HR	Heart rate	Direct measurement	65–80	beats/min
Temp	Temperature	Direct measurement	98–98.6; 37	°F; °C
O_2	O_2 availability	O_2 avail = CI × Ca_{O_2} × 10	500–700	ml/min/M^2
$\dot{V}_{O_2}$	O_2 consumption	$\dot{V}_{O_2}$ = CI × (Ca_{O_2} − $C\bar{v}_{O_2}$) × 10	180–200	ml/min/M^2
O_2 ext	O_2 extraction	$O_2 \text{ ext} = \dfrac{(Ca_{O_2} - C\bar{v}_{O_2})}{Ca_{O_2}}$	20–30	
V_D/V_T	Dead space/tidal ventilation	$V_D/V_T = \dfrac{Pa_{CO_2} - Pe_{CO_2}}{Pa_{CO_2}}$ or $\dfrac{Pa_{CO_2} - Pe_{CO_2}}{Pa_{CO_2}}$	0.30	
POsm	Plasma osmolality	Direct measurement	279–295	mOsm/kg
Pa_{O_2}	Alveolar oxygen tension	$Pa_{O_2} = (P_B - 47) Fi_{O_2} - \dfrac{Pa_{CO_2}}{R}$	5–20	mm Hg
$\dot{Q}s/\dot{Q}t$	Physiological shunt	$\dot{Q}s/\dot{Q}t = \dfrac{Cc_{O_2} - Ca_{O_2}}{Cc_{O_2} - C\bar{v}_{O_2}}$	3–5	percent

displacement with reasonable fidelity. Problems yet to be solved include artifacts from motion and from calibration errors because of tissue variation. Development is needed in sensor technology and physical mounting.[3,27]

Respiratory Rate. One of the earliest responses to a decrease in Pa_{O_2} or a rise in Pa_{CO_2} is an increase in respiratory rate. The normal range is 10–16/minute, and a rate over 20/minute should be viewed as abnormal, particularly if an upward trend continues. Rates over 30/minute indicate severe respiratory distress and may produce severe hypocarbia. A sudden increase in respiratory rate may be the first detectable sign of sepsis or a pulmonary embolization.

Recently, large intravenous carbohydrate loads administered as a part of total parenteral nutrition have been shown to markedly increase $\dot{V}_{CO_2}$ and require a much higher minute ventilation to excrete the excess carbon dioxide[2] (Fig. 4-1). This abnormality can be a significant physiological

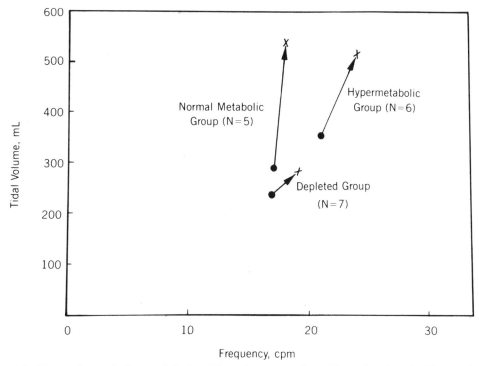

Fig. 4-1. Gas exchange before and during (X) total parenteral nutrition. (Reprinted with permission from Askanazi J, Rosenbaum SH, Hyman AL, et al: Respiratory changes induced by the large glucose loads of parenteral nutrition. JAMA 243:1444, 1980. Copyright 1980, American Medical Association.)

stress, especially to the patient with chronic obstructive lung disease who is already hypercapneic. Thus overfeeding may make weaning impossible and be manifested by tachypnea and dyspnea when the patient breathes spontaneously through a T-tube. Two alternatives are available: (1) decrease the caloric load; and (2) use fat emulsions as a source of nonprotein calories because they are associated with lesser degrees of CO_2 production than isocaloric amounts of glucose.[1]

Chest Inspection and Auscultation. Observation of chest movement often provides general assessment of ventilatory adequacy. Asymmetrical movement of the chest or asymmetrical breath sounds indicate unequal ventilation associated with abnormalities such as right mainstem bronchial intubation, atelectasis, or pneumothorax. Dysynchronous motion of the

chest and abdomen is also an indicator of diaphragmatic fatigue (Fig. 4-2).

The presence of crackles, wheezes, and dullness to percussion are usually late signs of pulmonary disease. Nevertheless, physical examination is important in detecting preoperative chronic pulmonary disease, failure of ventilation, and airway obstruction. Auscultation may also allow detection of an inadequately inflated cuff on an endotracheal or tracheostomy tube.

Body Weight. An accurate record of daily weight is often the most important indicator of fluid balance. Patients receiving only intravenous fluids usually lose 0.3–0.5 kg (0.6–1.1 lb) per day. If weight loss is greater than this amount, it is excessive. Unless a patient is receiving substantial intravenous or enteral alimentation, stable weight or a weight gain indicates retention of water.

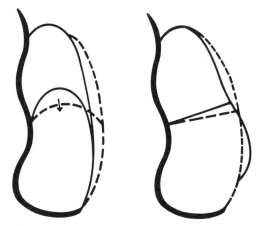

Fig. 4-2. During normal inspiration the diaphragm descends (left), and the thorax and abdomen move outward synchronously. On expiration, the chest and abdomen move inward synchronously. With asynchronous breathing (right), outward movement of the abdomen occurs during expiration. Asynchronous breathing probably results from an inefficient position of the diaphragm plus maximal use of accessory muscles of respiration. (Reprinted with permission from Bone RC: Treatment of respiratory failure due to advanced obstructive lung disease. Arch Intern Med 140:1018, 1980. Copyright 1980, American Medical Association.)

Radiological Examination

The chest roentgenogram may reflect late changes. However, it is very useful in following the treatment of respiratory failure. As PEEP is applied to patients with the adult respiratory distress syndrome (ARDS), the chest roentgenogram may assist in the evaluation of localized hyperinflation associated with unequal lung damage.[19,28] It is also useful to detect certain complications, e.g., atelectasis, pneumonia, right mainstem bronchial intubation, and pulmonary barotrauma.

The chest roentgenogram should be examined meticulously to ascertain the position of an artificial airway, remembering that the tube may move in and out of a main bronchus with respiration and flexion, or extension of the neck. An especially im-portant use of chest roentgenography is the recognition of pneumothorax from trauma, subclavian venous catheterization, or localized lung hyperinflation.

The recognition of a pneumothorax depends on the visualization of air separating the visceral and parietal pleurae. Usually a thin white line representing visceral pleura and a peripheral lucent space devoid of lung structures are seen. When only supine films are available for interpretation, the diagnosis may be more difficult. Two recently described findings on a supine film that should raise a suspicion of pneumothorax are: (1) an abrupt curvilinear change in density projected over the upper quadrant of the abdomen, with increased radiolucency over the upper quadrant; and (2) a deep lateral costophrenic angle on the involved side.[19,28] Either finding should prompt a follow-up cross-table lateral or decubitus film to confirm the diagnosis of pneumothorax.

Electrocardiogram

Visual systems for detection of dysrhythmias are an integral part of most monitoring systems. Computer programs are now available that can detect dysrhythmias with more accuracy and consistency than can human observers. Rhythm disturbances are usually late manifestations of respiratory problems and should not be relied on to detect early changes. Approximately 10 percent of patients receiving postoperative care have serious dysrhythmias, and about one-half of these are due to undetected respiratory complications.[24]

Laboratory Examination

Urine Output, Plasma and Urine Osmolality, Specific Gravity, Osmolar and Free Water Clearance. Renal failure complicating respiratory failure leads to a precipitous increase in mortality. Among 400-plus critically ill patients, Sweet et al. reported a mortality of 32 percent with respiratory failure alone, 44 percent with renal failure alone, and 65 percent with combined renal and respiratory failure.[34] A significant increase in the requirement for positive end-expiratory pressure (PEEP) was found in patients with combined renal-respiratory failure compared to those with respiratory failure alone. Alterations in renal hemodynamic and tubular functions occur in association with respiratory failure as a result of hypoxemia, acidosis, mechanical ventilation, and PEEP. Decreased urine output, decreased sodium excretion, and increased antidiuretic hormone secretion have been associated with mechanical ventilation and PEEP. Other factors implicated in the pathogenesis of renal failure are hypovolemia, hypotension, sepsis, and nephrotoxic drugs.

Renal failure in the critically ill patient can be classified into four types: prerenal azotemia, oliguric acute tubular necrosis, nonoliguric acute tubular necrosis, and obstructive uropathy. Patients with respiratory failure and prerenal azotemia have the greatest mortality compared to those with the other categories of renal failure despite a lower mean serum creatinine level.[34] Because respiratory failure combined with renal failure is associated with increased mortality, factors known to predispose to renal failure should be eliminated prophylactically or treated aggressively as they are detected.

Urine output provides a good estimate of the adequacy of renal perfusion, and urine specific gravity reflects renal concentrating ability. Serum creatinine and blood urea nitrogen (BUN) levels are traditionally used to monitor renal function; however, other less frequently used tests may also be useful. An early sign of relative hypovolemia may be a falling urine sodium concentration and/or a rising urine osmolality. Urine sodium less than 10–20 mEq/L or urine osmolality greater than 600 mOsm/L suggests hypovolemia.

Renal function also can be monitored by measurement of plasma (Posm) and urine (Uosm) osmolality as well as calculation of osmolar and free water clearance. The Uosm/Posm ratio is calculated, and if it is greater than 1.7 good concentrating ability is present. The osmolar clearance (Cosm) is calculated according to the following equation:

$$Cosm = \frac{Uosm}{Posm} \times urine\ output \quad (1)$$

The osmolar clearance reflects the rate of removal of solutes from plasma. Normal osmolar clearance is 120 ml/hr and is decreased in renal failure. Free water clearance is calculated by subtracting the Cosm from the urine output. The free water clearance (C_{H_2O}) usually is negative (-125 to -100 ml/hour), and values close to zero precede acute renal failure.

Normal osmolality of body fluids is 275–295 mOsm/L H_2O. Plasma osmolality is calculated by the following formula:

$$Posm\ (mOsm/L) = 2 \times sodium\ (mEq/L)$$
$$+ \frac{glucose\ (mg/dl)}{18} + \frac{BUN\ (mg/dl)}{2.8} \quad (2)$$

An osmolality above 320 mOsm/L generally is tolerated poorly, and levels greater than 350 mOsm/L may be fatal. The calculated serum osmolality is normally 5–8 mOsm less than the measured osmolality. This difference is called the osmolar discriminant and is due to the presence of anions, e.g., lactate or phosphate. An increased osmolar discriminant is usually associated with increased lactate production and a poorer prognosis.

Hematocrit and Hemoglobin. The hematocrit is a static measurement and is affected by gains or losses of red blood cells and plasma volume. After hemorrhage associated with trauma, the hematocrit gradually falls. This change results from transcapillary refilling of the plasma volume by extracellular fluid and reflects a compensatory reaction to, rather than a direct measure of, blood loss. Compensation requires time. Blood loss is replaced by interstitial water at an initial rate of 1 ml/minute. With severe hemorrhage, transcapillary refilling is more rapid. Serial hematocrit determinations at maximum 4-hour intervals should be performed on blood samples from patients with suspected hemorrhage.[32] Serial hemoglobin measurements are needed to calculate the oxygen content of the blood.

The hematocrit value for optimal oxygen delivery is disputed. For example, active changes in coronary arterial dilatation occur in response to changes in hematocrit. At normal blood pressure, maximum myocardial oxygen consumption is achieved over a wide range of hematocrit values (20–60 percent), and the optimal hematocrit is the same for the heart and the rest of the body.[20] However, during hemorrhagic hypotension, changes in hematocrit over a much narrower range adversely affect myocardial oxygen consumption. Here, the optimum hematocrit for the coronary circulation is lower.[20]

Arterial Blood Gas Analysis. Arterial blood gas tensions are determined by the composition of alveolar gas and the efficiency of gas transfer between the alveoli and pulmonary capillary blood. Alveolar gas tension depends on the mixture of inspired gas, ventilation and blood flow in the lungs, the matching of ventilation and blood flow ($\dot{V}/\dot{Q}$), and the composition of mixed venous blood gases. Because mixed venous Po_2 usually varies with cardiac output, significant arterial hypoxemia can result from shunting of venous blood with a low Po_2 through the pulmonary circulation. Failure to recognize this nonpulmonary cause of arterial hypoxemia may cause a clinician to falsely ascribe a falling Pao_2 to deteriorating pulmonary function.[43]

Pulmonary abnormalities which may result in hypoxemia, alone or in combination, include diffusion block, ventilation/perfusion inequality, intrapulmonary shunting, and hypoventilation. Diffusion abnormalities lead to hypoxemia if pulmonary end-capillary blood fails to equilibrate fully with alveolar gas. Such conditions are probably a very uncommon cause of hypoxemia except in patients with chronic lung disease during exercise or exposure to a decreased Fio_2 at high altitude.[39,40]

Although bulk oxygen is carried in combination with hemoglobin, delivery to tissue depends on its partial pressure in the blood, which also reflects the amount of oxygen available to be delivered from hemoglobin. A fall in Pao_2 without a change in $Paco_2$ suggests that blood oxygenation is deteriorating despite constant alveolar ventilation. In the acutely ill patient, this finding usually is due to ventilation-perfusion imbalance or intrapulmonary shunting. An important feature of shunting is that hypoxemia cannot be abolished by the administration of 100 percent oxygen because shunted blood totally bypasses ventilated alveoli. A shunt usually does not result in a raised $Paco_2$ because the chemoreceptors sense any elevation in $Paco_2$ and reflexly induce an increase of ventilation.

When patients hypoventilate while breathing ambient air, hypoxemia results from an increase in alveolar Pco_2. Calculation of the alveolar oxygen tension and determination of the alveolar-arterial (A-a) oxygen tension difference allows separation of hypoventilation from other causes of hypoxemia. With hypoventilation, the A-a oxygen gradient is normal; with other causes of hypoxemia, it is increased. The alveolar oxygen tension can be estimated from the following abbreviated formula which is adequate for clinical purposes:

$$P_{AO_2} = P_{IO_2} - \frac{Paco_2}{R} \qquad (3)$$

P_{IO_2} is equal to the barometric pressure (P_B) minus the water vapor pressure (47 mm Hg at 37°C) multiplied by the F_{IO_2}. The respiratory quotient (R) is approximately 0.8 in the steady-state resting condition. It is assumed to be 0.8 in respiratory failure, although this assumption is not always valid.

The correction for R varies depending on the inspired oxygen concentration (F_{IO_2}), as can be seen from the nonsimplified alveolar air equation:

$$P_{AO_2} = F_{IO_2}(P_B - 47)$$
$$- P_{ACO_2}\left(F_{IO_2} + \frac{1 - F_{IO_2}}{R}\right) \quad (4)$$

Although this equation appears formidable, if P_{aCO_2} is used rather than P_{ACO_2}, and 100 percent oxygen is inhaled, solution of the equation is simply the difference between inspired P_{O_2} and P_{aCO_2}. For clinical purposes, it is important to appreciate the small but definite error if P_{AO_2} is calculated using the abbreviated formula at different inspired oxygen concentrations.

The arterial oxygen tension divided by the alveolar oxygen tension is called the a/A ratio. This ratio is relatively stable with a varying F_{IO_2}, unlike the classic alveolar-arterial gradient. Thus it is a useful index of changes in lung function when a patient's inspired oxygen concentration is changed. The normal a/A ratio is > 0.75. The ratio can also be used to predict the new P_{aO_2} that results from a change in inspired oxygen concentration.[17]

Another nonpulmonary factor that can significantly affect gas exchange is the level of CO_2 production ($\dot{V}CO_2$). The amount of CO_2 produced by the body is a function of the metabolic rate and the substrate(s) used as fuel. CO_2 production varies from 70 to 100 percent of the O_2 consumption as the fuel is switched from fat to carbohydrate. When caloric input exceeds metabolic needs, excess calories are converted to fat, which further increases CO_2 production. Askanazi et al. have shown that hospitalized patients receiving parenteral hyperalimentation can increase their $\dot{V}CO_2$ as much

as 50 percent.[1] To excrete this excess CO_2, an increased minute ventilation is needed which might be impossible in a patient with chronic obstructive pulmonary disease (COPD) or cause failure to wean from mechanical ventilation.[1]

Monitoring P_{50} (P_{O_2} at 50 percent oxyhemoglobin saturation) may also be helpful in assessing oxygen delivery. As shown in Figure 4-3, a right-shifted curve (e.g., higher P_{50}) assists in delivery of oxygen to tissues. The significance of shifts of the oxyhemoglobin curve on overall tissue oxygenation remains a topic of active investigation. Rightward shifts are commonly seen in conditions associated with decreased oxygen delivery, e.g., anemia and chronic hypoxemia. Beneficial effects of decreased oxygen affinity are difficult to demonstrate experimentally. Increased mortality and decreased oxygen consumption and cardiac output have been associated with a low P_{50} in experimental studies. These findings are of clinical significance to patients receiving large transfusions of stored blood or others who develop respiratory alkalemia or metabolic alkalosis, a resultant leftward shift of the oxyhemoglobin dissociation curve and decreased P_{50}. As these patients are more likely to have limited cardiac reserve because of acute illness, they are least able to compensate by an increase in cardiac output or a shift in blood flow to tissues utilizing high extraction ratios to meet required oxygen demands. Organs such as the heart and brain are particularly vulnerable.

Marked changes in P_{aO_2} in critically ill patients that may be missed by intermittent sampling occur during the administration of drugs, suctioning, and changes in body position. Continuous monitoring of P_{aO_2} by electrodes in the femoral, radial, and brachial arteries as well as the P_{O_2} in mixed venous blood in the pulmonary artery has been reported.[18] Obviously these techniques have the same problems as other invasive techniques, and further experience is needed before it can be concluded that

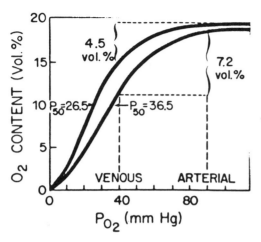

Fig. 4-3. The shape of the oxyhemoglobin dissociation curve results in 90 percent hemoglobin saturation at a Pao$_2$ of 60 mm Hg. At a Po$_2$ of 60 mm Hg, approximately 90 percent of total oxygen content found at a Po$_2$ of 100 mm Hg is present in the blood. The position of the oxyhemoglobin dissociation curve is expressed as the P$_{50}$. The P$_{50}$ is the Po$_2$ at which hemoglobin is 50 percent saturated. The left curve represents normal cells with a P$_{50}$ of 26.5. The right curve has a P$_{50}$ of 36.5. The arterial oxygen tension displayed is 90 mm Hg, almost complete saturation. The mixed venous oxygen tension is 40 mm Hg. The left curve is capable of releasing an oxygen content of 4.5 ml/dl. The right curve, however, is capable of releasing 7.2 ml/dl, a 60 percent increase in the amount of oxygen available to the tissues. It is apparent that the right-shifted curve, with its property of enhanced unloading of oxygen at the tissue-capillary level, is much more advantageous at this saturation. (Reprinted with permission from Murphy EM, Bone RC, Diederich DA, et al: The oxyhemoglobin dissociation curve in type a and type b chronic obstructive pulmonary disease. Lung 154:299, 1978.)

such monitoring is indicated in the management of critically ill patients.

Because of the intermittent nature of blood gas measurement and the lag in reporting results, considerable effort has been directed to developing noninvasive continuous monitoring of blood and tissue gas values. Ear oximetry is the most widely used technique. Advances in oximeter technology have eliminated early problems with this technique and now allow accurate calibration and measurement of oxygen saturation. A beam of light of appropriate wavelength shines through the earlobe; change in transmittance is measured, and hemoglobin saturation is electronically calculated. The disadvantages of the technique are that the sensor must be maintained in position on the earlobe, and it is difficult to use if the skin is deeply pigmented. Accuracy in patients with low cardiac output has been questioned. Reproducibility in other situations has generally been good. Ear oximetry is most accurate in the steep portion of the oxyhemoglobin dissociation curve when changes in Pao$_2$ are accompanied by significant changes in oxygen saturation. This is not a major problem in monitoring the patient with respiratory failure because the range of greatest clinical interest falls on the steep portion of the oxygen-hemoglobin dissociation curve where saturation is a sensitive index of oxygen tension.

Another approach that has proved to be effective in monitoring infants with respiratory failure is transcutaneous blood gas analysis. Warming the skin underneath an appropriate electrode causes blood flow to the skin to increase out of proportion to its need in order to eliminate heat. Thus capillary gas tensions are minimally affected by tissue metabolism. Under most circumstances, transcutaneous values in infants accurately reflect arterial blood gas tensions.[25,38] Situations associated with changes in oxygen delivery to the skin (changes in cardiac output, blood volume, hematocrit, and acid-base status) may cause considerable differences between directly measured arterial gases and transcutaneous values.[35,36] In fact, in some adults monitored continuously with an intraarterial electrode, transcutaneous Po$_2$ correlated better with changes in blood pressure than did Pao$_2$.

In patients with leukocytosis and thrombocytosis, spurious hypoxemia can occur in

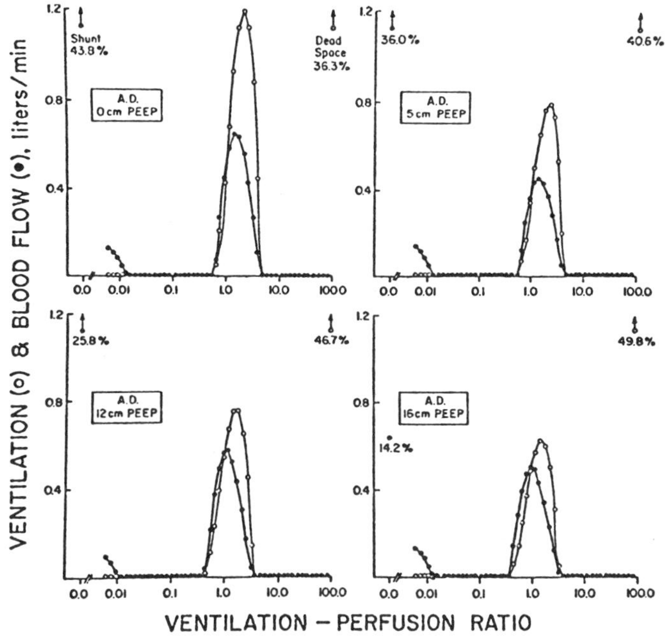

Fig. 4-4. Ventilation-perfusion distribution in a patient with adult respiratory distress syndrome. The blood flow is divided between well-ventilated and shunt lung units. (Reprinted with permission from Dantzker DR: Gas exchange in the adult respiratory distress syndrome. Clin Chest Med 3:59, 1982.)

arterial or mixed venous blood due to consumption of oxygen by leukocytes and platelets before laboratory analysis. With extreme leukocytosis, this decrease in Po_2 can be as much as 72 mm Hg within the first 2 minutes after the blood is drawn. Spurious hypoxemia is prevented by the addition of potassium cyanide and blunted by placing the blood sample in ice. Because these patients often have respiratory complications, spurious hypoxemia must be differentiated from true hypoxemia to avoid unnecessary diagnostic and therapeutic intervention.[16]

The most elegant evaluation of ventilation and perfusion relationships is that developed by Wagner et al., who studied gas exchange with a multiple gas elimination technique.[41] With this method, the distribution of blood flow and ventilation is related to the ventilation/perfusion ratio ($\dot{V}A/\dot{Q}$) (Fig. 4-4). True shunt is quantified and separated from units with low $\dot{V}A/\dot{Q}$ ratios. This multicompartmental model of the lung, despite its complexity, has added insights not available from the traditional three-compartment analysis of Riley and Cournand (Fig. 4-5).

Intraarterial Monitoring

Intraarterial monitoring is usually accomplished by cannulation of the radial or brachial artery. One should ensure that adequate collateral circulation exists when arterial cannulation is performed. Before radial cannulation, an Allen test should be performed to ensure adequacy of collateral circulation. With the Allen test, the hand is blanched by firm pressure on the radial and ulnar arteries. A well-developed collateral circulation exists if release of the ulnar artery is accompanied by suffusion of the hand within 5 seconds. Arterial cannulation in the ICU allows pressure monitoring and permits sampling of arterial blood, thereby avoiding repeated arterial puncture.

Pressure transducers used in monitoring arterial pressure have been identified as a source of nosocomial bacteremia. Bacteremia resulted from faulty sterilization of the transducer dome. Recently a change in transducer design has been initiated. A disposable diaphragm has been added to isolate the sterile fluid chamber from the proximal portion of the dome which is attached

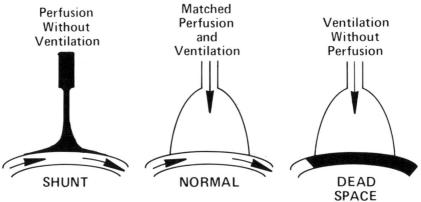

Perfusion Without Ventilation   Matched Perfusion and Ventilation   Ventilation Without Perfusion

SHUNT   NORMAL   DEAD SPACE

Fig. 4-5. Hypoxemia in the adult respiratory distress syndrome (ARDS) results from intrapulmonary shunting. Shunting results from perfused but unventilated alveoli, as shown on the left. In ARDS many alveoli are also ventilated but not perfused, resulting in an increased physiological dead space, as seen on the right. Both shunt and physiological dead space may exceed 50 percent in severe ARDS. (Reprinted with permission from Bone RC: Treatment of respiratory failure due to advanced obstructive lung disease. Arch Intern Med 140:1019, 1980. Copyright 1980, American Medical Association)

to a nonsterile transducer. Despite a decreased infection risk with transducers utilizing disposable domes, nosocomial bacteremia still has been reported.

Regular procedures are necessary to evaluate the accuracy of the pressure-measuring system in use. The transducer should be placed as close to the patient as possible, and air bubbles should be assiduously eliminated from the system. Long extension tubes increase resonant frequency and artifactually amplify systolic pressure, while trapped air bubbles "damp" the system and record an erroneously low systolic pressure.[29]

Tidal Volume, Expired Minute Volume, and Inspiratory Force

In addition to spirometry, a waterless volume displacement spirometer and a variety of electronic spirometers are readily available. Also, dry gas meters are available to measure exhaled volumes. Two of the most practical and useful instruments for clinical work are the Wright and Drager respirometers.

Low tidal volumes associated with tachypnea increase dead space ventilation and decrease alveolar ventilation. The product of rate and tidal volume is minute volume, a useful measure of total ventilation. High minute ventilation suggests severe hypocarbia or increased dead space and respiratory work which may lead to exhaustion. A tidal volume greater than 5 ml/kg and a vital capacity greater than 10 ml/kg may be useful guidelines for predicting successful weaning from mechanical ventilation. Measurement of minute volume and maximum inspiratory pressure are also employed. Sahn and Lakshminarayan showed that a resting minute volume of less than 10 L and the ability to double the resting minute volume on command predicts success in weaning. A maximum "negative" inspiratory pressure greater than 20 cm H_2O is also used.[30]

Physiological Dead Space

Physiological dead space is the portion of tidal volume that does not participate in gas exchange. In healthy adult subjects the physiological dead space is approximately 150 ml at rest (about 20–30 percent of each tidal volume). This value represents the anatomical dead space from the mouth, pharynx, larynx, trachea, bronchi, and bronchioles as well as the contribution of any alveoli that are overventilated with respect to perfusion. Positive-pressure ventilation alone can increase dead space.[33] With respiratory failure the physiological dead space is increased because of continued ventilation of alveoli whose perfusion is either absent or decreased. Varieties of dead space and the expired CO_2 curve resulting from series and parallel dead space are shown in Figure 4-6. The ratio of dead space to tidal volume (V_D/V_T) can be calculated by measuring the arterial and mixed expired CO_2 tension ($P\bar{E}CO_2$) by the Bohr equation:

$$\frac{V_D}{V_T} = \frac{P_{ACO_2} - P\bar{E}CO_2}{P_{ACO_2}} \qquad (5)$$

The Enghoff modification of the Bohr equation is often used clinically:

$$\frac{V_D}{V_T} = \frac{P_{ACO_2} - P\bar{E}CO_2}{P_{ACO_2}} \qquad (6)$$

If the end tidal P_{CO_2}(P_{ETCO_2}) is substituted for the P_{ACO_2}, anatomical dead space can be calculated, requiring only expired air (arterial blood sampling is eliminated). Changes of physiological dead space during respiratory failure from the adult respiratory distress syndrome show a striking relationship to survival[31] (Fig. 4-7).

The breathing circuit to collect exhaled gas is used at the patient's bedside. Calculations are made with measured P_{ACO_2} or P_{ETCO_2} and a sample of exhaled gas. This method is applicable to both mechanically ventilated and spontaneously breathing patients. Correction for dead space due to expansion of the tubing in the mechanically ventilated patient should be made. In the spontaneously breathing patient, the exhaled gas can be collected from a mouthpiece through a one-way valve into a Douglas bag or other suitable apparatus to

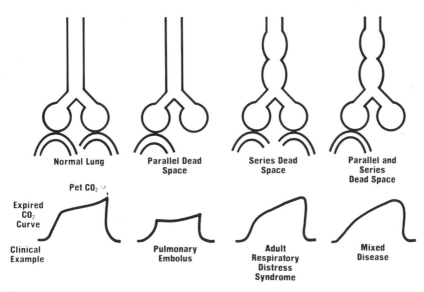

Fig. 4-6. Physiological dead space can be increased by diseases causing ventilation that exceeds perfusion. Graphic representation of diseases producing increased dead space and the resulting expired carbon dioxide curve is shown. (Reprinted with permission from Bone RC: Monitoring patients in acute respiratory failure. Respir Care 27:700, 1982.)

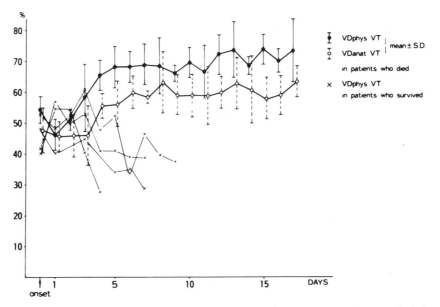

Fig. 4-7. The time course of change in physiological dead space (V_D/f) and anatomical dead space (V_D anat) to tidal volume (V_T) ratios in patients with the adult respiratory distress syndrome. (Reprinted with permission from Shimada Y, Yoshiga I, Tomala I, et al: Evaluation of the progress and prognosis of adult respiratory distress syndrome, simple physiologic measurements. Chest 76:180, 1979.)

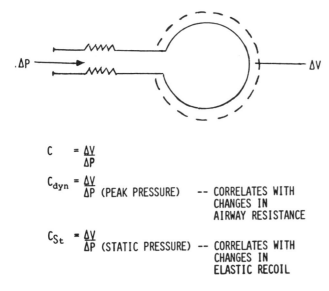

Fig. 4-8. Mechanical analog of the lung. Pressure at the mouth is dissipated in overcoming airway resistance and elastic recoil of the lung and chest wall. From Bone RC: Monitoring patients in acute respiratory failure. (Reprinted with permission from Bone RC: Monitoring respiratory function in the patient with the adult respiratory distress syndrome. In Decker BC (ed): Adult Respiratory Distress Syndrome. Seminars in Respiratory Medicine. Vol. 2. pp. 140–150, Georg Thieme Verlag, Stuttgart, 1981.)

measure the mixed expired CO_2. Because a spontaneously breathing patient may not breathe with consistent tidal volumes, collection must be continued for 3–4 minutes.

Bedside Measurement of Mechanics

Volume change per unit of pressure change is compliance, a useful measure of the elastic properties of a body. The compliance of the normal lung is about 200 ml/cm H_2O. If one follows the pressure dial on a ventilator, a rapid rise of airway pressure with a peak at the end of inspiration is noted, followed by a rapid fall to the resting or baseline pressure. This peak pressure is required to overcome the elastic properties of the lung and chest wall and the flow-restrictive properties of the airway (Figs. 4-8 and 4-9). The volume delivered by the ventilator divided by the peak pressure is called *dynamic characteristic*.[6] It is not correct to call this value dynamic compliance because it is actually an impedence measurement and includes compliance and resistance components. If the outflow limb of the ventilator circuit is occluded momentarily by pinching the tubing to control the expiratory valve opening (or dialing in "expiratory retard" or inspiratory hold), the pressure reading will show a momentary plateau during which time no air is flowing. Normal compliance of the lung and chest wall in the mechanically ventilated patient is about 70 ml/cm H_2O. When the static compliance of the lung and chest wall is less than 25 ml/cm H_2O, as in severe respiratory failure, difficulties in weaning are common because of the high work of breathing.[13,22,23]

The term "chest wall" includes all structures outside the lungs that move during breathing. Pressure usually is measured from the ventilator anaeroid gauge, which is sufficiently accurate for clinical purposes if the pressure tubing is connected to the proximal airway. The plateau pressure di-

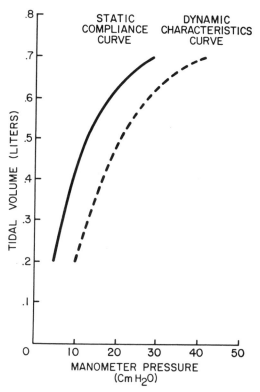

Fig. 4-9. Pressure-volume measurements at various tidal volumes. These measurements are made from many breaths and differ from the compliance measurements made in the pulmonary function laboratory, which are measured during a single breath. From Bone RC: Monitoring patients in acute respiratory failure. (Reprinted with permission from Bone RC: Monitoring respiratory function in the patient with the adult respiratory distress syndrome. In Decker BC (ed): Adult Respiratory Distress Syndrome. Seminars in Respiratory Medicine. Vol. 2. pp. 140–150, Georg Thieme Verlag, Stuttgart, 1981.)

vided by the tidal volume represents the combined static compliance of the lungs and chest wall. If one ventilates the lungs at various tidal volumes and records the peak and plateau pressure for each volume, dynamic and static curves can be quickly graphed; the former correlates with airway resistance, and the latter is a measure of lung stiffness (Fig. 4-10). The method is as follows:

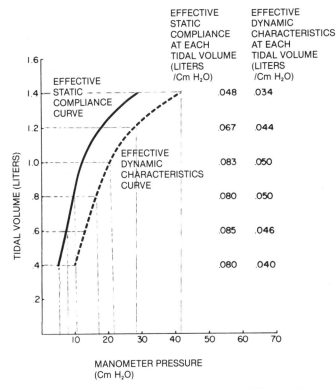

Fig. 4-10. Pressure-volume curves with static compliance and dynamic characteristics calculated at each tidal volume. (Reprinted with permission from Bone RC: Monitoring respiratory function in the patient with the adult respiratory distress syndrome. In Decker BC (ed): Adult Respiratory Distress Syndrome. Seminars in Respiratory Medicine. Vol. 2. pp. 140–150, Georg Thieme Verlag, Stuttgart, 1981.)

1. Explain the procedure to the patient if he/she is awake.
2. Ensure adequate tracheal tube cuff inflation during the procedure to prevent leaks.
3. Set maximal expiratory retard (if available); otherwise, after each delivered V_T, cross-clamp the exhalation tube until a pressure plateau is seen.
4. Select a series of V_T settings to be used, e.g., 7, 10, 13, and 16 ml/kg body weight or 400, 600, 800, 1000 ml.
5. For each breath, record:
   a. Spirometer volume.
   b. Peak airway pressure.
   c. Plateau pressure.
   When PEEP is used, the value must be subtracted from peak and plateau pressures before charting.

Static compliance

$$= \frac{\text{spirometer volume} - \text{tube expansion volume}}{\text{plateau pressure} - \text{PEEP}} \quad (7)$$

6. Repeat this step for each volume setting selected.
7. If at any setting the pressure increases markedly, do (not) go to larger volumes as pulmonary barotrauma may result.
8. Remove expiratory retard.
9. Readjust cuff pressure.
10. Carry out a complete ventilator check.
11. Chart data on graph (six such charts can be printed on an 8 × 11 inch sheet).

These measurements can be made at one volume and followed numerically. A simpler method plots static and dynamic pressures graphically at a constant tidal volume, a useful and faster monitoring tool. At higher tidal volumes and/or PEEP, decreasing static compliance often heralds lung hyperinflation. The decrease in static compliance is most pronounced when large tidal volumes are combined with PEEP (Fig. 4-11).

More information is available from inspection of the graphic measurement of the

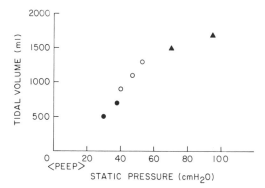

Fig. 4-11. Static pressure-volume relationship of the lungs and thorax. Each observation represents the inflation hold manometer pressure of the ventilator on the horizontal axis, which relates to the tidal volume indicated on the vertical axis. Static compliance = tidal volume/inflation hold pressure − PEEP pressure. In this example, PEEP pressure is 10 cm H_2O. Compliance for tidal volumes indicated by 0 = 25 ml/cm H_2O; 0 = 30 ml/cm H_2O; 0 = 25 and 20 ml/cm H_2O). Tidal volumes above this level produce "optimal compliance." (Reprinted with permission from Bone RC: Monitoring respiratory function in the patient with the adult respiratory distress syndrome. In Decker BC (ed): Adult Respiratory Distress Syndrome. Seminars in Respiratory Medicine. Vol. 2. pp. 140–150, Georg Thieme Verlag, Stuttgart, 1981.)

curves at multiple volumes. Figure 4-12 indicates that conditions which increase airway resistance shift the dynamic curve to the right and flatten it (higher pressure per volume increase). Those conditions producing increased lung or chest wall stiffness flatten and shift both the static and dynamic curves to the right.[6] If the patient is hypoxemic and the compliance curves are unchanged, pulmonary embolization should be suspected.

Two errors in these measurements are possible with unrelaxed respiratory muscles. If the patient is resisting mechanical ventilation, the total pressure developed by the ventilator will be greater than that required to inflate the lungs of the relaxed patient. Also, if the patient is actively inspiring, the pressure developed by the ventilator will be less than the total pressure required.

Factors which are important clinically in respiratory failure produce mechanical changes in lung function that can be detected by the above measurements. The advantage of the method cited is that it requires no special equipment, takes only a few minutes, and can be done routinely by the respiratory therapist. The serial curves give warning of decreasing compliance and help to differentiate airway from parenchymal disease. Further, when the compliance decreases, hyperinflation (or barotrauma) may be present. The difference between peak (Pp) and static pressure (Pst) is the pressure required to overcome flow resistance. If flow is measured, airway resistance (Raw) can be calculated:

$$Raw = \frac{Pp - Pst}{\dot{V}} \qquad (8)$$

Flow is measured at end-inspiration at the time of peak pressure.[22] From Figure 4-13:

$$Raw = (40 - 20)/2$$

$$= 10 \text{ cm } H_2O/L/\text{second}$$

Alternatively, Raw can be calculated at other points during inspiration. For example, the flow at 0.5 L/second is corrected for static compliance, which equals the tidal volume divided by the static pressure minus PEEP. Thus:

$$Cst = \frac{500}{20 - 10} = 50 \text{ ml/cm } H_2O$$

Assuming a constant Cst, the pressure at a volume of 200 ml is 4 cm H_2O. The Raw at 0.5 L/sec flow can then be calculated:

$$Raw = \frac{20 - PEEP - Pst}{\dot{V}}$$

$$= \frac{20 - 10 - 4}{0.5}$$

$$= 12 \text{ cm } H_2O/L/\text{second}$$

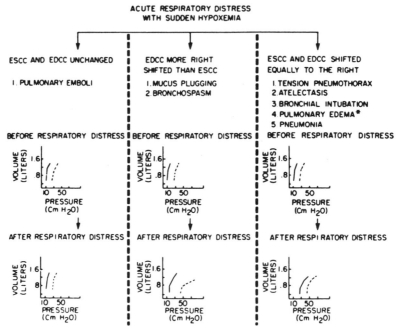

Fig. 4-12. Pressure-volume measurements before and after respiratory distress, taken from reference 1. ESCC is effective static compliance curve. EDCC is effective dynamic characteristics curve. (Reprinted with permission from Bone RC: Monitoring respiratory function in the patient with the adult respiratory distress syndrome. In Decker BC (ed): Adult Respiratory Distress Syndrome. Seminars in Respiratory Medicine. Vol. 2. pp. 140–150, Georg Thieme Verlag, Stuttgart, 1981.)

In healthy subjects, <u>Raw ranges between 2 and 3 cm H_2O/L/second</u>. When measured at flow rates of 1 L/second, approximately 10 percent of the calculated Raw is due to turbulence. With bronchospasm or airway inflammation, Raw may be 10 times that seen in healthy individuals.

HEMODYNAMIC MONITORING

The major purposes of hemodynamic monitoring are to: (1) determine the magnitude of pulmonary congestion and peripheral hypoperfusion; (2) assess left ventricular pump performance; and (3) determine the magnitude of the vascular resistance. Terms important in understanding hemodynamic monitoring include:

1. Preload—the filling pressure or volume in the ventricle at end-diastole.

2. Afterload—the impedence against which the heart works.

3. Contractility—intrinsic muscle power which allows the heart to increase the extent and force of shortening independent of the Starling mechanism.

The most important measurement is the relationship between these factors. Because the heart is a dynamic pump, it must vary the stroke volume with the volume it receives. The degree that the myocardial cell is stretched during diastole (preload) is related to the force developed during systole. Starling's law states that increased myocardial fiber stretching during diastole is associated with increased shortening in systole. Preload (filling pressure) cannot be measured directly in the left ventricle, but it can be measured by a catheter wedged in a small pulmonary artery. This measure-

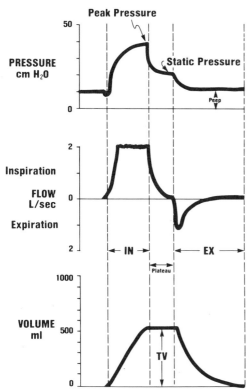

Fig. 4-13. Monitoring pressure, flow, and volume in a patient requiring mechanical ventilation. (Reprinted with permission from Bone RC: Monitoring respiratory function in the patient with the adult respiratory distress syndrome. In Decker BC (ed): Adult Respiratory Distress Syndrome. Seminars in Respiratory Medicine. Vol. 2. pp. 140–150, Georg Thieme Verlag, Stuttgart, 1981.)

ment is called the pulmonary capillary wedge pressure (PCWP) or pulmonary artery occlusion pressure. The central venous pressure (CVP) is an unacceptable measure of left ventricular preload because of damping of left-sided pressures by variable resistance in the pulmonary circuit and the interposition of the right ventricle, tricuspid, and pulmonary valves downstream from the central venous catheter. An increased PCWP (even in the normal range) in the patient with respiratory failure can be harmful because it induces a large flux of water and solute across the damaged pul-

monary capillary. Thus even though "normal," PCWP should be monitored.

Afterload is determined by the volume of blood ejected from the left ventricle and is related to the compliance and total cross-sectional area into which the volume is ejected. The clinical measurement of afterload is the systemic vascular resistance (SVR), the formula for which is shown in Table 4-4.

Contractility is the intrinsic property which allows the heart to increase its force of shortening, independent of preload and afterload. One assumes that an increase in contractility has occurred when the stroke volume increases at the same or lesser preload and the same or greater afterload.

A Starling curve provides a graphic presentation of ventricular performance in terms of stroke work and preload. The Starling curve allows a mapping of ventricular performance with time and provides an indication of the optimal preload resulting in optimal cardiac output and stroke work.

Afterload reduction by pharmacological means is useful in patients with high systemic vascular resistance and decreased forward flow not attributable to hypovolemia or myocardial ischemia. Stroke volume often increases with afterload reduction so that little or no reduction in arterial pressure may occur.

TECHNIQUES OF PULMONARY ARTERY CATHETERIZATION

The first balloon flotation catheter contained two lumens. The central lumen measured intravascular pressures through a fluid-filled system connected to a pressure transducer, and the other was used to inflate or deflate a balloon at the catheter tip. When inflated, the balloon acts like a sail to "flow-direct" the catheter tip through the right atrium and ventricle, and into the pulmonary artery. The inflated balloon also surrounds the catheter tip in such a manner that injury to the vessels and heart is less likely and the incidence of catheter-induced dysrhythmias is reduced.

The balloon-flotation catheters are 5 or 7 French double-lumen and triple-lumen (for CVP and pulmonary artery pressure measurements), or 7 French quadruple-lumen, thermodilution cardiac output types. Monitoring equipment includes a strain-gauge pressure transducer, connecting tubing and three-way stopcocks, electrocardiogram (ECG) monitor, pressure recorder, and heparinized saline (1000 U/100 ml). The pressure transducer is calibrated so that a deflection of 1 cm is equivalent to a pressure increment of 5 mm Hg. A fluoroscope may facilitate passage of the catheter but usually is not essential.

The catheter is inserted into the antecubital vein through a variety of commercially available introducer kits. The external jugular vein can be catheterized if a J-wire is used to facilitate introduction.[14] The subclavian, internal jugular, and femoral veins are also frequently used. The femoral vein is easily cannulated and anatomically provides the most direct access to the pulmonary artery. When the antecubital fossa is used, the patient is supine with the arm abducted 90 degrees. The catheter is advanced centrally about 35–40 cm from the right antecubital fossa and 45–50 cm from the left antecubital fossa. The left antecubital fossa is preferred because of the unidirectional arc construction of the catheter. When respiratory fluctuations are seen in the pressure recording, intrathoracic positioning is indicated. The balloon is fully inflated during passage through the right heart. If multiple ectopic beats are seen, the balloon is deflated and the catheter pulled back. Otherwise, it is advanced until a PCWP tracing is obtained (similar to a CVP trace).

Proper positioning of the catheter is confirmed if: (1) the PCWP is lower than the pulmonary artery pressure (PAP); and (2) the change to PAP configuration consistently occurs upon deflation of the balloon.

The PCWP waveform is characteristic, and "arterialized" (pulmonary venous) blood can be obtained when the catheter is in the wedged position. A portable chest roentgenogram should be obtained at completion of the procedure to ensure that the tip of the catheter lies in the main pulmonary artery. Accurate reference to zero (atmospheric) pressure is important. This level is arbitrarily taken in the middle of the chest or a point 5 cm below the sternal angle (angle of Lewis). All subsequent readings should be made at the same reference point. A constant heparin-saline flush of 2–3 ml/hr is maintained (0.9 percent saline with 1000 U heparin/100 ml). The balloon should never be left inflated after measurement of the PCWP. At body temperature, the catheter softens and the transcardiac loop may shorten and allow distal catheter migration. This complication is detected by a constant PCWP rather than a PAP recording, and a saturated, arterialized rather than mixed venous blood specimen obtained upon aspiration through the distal lumen. This complication must be detected to prevent pulmonary infarction (Fig. 4-14). If the PAP tracing is damped, the catheter should be flushed; if still damped after the flushing, the catheter should be withdrawn 1–2 cm.

Rare complications include pulmonary artery rupture or perforation of the pulmonary artery and cardiac tamponade.[15] Rupture of the pulmonary artery is produced by overinflation of the balloon in a distal vessel. This problem is prevented by *not* using fluid as the inflation medium, never inflating the balloon beyond the recommended amount, and stopping balloon inflation whenever resistance is encountered. Balloon rupture is also caused by overinflation of the balloon and reuse of the catheter after gas sterilization. For this reason, each catheter should be used only once. Perforation of the pulmonary artery is usually caused by advancement of the catheter with the balloon uninflated. Cardiac tamponade results from perforation of

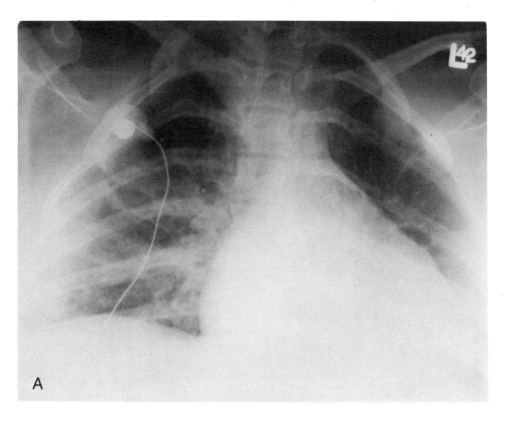

A

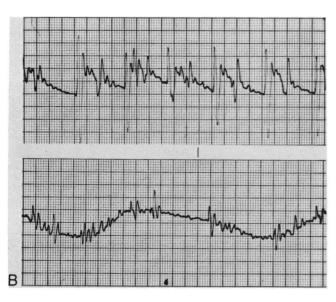

B

Fig. 4-14. (A) Pulmonary infarction. Chest roentgenogram of a patient before insertion of a pulmonary artery catheter. (B) Pressure readings from the pulmonary artery catheter. Upper tracing is the pulmonary artery pressure. The lower tracing is similar to one obtained from a pulmonary capillary wedge pressure from the same patient, resulting from peripheral wedging of the catheter with the balloon in the noninflated position (Figure continues).

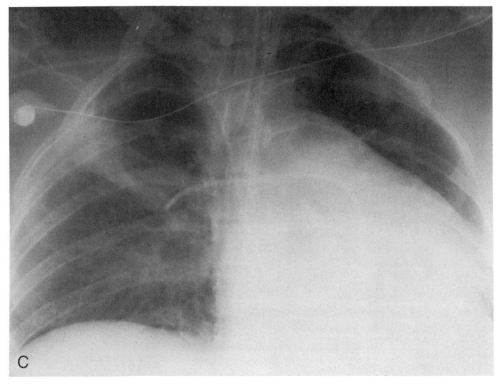

Fig. 4-14 (Continued). C. An iatrogenic pulmonary infarction resulting from peripheral wedging of a pulmonary artery catheter. Careful attention to the pressure readings in B shows that a wedge reading when the balloon of the catheter was in the noninflated position could have prevented this complication. (Reprinted with permission from Bone RC: Monitoring patients in acute respiratory failure. Respir Care 27:700, 1982).

the right ventricle by the catheter tip as well as from advancement of the catheter with the balloon uninflated. Hence the catheter should be advanced only when the balloon is inflated.

Catheter kinking or knotting usually is due to insertion of an excessive length of the catheter too rapidly. This problem is avoided by using fluoroscopy, if possible, and not advancing the catheter beyond a distance where ventricular entrance is anticipated.

Septic phlebitis is minimized by rigid adherence to a sterile protocol during insertion, suturing of the catheter to prevent movement in and out of the skin insertion site, and removal as soon as possible. In one

prospective study, 29 of 153 pulmonary artery catheter tips had a positive bacteriological culture.

Catheter malfunction occurs in up to 24 percent of insertions and maintenance, and includes balloon rupture, thermistor malfunction, and luminal obstruction—the incidence of problems being related directly to the duration of the catheterization. Avoiding technical sources of error is important in hemodynamic monitoring. Equipment failure is minimized if the electronic monitors are checked before insertion of the catheter and preventive maintenance of equipment is performed frequently by medical bioengineering personnel. Despite the variety of systems for intravascular monitoring, each employs a closed fluid system interconnected to a pressure transducer which converts a mechanical signal to an electrical one. The fluid pathway must be inspected for air bubbles which dampen the signal. Pressure waveform damping can also be caused by clotting at the catheter tip, loose connections, excessive or asymmetrical balloon inflation, catheter tip impingement on a vessel wall, and peripheral placement of the catheter. Abrupt changes in airway and pleural pressure can alter pressure readings from the pulmonary artery catheter strikingly. Pressure readings should be made at end-expiration to reduce respiratory waveform artifact.

The determination of cardiac filling pressures in patients treated with PEEP is often difficult. If the catheter tip is in the base of the lung (West zone 3) (Fig. 4-15), the PCWP reflects left atrial pressure accurately. Because the catheter is flow-directed, one anticipates that it will usually go toward the lung base. Increased alveolar pressure (with PEEP) or decreased pulmonary venous pressure associated with hypovolemia may "convert" a zone 3 area to a zone 1 or 2, and the pressure recorded is not truly indicative of that in the left atrium. If one suspects artifactual pressure transduction, guides to assessment include: ① identification of a, c, or v waves in the wedge pressure tracing, which if present indicate left atrial rather than alveolar pressure; and ② obtaining a <u>cross-table lateral chest film</u> to determine the location of the catheter placement. If the artifacts persist despite the fact that the catheter is properly located in the lower half of the lung, a fluid challenge may be administered in cases of suspected hypovolemia; or the PEEP level may be <u>decreased transiently</u> (but not removed) if high levels are required. Total discontinuation of PEEP can be dangerous and, additionally, does not provide an accurate estimation of PCWP because of the

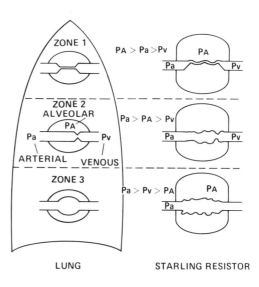

LUNG   STARLING RESISTOR

Fig. 4-15. The pulmonary capillary bed has flow characteristics of a Starling resistor, which consists of a length of flaccid collapsible tubing passing through a rigid chamber. In the Starling resistor, when chamber pressure (PA) exceeds the downstream pressure (pv), flow is independent of downstream pressure. However, when downstream pressure exceeds the chamber pressure, flow is determined by the upstream-downstream difference. The alveolar pressure is the same throughout the lung. The pulmonary artery pressure (Pa) increases down the lung. Zone 1 exists when alveolar pressure exceeds pulmonary arterial pressure and no blood flow occurs. This might occur when the pulmonary arterial pressure is decreased, as in hypovolemia, or when alveolar pressure is increased, as with the application of positive end-expiratory pressure. Zone 1 functions as alveolar dead space. In zone 2, pulmonary arterial pressure increases and exceeds alveolar pressure. In zone 2, blood flow is determined by the difference between arterial and alveolar pressures. In zone 3, blood flow is determined by the arteriovenous pressure difference. (Reprinted with permission from Bone RC: The treatment of severe hypoxemia due to the Adult Respiratory Distress Syndrome. Arch Intern Med 140:85–89, 1980).

acute hemodynamic fluctuations generated by the sudden change in airway pressure.[12]

Physiological Shunt and Oxygen Delivery

One useful index of ventilation-perfusion inequality is the physiological shunt (also called venous admixture or wasted blood flow). The shunt equation can be used in the following form:

$$\frac{\dot{Q}sp}{\dot{Q}t} = \frac{C\dot{c}o_2 - Cao_2}{C\dot{c}o_2 - C\bar{v}o_2} \qquad (9)$$

where $\dot{Q}sp$ refers to the physiological shunt, $\dot{Q}t$ to the total lung blood flow, and $C\dot{c}o_2$, Cao_2, and $C\bar{v}o_2$ to, respectively, the oxygen content of ideal pulmonary capillary, arterial, and mixed venous blood.[21] The normal value is less than 5 percent. If a physiological shunt is determined on other than a F_{IO_2} of 1.0, hypoxemia due to $\dot{V}/\dot{Q}$ inequality contributes to the calculated shunt. "True" shunt is determined during 100 percent oxygen breathing, and overestimation may result if inadequate time is given to completely wash out poorly ventilated alveoli.[12] Po_2 electrodes may underestimate the true Po_2 at high levels when compared to blood tonometered with 100 percent O_2.[11] The magnitude of the physiological shunt is related to cardiac output. A decrease in flow or cardiac output often (but not always) decreases the shunt. Conversely, an increased cardiac output resulting from volume expansion or pharmacological intervention increases the shunt in septic shock.[11] Thus the magnitude of the shunt should be interpreted in relation to cardiac output. The arteriovenous oxygen difference often is estimated rather than measured in the critically ill patient. This "shortcut" may lead to considerable inaccuracy in the estimation of the physiological shunt. A clinical example of the determination of maximal oxygen delivery follows.

Table 4-5. Hemodynamic Profile for "Optimum" PEEP

Measurement	Unit	PEEP 5 cm H₂O	10 cm H₂O	15 cm H₂O
Blood pressure	mm Hg	140/80	132/82	112/82
Pulse	/min	100	90	103
Wedge pressure	mm Hg	10	13	15
Pulmonary artery pressure	mm Hg	45/22	37/17	51/15
Cardiac output	L/min	5.9	5.8	4
Blood gases				
pH	–	7.3	7.39	7.32
Paco₂	mm Hg	28	38	32
Pao₂	mm Hg	50	80	55
Sat	percent	85	95	82
Hemoglobin	g	12	12	12
Urine	ml/hr	50	50	30
Oxygen delivery	ml O₂/min	847	933.4	544

A 24-year old female with ARDS secondary to thrombotic thrombocytopenic purpura requires PEEP. The initial hemodynamic profile is outlined in Table 4-5. The optimum level of PEEP is 10 cm H_2O because it is associated with the best tissue oxygen delivery of 933.4 ml O_2/minute. Necessary calculations at 10 cm PEEP are, where Hgb = hemoglobin:

Tissue delivery of oxygen

$$= \text{cardiac output} \times Cao_2 \qquad (10)$$

$$Cao_2 = \text{Hgb (g)} \times 1.39 \text{ ml } O_2/\text{g Hgb}$$

$$\times So_2 + (0.003 \times Pao_2)$$

$$= 16.1 \text{ ml } O_2/100 \text{ ml blood} \qquad (11)$$

$$CO \times Cao_2 = \frac{5800 \text{ ml/min} \times 16.1 \text{ ml } O_2}{100 \text{ ml blood}}$$

$$= 933.4 \text{ ml } O_2/\text{minute}$$

The mixed venous oxygen tension ($P\bar{v}o_2$) has gained popularity as an index of tissue oxygenation, a trend facilitated by the relative ease with which $P\bar{v}o_2$ measurements can be made from the pulmonary artery catheter (Fig. 4-16). Blood drawn from a central venous catheter is not a mixed specimen; a pulmonary artery catheter sample is necessary. At best, the $P\bar{v}o_2$ reflects a weighted mean of tissue oxygenation because of variable flow rates and extraction in different organs. A $P\bar{v}o_2$ of less than 30 mm Hg is a sign of severe tissue hypoxia. We usually determine the $P\bar{v}o_2$ together with the Pao_2 when a pulmonary artery catheter is in place; we recently showed that $P\bar{v}o_2$ is an accurate assessment of the tissue oxygen in patients with hemorrhagic and hypoxic shock but is falsely high in those with endotoxin shock because of peripheral

arteriovenous shunting. Others have shown that the $P\bar{v}o_2$ at which blood lactate increases is different for patients with anemia and hypoxic hypoxia. Danek et al. suggested that $P\bar{v}o_2$ may not be quite as useful as previously assumed to estimate oxygen delivery during PEEP.[10]

When the patient is in a basal state with a constant oxygen consumption, cardiac output is inversely related to the $Cao_2 - C\bar{v}o_2$, as shown by the Fick equation:

$$\frac{O_2 \text{ consumption}}{\text{cardiac output}} = CaO_2 - C\bar{v}O_2 \quad (12)$$

Simultaneous measurement of Pao_2, $P\bar{v}o_2$, cardiac output, and hemoglobin allows ox-

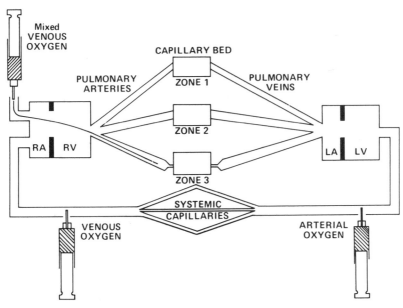

Fig. 4-16. Oxygen determinations can be obtained from the arterial, peripheral venous, or mixed venous blood. Arterial blood provides essential information about lung function. In certain circumstances, the Pao_2 might increase but be accompanied by a deterioration in oxygen delivery to tissue. For example, the application of PEEP in a relatively hypovolemic patient with ARDS might increase Pao_2 but depress cardiac output. In this situation, the arterial-mixed venous oxygen content difference increases, reflecting decreased cardiac output. Peripheral venous oxygen measurements are unreliable because they do not reflect changes from vital organs. $P\bar{v}o_2$ gives important information about decreased oxygenation despite improvement of arterial oxygenation. A $P\bar{v}o_2$ of less than 30 mm Hg suggests critical impairment of oxygen delivery. $P\bar{v}o_2$ is obtained from the pulmonary artery, as shown in this example. Also, the flow-directed pulmonary artery catheter is more likely to locate in better perfused lung regions (zone 2 or 3). In the supine patient, zone 3 is posterior, and in the upright patient it is inferior.

ygen consumption to be calculated. Danek et al. showed that as oxygen delivery decreases in patients with ARDS treated with PEEP a decrease in oxygen consumption results which may not be reflected by $P\bar{v}_{O_2}$ or even $Ca_{O_2} - C\bar{v}_{O_2}$.[10]

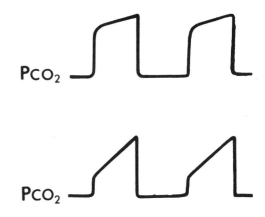

Fig. 4-17. End-tidal carbon dioxide in normal lungs and with ventilation-perfusion mismatching.

CARDIAC OUTPUT

Cardiac output is usually calculated by one of three methods: (1) Fick; (2) indicator dye dilution; and (3) thermodilution. The Fick method involves measurement of oxygen consumption and arterial-venous oxygen content difference (Eq. 12). With the indicator dye dilution method, a dye of known concentration and volume is injected into the blood. The concentration of the dye is then measured at a "downstream" site. The thermodilution method employs injection of a solution of known temperature into the right atrium or superior vena cava. Blood temperature change is measured in the pulmonary artery by a thermistor near the tip of the thermodilution catheter, and the change in resistance across a Wheatstone bridge is converted into liters per minute by a cardiac output computer.

In patients with severe respiratory failure, improvement in tissue oxygenation may require PEEP. Because oxygen delivery is the product of cardiac output and arterial oxygen content, the cardiac output or some index of changes of cardiac output should be followed as the PEEP is changed. Several studies have shown that even when Pa_{O_2} increases, significant reduction in cardiac output can result from PEEP in combination with mechanical ventilation. If cardiac output falls, the patient may be hypovolemic and cardiac filling pressure too low to be maintained in the presence of PEEP. In this case, intravascular volume repletion is indicated. Alternatively, the patient may have primary cardiac dysfunction and require inotropic agents.

Inspired and Expired Gas Analysis

The analysis of expired air has definite appeal for monitoring because of its continuous noninvasive applicability. Both the respiratory mass spectrometer[26] and new O_2 and CO_2 analyzers[5] have increased the attractiveness of such measurements. Capnography is the recording of CO_2 waveforms during the respiratory cycle and can be an important diagnostic tool. The peak expired pressure of CO_2 is directly related to the Pa_{CO_2}, which in turn is primarily dependent on CO_2 production, alveolar ventilation, and pulmonary capillary blood flow.

Measurement of expired CO_2 may be advantageous in ventilator management. Alveolar ventilation ($\dot{V}_A$) is inversely related to alveolar carbon dioxide tension (Pa_{CO_2}) as defined by the following equation:

$$\dot{V}_A = \frac{\dot{V}_{CO_2} \times 0.863}{Pa_{CO_2}} \qquad (13)$$

With continuous measurement of the expired CO_2 waveforms, end-tidal CO_2 can be measured (Fig. 4-17). The end-tidal CO_2 closely approximates Pa_{CO_2} and can serve as a readily available noninvasive estimate of the Pa_{CO_2}. Thus $P_{ET_{CO_2}}$ increases if alveolar ventilation decreases or CO_2 production increases. Access to breath-by-breath P_{ETCO_2} analysis allows the clinician to change Pa_{CO_2} gradually during mechanical ventilation. Because P_{ETCO_2} has a rather consistent relationship to Pa_{CO_2}, its measurement may decrease the amount of blood normally drawn to assess the adequacy of ventilator adjustment.[37,42] Nonintubated patients may be monitored continuously by placing the mass spectrometer probe through an oxygen catheter into the posterior nasopharynx. Such monitoring may be of help in following the progress of recently extubated patients. End-tidal CO_2 can be monitored satisfactorily on a breath-by-breath basis with infrared techniques or with a mass spectrometer. P_{ETCO_2} is dependent on tidal volume (at a constant $\dot{V}_A$). Unfortunately, the presence of $\dot{V}_A/\dot{Q}$ inequality and shunt in lung disease leads to a divergence of P_{ETCO_2} and Pa_{CO_2}. As the distribution of $\dot{V}_A/\dot{Q}$ increases, the expired air is weighted by lung units with high $\dot{V}_A/\dot{Q}$ and dead space, and the arterial blood is weighted by regions with a low $\dot{V}_A/\dot{Q}$ and shunt. This problem may be managed by doing an initial measurement to establish the arterial end-tidal difference and then adjusting for the magnitude of $\dot{V}_A/\dot{Q}$ abnormality demonstrated.

MASS SPECTROMETRY

A mass spectrometer is an instrument which determines components and measures component concentrations of a substance. The type of mass spectrometer most commonly used to measure gases is the magnetic sector mass spectrometer[26] (Fig. 4-18). Gases (oxygen, carbon dioxide, and nitrogen) are converted into a beam of ionic particles by the spectrometer, passed into a magnetic field, and deflected to a collector plate according to ionic weight. The deposited ions give up an electrical charge and establish a current proportional to the number of ions in the sample. Assuming there

are collectors present for all ions formed from the sample, the mass spectrometer measures the concentration of each gas in the sample. Inspired and expired oxygen are best measured by the mass spectrometer because most other techniques of gas analysis have a slow response time. (Some investigators have reported that the hot ceramic oxygen polarograph has a rapid enough response for breath-by-breath measurements). For computer-based calculations, a response time of 90 percent in 200 milliseconds is adequate. Most mass spectrometers and carbon dioxide analyzers and some oxygen polarographs fulfill this requirement.

If a number of beds are to be monitored, the mass spectrometer may be more cost-effective because a single unit can be multiplexed to multiple beds (Fig. 4-19). The mass spectrometer also has a faster response time, requires a smaller sampling volume, and can detect a variety of gases.[26] In practice, most difficulties with spectrometric measurements have been primarily related to obstruction of probe catheters by moisture and secretions, other problems of gas sampling, and instrument failure.

Coupling of other pulmonary measurements, e.g., flow rate, volume, and airway pressure with mass spectrometry, has proved technically troublesome at the present time for on-line computation.

If information is desired simultaneously from both the mass spectrometer and gas flow and pressure, the signals must be matched in time.[37] This problem may be difficult to solve because gas flow depends on viscosity and temperature, both of which can change. Temperature change results from the use of heated humidifiers or because the patient is hypo- or hyperthermic. The F_{IO_2} is also important because a 16 percent change in calibration occurs between air and 100 percent oxygen.[37]

Potential disadvantages to many institutions are the size of the mass spectrometer, its high initial cost, and the technical ina-

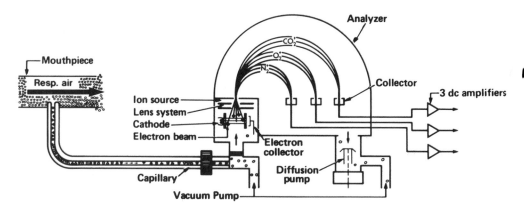

Fig. 4-18. A magnetic, respiratory-gas mass spectrometer. See text for description of operation. (Reprinted with permission from Bone RC: Monitoring patients in acute respiratory failure. Respir Care 27:700, 1982).

bility to measure carbon monoxide because of its molecular weight equivalency with nitrogen. In general, many of the claimed capabilities of the respiratory mass spectrometer in the ICU have not yet been substantiated. Literature describing the clinical applications of mass spectrometry notes that it is best viewed as a research tool with potential clinical usefulness.

On-Line Mechanics

The respiratory system behaves mechanically as a pump with flow-resistive and volume-elastic components connected in series.[44] According to Newton's third law of motion, opposing forces must be overcome to produce a volume change. An increase in pressure at the mouth (Fig. 4-8) causes a

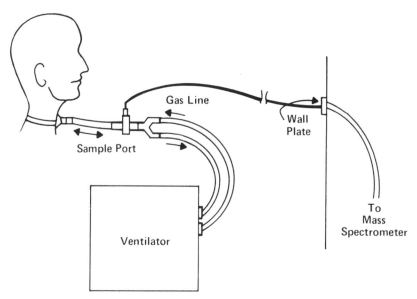

Fig. 4-19. A mass spectrometer can be multiplexed to multiple beds in a time-sharing arrangement or devoted to a single patient. (Reprinted with permission from Bone RC: Monitoring patients in acute respiratory failure. Respir Care 27:700, 1982).

flow of gas through the airways, which exhibit resistance to flow. The pressure not utilized to overcome airway resistance is dissipated by the volume elastic component (lungs and chest wall) that is capable of deformation and volume change. The total pressure applied must overcome elastic forces (1/C) to produce a volume change (V), resistive forces (R) to produce flow ($\dot{V}$), and inertial forces (I) to produce acceleration (V). These components are combined to form the equation of motion for the respiratory system:

$$P = (1/C \times V)$$
$$+ (R \times \dot{V}) + (I \times V) \quad (14)$$

Changes due to inertia (I) are small and for clinical use can be ignored.

Elucidation of the mechanical function of the lung requires the continuous recording of pressure and flow during the respiratory cycle.[37,42] Flow usually is measured by a pneumotachograph, which senses the differential pressure across a resistance in most cases. Inspiratory and expiratory pneumotachographs are a part of some single-patient monitoring systems, as in the Siemens-Elema ventilator. With in-line pneumotachographs, expired volume measurements that include volume expended by compression in and expansion of the ventilator circuit are less of a problem. However, incorporation of pneumotachographs into the ventilator system introduces an entirely new set of problems, ranging from incorrect information because of mucous plugging of the pneumotachograph to problems of calibration changes caused by varying gas concentration. Because of problems with constant measurements using the Fleish pneumotachograph, other flow-measuring devices have been developed, including the variable-orifice flowmeter, ultrasonic flowmeter, and turbulent flowmeter. These flowmeters are presently undergoing clinical trials, and their accuracy and durability are still to be determined.

The pneumotachograph must be frequently calibrated to avoid error, usually with a 1- to 3-L syringe in line with a standard spirometer. Because pneumotachographs are sensitive to temperature, humidity, and flow, they should be calibrated under clinical conditions for reliable results. Flow rates should be linear over a range of 0–3 L/second for mechanically ventilated patients. Some patients with respiratory failure may have expiratory flow rates exceeding 5 L/second, and appropriate pneumotachographs should be used in those patients.[13] In automated systems, airway pressure is measured by reliable strain gauges which provide a linear electrical output spanning a range of 0–200 cm H_2O.

A Fleish pneumotachograph with pressure and gas sampling lines leading to a mass spectrometer and computer allows simultaneous measurement of inspired and expired gases and mechanics (Fig. 4-20).

To measure lung compliance rather than lung and chest wall compliance, transpulmonary pressure must be determined. Respiratory pressure fluctuations reflected by an esophageal balloon or from the proximal port of a thermodilution Swan-Ganz catheter or a central venous catheter can be used for this purpose. Esophageal balloons are now available that attach to standard nasogastric tubes. If an esophageal balloon is used, a differential pressure transducer is needed to measure intrapleural pressure relative to mouth pressure. Lung plus chest wall compliance measured from airway pressure of the ventilated patient is affected by muscle contractions. The direct measurement of lung compliance thus adds both specificity and resolution.

Static compliance curves plotted in the pulmonary physiology laboratory are measured on a static deflation from total lung capacity. The plot of static transpulmonary pressure against lung volume is curvilinear; compliance is equal to the slope of the curve at a particular point. Unless functional residual capacity is measured and the compliance curve plotted at multiple volumes

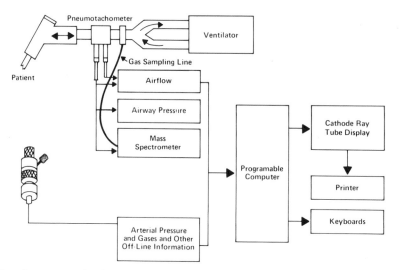

Fig. 4-20. Respiratory monitoring system. Air flow, pressure, and gas concentrations are measured simultaneously. Calculations are made by a computer utilizing these signals and off-line information. (Reprinted with permission from Bone RC: Monitoring patients in acute respiratory failure. Respir Care 27:700, 1982).

on deflation from a single breath, static compliance determinations in the ICU are not equivalent to those obtained in the pulmonary function laboratory. In the ICU the lung volume usually is unknown, and a decrease in compliance can result from a true increase in elastic recoil (pulmonary edema) or the same elastic recoil exerted on a small volume (atelectasis). Regardless of the mechanism of decrease in compliance, the knowledge that it is decreased is important and should not be ignored because of the lack of knowledge of absolute lung volume before and after the development of atelectasis or pulmonary edema.[6]

COMPUTERS

Terminology important in understanding computers is listed in the Glossary at the end of the chapter. Computer-based monitoring systems allow the rapid computation of multiple physiological variables and provide a trend analysis of changing variables. A properly programmed computer-based system assists in gathering, processing, and displaying pertinent information. With this type of information, critical care personnel are freed from repetitive duties and have more time for patient contact and decision-making. Analog signals are fed to a microcomputer after they are sorted and arranged in an order easily accepted for the computer by an electronic device called the multiplexer. The minicomputer serves as a storage and processing unit and can be programmed to perform computations automatically. It is relatively expensive. The microcomputer, conversely, is inexpensive enough to be dedicated to continuous respiratory monitoring, an advantage because the time-sharing arrangement necessary for use of central computers precludes their satisfactory utilization in monitoring rapidly changing respiratory variables.

Despite many advances in electronic, computer, and engineering technology, sophisticated monitoring of respiratory function in the critically ill patient has advanced slowly. Experience with mass spectrometry and on-line measurements of mechanics is largely anecdotal. The usefulness of these tools depends on their ability to provide information in a cost-effective and dependable fashion. Some automated monitors, e.g., those which regulate intravenous infusion rates based on physiological information, may decrease the time expended by the staff for this purpose. It is unlikely that respiratory monitoring will reach that stage of sophistication in the near future. To the contrary, the use of a mass spectrometer and continuous measurements of mechanics probably will require more staff time, rather than less, to analyze and interpret the new information. It will also require access to sophisticated bioengineering skills to keep the machinery functioning. Personnel must be trained thoroughly in the calibration, use, and maintenance of the new equipment. It is demoralizing to staff and hospital administrators to purchase an expensive piece of equipment which is "down" most of the time. These considerations are essential before purchasing such a system. Respiratory monitoring equipment will not function continuously without dedicated attention.

DEVELOPMENT OF NEW MONITORING TECHNIQUES

Special scrutiny should be applied to two areas when assessing the potential value of new monitoring techniques. The first question to be asked is: Can the technique provide the information it claims in a reliable manner under usual clinical conditions? If a method is proved in the technical sense, we must still ask: Of what value to patient management are the data produced?

Few convincing data are available to answer these questions with regard to newer, more sophisticated respiratory monitoring methods. Economic considerations demand that resources not be devoted to gathering useless information, although some redundant information is valuable for detecting errors. Possibly the most serious danger of adopting monitoring techniques uncritically

is to drown clinicians in a flood of numbers. The presentation of more data than can be assimilated can contribute to incorrect clinical decisions. This factor is too often ignored when assessing the utility of new measurements.

Electronic computers have the potential for alleviating some of these problems.[42] They can perform much of the tedious work of analyzing large amounts of data, reducing them to a form useful for making decisions. For example, they can produce summaries which list only aberrant values, reduce long lists of numbers to graphic form, or display only data considered relevant according to predetermined criteria. Even though the availability of inexpensive, powerful microcomputers makes such applications feasible, little has been done toward determining how they can best perform such clerical functions. Thus far, most effort has been devoted to overcoming difficulties associated with on-line data acquisition and to solving various technical problems. As the quantitative data generated in the ICU increase, it will become increasingly important to have machines do what machines can do best in order to spare people for tasks requiring uniquely human abilities.

WHAT BIOLOGICAL VARIABLES SHOULD BE MONITORED?

The generally accepted therapeutic goal of maintaining biological variables in the normal range is being questioned. For example, the blood pressure and cardiac output can be restored to normal values after shock in most patients, yet many still die. Survivors often show supernormal values, reflecting their stress response to a critical illness and the subsequent metabolic and circulatory adjustment. Bland et al. monitored the 20 most common variables in a series of 113 critically ill patients.[4] For arterial pressure, heart rate, central venous pressure, and cardiac output, normal values were restored in 75 percent of the survivors and 76 percent of the nonsurvivors. The authors suggest that we may not have the correct therapeutic goals or that we may not be monitoring the correct variables. The ability of commonly monitored variables, e.g., vital signs, heart rate, and hemoglobin, to predict outcome were poor.[4] Perfusion-related variables which express the interrelationship of O_2 transport to red blood cell volume and flow correlated best as predictors of outcome. Perfusion-related variables reflecting the maldistribution of systemic circulation should receive at least as much attention as variables reflecting maldistribution of the pulmonary circulation in future research.

ACKNOWLEDGMENT

This work was supported by NIH Academic Career Award 1K07 HL00518-01.

GLOSSARY: TERMINOLOGY COMMONLY USED IN AUTOMATED DATA HANDLING

Analog input: Electronic signal from a spirometer, gas analyzer, plethysmograph or pneumotachometer.

A/D converter: Analog-to-digital converter; changes electronic signals into computer language.

Bit: A single digit in a binary number system.

Byte: Includes eight bits.

Computer: An electronic device that is centrally located and is capable of performing high-speed calculations and assembling and storing information in a memory; computers can correlate and cross-reference by means of a logic or processor unit.

CRT: A video control terminal (cathode ray tube) which consists of a typewriter keyboard and viewing screen that allows the operator to manually supply information to the computer and to initiate and terminate procedures.

Hardware: The physical equipment comprising the computer and memory.

Language: A system of symbols that allows a programmer to instruct the computer to perform a certain task.

Memory: An electronic or mechanical device used to store data and programs; types of memory include magnetic core, floppy disk, magnetic tape, and tape cassettes; the amount of information that can be stored is described in bits, each of which approximates one character; memory size is usually classified in K (thousands of bits) or mega (millions of bits).

Microprocessor: A single electronic component that is hardwired or contained on chips; microprocessors usually have fixed programs and can be built into testing systems to perform calculations, do some assembly, and have a limited storage or memory.

On-line: A descriptive term denoting a direct connection between the testing instrument and the computer.

Peripherals: Devices that allow communication with computer and other devices, e.g., terminals, printers, and plotters.

Plotter: An electromechanical device that converts digital outputs into tracings.

Printer: An electromechanical device that reports data in hard-copy form on paper.

Real time: A descriptive term denoting direct user response by the computer

Shared time: A descriptive term denoting a computer with multiple users, working one at a time; the most sophisticated systems use a combination of real-time and shared-time modes.

Software: All programs including those that control computer functions and those that process input data.

Word: A specified number of bits.

REFERENCES

1. Askanazi J, Norderstrom J, Rosenbaum SH, et al: Nutrition for the patients with respiratory failure: glucose vs. fat. Anesthesiology 54:373, 1981
2. Askanazi J, Rosenbaum SH, Hyman AL, et al: Respiratory changes induced by the large glucose loads of parenteral nutrition. JAMA 243:1444, 1980
3. Bahr DE, Clark KR: Continuous arterial tonometry in essential noninvasive monitoring in anesthesia. In Gravenstein JS, Newbower RS, Ream AK, et al (eds): Monitoring Surgical Patients in the Operating Room, pp. 25–33. Grune & Stratton, New York, 1980
4. Bland R, Shoemaker WC, Czor LSC: Evaluation of the biological importance of various hemodynamic and oxygen transport variables. Crit Care Med 7:424, 1979
5. Blumenfeld W, Wolf S, McCokuggage R, et al: On-line respiratory gas monitoring. Comput Biomed Res 6:139, 1973
6. Bone RC: Diagnosis of causes for acute respiratory distress by pressure-volume curves. Chest 70:740, 1976
7. Bone RC: Monitoring patients in acute respiratory failure. Respir Care 27:700, 1982
8. Bone RC: Monitoring respiratory function in the patient with the adult respiratory distress syndrome. In Decker BC (ed): Adult Respiratory Distress Syndrome. Seminars in Respiratory Medicine. Vol. 2. pp. 140–150. 1981
9. Bone RC: Treatment of respiratory failure due to advanced obstructive lung disease. Arch Intern Med 140:1018, 1980
10. Danek SI, Lynch JP, Weg JG, et al: The dependence of oxygen uptake on oxygen delivery in the adult respiratory distress syndrome. Am Rev Respir Dis 22:387, 1980
11. Dantazker D: Abnormalities of oxygen transfer. In Bone RC (ed): Pulmonary Disease Reviews. Vol. 1. p. 1. Wiley, New York, 1980
12. Downs JB, Douglas ME: Assessment of cardiac filling pressure occurring in continuous positive pressure ventilation. Crit Care Med 8:285, 1980
13. Fallat RJ: Bedside testing and intensive care monitoring of pulmonary function. In: Standards and Controversies in Pulmonary Function Testing. California Thoracic Society Annual Postgraduate Course, January 1980
14. Fitzpatrick GF: Pulmonary artery catheterization with balloon flotation (Swan-Ganz) catheter. In Salem TJV, Cutler BS, Wheeler HB (eds): Atlas of Bedside Procedures. pp. 105–117. Little, Brown, Boston, 1979
15. Foote GA, Schabel I, Hodges M: Pulmonary complications of the flow-directed balloon-tipped catheter. N Engl J Med 290:927, 1974
16. Fox MG, Brady JS, Weintraub LR: Leukocyte larceny: a case of spurious hypoxemia. Am J Med 676:742, 1979
17. Gilbert F, Keightley JF: The arterial/alveolar oxygen tension ratio: an index of gas exchange applicable to varying inspired concentrations. Am Rev Respir Dis 109:142, 1974
18. Goecbenjan G: Continuous measurement of arterial P_{O_2}—significance and indications in intensive care. Biotel Patient Monitor 6:51, 1979
19. Gordon R: The deep sulcus sign. Radiology 136:25, 1980
20. Ian EM, Heldman JJ, Chen SS: Coronary hemodynamics and oxygen utilization after hematocrit variations in hemorrhage. Am J Physiol 243:H325, 1980
21. Jordan E, Eveleigh MC, Gurdjion F, et al: Venous admixture in human septic shock: comparative effects of blood volume expansion, dopamine infusion, and isoproterenol infusion on mismatching of ventilation and pulmonary blood flow in peritonitis. Circulation 60:155, 1979
22. Luterman A, Horovitz JH, Carrico PC, et al: Withdrawal from positive end-expiratory pressure. Surgery 83:328, 1978
23. Newell JC, Shah DM, Dutton RE, et al: Pulmonary pressure-volume relationships in traumatized man. J Surg Res 26:114, 1979
24. Osborne JJ, Raison CA, Beaumont JD, et al: Respiratory causes of "sudden unex-

plained arrhythmia'' in post-thoracotomy patients. Surgery 69:24, 1971

25. Peabody JL, Willis MM, Gregory GA, et al: Clinical limitations and advantages of transcutaneous oxygen electrodes. Acta Anesth Scand [Suppl] 68:76, 1978

26. Popovich J, Bone RC, Wilson F, et al: Mass spectrometry. Respir Ther 10:50, 1980

27. Ream AK: Systolic, diastolic, mean or pulse: which is the best measurement of arterial pressure. In Gravenstein JS, Newbower RS, Ream AK, et al (eds): Monitoring Surgical Patients in the Operating Room, pp. 53–73. Grune & Stratton, New York, 1980

28. Rhea JT, Sonnenberg EV, McLoud TC: Basilar pneumothorax in the supine adult. Radiology 133:593, 1979

29. Rothe CF, Kim KC: Measuring systolic arterial blood pressure: possible errors from extension tubes or disposable transducer domes. Crit Care Med 8:683, 1980

30. Sahn SA, Lakshminarayan S: Bedside criteria for discontinuation of mechanical ventilation. Chest 63:1002, 1973

31. Shimada Y, Yoshiga I, Tamala K, et al: Evaluation of the progress and prognosis of acult respiratory distress syndrome: simple physiologic measurement. Chest 76:180, 1979

32. Skillman JJ, Awwad HK, Moore FD: Plasma protein kinetics of the early transcapillary refill after hemorrhage in man. Surg Gynecol Obstet 123:983, 1967

33. Suwa K, Hedley-White J, Bendixen HH: Circulation and physiological dead space changes on controlled ventilation of dogs. J Appl Physiol 231:1855, 1966

34. Sweet SJ, Glenney JP, Fitzibbons JP, et al: Effect of acute renal failure and respiratory failure in the surgical intensive care unit. Am J Surg 141:492, 1981

35. Tremper KK, Waxman K, Bowman R, et al: Transcutaneous oxygen monitoring during arrest and CPR. Crit Care Med 8:377, 1980

36. Tremper KK, Waxman K, Shoemaker WC: Effects of hypoxia and shock on transcutaneous P_{O_2} values in dogs. Crit Care Med 7:526, 1979

37. Turney SZ, McAslan TC, Cowley RA: The continuous measurement of pulmonary gas exchange and mechanics. Ann Thorac Surg 13:229, 1973

38. Versmold HT, Linderkamp O, Holzmann M, et al: Limits of tcP_{O_2} monitoring in sick neonates: relation to blood pressure, blood volume, peripheral blood flow and acid base status. Acta Anaesth Scand [Suppl] 68:88, 1978

39. Wagner PD: Diffusion and chemical reaction in pulmonary gas exchange. Physiol Rev 57:257, 1977

40. Wagner PD, West JB: Effects of diffusion impairment on O_2 and CO_2 time courses in pulmonary capillaries. J Appl Physiol 33:62, 1972

41. Wagner PD, Saltzman HA, West JB: Measurement of continuous distributions of ventilation-perfusion ratios: theory. J Appl Physiol 36:588, 1974

42. Wald A, Jason D, Murphy TW, et al: A computer system for respiratory parameters. Comput Biomed Res 2:411, 1969

43. West JB, Wagner PD: Pulmonary gas exchange. In: West JB (ed): Bioengineering Aspects of the Lung. Marcel Dekker, New York, 1977

44. Wilson RS: Monitoring the lung: mechanics and volume. Anesthesiology 45:135, 1976

45. Zwillich CW, Pierson DJ, Creach CE, et al: Complications of assisted ventilation. Am J Med 57:161, 1974

5

Pulmonary Hygiene and Artificial Airway Management

Robert R. Demers
Richard S. Irwin

Art is the only clean thing on earth . . .
Les Foules de Lourdes, 1906 Joris Karl
Huysmans

Hygiene is defined as "conditions or practices that are conducive to health."[153] This presentation dealing with pulmonary hygiene and artificial airway management therefore begins with a consideration of the function of the normal, healthy airway and proceeds to a discussion of altered physiological states.

NORMAL FUNCTIONS

Heat and Moisture Exchange

The upper airway is admirably suited to its task of warming inspired gases to body temperature and saturating those gases with water vapor.[91] This function is facilitated by exposing the inspirate to a moist and richly vascular membrane. In a canine model, inspiration through an intact upper airway results in a gas mixture that approaches body temperature and full saturation at the car-

ina. However, complete warming to body temperature and full saturation do not occur until the airways fully 15 cm below the carina are reached.[46] These findings probably apply to heat and moisture exchange prevailing in the human respiratory tract.

The properties of the lung parenchyma qualify it as a nearly perfect heat source and heat sink. Clinically, it has been observed that the inhalation of superheated air or even flames sufficiently hot to singe the nasal hairs cause tracheal burns but no grossly observable burns of the mucosa lining the peripheral airway. It seems that only steam is able to overwhelm the heat-exchanging capacity of the lung parenchyma and produce frank burns at the level of the peripheral airways.

The conducting airways also seem to be surprisingly efficient as a moisture exchanger. Complete saturation of inspired gases persists even in the face of marked systemic dehydration.[17] The quantitative moisture exchange characteristics of the respiratory tract seem to be widely misunderstood by clinicians. On occasion, insensible water loss via the respiratory tract is invoked as a possible mechanism for substantial variations in the body weight of critically ill patients. As the following calculations indicate, however, volumetric water losses over a 24-hour period are rather modest and are therefore unlikely to account for appreciable variations in body weight. Insensible water loss from the respiratory tract depends, of course, on the relative humidity of the inspired air. One can calculate the maximum insensible water loss as follows:

Assuming a minute ventilation of exactly 6 L of absolutely dry air at sea level (where barometric pressure equals 760 torr) and a normal body temperature of 37°C (310° Kelvin, at which water vapor pressure equals 47 torr), water vapor excretion is:

$$(6 \text{ L}) \times (47/760) = 0.371 \text{ L/minute}$$

Over a 24-hour period, water vapor production would be:

$$(0.371 \text{ L/minute}) \times (60 \text{ minute/hour}) \times (24 \text{ hour/day}) = 534 \text{ L/day}$$

This volume of water vapor is referenced to body temperature and pressure (BTP). The corresponding water vapor volume at standard temperature and pressure (STP) can be calculated by the appropriate temperature correction factor:

$$(534 \text{ L}) \times (273°\text{K}/310°\text{K}) = 470 \text{ L}$$

As 1 mole of any gas at standard temperature and pressure occupies 22.4 L, the number of moles of water vapor represented by this volume is:

$$(470 \text{ L})/(22.4 \text{ L/mole}) = 21 \text{ moles}$$

The mass of 21 moles of water is:

$$(21 \text{ moles}) \times (18 \text{ g/mole}) = 378 \text{ g}$$

This is, of course, equivalent to a volume of 378 ml of water. Naturally, to the extent that inhaled gases are partially saturated with water vapor, this figure will decrease. As a limiting case, if inhaled gases are fully saturated at body temperature before being drawn into the respiratory tract, insensible water loss will be zero.

Protection of the Lower Respiratory Tract

The lower respiratory tract is protected from the inhalation of noxious fumes and particles by nonimmunological and immunological mechanisms. Together these defenses keep the lower respiratory tract (below the vocal cords) sterile in normal, conscious man. This fact is particularly impressive when one considers the number of bacteria normally present in the naso- and oropharynges. The density of bacteria approaches 10^5/ml on tooth surfaces, 10^6/ml from gingival scrapings, 10^7/ml in saliva, and up to 10^9/ml within the gingival crypts.[66,70] This latter concentration seems to represent the upper limiting population density for bacteria or, quite literally, "wall-to-wall bugs."

An attempt to catalogue each of the species of organism that inhabits the respiratory tract is hopelessly time-consuming. However, it is useful to consider the major components of what constitutes "normal flora." *Staphylococcus* species predominate in the nose, whereas oral flora consists primarily of *Streptococcus* (anaerobes and *Strep. Viridans*) and *Neisseria* species. Viridans group streptococci and *Neisseria* species predominate in the normal pharynx just as they do in the mouth. Despite the fact that we all "silently" aspirate oropharyngeal secretions during sleep,[68] lower respiratory tract secretions sampled by transtracheal aspiration are free of bacteria.[66] This almost certainly must be due to efficient clearance and detoxification.

Nonimmunological Mechanisms. *Aerodynamic Filtration.* Particulate pollutants are scrubbed from inhaled air through the mechanisms of mechanical filtration, inertial impaction, sedimentation, and diffusion.[143] Particles larger than 10 μm in diameter are filtered out in the nose (nasal fibrissae and turbinates), mouth, pharynx, and larynx. Most particles that are smaller than 1 μm in diameter are not deposited at all within the respiratory tract but, rather, are expelled in exhaled gas. The small percentage of submicronic particles that deposit themselves within the respiratory tract, however, do so between the nose and the larynx. Particles 5 to 10 μm in diameter impact in the airways where turbulent flow occurs (at bifurcations that define the successive generations of airways). Only particles 1–3 μm in diameter actually reach the alveoli.

Laryngeal Reflex. This reflex protects against inhalation of fluid, food, other foreign bodies (i.e., suction catheters), and noxious fumes. When pharyngeal swallowing begins to push an ingested bolus through the relaxed upper esophageal sphincter (the cricopharyngeus muscle), the vocal cords immediately close. Similarly, the cords close as soon as a noxious fume is detected in the inhaled air. Normally, this reflex becomes sluggish with advancing years, with sedation, and during sleep.[68] Sleep provides a potential for double jeopardy for clinically significant aspiration because the cough reflex is depressed during non-rapid-eye-movement (REM) sleep and virtually absent during REM sleep.[68]

Mucociliary Clearance. Particles that reach the tracheobronchial tree are cleared and detoxified by a moving, thin continuous sheet—the "mucous blanket." Normally, about 100 ml of mucus is produced in 24 hours by submucosal glands (under parasympathetic nervous control) and by goblet cells that produce mucus when directly irritated. Mucus consists of a mixture of water and complex polysaccharides that are moved along toward the pharynx by the coordinated rhythmic motion of the cilia; it contains lysozymes and other proteases that detoxify particles as they are being cleared. Once it reaches the pharynx, the mucus is swallowed along with whatever materials were trapped on its sticky surface. The transport velocity of the mucous blanket varies according to the site of measurement; transport velocity is slowest in the terminal bronchioles, gradually increases at the intermediate airways, and is highest in the central airways and trachea where mucus is mobilized toward the pharynx at a rate of 6–18 mm/minute.[128]

Mucociliary clearance is not normal in the presence of the following depressant influences: (1) long-term cigarette smoke exposure; (2) atmospheric pollutants, e.g., sulfur dioxide and nitrogen dioxide; (3) hyperoxia; (4) severe hypoxia; (5) hypercapnia; and (6) general inhalational anesthesia.[150] Aside from these influences, mucociliary clearance is depressed in patients with asthma, cystic fibrosis,[158] and chronic bronchitis.

Alveolar Macrophages. Particles that reach the alveoli are phagocytized by the alveolar macrophage,[31] which is virtually omnivorous and ingests any organic or inorganic particulate debris or bacteria it encounters. Once the macrophage engulfs its prey, the material is digested by powerful enzymes that are contained in intracellular organelles called lysosomes. The pulmonary alveolar macrophage is the most important bactericidal defense. It does not function normally when exposed to the following influences: (1) lower respiratory tract viral infection; (2) corticosteroids; (3) alcohol; (4) chronic liver disease; (5) an arterial pH ≤7.2; (6) cigarette smoke exposure; and (7) an alveolar oxygen tension <25 torr.

Cough. Normal subjects rarely cough unless mucociliary clearance is inadequate or overwhelmed. The act of coughing involves a complex reflex arc that begins with irritation of a receptor. Once the reflex is initiated, it proceeds according to a fixed pattern.[71] Impulses from the receptor are conducted to a central area via afferent nerves and then transmitted down appropriate efferent nervous pathways to the expiratory musculature. The cough is comprised of three phases. During the inspiratory phase the vocal cords open widely, a deep inspiration occurs, and high lung volumes are achieved. The compressive phase of cough begins with closure of the vocal cords, continues with the active contraction of expiratory muscles, and concludes with sudden opening of the vocal cords.

Although closure of the vocal cords is an integral part of the compressive phase in the intact airway, it is not mandatory for the production of an effective cough because the muscles of expiration are capable of producing extremely high intrathoracic pressures even with the vocal cords open.

The final, expiratory phase of cough consists of coordinated movements of the vocal cords, respiratory muscles, and tracheobronchial tree. The phase begins with opening of the vocal cords and explosive release of trapped intrathoracic gas. Striking dynamic changes occur during the expiratory phase of cough: The vocal cords and the membranous posterior aspect of the laryngeal wall vibrate forcefully, literally shaking secretions loose from the larynx.[149] Simultaneously, the abdominal muscles that were recruited during the compressive phase of cough contract yet further. The progressive shortening of these muscles after the opening of the vocal cords serves to maintain a high linear velocity.

Clinically, the crucial role of the expiratory musculature is manifested by the vigorous cough that may be elicited from patients whose vocal cords are kept open by indwelling endotracheal tubes. A careful consideration of the "equal pressure point" concept [99] suggests that coughing at large lung volumes results in dynamic compression of large airways, and coughing at small lung volumes dynamically compresses smaller airways. Thus, during a series of coughs starting with a full inspiration, secretions are first cleared from the larger airways. As lung volume decreases with successive coughs, secretions are moved from smaller, peripheral bronchi to the central airways. After another deep breath and series of coughs, secretions from all of the airways can be eventually cleared. It is useful to note that those airways in which cough is most effective in clearing secretions are precisely the same airways in which cough receptors are most richly distributed.

Immunological Mechanisms. Local and systemic immunity enhance the nonspecific, nonimmunological defense mechanisms cited earlier.[59] For instance, immunoglobulin G (IgG) and complement opsonize bacteria for the pulmonary alveolar macrophage; secretory IgA, the most important mechanism to neutralize viruses, also renders bacterial antigenic material nonimmunogenic. The T and B lymphocytes modulate the activity of alveolar macrophages and neutrophils in various infections (especially tuberculosis, viral infections, and fungal infections).

FACTORS THAT AFFECT NORMAL FUNCTIONS

Nasotracheal Suctioning

Nasotracheal suctioning involves the introduction of a suction catheter into the trachea by way of the nose in a nonintubated patient. The procedure is performed for the purpose of evacuating secretions from a patient whose normal defense functions have failed. The patient may or may not have a nasopharyngeal airway in place. This procedure may also adversely affect a patient's normal functions.

Adverse Effects on Nonimmunological Functions. Any foreign material, including liquids, foodstuffs, or a suction catheter may elicit a vagally mediated laryngeal reflex. This reflex may take the form of coughing, subtotal obstruction secondary to stimulation of the laryngeal musculature (this usually presents in the form of stridor, a high-pitched "crowing" sound during inspiration), or total obstruction of the airway secondary to glottic adduction (laryngospasm, the forceful closing of the vocal cords), which completely obstructs both inspiratory and expiratory air flow. Although respiratory impulses are no doubt being propagated down the phrenic nerves, the patient is effectively in respiratory arrest.

Laryngospasm. Laryngospasm may terminate spontaneously if the offending instrument is immediately withdrawn. However, if laryngospasm occurred only after the catheter was introduced through the cords, one may not be able to withdraw the catheter; in fact, one should not attempt to do so forcefully because vigorous stimulation can be expected to provoke a persistent episode. Of course, the laryngospasm is self-limiting to the extent that the patient sustains a sufficient degree of cerebral hypoxia to cause syncope. Unfortunately, cardiac dysrhythmias and asystole frequently supervene, necessitating cardiopulmonary resuscitation. The threat of laryngospasm secondary to nasotracheal suctioning is sufficiently real to justify the following safeguards:

1. A self-inflating resuscitator bag capable of delivering high concentrations of oxygen, fitted with an appropriate mask, oxygen reservoir, and oxygen source, should be available. In the event that the suction catheter is trapped between the vocal cords, preparations to ventilate the patient with virtually 100 percent oxygen should be instituted immediately. The face mask should be fitted as snugly as possible to the patient's face and moderate pressure applied to the bag. Until the vocal cords open, of course, it is impossible to ventilate the patient. However, one should be prepared to ventilate as soon as the cords relax so as to prevent or minimize undesirable cardiac side effects. Cardiac rhythm disturbances, it must be noted, may be present on the basis of cardiac inhibition secondary to vagal stimulation as well as myocardial hypoxia.

2. Oxygen administration through the suction catheter should NOT be attempted. Such attempts are bound to be time-consuming and largely ineffective because of the small caliber of the catheter and the requirement that it serve as a route for the expired as well as the inspired gas. Furthermore, the already small lumen of the suction catheter is likely to be compromised because of the external pressure of the constricted vocal cords.

3. Some institutions require that nasotracheal suctioning be performed only by a physician. The reason for this policy resides in the realization that cardiopulmonary resuscitation is optimal in the presence of a physician, and the only way to ensure that one is present is to insist that the procedure be performed only by the physician.

4. Inadvertent stimulation of the vagal reflex is aggravated by such factors as preexisting hypoxemia, inappropriately vigorous advancement of the suction catheter, or application of high suction while the catheter is being introduced. Prophylactic measures aimed at minimizing vagal stimulation include: prior administration of oxygen; smooth, gentle introduction of the catheter through the cords; and the avoidance of active suction until the catheter is in the appropriate position.

Colonization/Infection of the Lower Respiratory Tract. The performance of nasotracheal suctioning obliges one to pass the catheter through the upper airway, which is teeming with microorganisms even in healthy subjects. In hospitalized patients the flora changes to predominantly facultative, gram-negative enteric bacilli.[73,130] Advancement of the catheter through the vocal cords compromises the role of the larynx as a guardian of the lower respiratory tract. Any procedure which results in the introduction of a device through the vocal cords (i.e., fiberoptic bronchoscopy, tracheal intubation, or nasotracheal suctioning) is certain to cause colonization of the lower respiratory tract and potentially set the stage for subsequent frank infection. Whether infection actually occurs in the wake of colonization depends on multiple factors, including the prevailing status of the host's natural defenses and the species, concentration, and virulence of the organism(s) involved.

Impairment of Mucociliary Escalator. The local trauma caused by a suction catheter has been shown to abolish ciliary activity in the area of trauma with subsequent stasis of secretions.[156] This effect, termed "puddling," is not peculiar to nasotracheal suctioning but can occur in association with endobronchial trauma from any cause. In view of the fact that the reason for performing nasotracheal suctioning is to clear secretions, traumatization of the airway mucosa and puddling are singularly counterproductive. Here again, frequent repetition, lack of skill or delicacy on the part of the operator, and/or high levels of "negative" pressure during suctioning predispose to impairment of mucociliary clearance.

Impairment of Cough. Impingement of the suction catheter on those parts of the airway supplied with cough receptors (which includes the nasopharynx, oropharynx, hypopharynx, larynx, trachea, carina, and bronchi) frequently triggers an involuntary series of coughs. This may actually be advantageous in patients who cannot be coached to cough otherwise. On the other hand, it may cause mild discomfort or pain. Relative contraindications to stimulating a cough may be the presence of fractured ribs, systemic hypotension (wherein a modified Valsalva maneuver may cause circulatory embarrassment), or intracranial hypertension (which may be aggravated by the transmission of elevated intrathoracic pressures to the cranial vault).

Other Complications and Their Prevention. *Bacteremia.* Transient bacteremia has been documented in association with a wide variety of procedures, including dental manipulation, genitourinary instrumentation, sigmoidoscopy, bronchoscopy, barium enema, percutaneous liver biopsy, and tonsillectomy. Bacteremia has also been reported in association with nasotracheal suctioning.[86] Any procedure which inflicts trauma on a membranous surface that harbors a dense population of resident organisms predisposes to such a result. It is well appreciated that nasotracheal suctioning or analogous procedures, e.g., fiberoptic bronchoscopy, are associated with parenchymal infiltration, fever, and pneumonitis.

Practitioners should use appropriately supple catheters and introduce them smoothly by the use of gentle yet firm pressure. When introducing the catheter through the nostril, the distal tip should be directed inferiorly and medially along the floor of the nasal cavity; improper direction of the catheter along a superior and lateral course may cause it to "hang up" in the area of the nasal turbinates.[44] Soon after the catheter is introduced into the nostril, one usually encounters resistance because the catheter impinges on the posterior wall of the nasopharynx. At this point, forceful poking should be avoided because this portion of the nasopharynx is exquisitely sensitive. Steady, gentle pressure coupled with rotation of the catheter between the fingers usually succeeds in deflecting it toward the hypopharynx. If difficulty is encountered at this point, insertion of a soft polyvinyl chloride or latex nasopharyngeal airway facilitates introduction of the catheter.[123] These airways also serve to shield the pharynx from avulsion, abrasion, or traumatic perforation.[146]

Mucosal Trauma. Mucosal hemorrhage and erosion can occur during nasotracheal suctioning, endotracheal suctioning (through an endotracheal or tracheostomy tube),[1] or suctioning through a bronchoscope. Entrapment of the mucosa and unintentional biopsy are likely to occur when an excessive amount of negative pressure is applied and when the catheter's thumb port is occluded continuously. The wisdom of using unregulated suction or, indeed, any suction level in excess of 100 torr subatmospheric pressure is open to question. The results of one animal study[84] convincingly demonstrated that tracheobronchial trauma was likely to occur when a negative pressure of 200 torr was used to suction simulated mucus from the airway. The same study revealed that a subatmospheric pressure of 100 torr was far less likely to inflict damage, yet was as effective in terms of aspiration efficiency.

Various configurations of suction catheter distal tips have been devised in an effort to prevent direct impingement of the aspiration channels on the mucosa.[124] However, the results of a clinical study wherein patients' airways were directly visualized with a fiberoptic bronchoscope suggests that catheter design is of only minor importance.[74] Rather, mucosal trauma during suctioning seemed to be related to repetition, vigor, and amount of suction applied regardless of the type of catheter used. Furthermore, the distal tip of "atraumatic" catheters is rather bulky and very difficult to introduce through the nasopharynx. In summary then, operators are well advised to use regulated suction and to occlude the thumb port intermittently instead of continuously.

Hypoxemia. Potentially serious degrees of arterial desaturation have been documented during nasotracheal[114] and orotracheal[16] suctioning. Decreases in arterial saturation are rather predictable in view of the fact that suctioning evacuates large amounts of gas from the airway along with secretions. Prior administration of a gas mixture that is rich in oxygen is advisable before nasotracheal suctioning is actually performed.

Cardiac Dysrhythmias. If preoxygenation is either neglected or inadequate, nasotracheal suctioning is accompanied by arterial hypoxemia, placing the patient at risk for development of cardiac dysrhythmias or cardiac arrest.[3,133] The mechanical stimulation of the vocal cords by the catheter itself constitutes an additional stimulus that may provoke cardiac rhythm disturbances.[55] Actually, it is rather surprising that cardiac dysrhythmias, laryngospasm, and cardiac arrest do not occur even more frequently from nasotracheal suctioning when one considers, for example, that they occur during transnasal flexible fiberoptic bronchoscopy, another nasotracheal instrumentation procedure. Even though the patient inhales an anesthetic aerosol and topical anesthetic is squirted directly onto the vocal cords, cardiac dysrhythmias and laryngospasm are still observed with the latter procedure.[38] These sobering observations should temper the prudent practitioner's enthusiasm for nasotracheal suctioning and emphasize that the procedure is contraindicated for patients who demonstrate profound refractory hypoxemia or an irritable myocardium.

TRACHEAL INTUBATION*

Tracheal intubation is the placement of a flexible tube, usually a thermoplastic polymer, e.g., polyvinyl chloride, into the trachea by way of either the mouth or the nose. Successful intubation of the trachea with a

---

* This section draws heavily from the excellent review by Stauffer and Silvestri.[140]

cuffed endotracheal tube serves to isolate the trachea, permitting positive-pressure inflation of the lungs and allowing delivery of a precisely controlled mixture of gases without fear of admixture with entrained air. The presence of a properly inflated cuff also protects the patient against aspiration of gastric and pharyngeal material, which is especially important in patients whose laryngeal or "gag" reflex is impaired or absent. Finally, the endotracheal tube provides direct access to the lower respiratory tract and allows repeated suctioning of the lower airway without invoking the hazards associated with vagal stimulation of those portions of the airway lying above the trachea.

In general, tracheal intubation is relatively easy, rapid, and safe. Only a minimal amount of equipment is necessary, and this equipment is easily assembled and transported. A skilled intubator can perform the procedure almost anywhere, even in the field, establishing an airway within a minute or less. The surgical risks and expense of a tracheostomy are avoided. Although morbidity is a significant problem (see below), the mortality associated with tracheal intubation is very low. The procedure is easily reversible so that if the patient's clinical status should abruptly improve extubation can be performed immediately.

The disadvantages of tracheal intubation, however, are numerous and noteworthy. Traumatic complications encountered during intubation are usually the result of inexperience, poor technique, or poor judgment. Tooth avulsion has been reported to occur in up to 2 percent of oral intubations, and nasal bleeding was observed in 54 percent of nasal intubations in a prospective study.[138] Vasoconstrictive agents are useful to prevent nasal bleeding, and topical anesthetics (sprays and water-soluble jellies) are useful to prevent the pain associated with nasotracheal intubation. Retropharyngeal and hypopharyngeal perforation have been reported which may lead to ab-

scess formation, subcutaneous emphysema, and mediastinitis.[65,139] Additional complications occur in the form of vocal cord hematomas, dislocation of the arytenoid cartilages,[21] pulmonary aspiration (in up to 19 percent of intubations of critically ill adults)[145] inadvertent intubation of the right mainstem bronchus (in about 9 percent of intubations performed in the ICU of a teaching hospital),[160] cardiac dysrhythmias (seen in 58 percent of nasal intubations and 32 percent of oral intubations in one study),[94] and cardiac arrest (in less than 1 percent of ICU intubations).[138]

Numerous complications may occur after intubation has been performed. The most common and most severe are referable to the larynx and trachea. Laryngeal injury takes the form of laryngeal edema (an inflammatory response), laryngeal ulceration, and laryngeal hematoma. Whereas mild to moderate laryngeal inflammation is unavoidable, severe inflammation and edema was reported in 29 percent of patients examined at autopsy.[138]

Laryngeal ulceration is also common, uniformly occurring at the posterior rim of the glottis where the shaft of the tube exerts persistent pressure on the mucosa. The incidence of ulceration ranges from 50 to 100 percent, depending on the duration of the intubation and other factors.[47,48] Ulceration may even occur after anesthetic intubation of only a few hours' duration. Hematoma of the larynx has been observed in up to 10 percent of tracheal intubations.[82]

Laryngeal injuries classified as severe were seen in 62 of 1000 patients after controlled anesthetic intubation; vocal cord hematoma was found in 45 of these 62 patients.[75] In intubated children, subglottic stenosis is common and constitutes a serious complication owing to the smaller size of the airway and its poor tolerance of a further reduction in the size of the lumen. On the other hand, serious and persistent sequelae of postintubation laryngeal injury are quite uncommon in adults.[89,132,154] Lindholm's study impressively demonstrates that laryngeal granulomas are a virtually universal finding after extubation in adults and that these lesions heal spontaneously and without incident in the vast majority of patients.[89] In addition to damage inflicted at the level of the vocal cords, endotracheal tubes may also cause injury at the site of the inflatable cuff and at the level of the tip of the endotracheal tube. Pressure-mediated cuff injury is far more common and more serious than the damage observed at the tube tip.

The incidence of mechanical problems related to the maintenance of the endotracheal tube have been reported in 6 percent of intubations.[138] These include accidental disconnection from the ventilator; obstruction of the tube's lumen secondary to kinking, intraluminal secretions, or clots; occlusion of oral tubes by biting; encroachment on the lumen of the endotracheal tube by integral cuffs; herniation of the cuff over the tip of the endotracheal tube; laceration of the cuff/cuff filling line/pilot balloon; or failure of inflating valves.[14,67,78,87,117] A prospective study of ICU patients revealed that patients extubated themselves 13 percent of the time.[138] Self-extubation is more frequent with oral tubes than with nasal tubes, probably because the former are less comfortable for the patient.[119] Lip ulceration has been reported in 5 percent of patients with oral tubes.[138]

Miscellaneous injuries ascribed to nasotracheal tubes cover a broad spectrum and include alar [159] and septal necrosis, purulent infection and bacteremia[13] (which is not seen with orotracheal tubes[12]), sinusitis,[5,60] and otitis media,[10] presumably caused by obstruction of the eustachian tube with the nasotracheal tube. Pulmonary aspiration in the presence of cuffed tubes has been seen in up to 20 percent of critical care patients.[11] Several other complications of tracheal intubation are very common although virtually never documented objectively. These include inadequate nutrition, pain and dis-

comfort, and an inability to speak. Certainly the latter must be extremely distressing to a patient who finds himself thrust into a completely foreign and ominous environment. Such patients would surely have many questions to ask and feelings to share if they could speak. One of the most surprising facts about intensive care psychosis and depression is that it does not occur much more frequently.

The act of extubation is associated with complications of its own, including pain and discomfort, sore throat,[90] dysphagia, stridor[93] (seen in less than 1 percent of cases and usually caused by laryngeal edema), bronchoconstriction, laryngospasm,[15] respiratory obstruction, aspiration, and cardiac arrest.[87]

Postextubation complications are usually related to laryngeal or tracheal injury inflicted during the period of intubation. Hoarseness is virtually universal,[138] sometimes persisting for several weeks.[154] The differential diagnosis for persistent hoarseness includes vocal cord paresis or paralysis or a structural lesion of the larynx. Sore throat and dysphagia are fairly common after extubation but rarely persistent.[87] Although vocal cord granulomas are absorbed uneventfully in the vast majority of patients, they may rarely enlarge after extubation, necessitating surgical extirpation.[89] Laryngeal synechiae (cicatricial webs) may similarly present with signs of upper airway obstruction as does laryngeal stenosis.[132] Fortunately, severe and persistent laryngeal complications secondary to tracheal intubation are extremely rare.[40,89] Subclinical degrees of tracheal stenosis are traceable to circumferential granulation tissue at the cuff site or at the level of the cricoid cartilage. Stauffer et al. found greater than 10 percent airway narrowing in 5 of 27 adult ICU patients after intubation.[138] Laryngeal incompetence with resultant aspiration is a rather common finding in patients extubated after anesthesia,[20] but its incidence after prolonged intubation has not been studied.

Orotracheal Versus Nasotracheal Intubation

Orotracheal intubation is preferred in most emergencies because it is easier and faster than nasotracheal intubation. Although an indwelling orotracheal tube stimulates the gag reflex and is less comfortable than a nasotracheal tube, the act of placing an orotracheal tube is far less painful than placement of a nasotracheal tube. Unconscious patients may be intubated within seconds with an orotracheal tube in the hands of a skilled practitioner. Oral intubation is easier to learn, and the tube is less likely to kink (although more likely to be occluded by biting) than its nasal counterpart because of its lesser angle of curvature. The lesser curvature and shorter length of an oral tube affords less air flow resistance (to the ventilator during mechanical ventilation or to the patient during spontaneous ventilation) and offers less resistance to the passage of secretions, suction catheters, or a fiberoptic bronchoscope. Bronchoscopists also prefer an oral endotracheal tube because, for a given patient, it is usually one full size larger than the corresponding nasal tube. This difference may prove to be crucially important if one is contemplating bronchoscopy for the purpose of suctioning secretions or performing a biopsy. On the other hand, if bronchoscopy is being performed merely to visualize the airways or the cuff site, a pediatric flexible fiberoptic bronchoscope can be used with even the smallest adult tubes (providing, of course, that such an instrument is available).

Orotracheal intubation is associated with several disadvantages, including the labial, dental, oral, and oropharyngeal complications related to direct trauma mentioned earlier. Oral intubation requires that a laryngoscope be available. Laryngoscopy and oral intubation are not well tolerated by the conscious patient, and sedative drugs usually must be administered.

Nursing care of the patient with an indwelling orotracheal tube is more time-consuming, the position of the tube within the mouth must frequently be changed, and the mouth must be carefully inspected for complications. It is difficult for a patient with an oral tube to swallow secretions and virtually impossible to swallow food. Oral intubation most often requires an oropharyngeal airway or a bite block, either of which may be unpleasant. Oral tubes are aesthetically unpleasant because of odor, secretions, and the elaborate taping necessary to hold the tube in place. Talking is impossible with either a nasotracheal or an orotracheal tube, but with the latter the patient finds it difficult to communicate even by lip motion. The tape securing the tube may itself produce or obscure dental, mucosal, and lingual complications.

Nasotracheal intubation enjoys many advantages over oral intubation. Because the nasotracheal tube is not inserted through the retromolar triangle where gag and vomiting reflexes are initiated, it is far more comfortable for the conscious patient. Similarly, nasal intubation is advantageous in patients with full stomachs who may aspirate gastric secretions if vomiting is triggered by orotracheal intubation. Nasotracheal intubation can often be performed by the "blind" technique if a laryngoscope is not available or if laryngoscopy is not tolerated by the hyperreflexic patient. Nasal intubation is indicated if the oral route is difficult, hazardous, or obstructed by an oral or oropharyngeal lesion (in the setting of mandibular or maxillofacial trauma, trismus, patients with short "bull" necks, or uncooperative patients). Patients with nasotracheal tubes in place can usually swallow saliva, and some patients can even sip liquids. Mouth care is far easier, and an oropharyngeal airway or bite block is not required because the nasal tube cannot be obstructed by biting (this advantage makes nasotracheal intubation preferable for patients with seizure disorders, trismus, or decerebrate rigidity). Nasal tubes are better tolerated for extended periods of intubation because there is far less gagging, pain, and discomfort than with their oral counterparts. Laryngeal ulceration is only about half as common with nasal intubation as with oral intubation,[48] presumably because the nasal tube exerts less leverage and pressure on the cords. Nasal tubes are easier to anchor, thus rendering self-extubation and migration of the tube into the mainstem bronchus less likely.

Nasotracheal intubation does carry some notable disadvantages. The procedure is not suitable for emergency intubation because preparation of the nasal mucosa with analgesic and vasoconstrictive agents is not possible. If the patient is not properly prepared in this manner, epistaxis and septal or turbinate injury are likely to be severe, whether the patient is conscious or unconscious. Septal injury by the nasotracheal tube is particularly likely to occur if a large and/or rigid nasogastric tube is in place within the opposite nostril.

Tracheostomy

Many clinicians believe that tracheostomy provides the optimal route for long-term airway maintenance, tracheal toilet, and mechanical ventilation. The procedure dates back to the sixteenth century[56] but was rarely performed until the diphtheria epidemics of the last century when it gained favor as a definitive operation to relieve upper airway obstruction. It has only been over the last three decades that substantial literature has accumulated relative to tracheostomy, and much of this literature has focused on complications and limitations of the procedure.[110]

Complications. The overall complication rate of tracheostomy is substantial. Operative complications include subcutaneous or mediastinal emphysema[138] (13 percent incidence); hemorrhage[39,100,106] (5–10 percent incidence); pneumothorax[100] (5 per-

cent incidence); injury to the recurrent laryngeal nerve, thyroid gland, or carotid sheath; mechanical problems secondary to placement of the tracheostomy stoma inappropriately high or low in the trachea; and cardiac arrest.[140] In one instance, cardiac arrest was noted after the tracheostomy tube was accidentally placed in the pretracheal space.[138] The cuff may be lacerated by sharp edges of the tracheal cartilage during insertion. Tracheoesophageal fistula may occur because of incision of the posterior membranous aspect of the trachea during formation of the stoma. Mortality is distinctly unusual when an experienced and skillful surgeon performs the operation over an indwelling endotracheal tube in a controlled setting.

Numerous complications have been observed with the tracheostomy tube in situ. Complications ascribed to the intratracheal inflatable cuff are considered separately below; other complications relate to the surgical stoma or to miscellaneous factors. The most commonly seen stomal complications are infection and bleeding.[138] Mild infection of the stoma is very common, and signs of more serious infection, e.g., cellulitis and purulent stomal exudate, may be seen in more than one-third of cases.[138] Likewise, mild stomal bleeding is commonplace, whereas moderate to severe bleeding can occur in more than one-third of the patients.[138]

Miscellaneous problems that may arise while the tracheostomy tube is in place are similar to those seen with translaryngeal intubation. Discomfort is a rare finding. Health care personnel, we suspect, often impute more pain and discomfort to the procedure than is perceived by the patient. One of us (RRD) was acquainted with a young man who was resuscitated and intubated after an episode of near-drowning. This patient revealed that the single biggest relief of his hospitalization came when a tracheostomy was performed, permitting removal of the oral endotracheal tube. Thus, although a tracheostomy may look uncomfortable to observers, it is generally far more comfortable for the patient than translaryngeal intubation.

Pulmonary aspiration is seen despite the presence of an inflated cuff, as is dislocation of the tube and even self-decannulation, although the latter two problems are unusual. Pneumonitis and atelectasis are sometimes seen, with an incidence of 15 and 8 percent, respectively.[100] Inadequate nutrition is far less common after tracheostomy than with prolonged endotracheal intubation because most patients can swallow liquid and solid food after the tracheostomy tube has been in place for a few days.

Tracheostomy decannulation is usually benign except for patient discomfort. Discomfort or pain, however, may be appreciable in those instances where the decannulation is rendered more difficult by the tightness of the stoma or by defective cuffs.[111] McClelland observed a 5.5 percent frequency of difficulty during tracheal decannulation.[97]

Tracheal stenosis at the stoma site is seen with an incidence ranging from 0 to 85 percent.[2,138,142,151,152] The wide variation in the incidence of this complication is largely due to the degrees of tracheal narrowing used as a criterion for stenosis. Suffice it to say, a prospective study disclosed that 8 percent of tracheostomy patients sustained symptomatic stomal stenosis severe enough to require resection.[39] Subglottic stenosis is occasionally seen after tracheostomy; it is unclear, however, if this complication is related to tracheostomy or to antecedent translaryngeal tracheal intubation. Other sequelae of tracheostomy after decannulation correspond to those seen after tracheal extubation and include tracheal granuloma, tracheal dilation, and tracheomalacia. The formation of incisional keloids or persistence of an open stoma are occasionally seen. Dysphagia is a more common yet less severe consequence of tracheostomy compared to translaryngeal tracheal intubation.

Tracheostomy Versus Translaryngeal Intubation

Several major advantages are associated with tracheostomy. Obviously, tracheostomy avoids the oral, nasal, pharyngeal, and laryngeal complications of oral or nasal intubation that were enumerated earlier. A tracheostomy tube is a much more aesthetically acceptable airway. Once the surgical wound has healed, the tracheostomy tube is tolerated with little or no discomfort. Because the tracheostomy tube is shorter, wider, and less curved than an endotracheal tube, it affords less resistance to air flow, the passage of suction catheters, and the introduction of a fiberoptic bronchoscope. The patient is able to swallow secretions and nourishment easily. He can communicate fairly easily with his lips and may even talk and breathe through the upper airway with a fenestrated tube in place. If accidental decannulation should occur, the tracheostomy tube may be reinserted into the stoma with ease, providing it is not fresh. By contrast, reintubation after accidental removal of an endotracheal tube may be extremely difficult. Tracheostomy tubes are well tolerated for months or even years, and the patient does not require the services of an acute care facility.[110]

The disadvantages of a tracheostomy cannot be ignored, however. Clearly, tracheostomy carries a greater morbidity and mortality than does endotracheal intubation. A high rate of complications can be anticipated when the tracheostomy is performed on an emergency basis and in an uncontrolled setting. The surgical operation is more expensive than intubation and requires the services of an operating room. The complications of tracheostomy may be life-threatening, whereas severe complications of intubation are unusual. Although the tracheostomy makes long-term cannulation possible, it does not make it necessary. Tracheostomy tubes, like endotracheal tubes, should be removed as early as practicable if long-term complications are to be minimized.

The duration of translaryngeal tracheal intubation generally conceded to be "safe" has increased progressively over the past three decades. During the 1950s the longest tolerable period of intubation was said to be 12 hours.[88] By 1969 the "safe" period had increased to 3 days[89] and by 1976 to 11 days.[53] It has been suggested that some patients may tolerate tracheal intubation quite well for as long as 3 weeks.[138] However, no prospective studies have examined the relationship of complications to intubation durations exceeding 3 weeks, and only three studies have been performed in patients intubated for longer than 10 days.[40,41,138] A single report exists of a patient in whom oral tracheal intubation was maintained for 2 months without significant pathological sequelae.[148] If attention is confined to injury at the cuff site, data suggest that any difference between endotracheal and tracheostomy tubes is a function of duration of use.

In summary, a tracheostomy should not be performed routinely simply because an arbitrary duration of intubation has elapsed. Therapy must be tailored to the patient, and the decision to perform a tracheostomy should be based on factors related to the individual patient, e.g., the estimated period for which an artificial airway will be needed, the patient's level of tolerance for the endotracheal tube, the likelihood that airway care and total patient care will be improved by tracheostomy, and the likely morbidity and mortality for the patient involved. Unless specific contraindications prohibit, tracheostomy should be performed only after an endotracheal tube has been inserted to establish and control the airway.

INFLATABLE CUFFS*

The trachea displays the smallest cross-sectional area in infants and young children. Thus endotracheal tubes that fit snugly within the trachea can be introduced through the infant's vocal cords with ease. For this reason, such endotracheal tubes need not be fitted with inflatable cuffs for an airtight seal to be obtained.

In contradistinction, the area of the vocal cords of an adult is the portion of the respiratory tract having the smallest cross section. The shape of the glottic opening does not even roughly approximate the geometry of the endotracheal tube. Furthermore, any appreciable pressures exerted on the vocal cords can be expected to inflict damage. For these reasons, adult endotracheal and tracheostomy tubes are fitted with inflatable cuffs to secure an airtight seal. In the absence of a cuff, some or most of the volume delivered to an adult through the tube by a positive-pressure ventilator leaks out around the tube's outer walls. A properly designed and properly inflated cuff not only prevents losses of tidal volume but also effectively isolates the trachea from the pharynx. This feature prevents aspiration of almost all material that may lie in the pharynx, e.g., saliva, pharyngeal secretions, or regurgitated gastric contents.

Complications

Until the mid-1970s most cuffs were fabricated of stiff rubber, required high pressures to inflate, and accommodated low cuff volumes. Such cuffs were designated "high-pressure, low-volume" cuffs or simply "high-pressure" cuffs. These cuffs were subject to several serious shortcomings. Because the thickness of the cuff walls was

---

*This section is drawn from a review of this topic by Demers and Saklad.[43]

usually not uniform, they displayed a propensity to inflate eccentrically.[25] Tubes on which they were fitted were often displaced away from the center of the trachea and toward the tracheal wall. The rigid tube could then impinge on the fragile tracheal mucosa and produce serious damage as the mucosa moved to and fro during tidal breathing.[34] If inflation was especially asymmetrical, the cuff could herniate over the distal end of the tube, resulting in partial or even complete obstruction of expiratory flow.[64,101]

An even more prevalent hazard associated with high-pressure cuffs was their tendency to exert dangerously high pressures on the tracheal wall because of inadvertent overinflation. However, if practitioners were meticulous in managing such cuffs and scrupulously avoided overinflation, tracheal damage could be avoided. Jenicek et al. managed 583 patients for prolonged periods without observing a single serious complication.[72] However, the study of Knowlson and Bassett indicates that the high-pressure cuff was a very unforgiving device in that the pressure between the cuff and the trachea—"cuff-tracheal pressure"—increased precipitously when the cuff was even slightly overinflated.[81] These authors were able to measure cuff-tracheal pressures directly through the use of an ingenious open-ended polyethylene envelope placed at selected positions around the cuff. In this manner, they documented differences in cuff-tracheal pressures between anterior, posterior, and lateral sites. With the patient's head in the neutral position, the cuff-tracheal pressure was least at the posterior aspect of the membranous trachea. The anterior and lateral aspects of the trachea derive fairly rigid support from rings of tracheal cartilage. During hyperextension of the head, however, posterior cuff-tracheal pressures rise to a point at which they may exceed either anterior or lateral pressures. This phenomenon results from referred pressure on the posterior as-

pect of the trachea from the very rigid subjacent vertebral column. It has been observed that overzealous hyperextension of the head in infants can cause tracheal obstruction by the same mechanism. Documented variations in cuff-tracheal pressure also are associated with changes in the patient's level of consciousness.[81] Cuff-tracheal pressure may change as a result of variations in end-inspiratory upper-airway pressure in patients with changing compliance and/or airway resistance.[37,92] An increase in end-inspiratory pressure results in an increase in the cuff inflation volume necessary to obtain a seal.

Carroll et al.[27] recounted the history of tube and cuff design in an excellent paper, tracing the development of the large-bore cuffless tube[105] through modifications that included cuffs that inflated only during positive-pressure inflation[80] (and forfeited the ability to prevent aspiration), double-cuffed tubes[24] (that promoted double, often confluent areas of injury), prestretched cuffs,[58] and the most recent design—thin walled, easily inflated devices that accommodate high cuff volumes at low inflation pressures.[26,32,33,61,98] This type of cuff has come to be known as the "low-pressure, high-volume" cuff or simply the "low-pressure" cuff. Such cuffs are likely to exert much lower cuff-tracheal pressures than their high-pressure forerunners.[29,95,104] The cuff designed by Cooper and Grillo was the first to be marketed commercially (Soft-Cuf, Foregger Division, Air Products and Chemicals, Allentown, PA); many other manufacturers have followed suit in offering cuffs of similar configuration. It must be emphasized, however, that even cuffs that are billed as low-pressure designs can inflict severe and even fatal damage.[79,85] The following clinical rule must always be borne in mind: The cuff should never be maintained at a volume in excess of that necessary to just prevent leakage (the "minimum occlusive volume"[81]). Maintaining a cuff at a volume larger than this renders the patient vulnerable to a wide spectrum of tracheal damage that has been vividly described and documented in the literature.[33,85]

The perfusion pressure of tracheal tissue in a normotensive patient has been estimated at about 30 torr.[57] Ischemia results whenever the cuff-tracheal pressure exceeds the perfusion pressure. If this excessive cuff-tracheal pressure is maintained over a prolonged period, the tracheal capillary network may actually be obliterated after several hours. Dunn and co-workers have documented this damage in dogs using an elegant radiographic technique.[50]

Tracheitis, the next phase of tracheal damage, is characterized by the appearance of petechial hemorrhages on the mucosal surface. This damage may subsequently extend into the submucosa, resulting in frank ulceration and sloughing of mucosal layers. Microscopic examination of the involved tissue at this stage reveals the presence of granulation tissue in most patients. It is not uncommon to note that granulation, the result of natural reparative processes, can be observed in one area of the tissue even as damage is being extended in closely adjacent tissue.

Ulceration, necrosis, and sloughing of tissue results in exposure of the cartilaginous rings that provide anterior and lateral support to the trachea. Softening of these rings (tracheomalacia), fragmentation, and eventual absorption of the cartilaginous structures represent the next stage of pressure-related injury. Even if the process of injury is arrested at this stage, the collapsible tracheal segment produced by absorption of the cartilage represents a severely limiting functional defect in that the involved segment demonstrates dynamic collapse during forced expiration or coughing. Erosion of the posterior membranous aspect of the trachea may result in tracheoesophageal fistula. Because the fistula provides a pathway

for chronic aspiration, it must be surgically repaired.

Several case reports have described erosion through the lateral tracheal wall and into the innominate artery.[85,102,106,107,134] Hyperextension of the head secondary to improperly applied skull-tong traction seems to potentiate this complication.[102] A self-limiting, premonitory hemorrhage has been observed in some cases several hours before the ultimate massive hemorrhage.[107] Similar episodes of bleeding have rarely been observed to occur secondary to severe tracheitis,[106] which carries a fairly benign prognosis. Therefore diagnostic bronchoscopy is indicated in patients observed to pass small amounts of frank blood from their endotracheal or tracheostomy tube (see section on Bronchoscopy).

In those patients in whom bleeding is the result of innominate artery perforation, immediate surgical repair is necessary. By promptly inflating the cuff further, one may sometimes reduce bleeding enough so that the patient can be brought to the operating room for definitive repair of the lesion. It seems paradoxical that further inflation of the cuff is indicated in this setting, in view of the fact that previous long-term overinflation of the cuff caused the lesion in the first place; however, this maneuver provides tamponade of the perforated vessel and temporary hemostasis until surgical repair can be performed. One must exercise care not to inflate the cuff excessively when using this technique, however, or cuff rupture may occur with disastrous results. The addition of 5 ml to the cuff volume usually provides more than enough additional pressure for tamponade.

Tracheal stenosis is a very late complication of intubation, usually not occurring until several months after the cuffed tube has been removed. Severe tracheal stenosis produces dyspnea and stridor. Resected specimens of these circumferential lesions exhibit extensive deposition of granulation tissue at the site formerly occupied by the cuff. Encroachment on the tracheal lumen is often dramatic: The tracheal cross section may be reduced to a few square millimeters.

Proper Cuff Use

In an effort to reduce or eliminate the incidence of tracheal damage by cuffs, routine deflation of the cuff for several minutes at hourly intervals was once advocated. However, it is doubtful that periodic deflation for a few minutes out of each hour was ever worthwhile,[18,27,116,147] especially if the cuff was overinflated for the balance of the hour. The findings of Jenicek's group[72] demonstrate that careful attention to proper inflation is much more important than periodic deflation according to any preselected schedule. Proper cuff inflation technique is neither difficult nor complicated. A detailed description follows:

1. With the cuff partially deflated, listen at the patient's mouth for leakage around the cuff. If the patient is awake and cooperative, request that he keep his mouth open for the brief period required to reinflate the cuff.
2. As the positive-pressure ventilator cycles into the inspiratory phase and leakage is heard, slowly inject air into the cuff. Discontinue cuff inflation during the expiratory cycle.
3. Resume slow cuff inflation during the subsequent inspiratory cycle(s).
4. Terminate cuff inflation when leakage *just* stops; this is the minimum occlusive volume. DO NOT inject an extra milliliter or two "for good measure" as this potentiates the likelihood for tracheal damage.
5. A small amount of air (about 0.1 ml) may be withdrawn from the cuff at this point, if preferred. This creates a very small amount of leakage past the cuff which some operators prefer to maintain to provide audible evidence that the cuff is not overinflated. A very small leak may be barely audible at the patient's mouth. Auscultation of the trachea at the level of the cuff is useful in determining the presence of even a tiny leak. Aspiration protection is still provided when using this "minimal leak" technique because the leakage proceeds in a retrograde direction only, from the trachea and toward the oropharynx. Also, the leakage occurs only at end-inspiration when tracheal pressure is highest; a competent seal is restored immediately as tracheal pressure falls.
6. A cuff inflated in the manner outlined in steps 1–4 contains the minimum occlusive volume; no leakage is evident during delivery of a normal tidal volume. A small amount of leakage past the cuff is heard during the latter part of hyperinflation ("sigh"), however.

If one anticipates a vigorous inspiratory effort on the part of the patient, the cuff should be *temporarily* overinflated with about 2 ml of additional air to prevent aspiration during the inspiratory effort.[51] This precaution should always be employed before one performs an "inspiratory force (peak negative pressure; PNP) maneuver."[125,126] Of course, restoration of the minimum occlusive volume or minimal leak must be carried out after the inspiratory force maneuver is completed. Unfortunately, some cuff systems (e.g., the Shiley) incorporate a pressure-limiting valve that *may* make temporary overinflation impossible. Because one cannot manually override this system, we do not recommend such valves, despite their obvious advantages in the hands of uneducated operators.

If the minimum occlusive volume (MOV) is used in lieu of the minimal leak technique, the cuff should be *partially* deflated at least every few hours and the minimum occlusive volume empirically redetermined according to the procedure outlined previously. The duration of partial cuff deflation need not be prolonged. Deflation is performed merely to permit a new determination of the MOV, which is subject to some degree of variation. One must exercise care in ensuring that the cuff is only partially deflated during this procedure so that the chance that secretions above the cuff are aspirated is minimized. Partial deflation to redetermine the MOV actually renders pharyngeal secretions more accessible to suctioning as they are blown into the oropharynx. This advantage also obtains when one employs the minimal leak technique. Pharyngeal suctioning should be routinely performed because pooled secretions provide a favorable medium for the growth of multiple species of pathogenic organisms.

Listing the MOV in the patient's medical record may be advantageous during long-term intubation or tracheostomy. Despite the best efforts, an occasional patient suffers tracheal damage; debilitated, hypotensive patient are especially at risk. Gradual increases in the MOV, if they are of appreciable magnitude, may serve to alert the clinician to the possibility of tracheomalacia. If one wishes to compare successive readings of the MOV, the patient must be in the same position and posture because substantial changes in the MOV (and minimal leak) are frequently observed to occur when the patient is turned onto his side from the supine position. For those patients in whom a significant upward trend in the MOV is noted with time, aggressive therapy and early extubation are especially important. On occasion, a cuff-inflation volume is charted by an operator who has used improper technique and has himself overinflated the cuff. If those who subsequently inflate the cuff refer to the original entry in the patient's chart and religiously follow this lead, the hazard of tracheal damage is perpetuated. Obviously, this practice is to be avoided. The MOV or minimal leak should be redetermined *every time the cuff is inflated*.

Despite recent advances in design represented by the low-pressure cuff, the search for the ultimate fail-safe device continues. The Lanz cuff system (Extracorporeal Medical Specialities, Inc., King of Prussia, PA), though not foolproof, is an ingenious design. This system incorporates an external reservoir that communicates with the cuff and is enclosed by a stiff rubber shield. The design of this system is such that the reservoir preferentially fills at the expense of the cuff volume if the system is inflated beyond a certain critical volume. If the cuff volume and cuff-tracheal pressure prevailing at that critical system volume are less than that required for a seal, further attempts to inflate the system succeed in *deflating* the cuff. That is, the newly injected air is all mobilized into the reservoir, and an additional increment of air leaks from the cuff to the reservoir in retrograde fashion. An operator who is unfamiliar with the principle of operation of the Lanz system might then proceed to inflate the system even further in an attempt to effect a seal. With progressive overinflation, the reservoir eventually expands until it comes into contact with the stiff rubber shield. At this stage the reservoir becomes incarcerated within the shield, and the cuff can then be overinflated. One of our colleagues discovered a Lanz system in use that had adhesive tape firmly wrapped around the external reservoir and its shield. Such a maneuver likewise frustrates the controlled-pressure feature of the Lanz system.

Such problems are, of course, attributable to a lack of operator education in the use of the device and not to any basic design fault. Pavlin et al., however, reported another hazard of the Lanz system that is related to its design.[112] The resting diameter of the inflated Lanz cuff is so large it is prevented from inflating to its full diameter when placed in the trachea. As a result, invaginations and wrinkles appear on the surface of the cuff as it resides in the trachea. The involutions formed on the cuff's surface provide channels through which aspiration may occur. In a laboratory model, we have found that the Foregger Soft-Cuf displays similar infolding but to a lesser degree than the Lanz cuff. Aspiration around these cuffs may not be a problem if the patient is treated with a positive-pressure ventilator (where cyclical increases in pressure below the cuff may prevent lungward migration of secretions) or in patients whose pharyngeal secretions are sufficiently viscous.

Several bizarre and dangerous malfunctions have been reported with some commercial cuffs. These include solidification of the cuff after a few hours' incubation at body temperature[111] and collapse of a disposable endotracheal tube by its integral high-pressure cuff.[78] The Kamen-Wilkinson cuff (Fome-Cuff, Bivona Surgical Instruments, Chicago, IL) represents a novel approach to cuff design.[76] This cuff assumes an inflated configuration at ambient pressure because of a foam rubber insert within the cuff. The cuff requires the application of subatmospheric pressure to the filling line in order to deflate it. Modest pressures are exerted on the endotracheal mucosa as the cuff is allowed to expand and produce a seal. Nevertheless, one study demonstrated that certain conventional low-pressure cuffs may produce a seal at even lower pressures than the Kamen-Wilkinson Cuff.[92] Portex has marketed a system (Soft-Seal system, Portex Division, Smith's Industries, Inc., Wilmington, MA) that incorporates a pressure gauge in the cuff inflation line to allow intracuff pressures to be read directly. The data of MacKenzie et al.[92] indicate that the Portex cuff exerts very low cuff-tracheal pressures when managed properly. One potential drawback of the system exists, however. The pressure range of 0–25 torr on the gauge is labeled as a safe zone. The unwary operator might be tempted to pay little heed to the MOV or minimal leak and instead inflate the cuff progressively until a given "safe" pressure is displayed on the gauge. However, whereas intracuff pressures of less than 25 torr would be safe in a healthy subject, ap-

Table 5-1. Recommended Sizes for Endotracheal Tubes

Age	Endotracheal Tube Internal Diameter (mm)*
Newborn	3.0
6 Months	3.5
18 Months	4.0
3 Years	4.5
5 Years	5.0
6 Years	5.5
8 Years	6.0
12 Years	6.5
16 Years	7.0
Adult female	8.0–8.5
Adult male	8.5–9.0

* One size larger and size smaller should be allowed for individual intraage variations.

(Reprinted from the Supplement to Journal of The American Medical Association, August 1, 1980. Copyright 1980, The American Medical Association. Reprinted with permission from The American Heart Association.)

preciably *lower* pressures may be *unsafe* in certain patients (e.g., those with systemic hypotension[89]).

It is crucially important to note that very modest cuff-tracheal pressures may be sufficient to obtain a seal during positive-pressure ventilation. In a fresh human cadaver model, cuff-tracheal pressures of only 2–7 torr were observed to be sufficient to prevent leakage until ventilator cycling pressure exceeded 30 cm H_2O.[76] Therefore the empirical determination of the MOV or minimal leak remains the method of choice for cuff inflation in the presence or absence of devices that furnish intracuff pressure readings. We have been favorably impressed

Table 5-2. Inside and Outside Diameters of Shiley Tracheostomy Tubes

Size No.	Inside Diameter (mm)	Outside Diameter (mm)
4	5.0	8.5
6	7.0	10.0
8	8.5	12.0
10	9.0	13.0

with the Shiley cuff system (Shiley Laboratories, Inc., Santa Ana, CA) over the past 8 years that we have employed it. The cuff inflates evenly and cylindrically, centering the tube within the tracheal lumen. MacKenzie's group found that the Shiley cuff exerted the lowest cuff-tracheal pressure at seal of any of the cuffs they tested.[92] With careful management, it has proved itself a safe and reliable cuff system in our institution. However, because this cuff, as well as some other commercially available designs, may revert to a relatively high-pressure cuff if overinflated, care must be exercised in the choice of a proper size. Proper tube sizes for patients of various ages are listed in Table 5-1.[137] The reader is cautioned, however, not to assume that the size number for a given tube corresponds to its internal diameter. Table 5-2 lists the outer and inner diameters for various sizes of Shiley tracheostomy tube.

Commercial introduction of low-pressure cuffs has fostered a false sense of security among some medical and allied health personnel. It seems to be widely (and erroneously) believed that the low-pressure, high-volume cuff designs that are currently available preclude the necessity for continued diligence and meticulous attention to cuff inflation technique. On the contrary, careful inflation of intratracheal cuffs with the minimum occlusive volume or with a volume that produces a minimal leak is still required. The knowledgeable and meticulous management of intratracheal inflatable cuffs remains an important component of better patient care.

ENDOTRACHEAL SUCTIONING*

In spite of the fact that most practitioners consider suctioning a benign procedure, it can be accompanied by numerous complications.[42] In this section, we focus on spe-

---
* This section has been adapted from a recent review of the topic.[42]

cific categories of complications and discuss elements of technique that place a patient at increased risk from such complications. Methods of prophylaxis are also discussed.

Complications

Tissue Trauma. Although endotracheal suctioning is meant to be therapeutic, the suction catheter all too often serves as an instrument of direct mechanical insult to the pharyngeal and endobronchial mucosa. Some catheters, i.e., those with appreciable "memory" (that retain the shape in which they were stored), are fabricated of rather stiff material. This stiffness and any rough poking or prodding movements imparted to the catheter during introduction can be expected to traumatize delicate mucosa. An appropriately supple catheter and its smooth introduction by the use of firm but gentle pressure are optimal. Naturally, a tradeoff exists in that excessively limp catheters are difficult to direct along the course one chooses. Although particular catheter configurations have been billed as atraumatic, direct visualization by fiberoptic bronchoscopy suggests that the mucosal trauma seen with tracheobronchial suctioning is more likely due to repetition, vigor, and amounts of suction applied, regardless of the type of catheter used.[74] Therefore when one is suctioning any part of the airway, he should use a relatively supple catheter; introduce the catheter by means of smooth, firm, yet gentle, pressure; rotate the catheter between the fingers when resistance is encountered; employ intermittent rather than continuous occlusion of the thumb port; and use a suction pressure that has been regulated to 100 torr subatmospheric pressure or less.

Hypoxemia. Hypoxemia has long been recognized as a potential problem of endotracheal suctioning. Such a hazard is predictable because suctioning evacuates large amounts of gas from the airway as well as secretions. Hypoxemia has been shown to be more pronounced after apnea with suction than after apnea alone.[16] Also, further degrees of hypoxemia are to be anticipated in patients for whom mechanical ventilation must be interrupted during the suctioning procedure. Yet in another study, similar degrees of hypoxemia during apnea with or without suctioning were observed in an animal model.[52] These variable findings might be explained by the differences in the diameters of the artificial airways and the suction catheters used in the two studies[6] and serve to underscore the importance of using the smallest catheter that is adequate for the task at hand. One rule of thumb stipulates that the diameter of the suction catheter should be no greater than half the inner diameter of the airway into which it is being inserted.[44]

The most effective way to prevent intercurrent hypoxemia is to ventilate the patient with very high concentrations of oxygen for a minute or more before the suction catheter is actually introduced into the airway.[54,108] This is easily accomplished in mechanically ventilated patients by raising the dial setting that governs the inspired oxygen fraction (F_{IO_2}) on the ventilator's control panel. A variable lag time elapses before the delivered inspirate actually reflects the new setting owing to the "washout" time of the ventilator system.[9] Therefore if this method is to be used, the adjustment should be made as soon as the practitioner decides to suction the patient, so that the F_{IO_2} can be rising toward the new setting while other preparations, e.g., handwashing and gloving, are being carried out. Of course, one must remember to return the F_{IO_2} setting to baseline after suctioning is complete.

If a second person is available, preoxygenation can be carried out by using a self-inflating resuscitator bag fitted with an oxygen reservoir. This method obviates the need to make any changes in ventilator setting and requires no lead time for the F_{IO_2}

to increase. Preoxygenation is especially important in patients who are being treated with mechanical ventilation and positive end-expiratory pressure (PEEP) because rapid and dramatic decreases in arterial oxygen tension have been documented after discontinuation of PEEP in these patients. In one study of eight patients with severe respiratory failure, a prompt and profound decrease in arterial oxygen tension (Pa_{O_2}) from 304 torr with PEEP to 143 torr after discontinuation and conversion to intermittent positive-pressure ventilation (IPPV) alone was documented.[83] Eighty percent of the reduction in Pa_{O_2} occurred *within the first minute* after discontinuation of PEEP. Clearly then, one must be extremely cautious in discontinuing PEEP even for short periods.

Devices are available which incorporate specially designed irises to allow introduction of a suction catheter into the patient's airway while the patient is still connected to the ventilator. Unfortunately, the irises that are an integral part of the special suction adaptors are not airtight and do not allow maintenance of a stable PEEP level. However, they may be useful in that they permit positive-pressure mechanical ventilation to continue uninterrupted while suctioning is performed. We have found them to be very useful for performing bronchoscopy in patients who are mechanically ventilated. They allow the procedure to continue at a much more deliberate pace, although we usually remove the bronchoscope at intervals to permit periods of normal ventilation.

Limiting the duration of suctioning is important in preventing hypoxemia even when preoxygenation has been performed. As a rule of thumb, one should limit each pass of the suction catheter to no longer than 20 seconds. Some clinicians advise that the operator hold his breath while suctioning the patient. Although this may be a useful technique to remind operators that the duration of suctioning should be limited, it is best to time the suctioning procedure by the clock. Otherwise, the operator may be too liberal in allocating time for the suctioning attempt because most healthy individuals can hold their breath for far longer than 20 seconds. Of course, oxygen should be administered again if one contemplates making a subsequent pass with the catheter. This maneuver succeeds in raising the PaO_2 to a high level such that the subsequent predictable fall in oxygenation does not place the patient in a profoundly hypoxemic range.

In summary, to prevent hypoxemia one should increase the dial setting that governs FIO_2 on the control panel of mechanically ventilated patients a few minutes before suctioning is to be carried out; alternatively, a second operator can ventilate the patient with oxygen by means of a self-inflating resuscitator bag before each pass of the suction catheter and limit individual suctioning attempts to 20 seconds' duration. Reports have appeared in the literature describing the use of jet ventilation for profoundly hypoxemic patients.[62,136]

Cardiac Dysrhythmias. Systemic hypoxia places a patient at risk of cardiac dysrhythmias or arrest. Thus adequate preoxygenation is crucial if one is attempting to prevent cardiac rhythm disturbances. As mentioned in the discussion of nasotracheal suctioning, mechanical stimulation of the vocal cords constitutes an additional stimulus that may provoke dysrhythmias. The presence of an endotracheal or tracheostomy tube prevents direct stimulation of the vocal cords, yet mechanical stimulation of the carina or bronchi can inhibit cardiac activity.

Atelectasis. The "negative" pressure supplied to the proximal end of a suction catheter is diverted to the catheter's thumb port. Large quantities of air are entrained through the thumb port so long as it is open, but when the operator's thumb occludes it the catheter entrains air through the distal aspiration channels. Gas can flow down the airway in a retrograde direction from the upper airway toward the lung, providing the catheter resides within a tube whose inner diameter exceeds the catheter's own outer diameter. However, if the suction catheter should become impacted in the airway while the thumb port is occluded, all negative pressure supplied to the proximal end of the catheter is transmitted to its distal end. Because gas can no longer be entrained in retrograde fashion around the catheter's outer walls, it promptly and completely evacuates the portion of the lung served by the airway within which it is impacted, resulting in atelectasis.[44]

The operator should avoid occlusion of the thumb port so that the catheter can be advanced into the airway *without active suction*. At the point of impaction, it should be withdrawn several centimeters into the larger, more central airways. Only then should active suction be applied and, even then, only by intermittent occlusion of the thumb port. During subsequent withdrawal, the catheter should be rotated between the fingers to entrain secretions that may adhere to the tracheal wall at various points on its circumference.

Although this meticulous technique is important, microatelectasis of some degree almost always results as slight to moderate degrees of negative pressure are transmitted to unstable airways. Atelectasis can be reversed by hyperinflating the lungs, either actively by coaching a cooperative patient or passively by a mechanical ventilator or resuscitator bag. Sustained deep breaths represent the optimum maneuver if one is attempting to reexpand collapsed alveoli.[7,45] One should attempt to hyperinflate the lung with a gas mixture that approximates the composition of gas the patient will receive during subsequent ventilation. This precaution is necessary in order to avoid "absorption atelectasis."[45]

Note that hyperinflation performed after the suctioning procedure is utilized for distinctly different reasons than preoxygenation. The preoxygenation maneuver, although it may be carried out with the same instrument (self-inflating resuscitator bag or mechanical ventilator), is employed to raise the Pa_{O_2} so as to prevent hypoxemia. After suctioning, hyperinflation is employed to expand atelectatic alveoli and to promote their stability. Obviously, if one uses a resuscitator bag the F_{IO_2} cannot be precisely determined and therefore cannot be matched perfectly to the composition of the gas mixture the patient will subsequently receive. A precise and exact duplication of that gas composition is not necessary, however. In contrast, the use of a mechanical ventilator which incorporates a "sigh" mode provides a gas mixture that corresponds exactly to the subsequent F_{IO_2} (provided the dial has been left at the appropriate setting for at least several minutes).

Even ventilators that deliver sigh volumes, however, do not *sustain* the sigh. Rather, they deliver a large tidal volume and then cycle immediately into exhalation. Therefore if the operator wishes to use the ventilator as a means of hyperinflation after suctioning, the sigh volume and pressure limits should be set appropriately, the sigh control depressed manually, and the sigh sustained. This can be accomplished in either of two ways: The operator can cap the expiratory limb of the ventilator with the hand, keeping the volume of gas just delivered to the patient in the lung until the hand is removed, or the tubing that leads to the ventilator's exhalation manifold can be occluded while the sigh volume is being delivered, which will have the same effect as capping the expiratory limb. After the inflation hold, removing the pressure from this line allows the patient to exhale.

Pneumonia. The insertion of an endotracheal tube through the nose or mouth transports bacteria-laden secretions into the lower airway. In addition, the elaborate antimicrobial defense mechanisms centered in the host's upper airway is bypassed.[113] On the other hand, placement of a tube might be expected to minimize the incidence of iatrogenic pneumonia related to catheter penetration because the endotracheal tube shields the catheter from the grossly contaminated nasopharynx. The study of Bryant et al. revealed that bacterial colonization and tracheobronchitis are virtually ensured once tracheal intubation or tracheostomy is performed[19]; moreover, subsequent pneumonia is frequent. Some of this bacterial invasion results from breaches of strictly aseptic technique. Strict observation of asepsis is imperative in intubated and tracheostomized patients because the presence of the tube itself compromises host defenses. Some practitioners persist in dipping the catheter into water before inserting it into the tube. This move is thought to lubricate the catheter and facilitate catheter entry. However, most suction catheters are fabricated of siliconized plastic which, in addition to being slippery, is highly water-repellent. The instant a catheter of this type is withdrawn from water, one can observe that virtually none of the water is retained on the catheter's surface. Actually, in addition to being useless, this practice may be hazardous if the water used as a lubricant is not sterile. Immersing the catheter in contaminated water immediately before it is inserted into the patient's airway has nothing to recommend it, and we are inclined to view this practice with a jaundiced eye.

It is useful to have a container of water at hand when one is finished suctioning the patient. This water is used to flush the suction line *after* the procedure is complete in order to cleanse tenacious and septic secretions from the inner lumen of the suction tubing that is fitted to the catheter's proximal end. This flushing solution does not have to be sterile or distilled; simple tap water will do.

Some nurses and respiratory therapists fit the proximal end of a new suction catheter to the suction tubing (while the distal portion of the catheter remains enclosed within its sterile sheath) just before leaving the bedside. It is reasoned that this practice is desirable so that the suction catheter will be instantly available if the patient should subsequently demonstrate a need to be suctioned quickly. Although such an intention to assist the subsequent operator might otherwise be considered laudable, this practice must be condemned. Connecting a sterile catheter to contaminated suction tubing may serve to contaminate the catheter by contiguous extension of the bacterial colonies.

Many suctioning kits are commercially available from various manufacturers. The contents of these kits vary from one manufacturer to another, and in fact some kits can be assembled with various components at the specific request of a particular institution. Aseptic technique demands that the hand used to guide the distal tip of the catheter into the airway be clothed with a sterile glove. The operator's other hand is used to occlude the thumb port intermittently. Many kits are now appearing on the market that contain only one glove for the "clean" hand that contacts the distal end of the sterile catheter. The operator's other hand virtually always becomes contaminated when it is used to manipulate the patient's swivel adaptor or to disconnect the patient from the ventilator; this is commonly termed the "dirty" hand. We strongly urge that gloves be donned over both hands in order to protect the operator from organisms that reside within the aspirated secretions. Herpetic paronychia (herpetic whitlow) is a herpes virus infection that is assuming increasing importance as an occupational hazard among personnel who perform endotracheal suctioning. Safeguards are definitely indicated to protect operators from this painful condition, both because its contraction can result in extended periods of inability to work and because cross infection to other patients or personnel is a distinct possibility.[49,120,141]

The importance of hand-washing by any and all personnel who perform suctioning cannot be overestimated. Numerous reports have identified respiratory equipment as either vectors or reservoirs of nosocomial infection. The types of equipment that have been implicated include pneumatic[36,77] and ultrasonic[118] nebulizers, multidose vials of medication,[127] mechanical ventilators,[22] and room humidifiers.[135] We reported an outbreak of *Acinetobacter* infection that was traced to the contamination of the expiratory, rather than inspiratory, limb of ventilator systems.[69] Patients did not acquire the organism directly from the machine; rather, the outbreak was similar to other nonventilator-associated infections in that the mode of transmission was from the contaminated hands of personnel.[129] The spirometer bellows housing served as a reservoir that contaminated their hands.[129] We concluded that antibiosis in the intensive care environment and a deterioration in aseptic awareness served to make *Acinetobacter* an environmental opportunist.

Coughing. As mentioned earlier, intubation and tracheostomy impair but do not abolish the cough reflex. To the extent that the patient is able to cough, he can mobilize secretions from his own airway and obviate the need for suctioning. However, coughing can be extremely tiring, often painful, and even traumatic. The act of coughing can generate intrathoracic pressures of sufficiently high magnitude to fracture ribs.[71] Many patients experience severe fatigue and extreme soreness of the intercostal and abdominal muscles secondary to frequent paroxysms of coughing. Obviously then, the clinician must exercise judgment in determining when a patient's coughing has reached the point of diminishing returns. The cessation of a voluntary cough may make suctioning at more frequent intervals a necessity. The suctioning procedure may itself provoke a cough, and the operator is well advised to exercise care during introduction of the catheter so as not to provoke excessive coughing.

Bronchoconstriction. Direct mechanical stimulation of the respiratory mucosa by a suction catheter frequently elicits bronchoconstriction that may persist for a variable time period after the initial stimulus is withdrawn. Because asthma is characterized by airway hyperreactivity, asthmatic patients are particularly vulnerable to bronchoconstriction induced by this mechanism. Therefore suctioning secretions from the airway of an asthmatic patient may represent a mixed blessing. Although it is certainly desirable to remove tenacious secretions from the airway lumen, active constriction of the smooth muscle that surrounds the airways may negate the beneficial effects of suctioning. If one suspects that a bronchoconstrictive response has occurred because of suctioning, administration of a bronchodilator aerosol might be considered.

Misdirection of the Catheter. The adult left mainstem bronchus angles away from the trachea more sharply than does the right mainstem bronchus. Consequently, it is more difficult to direct a suction catheter selectively into the left than into the right bronchial tree in adults.[4] The asymmetry of bronchial angles prevailing in adults is not seen in children less than 15 years old.[30] For adults in whom entry into the left mainstem bronchus is desired, certain maneuvers have been advocated. Turning the patient's head fully toward the right, either passively or through active coaching, has been reported to increase the success rate of left mainstem catheterization from zero to 100 percent.[63] The use of angle-tipped (Coudé) catheters was reported to be highly successful in the same study in selectively catheterizing the left mainstem bronchus. The "shoulder-dropping" technique, however, was found to be ineffective in facilitating successful catheterization. This technique consists of having the patient lower the left shoulder while the catheter is introduced.

Recommended Suctioning Technique

To minimize the incidence and the severity of suctioning complications, the

Table 5-3. Recommended Suctioning Technique

1. Preoxygenate the patient before suctioning begins, either by means of a mechanical ventilator or with the assistance of another person, using a self-inflating resuscitator bag.
2. Strictly observe aseptic technique by donning sterile gloves over freshly washed hands by using a sterile suction catheter from a newly opened package and by avoiding "prelubrication" with water.
3. Introduce the suction catheter smoothly by the use of firm yet gentle pressure without active suction.
4. Withdraw the catheter a few centimeters after it is observed to impact.
5. Apply active suction by intermittently occluding the thumb port as the catheter is withdrawn.
6. Limit each pass of the suction catheter to a duration of 20 seconds or less.
7. Turn the patient's head fully to the right when trying to access the left mainstem bronchus.
8. Reinstitute the baseline F_{IO_2} on the ventilator control panel if it had been altered during step 1.
9. Deliver sustained hyperinflations with approximately the same gas composition that will subsequently be used to ventilate the patient.

steps summarized in Table 5-3 are recommended.

EFFECTS OF INTUBATION AND TRACHEOSTOMY ON NORMAL DEFENSES

Heat and Moisture Exchange

Perhaps the most obvious interference with normal defenses posed by intubation/tracheostomy relates to the effects on heat and moisture exchange. Because the structures of the upper airway are bypassed, warming and humidification of inspired air is severely hampered. Therefore one must provide a means for adequately humidifying and warming the inspired gas when an artificial airway is in place. What constitutes "adequate" humidification is the subject of some controversy. Clinical studies have shown that gases which are less than saturated are still sufficiently moist to prevent mucosal dehydration and inspissation of secretions.

Aerodynamic Filtration

Because an endotracheal or tracheostomy tube bypasses the structures of the upper airway where turbulent air flow predominates, filtration of inspired air through the mechanism of inertial impaction is virtually abolished. Although the gas supply furnished through an endotracheal or tracheostomy tube should be devoid of materials that might elicit an unfavorable response from the airway, such is not always the case. Particulate aerosols, specifically those produced by ultrasonic nebulizers, constitute a bronchoprovocative challenge in patients with a history of chronic bronchitis or asthma.[28,96] If one is determined to deliver an ultrasonic aerosol to such a patient, a bronchodilator should be administered beforehand.[28] However, it should be noted that conventional pneumatic nebulizers are fully as efficient as ultrasonic devices in their ability to deliver dense concentrations of water to terminal airways.[23] The effluent of a conventional heated humidifier is tolerated far better by asthmatics and bronchitics, as well as by patients without preexisting lung disease.[28] Even normal volunteers are often observed to cough after inhalation of an ultrasonic aerosol, although bronchoconstriction is not seen in healthy individuals.

Laryngeal Reflex

Incompetence of the laryngeal reflex constitutes one of the indications for tracheal intubation. The presence of a properly functioning inflatable cuff isolates the trachea from the upper airway and theoretically should prevent aspiration of pharyngeal material or vomitus. Unfortunately, the design features of some cuffs leave much to be desired in terms of their ability to prevent aspiration[112]; small amounts of aspiration can and do occur even when cuffs are inflated. Also, patients can easily aspirate if and when the cuff is deflated.[103] For this

reason, we have always recommended careful suction of the area above the cuff before extubation to clear secretions that might subsequently be aspirated. More recently, we have made it a practice to withdraw the tube around a previously placed fiberoptic bronchoscope. This allows us to perform suction under direct visualization and to inspect the trachea for signs of damage that might have been incurred during the period of intubation. If the patient should have to be reintubated immediately for any reason, the tube can be reinserted around the indwelling bronchoscope far more easily than if the bronchoscope had not been used.

COLONIZATION

Colonization is defined as the appearance of any potential pathogen in tracheal cultures in the absence of purulent tracheobronchial secretions or clinical evidence of infection.[73] Severely ill, nonintubated patients admitted to ICUs acquire a gram-negative bacillary oropharyngeal flora.[19,130] Twenty-two percent become so colonized within 24 hours and 45 percent within 48 hours. This oropharyngeal flora change presumably takes place because the mucosa is more receptive to the adherence of gram-negative bacilli in the severely ill patient.[8] A similar change has also been observed in patients with a tracheostomy or endotracheal tube. All of these patients acquire gram-negative bacilli in their tracheas by the third day. Moreover, 43 percent of patients become colonized with two or more gram-negative organisms, and these organisms frequently change. The most likely source for these tracheal organisms is the oropharynx. Oropharyngeal secretions collect above the intratracheal inflatable cuff that lies below the open vocal cords. These organisms must spill into the lower respiratory tract around the indwelling cuff.

Tracheobronchitis can be distinguished from colonization when purulent secretions appear, but the patient does not manifest evidence of pneumonia by physical examination or chest x-ray.[59]

The actual physiological difference between colonization on the one hand and tracheobronchitis or pneumonia on the other is probably related to impairment of the alveolar macrophage in the latter situations. Alveolar hypoxia distal to inadequately cleared secretions presumably impairs macrophage function. Pneumonia is diagnosed when physical examination and/or chest x-rays are consistent with parenchymal disease. Because (1) all intubated patients eventually become colonized with potential pathogens, (2) most of these patients have fever referable to any number of sites, and (3) many develop pulmonary physical examination and chest x-ray abnormalities (i.e., edema), it may in fact become impossible to distinguish colonization from tracheobronchitis/pneumonia. Clinicians who are charged with the responsibility of treating intubated and tracheostomized patients in an ICU must strike a delicate balance between undertreatment and overtreatment. If the patient's condition is precarious, one might be forced to treat him aggressively, assuming that he has become infected with the "worst bug." Although this approach is admittedly aggressive, the results of a missed diagnosis might be lethal.

Mucociliary Clearance

Endotracheal and tracheostomy tubes or, more precisely, the inflatable cuffs attached thereto adversely affect the mucociliary escalator in two ways. First, the pressure exerted on the tracheal mucosa by the cuff, even for relatively short periods, impairs ciliary activity over the area of contact.[109] Secondly, the inflated cuff creates a barrier that completely blocks off the escalator such that secretions cannot be mobilized into the pharynx and swallowed as is usually the case. Instead, the patient must either cough the secretions out through the tube or have them suctioned. Sometimes patients are intubated in order to facilitate tracheal toilet. Somewhat paradoxically, then, we are forced to conclude that intubation not only makes suctioning possible, but often makes it necessary. If the integrity of the ciliated epithelial membrane is destroyed, stasis results at the site of such injury and persists until epithelial repair can occur.

Although mucociliary transport can be pharmacologically stimulated by theophylline[144] and terbutaline in patients with chronic obstructive pulmonary disease (COPD) and by terbutaline in patients with cystic fibrosis,[158] it is not known if the same effect can be achieved when an endotracheal tube is in place. Tenacious secretions that cannot readily be eliminated by cough can be liquified and more easily cleared with the use of mucolytic agents. The prototypical agent is acetylcysteine (Mucomyst). The effectiveness of this drug in reducing the viscosity of bronchial secretions in human subjects has been well demonstrated both in vivo and in vitro. The drug is usually administered by inhalation or instillation directly into the endotracheal tube. Mucolytics, however, should be used cautiously as they may produce a massive amount of secretions which overwhelm the patient's ability to clear his or her airways, and they occasionally induce bronchospasm in those patients most likely to need therapy (asthmatics).

Whereas mucolytics are useful drugs to augment clearance of lower respiratory tract secretions, expectorants seem to offer little benefit.[71] Expectorants are drugs that theoretically increase sputum volume, promoting the expulsion of secretions or exudates from the airways. They also may exert a demulcent action on irritated airway mucosa through the production of a greater amount of respiratory tract fluid. Perhaps with the exception of hydration (see below), there are no expectorants that are both effective and devoid of notable side effects. Maximum doses of glyceryl guaiacolate have been found to be no more effective than a placebo; the dosage of ammonium chloride used in most cough preparations is not sufficient to cause notable augmentation of respiratory tract fluid in man; the clinical usefulness of iodides is limited by side reactions that may warrant discontinuing the drug in approximately 14 percent of patients. The most common side effects are an unpleasant metallic taste in the mouth, skin eruptions, gastrointestinal upset, painful parotid swelling, and nodular enlargement of the thyroid that may occur in up to 50 percent of patients.[71]

Although water may suppress cough in upper respiratory tract disorders by its demulcent effect, the use of hydration as an expectorant is controversial. Experiments in animals have shown that oral administration of water has no effect on the volume or viscosity of respiratory tract fluid in the absence of severe systemic dehydration. Although the inhalation of steam is commonly considered an effective expectorant and is supported by one recent study of cough transport in mouth-breathing dogs, several other studies have shown that even with ultrasonic nebulization not enough water can be delivered to the lower respiratory tract to affect respiratory secretions. Further studies are necessary to settle the controversy.

Cough

It is surprising that many persist in their belief that an effective cough is impossible for an intubated or tracheostomized patient. This erroneous belief is based on the assumption that the compressive phase of cough—forced exhalation against a closed glottis—is necessary to generate adequately high intrathoracic pressures. However, the highest pressures observed during the cough reflex in normal volunteers occurs during the expiratory phase after the vocal cords have opened. Thus before one reflexly suctions a patient who is intubated or tracheostomized, the patient's ability to cough should be assessed through coaching and observation. If the patient is able to mobilize secretions out of the airway by coughing without encountering an undue amount of fatigue or pain, suctioning may be rendered unnecessary.

BRONCHOSCOPY*

Bronchoscopy, the endoscopic examination of the tracheobronchial tree, was initially developed as a method to recover foreign bodies that had become lodged within the airways. Although Green, O'Dwyer, and Kirstein played roles in developing an endoscopic method of examining the upper airways during the latter part of the nineteenth century, Killian and Jackson have been credited with the development of the method and instrumentation of translaryngeal rigid bronchoscopy in 1904.

Flexible fiberoptic bronchoscopy (FFB) has had a dramatic impact on the approach and management of patients with a wide variety of respiratory problems since its introduction in 1968 and has revolutionized the practice of clinical chest medicine.[122] The procedure: (1) is easily performed; (2) is associated with few complications; (3) is far more comfortable for the patient than rigid bronchoscopy; (4) exposes a far greater portion of the tracheobronchial tree (especially the upper lobes) to direct visualization than rigid bronchoscopy; (5) does not require general anesthesia or the use of an operating room; and (6) may be performed at the bedside. Consequently, FFB has replaced rigid bronchoscopy as the procedure of choice for most endoscopic eval-

---

* This section draws from Corwin and Irwin's recent review.[35]

uations of the airways.[122] Rigid bronchoscopy may still be the procedure of choice in certain settings, e.g., for brisk hemoptysis (greater than 200 ml/24 hours), the extraction of large foreign bodies, endobronchial resection of tumors or granulation tissue, and the biopsy of vascular tumors (e.g., bronchial adenomas) in which brisk bleeding can be controlled by packing.

Bronchoscopy, with either the flexible or the rigid instrument, is not a procedure that should be performed by the house staff; rather, the bronchoscope is a tool of the trained specialist familiar with all the indications, complications, and contraindications of the procedure.

Therapeutic Indications

Excessive Secretions/Atelectasis. When chest physiotherapy, incentive spirometry, and sustained maximum inspiration with cough fail to clear the airways of excessive secretions and to resolve lobar atelectasis, FFB may be successful. The direct instillation of acetylcysteine (Mucomyst) through the bronchoscope may occasionally be necessary to liquefy thick, tenacious, inspissated mucus. Asthmatics must be pretreated with a bronchodilator because acetylcysteine may induce bronchospasm. Although FFB may take longer to clear secretions than rigid bronchoscopy, it is clearly the method of choice.

Removal of Foreign Bodies. Although the rigid bronchoscope is currently the instrument of choice for removing large foreign bodies, this perception may change. Newer devices have become available which can be used to grasp large objects through the flexible fiberoptic instrument. Of course, these devices cannot then be withdrawn through the suction channel of the bronchoscope; rather, the grasping device and the bronchoscope must be removed as a unit.

Tracheal Intubation. The flexible fiberoptic bronchoscope may be used as an obturator to facilitate tracheal intubation of patients with ankylosing spondylitis or other anatomical problems of the neck.[121] An endotracheal tube can be passed over the bronchoscope, and the instrument can then be passed transnasally (after proper local anesthesia) through the vocal cords and into the trachea, after which the tube can be passed over the bronchoscope. The same technique can be employed in tetanus patients with trismus and in patients with acute epiglottitis. In the last two instances, the procedure should be done in the operating room with an anesthesiologist and otolaryngologist in attendance.

Hemoptysis. On rare occasions endobronchial tamponade of brisk bleeding may be lifesaving before definitive therapy can be given. The flexible bronchoscope is usually passed through a rigid bronchoscope, after which a balloon-tipped Fogarty catheter is passed through the channel of the fiberoptic bronchoscope into the bleeding lobar orifice. The patient can be transferred to surgery or angiography for bronchial arteriography and bronchial artery embolization once the balloon is inflated and wedged tightly.

Diagnostic Indications

Because FFB can be performed easily in intubated and nonintubated patients, the same indications apply in a general way to critically ill mechanically ventilated patients as to noncritically ill patients.

Hemoptysis. Hemoptysis is one of the most common clinical problems for which bronchoscopy is indicated. Whether the patient complains of merely blood streaking or of massive hemoptysis (expectoration of more than 600 ml in 48 hours), bronchoscopy should be considered to localize the site of bleeding and diagnose the cause. Localization is crucial if definitive therapy, e.g., surgery, becomes necessary. If FFB is performed before hemoptysis entirely ceases, the site and etiology of the bleeding can be determined in approximately 90 percent of patients. When performed after bleeding stops, the etiology can be determined only 50 percent of the time. Because hemoptysis can be caused by tracheobronchial tree disorders, cardiovascular disease, hematological conditions, and localized or diffuse pulmonary parenchymal disorders, clinical judgment will dictate if and when bronchoscopy is indicated. For example, FFB is not indicated in patients with obvious pulmonary embolism and infarction. Hemoptysis should always be evaluated in intubated patients or those with a tracheostomy as it may indicate potentially life-threatening tracheal damage. The flexible fiberoptic instrument, rather than the rigid bronchoscope, is the instrument of choice unless bleeding is massive.[131]

Atelectasis. Although atelectasis may be caused by mucous plugging, FFB should be performed to rule out endobronchial obstruction by carcinoma or foreign bodies. When atelectasis is seen in a critically ill patient whose initial chest film was normal, mucous plugging is the most likely cause. The position of the endotracheal tube should be verified by chest x-ray in intubated patients with atelectasis to rule out migration of the tube into the right mainstem bronchus and obstruction of the right upper lobe.

Diffuse Parenchymal Disease. Flexible fiberoptic and rigid bronchoscopes can be used to assess lung parenchyma as well as the airways. Lung biopsy performed through either of these instruments is called a transbronchoscopic lung biopsy (TBLB). The flexible instrument is vastly more comfortable for the conscious patient.

We perform TBLB only under fluoroscopic guidance. This procedure, performed with the flexible instrument, is associated with a 0.2 percent mortality rate and a 6–26 percent complication rate. Pneu-

mothorax and hemoptysis comprise most of the complications. Tissue is obtained approximately 95 percent of the time, and the diagnosis is made in 72–79 percent of cases. In order to avoid life-threatening complications, we do not perform TBLB on the following: (1) uncooperative patients; (2) uremic patients; (3) patients with abnormal bleeding, prothrombin, or partial thromboplastin times (4) patients with arterial oxygen tensions less than 70 torr with supplemental oxygen; and (5) patients receiving positive-pressure mechanical ventilation.

When TBLB is unlikely (by clinical judgment) to yield a diagnosis representing the diffuse lung process, or when TBLB is contraindicated, open lung biopsy should be performed. TBLB is extremely helpful in the immunocompromised host with a diffuse infection that can be identified only by histological means. For example, the procedure identifies *Pneumocystis carinii* infection about 90 percent of the time. The yield from bronchial brushing through the flexible fiberoptic instrument in the presence of disseminated *P. carinii* is about 60 percent. In studies combining both TBLB and bronchial brushing, the yield approaches 100 percent. In contrast, bronchoalveolar lavage during FFB identifies *Pneumocystis* only 21 percent of the time.

Acute Inhalation Injury. FFB may occasionally be indicated to identify the anatomical level and severity of injury in patients exposed to smoke inhalation.

Blunt Chest Trauma. Patients who present with an atelectatic lung, lobar atelectasis, pneumomediastinum, and/or pneumothorax after blunt chest trauma may have sustained a fractured airway. Because this lesion requires surgical intervention, bronchoscopy should be performed immediately. The fiberoptic bronchoscope allows a rapid yet thorough examination of the airways without necessitating general anesthesia.

Resectional Surgery. FFB is useful for identifying a disrupted suture line that may cause bleeding or pneumothorax.

Damage Caused by Intubation. Although the incidence of laryngeal and tracheal complications has been markedly reduced with the low-pressure cuffs of the newer, nonirritating endotracheal tubes, damage still does occur. In order to determine when a tracheostomy should be performed because of damage inflicted by the endotracheal tube, FFB with the adult instrument can be performed routinely so long as the endotracheal tube is at least 8 mm in its internal diameter. If the tube is smaller, the patient cannot be ventilated and bronchoscoped at the same time with the adult instrument. A pediatric bronchoscope can be used for patients with smaller tubes, but some degree of suctioning efficiency is forfeited.[157]

With patients who are nasotracheally or orotracheally intubated, one can routinely (at weekly intervals in our institution) deflate the cuff and withdraw the tube over the bronchoscope to check for subglottic damage. Subsequently, it can be withdrawn through the vocal cords over the instrument while glottic and supraglottic inspection proceeds. If the intubation procedure has not been traumatic, little damage will occur for up to 3 weeks in our experience. If subglottic ulcers/necrosis or glottic edema/ulcers are seen, tracheostomy is indicated. FFB can help differentiate aspiration from tracheoesophageal fistula in patients requiring long-term ventilatory assistance through cuffed tracheostomy tubes. The patient is asked to swallow a dilute solution of methylene blue with the bronchoscope within the distal trachea. The absence of methylene blue in the trachea and its presence leaking around and out of the tracheostomy stoma will accurately rule out a tracheoesophageal fistula and suggest a swallowing abnormality.

Microbiological Cultures. Transnasal or transoral FFB aspirates are no more reliable than nasotracheal suction aspirates or expectorated sputum specimens for culturing the routine aerobic and anaerobic organisms in the nonintubated patients. Each of these methods generates substantial amounts of false-positive and false-negative bacteriological data. FFB aspirates may, however, be extremely useful in identifying *Mycobacterium tuberculosis*, *Nocardia* species, pathogenic fungi, and *Legionella* species in those patients who are unable to expectorate adequate quantities of sputum.

Transtracheal aspiration, unless it is contraindicated, is the method of choice for sampling lower respiratory tract secretions in the nonintubated patient. A new sampling device has recently been marketed[155] which consists of a retractable sterile wire brush within two telescoping catheters plugged with gelfoam at the distal end. This device may improve the accuracy of FFB cultures, but too few data exist at this time to recommend its use over transtracheal aspiration in nonintubated patients. FFB aspirates are no better than endotracheal aspirates for culturing intubated patients. In this setting, the new sampling catheter may be superior to endotracheal suction; however, this application also has not been studied.

Complications

FFB is an extremely safe procedure when performed by a trained specialist. Mortality should not exceed 0.1 percent, and the overall complication rate should not exceed 8.1 percent. Those rare deaths that have been reported have occurred secondary to respiratory arrest from hemorrhage and laryngospasm or to cardiac arrest from acute myocardial infarction. Nonfatal complications occurring within 24 hours of the procedure include fever (1.2–16 percent), pneumonia (0.6–6 percent),[113] vasovagal reactions(2.4 percent), laryngospasm/bronchospasm (0.04–0.1 percent), hypotension and arrhythmias (0.06–0.9 percent), pneumothorax (0.04–0.2 percent), problems relating to anesthesia (0.08–0.1 percent), and aphonia (0.1 percent). The patients in whom complications are most likely to occur can be predicted: Asthmatics are prone to laryngospasm and bronchospasm; patients with cardiovascular diseases (angina, dysrhythmias, etc.) are at risk of developing cardiovascular problems; immunoincompetent hosts are prone to develop infections; patients with a history of hemoptysis are more likely to bleed; and patients with obstructing endobronchial lesions are more likely to develop pneumonia.

Contraindications

Bronchoscopy should not be performed: (1) when an experienced bronchoscopist is not available; (2) when the patient is unable or unwilling to cooperate; (3) when adequate oxygenation cannot be achieved (arterial oxygen tension must be at least 70 torr during the procedure); (4) when coagulation abnormalities cannot be corrected in patients for whom brush or forceps biopsies are planned; (5) in unstable cardiac patients; and (6) in untreated, symptomatic asthmatics. Although patients with stable hypercapnia can be safely bronchoscoped with the flexible instrument, premedication, sedation during the procedure, and supplemental oxygen administration must be monitored cautiously.

The Procedure

Preprocedure Considerations. The following checklist should be consulted:

1. Is the patient asthmatic?
2. Is cardiovascular disease present?
3. Is uremia present?
4. Is the patient immunocompromised?
5. Does the patient have a history of drug allergies?
6. Have a chest x-ray and an electrocardiogram (ECG) been done?
7. Have arterial blood gas analysis, plate-

let count, prothrombin time, and partial thromboplastin time been performed?
8. Has the patient recently been given a medication that will interfere with platelet function?
9. Has the patient fasted for at least 3 hours before the procedure?
10. Has the patient given informed consent?
11. Has premedication been ordered (e.g., intramuscular meperidine 1 mg/kg)?
12. Has an angiocath been placed in an arm vein?

Procedural Considerations. FFB can be performed in nonintubated patients via the transnasal route or by the transoral route with a bite block. The instrument can also be passed through an endotracheal tube or through a rigid bronchoscope. The majority of bronchoscopists in the United States favor the transnasal route in patients who have previously been anesthetized by hand-nebulized lidocaine with lidocaine jelly used as a lubricant. Lidocaine is absorbed by the mucous membranes, and significant blood levels may be reached after topical administration. However, only levels within the low therapeutic range (less than 2 $\mu g/ml$) are obtained if less than 200 mg (total) is used during the procedure. Patients who are receiving a lidocaine infusion should be given another anesthetic, e.g., topical cocaine. Lidocaine toxicity should be suspected in any patient who demonstrates a sudden change in mental status, tremulousness, hallucinations, increased level of sedation, or hypotension.

In intubated and mechanically ventilated patients, the flexible fiberoptic bronchoscope can be passed through a swivel adaptor incorporating a rubber iris, which prevents excessive loss of delivered respiratory gases. In this setting, the following points should be borne in mind (1) never introduce the adult instrument (5.5–5.7 mm external diameter) into a tracheal tube smaller than 8 mm because it will not be possible to deliver an adequate tidal volume and because inadvertent PEEP may result; (2) if PEEP is already being administered, it must be discontinued; (3) the inspired oxygen fraction (FIO_2) should be increased to 1.0 during the procedure; (4) the tidal volume setting on the ventilator generally must be increased substantially (a respiratory therapist should be in attendance to monitor expired volume and ensure that it is adequate); (5) suction should be used sparingly because suctioning decreases the tidal volumes being delivered; and (6) ECG monitoring should be used throughout the procedure.

Postprocedural Considerations. The following checklist should be consulted after performing the procedure: (1) obtain a chest x-ray to rule out pneumothorax after a transbronchoscopic lung biopsy in the nonintubated patient or after routine bronchoscopy in the intubated, mechanically ventilated patient; (2) restore the ventilator control settings (tidal volume, FIO_2, PEEP) to the level that prevailed before the procedure in mechanically ventilated patients; (3) continue supplemental oxygen for 2 hours after the procedure in the nonintubated patient; (4) obtain frequent vital signs until the patient is stable for 2 hours; and (5) do not allow the nonintubated patient to eat or drink until the effects of the local anesthetic have worn off. Approximately 1–2 hours after the procedure, allow the patient to sip some water. If he does not cough and sputter, eating and drinking are not contraindicated.

REFERENCES

1. Amikam B, Landa J, West J, et al: Bronchofiberscopic observations of the tracheobronchial tree during intubation. Am Rev Respir Dis 105:747, 1972
2. Andrews MJ, Pearson FG: Incidence and pathogenesis of tracheal injuries following cuffed tube tracheostomy with assisted ventilation: analysis of a two-year prospective study. Ann Surg 173:249, 1971
3. Anesthesia Study Committee of the New York State Society of Anesthesiologists. Clinical Anesthesia Conference: endotracheal suction and death. NY State J Med 68:565, 1968
4. Anthony JS, Sieniewicz DJ: Suctioning of the left bronchial tree in critically ill patients. Crit Care Med 5:161, 1977
5. Arens JF, LeJeune FE Jr, Webre DR: Maxillary sinusitis; a complication of nasotracheal intubation. Anesthesiology 40:415, 1974
6. Baier H, Begin R, Sackner MA: Effect of airway diameter, suction catheters, and the bronchoscope on airflow and endotracheal and tracheostomy tubes. Heart Lung 5:235, 1976
7. Bartlett RH, Gazzaniga AB, Geraghty TR: Respiratory maneuvers to prevent postoperative pulmonary complications. JAMA 224:1017, 1973
8. Beachley EH: Bacterial adherence: adhesion-receptor interactions mediating the attachment of bacteria to mucosal surfaces. J. Infect Dis 143:325, 1981
9. Benson MS, Pierson DJ: Ventilator washout volume: a consideration in endotracheal suction preoxygenation. Respir Care 24:832, 1979
10. Berman SA, Balkany TJ, Simmons MA: Otitis media in the neonatal intensive care unit. Pediatrics 62:198, 1978
11. Bernhard WN, Cottrell JE, Sivakumuran C, et al: Adjustment of intracuff pressure to prevent aspiration. Anesthesiology 50:363, 1979
12. Berry FA, Blakenbaker WL, Ball CG: A comparison of bacteremia occurring with nasotracheal and orotracheal intubation. Anesth Analg 52:873, 1973
13. Berry FA, Yarbrough S, Yarbrough N: Transient bacteremia during dental manipulation in children. Pediatrics 51:476, 1973
14. Bishop MJ: Endotracheal lumen compromise from cuff overinflation. Chest 80:1200, 1981
15. Blanc VF, Tremblay NAG: The complications of tracheal intubation: a new classification with a review of the literature. Anesth Analg 53:202, 1974
16. Boutros AR: Arterial blood oxygenation during and after endotracheal suctioning in

the apneic patient. Anesthesiology 32:114, 1970

17. Boyd EM, Boyd CE: Expectorant activity of water in acute asthma attacks. Ann J Dis Child 116:397, 1968

18. Bryant LR, Trinkle JK, Dubilier L: Reappraisal of tracheal injury from cuffed tracheostomy tubes. JAMA 215:625, 1971

19. Bryant LR, Trinkle JK, Mobin-Uddin K, et al: Bacterial colonization profile with tracheal intubation and mechanical ventilation. Arch Surg 104:647, 1972

20. Burgess GE, Cooper JR Jr, Marino RJ, et al: Laryngeal competence after tracheal extubation. Anesthesiology 51:73, 1979

21. Burns HP, Vayal VS, Scott A, et al: Laryngeotracheal trauma: observations on its pathogenesis and its prevention following prolonged orotracheal intubation in the adult. Laryngoscope 89:1316, 1979

22. Buxton AE, Anderson RL, Werdegar D, et al: Nosocomial respiratory tract infection and colonization with *Acinetobacter calcoaceticus*. Am J Med 65:507, 1978

23. Calderwood HW, Klein EF Jr, Modell JH, et al: Distribution of nebulized aerosols in spontaneously breathing puppies. Anesthesiology 41:368, 1974

24. Carroll RG: Evaluation of tracheal tube cuff designs. Crit Care Med 1:45, 1973

25. Carroll R, Hedden NM, Safar P: Intratracheal cuffs: performance characteristics. Anesthesiology 31:275, 1969

26. Carroll RG, Kamen JM, Grenvik A, et al: Recommended performance specifications for cuffed endotracheal and tracheostomy tubes: a joint statement of investigators, inventors and manufacturers. Crit Care Med 1:155, 1973

27. Carroll RG, McGinnis GE, Grenvik A: Performance characteristics of tracheal cuffs. Int Anesthesiol Clin 12:No. 3, 1974

28. Cheney FW Jr, Butler J: The effects of ultrasonically-produced aerosols on airway resistance in man. Anesthesiology 29:1099, 1968

29. Ching NP, Ayres SM, Paegle RP, et al: The contribution of cuff volume and pressure in tracheostomy tube damage. J Thorac Cardiovasc Surg 62:402, 1971

30. Cleveland RH: Symmetry of bronchial angles in children. Pediatr Radiol 133:89, 1977

31. Cohen AB, Cline MJ: The human alveolar macrophage: isolation, cultivation in vitro, and studies of morphologic and functional characteristics. J Clin Invest 50:1390, 1971

32. Cooper JD, Grillo HC: Analysis of problems related to cuffs on intratracheal tubes. Chest 62:215, 1973

33. Cooper JD, Grillo HC: Experimental production and prevention of injury due to cuffed tracheal tubes. Surg Gynecol Obstet 129:1235, 1969

34. Cooper JD, Grillo HC: The evolution of tracheal injury due to ventilatory assistance through cuffed tubes: a pathologic study. Ann Surg 169:334, 1969

35. Corwin RW, Irwin RS: Bronchoscopy. In Rippe JM, Csete ME (eds): Clinical Problems in Intensive Care. Little, Brown, Boston, in press (annotated with key references)

36. Covelli HD, Kleeman J, Martin JE, et al: Bacterial emission from both vapor and aerosol humidifiers. Am Rev Respir Dis 108:698, 1973

37. Crawley BE, Cross DE: Tracheal cuffs: a review and dynamic pressure study. Anaesthesia 30:4, 1975

38. Credle WR Jr, Smiddy JR, Elliott RC: Complications of fiberoptic bronchoscopy. Am Rev Respir Dis 109:67, 1974

39. Dane TEB, King EG: A prospective study of complications after tracheostomy for assisted ventilation. Chest 67:398, 1975

40. Deane RS, Mills EL: Prolonged nasotracheal intubation in adults: a successor and adjunct to tracheostomy. Anes Analg 49:89, 1970

41. Deane RS, Shinozaki T, Morgan JG: An evaluation of the cuff characteristics and incidence of laryngeal complications using a new nasotracheal tube in prolonged intubations. J Trauma 17:311, 1977

42. Demers RR: Complications of endotracheal suctioning procedures. Respir Care 27:453, 1982

43. Demers RR, Saklad M: Intratracheal inflatable cuffs: a review. Respir Care 22:29, 1977

44. Demers RR, Saklad M: Mechanical aspiration: a reappraisal of its hazards. Respir Care 20:661, 1975

45. Demers RR, Saklad M: The etiology, pathophysiology, and treatment of atelectasis. Respir Care 21:234, 1976

46. Dery R, Pelltier J, Jacques A, et al: Humidity in anesthesiology. III. Heat and moisture patterns in the respiratory tract during anaesthesia with the semi-closed system. Can Anaesth Soc J 14:287, 1967

47. Donnelly WH: Histopathology of endotracheal intubation: an autopsy study of 99 cases. Arch Pathol 88:511, 1969

48. Dubick MN, Wright BD: Comparison of laryngeal pathology following long-term oro- and naso-endotracheal intubations. Anesth Analg 57:663, 1978

49. Dunbar C: Herpetic whitlow: an occupational hazard for nursing personnel. Heart Lung 7:645, 1978

50. Dunn CR, Dunn DL, Moser KM: Determinants of tracheal injury by cuffed tracheostomy tubes. Chest 65:128, 1974

51. Egnatinsky J: Overinflating low-pressure cuffs to prevent aspiration. Anesthesiology 42:114, 1975

52. Ehrhart IC, Hofman WF, Loveland SR: Effects of endotracheal suction versus apnea during interruption of intermittent or continuous positive pressure ventilation. Crit Care Med 9:464, 1981

53. El-Naggar M, Sadagopan S, Levine H, et al: Factors influencing choice between tracheostomy and prolonged translaryngeal intubation in acute respiratory failure. Anesth Analg 55:195, 1976

54. Fell T, Cheney FW: Prevention of hypoxia during endotracheal suction. Ann Surg 174:24, 1971

55. Fineberg C, Cohn HE, Gibbon JH Jr: Cardiac arrest during nasotracheal aspiration. JAMA 174:410, 1960

56. Frost EAM: Tracing the tracheostomy. Ann Otol Rhinol Laryngol 85:618, 1976

57. Ganong WF: Review of Medical Physiology, 6th ed. Lange, Los Altos, CA, 1973

58. Geffin B, Pontoppidan H: Reduction of tracheal damage by the prestretching of inflatable cuffs. Anesthesiology 31:462, 1969

59. Green GM, Jakab GJ, Low RB, et al: State-of-the-art: defense mechanisms of the respiratory membrane. Am Rev Respir Dis 115:479, 1977

60. Gregory GA: Respiratory care of the child. Crit Care Med 8:582, 1980

61. Grillo HC, Cooper JD, Geffin B, et al: A low pressure cuff for tracheostomy tubes to minimize tracheal injury: a comparative clinical trial. J Thorac Cardiovasc Surg 62:898, 1971

62. Guntupalli K, Sladen A, Klain M: High frequency jet ventilation (HFJV) in the prevention of a decrease in Pao_2 during suctioning. Chest 80:381, 1981 (abstract)

63. Haberman PB, Green JP, Archibald C, et al: Determinants of successful selective tracheobronchial suctioning. N Engl J Med 289:1060, 1973

64. Harmel HD: Occlusion of endotracheal tube by overinflated cuff. NY State J Med 56:2125, 1956

65. Hawkins DB, Seltzer DC, Barnett TE, et al: Endotracheal tube perforation of the hypopharynx. West J Med 120:282, 1974

66. Hoeprich PD: Etiologic diagnosis of lower respiratory tract infections. Calif Med 112:1, 1970

67. Hoffman S, Freedman N: Delayed lumen obstruction in endotracheal tubes. Br J Anaesth 48:1025, 1976

68. Huxley EJ, Viroslav J, Gray WR, et al: Pharyngeal aspiration in normal adults and patients with depressed consciousness. Am J Med 64:564, 1978

69. Irwin RS, Demers RR, Pratter MR, et al: An outbreak of Acinetobacter infection associated with use of a ventilator spirometer. Respir Care 25:232, 1980

70. Irwin RS, Demers RR, Pratter MR, et al: Evaluation of methylene blue and squamous epithelial cells as oropharyngeal markers: a means of identifying oropharyngeal contamination during transtracheal aspiration. J Infect Dis 141:165, 1980

71. Irwin RS, Rosen MJ, Braman SS: Cough: a comprehensive review. Arch Intern Med 137:1186, 1977

72. Jenicek JA, Danner CA, Allen CR: Continuous cuff inflation during long-term intubation and ventilation: evaluation of technique. Anesth Analg 52:252, 1973

73. Johnson WG Jr, Pierce AK, Sanford JP, et al: Nosocomial respiratory infections with gram-negative bacilli: the significance of colonization of the respiratory tract. Ann Intern Med 77:701, 1972

74. Jung RC, Gottlieb LS: Comparison of tracheobronchial suction catheters in humans: visualization by fiberoptic bronchoscopy. Chest 69:179, 1976

75. Kambic V, Radsel Z: Intubation lesions of the larynx. Br J Anaesth 50:587, 1978

76. Kamen JM, Wilkinson CJ: A new low-pressure cuff for endotracheal tubes. Anesthesiology 34:482, 1971

77. Kelsen FG, McGuckin M, Kelsen DP, et al: Airborne contamination of fine-particle nebulizers. JAMA 237:2311, 1974

78. Ketover AK, Feingold A: Collapse of a disposable endotracheal tube by its high-pressure cuff. Anesthesiology 43:108, 1975

79. King K, Mandava B, Kamen JM: Tracheal tube cuffs and tracheal dilation. Chest 67:458, 1975

80. Kirby RR, Robison EJ, Schulz J: Intermittent cuff inflation during prolonged positive pressure ventilation. Anesthesiology 32:364, 1970

81. Knowlson GTG, Bassett HFM: The pressures exerted on the trachea by endotracheal inflatable cuffs. Br J Anaesth 42:834, 1970

82. Komorn RN, Smith CP, Erwin JR: Acute laryngeal injury with short-term endotracheal anesthesia. Laryngoscope 83:673, 1973

83. Kumar A, Falke KJ, Geffin B, et al: Continuous positive-pressure ventilation in acute respiratory failure: effects on hemodynamics and lung function. N Engl J Med 283:1430, 1970

84. Kuzenski BN: Effect of negative pressure on tracheobronchial trauma. Nurs Res 27:260, 1978

85. Lane EE, Temes GD, Anderson WH: Tracheal-innominate artery fistula due to tracheostomy. Chest 68:678, 1975

86. LeFrock JL, Klainer AS, Wu W-H, et al: Transient bacteremia associated with nasotracheal suctioning. JAMA 236:1610, 1976

87. Lewis RN, Swerdlow M: Hazards of endotracheal anaesthesia. Br J Anaesth 36:504, 1964

88. Lewy RB, Sibbitt JW: Tracheostomy and barbiturate poisoning. Am Pract Dig Treat 2:527, 1951

89. Lindholm C-E: Prolonged endotracheal intubation. Acta Anaesthesiol Scand [Suppl] 33:1, 1969

90. Loeser EA, Orr DL II, Bennet GM, et al: Endotracheal tube cuff design and postoperative sore throat. Anesthesiology 45:684, 1976

91. Lough M, Boat T, Doershuk CF: The nose. Respir Care 20:844, 1975

92. MacKenzie CF, Klose S, Browne DRG: A study of inflatable cuffs on endotracheal tubes: pressures exerted on the trachea. Br J Anesth 48:105, 1976

93. MacKenzie CF, Shin B, McAslan TC, et al: Severe stridor after prolonged endotracheal intubation using high-volume cuffs. Anesthesiology 50:235, 1979

94. MacKenzie RA, Gould AB Jr, Bardsley WT: Cardiac arrhythmias with endotracheal intubation. Anesthesiology 53:S102, 1980

95. Magovern GJ, Shively JG, Fecht D, et al: The clinical and experimental evaluation of a controlled-pressure intratracheal cuff. J. Thorac Cardiovasc Surg 64:747, 1972

96. Malik SK, Jenkins DE: Alterations in airway dynamics following inhalation of ultrasonic mist. Chest 62:660, 1972

97. McClelland RMA: Complications of tracheostomy. Br Med J 2:567, 1965

98. McGinnis GE, Shively JG, Patterson RL: An engineering analysis of intratracheal tube cuffs. Anesth Analg 50:557, 1971

99. Mead J, Turner JM, Macklem PT, et al: Significance of the relationship between lung recoil and maximum expiratory flow. J Appl Physiol 22:95, 1967

100. Meade JW: Tracheostomy—its complications and their management: a study of 212 cases. N Engl J Med 265:519, 1961

101. Meglio F: Hazard of removable tracheostomy cuffs. Respir Care 17:17, 1972 (letter)

102. Mehalic TF, Farhat, SM: Tracheoarterial fistula: a complication of tracheostomy in patients with brainstem injury. J Trauma 12:140, 1972

103. Mehta S: The risk of aspiration in the presence of cuffed endotracheal tubes. Br J Anaesth 44:601, 1972

104. Merav AD: Low-pressure "parachute" endotracheal cuff. NY State J Med 71:1926, 1971

105. Mörch ET, Saxton GA Jr, Gish G: Artificial respiration by the uncuffed tracheostomy tube. JAMA 160:884, 1956

106. Mulder DS, Rubush JL: Complications of tracheostomy: relationship to long-term

ventilatory assistance. J Trauma 9:389, 1969

107. Myers WO, Lawton BR, Sautter RD: An operation for tracheal-innominate artery fistula. Arch Surg 105:269, 1972

108. Naigow D, Powaser MM: The effect of different endotracheal suction procedures on arterial blood gases in a controlled experimental model. Heart Lung 6:808, 1977

109. Nordin U: The trachea and cuff-induced injury: an experimental study on causative factors and prevention. Acta Otolaryngol [Suppl] (Stockh) 345:1, 1977

110. Orringer MB: Endotracheal intubation and tracheostomy: indications, techniques and complications. Surg Clin North Am 60:1447, 1980

111. Pavlin EG, Nelson E, Pulliam J: Difficulty in removal of tracheostomy tubes. Anesthesiology 44:69, 1976

112. Pavlin EG, Van Nimwegan D, Hornbein TF: Failure of a high-compliance, low-pressure cuff to prevent aspiration. Anesthesiology 42:216, 1975

113. Pereira W, Kovnat DM, Kahn MA, et al: Fever and pneumonia after flexible fiberoptic bronchoscopy. Am Rev Respir Dis 112:59, 1975

114. Peterson GM, Pierson DJ, Hunter PM: Arterial oxygen saturation during nasotracheal suctioning. Chest 76:283, 1979

115. Pontoppidan H, Laver MB, Geffin B: Acute respiratory failure in the surgical patient. Adv Surg 4:163, 1971

116. Powers WE: Is periodic cuff deflation necessary? Respir Care 20:992, 1975

117. Redding GJ, Fan L, Cotton EK, et al: Partial obstruction of endotracheal tubes in children. Crit Care Med 7:227, 1979

118. Ringrose RE, McKeon B, Felton FG, et al: A hospital outbreak of Serratia marcescens associated with ultrasonic nebulizers. Ann Intern Med 69:719, 1968

119. Ripoll I, Lindholm CE, Carroll R, et al: Spontaneous dislocation of endotracheal tubes. Anesthesiology 49:50, 1978

120. Rosato F, Rosato EF, Plotkin SA: Herpetic paronychia—an occupational hazard of medical personnel. N Engl J Med 283:804, 1970

121. Rucker RW, Silva WJ, Worcester CC: Fiberoptic bronchoscopic nasotracheal intubation in children. Chest 76:56, 1979

122. Sackner MA: Bronchofiberoscopy. Am Rev Respir Dis 111:62, 1975

123. Sackner MA: Tracheobronchial toilet. In: Weekly Update: Pulmonary Medicine. Biomedia, Princeton, NJ, 1978

124. Sackner MA, Landa JF, Greeneltch N, et al: Pathogenesis and prevention of tracheobronchial damage with suction procedures. Chest 64:284, 1973

125. Sahn SA, Lakshminarayan S: Bedside criteria for discontinuation of mechanical ventilation. Chest 63:1002, 1973

126. Sahn SA, Lakshminarayan S, Petty TL: Weaning from mechanical ventilation. JAMA 235:2208, 1976

127. Sanders CV, Luby JP, Johanson WG, et al: Serratia marcescens infections from inhalation therapy medications: nosocomial outbreak. Ann Intern Med 73:15, 1970

128. Santa Cruz R, Landa J, Hirsch J, et al: Tracheal mucous velocity in normal man and patients with obstructive lung disease: effects of terbutaline. Am Rev Respir Dis 109:458, 1974

129. Schaberg DR, Alford RH, Anderson R, et al: An outbreak of nosocomial infection due to multiple resistant Serratia marcescens: Evidence of interhospital spread. J Infect Dis 134:181, 1976

130. Schwartz SN, Dowling JN, Benkovic C, et al: Sources of gram-negative bacilli colonizing the tracheae of intubated patients. J Infect Dis 138:227, 1978

131. Scully RE, McNeely BU: Weekly clinical pathologic exercises. N Engl J Med 291:464, 1974

132. Sellery GR, Worth A, Greenway RE: Late complications of prolonged tracheal intubation. Can Anaesth Soc J 25:140, 1978

133. Shim C, Fine N, Fernandez R, et al: Cardiac arrhythmias resulting from tracheal suctioning. Ann Intern Med 71:1149, 1969

134. Silen W, Spieker D: Fatal hemorrhage from the innominate artery after tracheostomy. Ann Surg 162:1005, 1965

135. Smith PW, Massanari RM: Room humidifiers as the source of Acinetobacter infections. JAMA 237:795, 1977

136. Spoerel WE, Chan CK: Jet ventilation for tracheobronchial suction. Anesthesiology 45:450, 1976

137. Standards for cardiopulmonary resuscitation (CPR) and emergency cardiac care (ECC). JAMA (Suppl) 227:854, 1974

138. Stauffer JL, Olson DE, Petty TL: Complications and consequences of endotracheal intubation and tracheotomy: a prospective study of 150 critically ill adult patients. Am J Med 70:65, 1981

139. Stauffer JL, Petty TL: Accidental intubation of the pyriform sinus: a complication of "roadside" resuscitation. JAMA 237:2324, 1977

140. Stauffer JL, Silvestri RC: Complications of endotracheal intubation, tracheostomy and artificial airways. Respir Care 27:417, 1982

141. Stern H, Elek SD, Millar DM, et al: Herpetic whitlow: a form of cross-infection in hospitals. Lancet 2:871, 1959

142. Stoeckel H: Late complications after tracheostomy. In Boulton, TB, Bryce-Smith R, Sykes MK, et al (eds): Progress in Anesthesiology: Proceedings of the Fourth World Congress of Anesthesiologists. p. 825. Excerpta Medica, Amsterdam, 1970

143. Stuart BO: Deposition of inhaled aerosols. Arch Intern Med 131:60, 1973

144. Sutton PP, Pavia D, Batemen JRM, et al: The effect of oral aminophyllin on lung mucociliary clearance in man. Chest (Suppl) 80:889, 1981

145. Taryle DA, Chandler JE, Good JT, et al: Emergency room intubations—complications and survival. Chest 75:541, 1979

146. Touloukian RJ, Beardsley GP, Ablow RC, et al: Traumatic perforation of the pharynx in the newborn. Pediatrics 59:1019, 1977

147. Trout C: Artificial airways: tubes and trachs. Respir Care 21:513, 1976

148. Vogelhut MM, Downs JB: Prolonged endotracheal intubation. Chest 76:110, 1979

149. VonLeden H, Isshiki N: An analysis of cough at the level of the larynx. Arch Otolaryngol 81:616, 1965

150. Wanner A: State-of-the-art: clinical aspects of mucociliary transport. Am Rev Respir Dis 116:73, 1977

151. Webb WR, Ozdemir IA, Ikins PM, et al: Surgical management of tracheal stenosis. Ann Surg 179:819, 1974

152. Weber AL, Grillo HC: Tracheal stenosis: an analysis of 151 cases. Radiol Clin North Am 16:291, 1978

153. Webster's New Collegiate Dictionary. Merriam, Springfield, MA, 1976

154. Whited RE: Laryngeal dysfunction following prolonged intubation. Ann Otol Rhinol Laryngol 88:474, 1979

155. Wimberly N, Faling LJ, Bartlett JG: A fiberoptic bronchoscopy technique to obtain uncontaminated lower airway secretions for bacterial culture. Am Rev Respir Dis 119:337, 1979

156. Wood PB, Nagy E, Pearson FG, et al: Measurement of mucociliary clearance from the lower respiratory tract of normal dogs. Can Anaesth Soc J 20:192, 1973

157. Wood RE, Fink RJ: Applications of flexible fiberoptic bronchoscopes in infants and children. Chest (Suppl) 73:737, 1978

158. Wood RE, Wanner A, Hirsch J, et al: Tracheal mucociliary transport in patients with cystic fibrosis and its stimulation by terbutaline. Am Rev Respir Dis 111:733, 1975

159. Zwillich C, Pierson DJ: Nasal necrosis: a complication of nasotracheal intubation. Chest 64:376, 1973

160. Zwillich CW, Pierson DJ, Creagh CE, et al: Complications of assisted ventilation: a prospective study of 354 consecutive episodes. Am J Med 57:161, 1974

6

Respiratory Failure in the Adult: Ventilatory Support

Michael J. Banner
T. James Gallagher

Hypoxia not only stops the machine but wrecks the machinery.

Haldane

PATHOLOGY AND PATHOPHYSIOLOGY

Hypoxemia

Mechanical ventilation treats three basic problems: (1) inadequate oxygenation—increased airway pressure therapy may eliminate hypoxemia; (2) inadequate alveolar ventilation, producing hypercapnea—augmentation of spontaneous minute ventilation often requires supplemental mechanical support; (3) loss of airway—some patients require an artificial airway and mechanical ventilatory support.

Many problems loosely grouped under the descriptive term adult respiratory distress syndrome (ARDS) cause acute hypoxemia and characteristically improve with positive end-expiratory pressure (PEEP) or continuous positive airway pressure (CPAP), usually coupled with mechanical ventilation. ARDS most often occurs in previously asymptomatic individuals with reasonably normal lungs as opposed to those with significant chronic obstructive or restrictive changes.

The major characteristic of ARDS is hypoxemia, which is often refractory to both supplemental oxygen therapy and mechanical ventilation. Progressive deterioration of arterial oxygen tension (Pao_2) and an increase of venous admixture and physiological shunt ($\dot{Q}sp/\dot{Q}t$) are the most sensitive indicators of ARDS. Confirmation of the diagnosis requires that other causes of hypoxemia must be ruled out, including decreased fractional inspired oxygen concentration (Fio_2), right mainstem bronchial intubation, pulmonary barotrauma, inadequate cardiac output ($\dot{Q}t$), and hypoventilation.

Patients with ARDS characteristically manifest a low Pao_2 that responds only minimally to an increase of Fio_2. A young, otherwise healthy patient with ARDS and breathing room air may have a Pa_{O_2} of 50–55 mm Hg that increases to 70 mm Hg after an increase in $F_{I_{O_2}}$ to 0.8. This response is considerably less than expected.

Tachypnea at rates up to 40 breaths/minute and hyperventilation (Pa_{CO_2}, 30–35 mm Hg) are commonly seen in patients with ARDS. Hypercapnia usually is seen only in late or advanced stages, in contrast to respiratory distress syndrome (RDS) of the newborn in which respiratory acidemia occurs relatively early because of an unstable chest wall. Functional residual capacity (FRC) is reduced, primarily as a result of a decrease in expiratory reserve volume (Fig. 6-1). Lung compliance (C_L) decreases and requires an increase in inspiratory transpulmonary pressure to maintain the same tidal volume (V_T). Chest roentgenograms are unreliable in the initial diagnosis. Deterioration of gas exchange often occurs long before significant roentgenographic change becomes evident. Characteristically, these changes lag behind the development of and recovery from ARDS.

Examination of the lungs in patients who die with ARDS reveals major pathological changes associated with increased lung water. The beefy, red, consolidated lungs emphasize the lack of viable gas exchange units. Interstitial pulmonary edema is prevalent, and the alveoli are filled with red and white blood cells and proteinaceous debris. Atelectasis is a late manifestation secondary to the other changes that have occurred.[67]

A number of clinical entities are associated with a high incidence of ARDS. Aspiration of gastric contents with a pH less than 2.5 is frequently a progenitor of respiratory failure (Mendelson's syndrome).[46] Acidic liquid not only fills the alveoli but also increases alveolar-capillary membrane permeability, which leads to additional fluid accumulation in the interstitial and alveolar spaces and further impairment of gas exchange.

When the possibility of aspiration exists, several measures may reduce its severity. Cimetidine decreases gastric volume and increases gastric pH. However, this drug requires at least an hour to take effect. Prophylactic antacids also have been advocated. However, alkaline solutions themselves can cause a substantial lesion[29] with significant deterioration of gas exchange. Steroids have no proved benefit in the treatment of aspiration syndromes.

Both seawater and freshwater near-drowning can cause respiratory failure.[47] Seawater aspiration is associated with severe interstitial and alveolar pulmonary

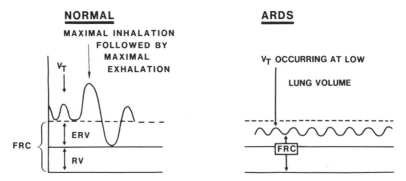

Fig. 6-1. Lung volume changes during ARDS. Lung volumes (including FRC and expiratory reserve volume [ERV]), except residual volume (RV), are diminished. Tidal volume (V_T) is also reduced at low lung volumes compared with normal (see text). Dotted line represents normal expiratory lung volume or FRC.

edema similar to that seen with congestive heart failure. Fresh water, however, inactivates surfactant and destroys the type II epithelial cells. Freshwater drowning usually requires a longer period of mechanical ventilation, probably because of surfactant inactivation and subsequent alveolar collapse.

The inhalation of noxious substances can cause ARDS. Most commonly, this problem is associated with combustion of synthetic materials (upholstery, plastics, etc.) in a closed environment. The primary insult probably involves direct action at the alveolar side of the alveolar-capillary interface. Inhalation of carbon monoxide is also a problem in such cases.

Injuries to several organ systems and direct thoracic injuries often cause ARDS. Diverse events—including release of free fatty acids, prostaglandins, endotoxin, and serotonin; complement activation; platelet and white blood cell aggregation and breakdown; massive homologous blood transfusion; and hemorrhage—have been implicated. Whatever the mechanism, the capillary membrane seems to be the ''target'' area of vulnerability.

Acute peritonitis, generalized sepsis, and pancreatitis are often grouped together as causes of ARDS. Each is associated with release of circulating toxic substances that interact with the alveolar-capillary membrane, increase capillary permeability, and promote fluid accumulation in the pulmonary interstitium. When fluid ingress exceeds the capacity of the pulmonary interstitium and the pulmonary lymphatics, alveolar flooding results.

Prolonged upper abdominal or thoracic surgical procedures may result in signs and symptoms suggestive of mild forms of ARDS. These operations usually are associated with decreased lung volume (FRC). Patients often respond to postoperative pain with splinted respirations and minimal diaphragmatic excursions.

Pulmonary edema, as a consequence of fluid overload or congestive heart failure, is thought by some to be a form of ARDS.[58] The vascular engorgement elevates microvascular pressures, promoting fluid egress from the vascular space into both the interstitial space and the alveoli.

Fat embolism, although a distinct entity, frequently produces ARDS after long bone fractures. Although fat globules may be elaborated from the fracture site, the release of free fatty acids seems to be the real culprit causing lung damage.[50] Interaction of these substances with the capillary membrane promotes eventually the same leaky capillary situation as in sepsis: endothelial damage, platelet aggregation at the site of injury, and release of serotonin. Pulmonary vasoconstriction raises microcapillary pressure and drives more fluid into the interstitium.

Segmental or lobar pneumonias do not cause ARDS. However, diffuse interstitial forms often cause a clinical picture characteristic of ARDS. Hypoxemia in such cases often responds to therapy that is successful for common forms of ARDS, which leads some clinicians to consider interstitial pneumonia a potential cause of the process.

In summary, a limited number of primary pathophysiological changes are associated with a number of clinical conditions and cause impaired oxygenation.[67] An excess of fluid movement into the pulmonary interstitium, over and above what can be removed by the lymphatics, is the element of major concern. This abnormality can be exacerbated by an increase in pulmonary hydrostatic pressure, a substantial decrease in colloid oncotic pressure, or further increases in pulmonary capillary permeability. As fluid accumulates, interstitial pressure increases, ultimately leading to terminal airway narrowing and collapse. The alveoli initially are unaffected. However, the narrowed terminal airways decrease the ventilation/perfusion ratio ($\dot{V}_A/$

$\dot{Q}$) in affected areas and the saturation of arterial blood with oxygen, which manifests as a fall in Pa_{O_2}.

Alveolar Ventilation

Inability to eliminate carbon dioxide normally is a second major problem which may require mechanical ventilatory support. Characteristically, patients respond with either an increase of Pa_{CO_2} or in the work of breathing required to maintain a normal Pa_{CO_2}. The respiratory rate usually increases up to approximately 40 breaths/ minute or more; however, unless V_T is sufficient (4–5 ml/kg), the increase in ventilation serves only to ventilate dead space (V_D) without any appreciable decrease in Pa_{CO_2} (in some instances Pa_{CO_2} actually increases).

Neuromuscular paralysis can lead to alveolar hypoventilation and hypercapnia. This problem usually occurs because of an overdose of an agent, e.g., pancuronium bromide (Pavulon), a neuromuscular blocking agent. Prolongation of blockade may be seen in hypothermic patients who are unable to metabolize such agents and/or to excrete them normally through the kidneys. If the drug has been given recently, immediate attempts to reverse its action will be to no avail.

Drug overdose with barbiturates and narcotics can lead to severe hypoventilation or cessation of breathing. With narcotics, the rate is depressed whereas V_T remains unaffected. The carbon dioxide response curve shifts to the right, and minute ventilation is depressed. Drug overdose may also occur with anesthetic agents. Most of the potent inhalational agents, including halothane, enflurane, and forane, decrease minute volume.

A common cause of hypercapnia is seen during acute ventilatory decompensation of patients with chronic obstructive pulmonary disease (COPD). In advanced stages, loss of normal airway architecture and function leads to chronic carbon dioxide retention and abnormally increased FRC. These patients have marginal pulmonary reserve, and any acute airway infection or event requiring pulmonary performance above normal often leads to acute decompensation. In normal individuals, spontaneous exhalation is a passive event. Patients with COPD must exhale actively and, in so doing, markedly increase the work of breathing and oxygen consumption ($\dot{V}_{O_2}$). Fatigue, additional air trapping, and CO_2 retention often result.

Severe restrictive lung disease with limited V_T and vital capacity can result in alveolar hypoventilation. With diffuse parenchymal involvement, these disease processes are often irreversible.

Airway Obstruction

Obstruction of the airway can occur as a result of tumors, foreign bodies, mucosal and submucosal edema, laryngeal spasm, epiglottitis, and tracheobronchial malacia. Many of these lesions can be acute or chronic, and most require artificial airway maintenance, usually with a translaryngeal or tracheostomy tube. Mechanical ventilatory support is frequently utilized adjunctively.

Altered levels of consciousness after surgery, especially in cases with neurological impairment, depress airway control. Often the gag reflex is impaired, and these patients require airway management identical to that described above until they can protect their own airway.

Lung Mechanics and Work of Breathing

Respiratory muscles must overcome three forces during breathing: (1) elastic forces, which result from deformations of pulmonary and thoracic tissues when their volumes change; (2) flow resistive forces, generated by resistance to gas flow in the airways and resistance of the inelastic elements of the lung and thorax during a change in volume; and (3) inertial forces, which depend on the masses of tissues and gases in the airways and lungs.[51] The last is a negligible factor at normal rates of breathing.

Respiratory work may be evaluated by simultaneously measuring the changes in lung-thorax volume and transpulmonary pressure (the difference between airway and intrapleural pressure). The relationship of respiratory work to changes in pressure and volume is described by the following expression:

$$W = \int P dV \qquad (1)$$

where W = work of breathing (kg·M/minute), P = change in transpulmonary pressure, and dV = rate of change in volume (flow).

The solution to the equation is represented by the circumscribed area of a pressure-volume diagram (Fig. 6-2). This method of describing respiratory work relates lung elasticity and flow resistance to the flow of gas. The work of breathing is a reflection of lung mechanical function as well as lung and chest wall expansibility and therefore is a measure of the energy required for ventilation. Total respiratory work during quiet breathing ranges from 0.3 to 0.8 kg·M/minute.

Proctor and Woolson[55] have reported that work of breathing values of 1.34 kg·M/minute or greater predict the dependence of postthoracotomy patients on mechanical ventilation. Peters and Hilberman[54] suggested the value to be 1.8 kg·M/minute. In another report by Henning et al.,[36] dependence on mechanical ventilation in patients with obstructive lung disease was likely when the work value was equal to or greater than 1.7 kg·M/minute. This report also demonstrated that patients could breathe spontaneously without the aid of a mechanical ventilator when the respiratory work was less than 1 kg·M/minute.

The work of breathing normally requires only 2–3 percent of total body oxygen consumption. However, in ARDS associated with decreased C_L, increased airway resistance, or both, the respiratory work and $\dot{V}O_2$ increase considerably. In such instances, respiratory work may be decreased by providing positive-pressure therapy, i.e., CPAP, to improve the C_L and restore the FRC.

Increased extravascular lung water (EVLW), decreased lung volume, and abnormal or absent surfactant predispose to a decreased C_L described by Downs.[14] The elastic work of breathing (Wel) is inversely related to C_L[13]:

$$Wel = \frac{\frac{1}{2}V_T^2}{C_L} \qquad (2)$$

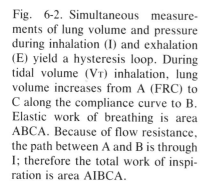

Fig. 6-2. Simultaneous measurements of lung volume and pressure during inhalation (I) and exhalation (E) yield a hysteresis loop. During tidal volume (V_T) inhalation, lung volume increases from A (FRC) to C along the compliance curve to B. Elastic work of breathing is area ABCA. Because of flow resistance, the path between A and B is through I; therefore the total work of inspiration is area AIBCA.

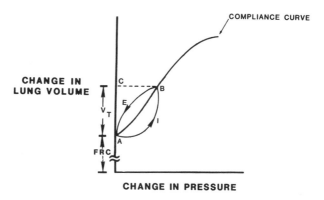

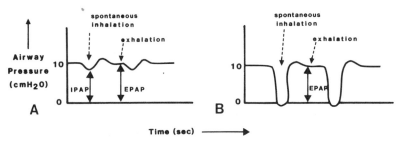

Fig. 6-3. (A) During CPAP when high rates of inspiratory flow are provided, airway pressure decreases slightly but remains positive during spontaneous inhalation (termed inspiratory positive airway pressure; IPAP). At exhalation, airway pressure increases to expiratory positive airway pressure (EPAP). (B) During positive end-expiratory pressure (PEEP), when the patient's inspiratory rate of flow exceeds that of the system, airway pressure decreases to zero or subambient levels during spontaneous inhalation. Airway pressure is positive during exhalation only, i.e., EPAP.

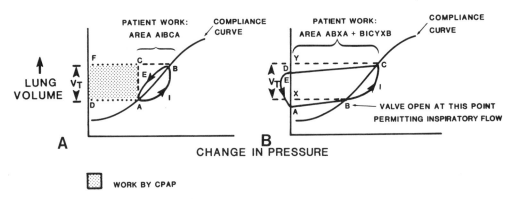

Fig. 6-4. Differences in work of breathing for (A) CPAP and (B) PEEP can be appreciated by assuming that both are applied at equal expiratory pressure levels. With CPAP, spontaneous inhalation begins at A through I to B, with exhalation following path BEA. Tidal volume (VT) change is from D to F. Spontaneous inspiratory work of breathing (elastic and flow resistance) is area AIBCA. The high rate of inspiratory flow (high IPAP) provides part of the force to perform the work of breathing, i.e., area ACFDA. With PEEP, spontaneous inhalation begins at A; however, during inspiration the patient must work to open the valve in order to obtain inspiratory flow (point B) (this point represents the airway pressure decrease to zero during spontaneous inhalation, as in Fig. 6-3B). Lung volume then increases along curve BIC; subsequently, the patient must work to exhale from point C to D. (This transition represents the airway pressure increase to EPAP during the beginning of exhalation as in Figure 6-3B.) At point D, the expiratory pressure valve opens and exhalation occurs along path DEA; point A is the level of EPAP. VT change is from X to Y. The inspiratory work of breathing is area ABXA (to open the inspiratory flow valve) plus area BICYXB. Quantitatively, a greater inspiratory work area occurs with PEEP than with CPAP. Thus inspiratory work of breathing is greater with PEEP than with CPAP. (Modified with permission from Douglas ME, Downs JB: Cardiopulmonary effects of PEEP and CPAP. Anesth Analg 57:347. (Copyright 1978 by the International Anesthesia Research Society)).

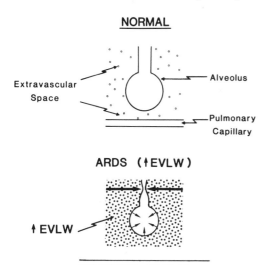

Fig. 6-5. Increased EVLW in ARDS compromises the patency of small airways and thus predisposes the patient to absorption atelectasis, loss of lung volume, and further edema.

In order to minimize the work of breathing, a patient with a decreased C_L compensates by breathing at a lower V_T. However, a higher respiratory rate is then needed for adequate gas exchange. Also, to maintain alveolar ventilation when C_L is decreased, peak inspiratory intrapleural pressure (Ppl) must be decreased significantly more than normal (increased change in transpulmonary pressure). Because

$$V_T = C_L \times \Delta Ppl \qquad (3)$$

further reduction of Ppl, of course, increases the work of breathing.

The work of breathing during CPAP compared with that during PEEP differs significantly.[12,14,28,37] From a physiological point of view, these spontaneous positive-pressure breathing patterns differ primarily in their pressure waveforms during inspiration (Fig. 6-3). With CPAP, airway pressure is positive during both spontaneous inspiration and expiration. CPAP therefore combines both inspiratory positive airway pressure (IPAP) and expiratory positive airway pressure (EPAP). With PEEP, airway pressure is positive only at end-expiration. Ap-

plying positive airway pressure to a spontaneously breathing patient without providing IPAP (i.e., PEEP) increases the work of breathing (Fig. 6-4). Because a fundamental goal in treating ARDS is to reduce respiratory work, careful attention must be paid to delivering CPAP with high IPAP. A low-resistance system providing a high flow on demand (usually greater than 60 L/minute) during spontaneous inspiration usually meets the requirements.

Lung Volume

Loss of lung volume is a hallmark of ARDS. FRC decreases specifically because of reduced expiratory reserve volume (ERV). The primary initial cause is increased extravascular lung water (EVLW)

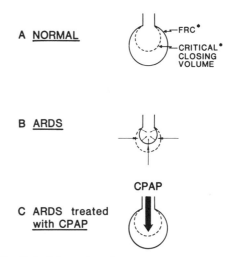

Fig. 6-6. When alveoli are normal (A), at end-exhalation the FRC is above critical closing volume. During ARDS (B) the expiratory volume (FRC) decreases below critical closing volume and predisposes the alveoli to collapse. CPAP as a treatment for ARDS (C) restores the FRC and prevents the alveolar volume from diminishing below critical closing volume. *Solid line represents FRC; dotted line represents alveolar critical closing volume, the expiratory volume below which alveolar instability and atelectasis occur.

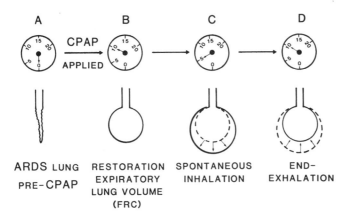

A   B   C   D

CPAP
APPLIED

ARDS LUNG   RESTORATION   SPONTANEOUS   END-
PRE-CPAP   EXPIRATORY   INHALATION   EXHALATION
              LUNG VOLUME
              (FRC)

Fig. 6-7. Pressure and volume changes in the lung during spontaneous ventilation with CPAP. (A) With ARDS, the lung characteristically has reduced expiratory lung volume or FRC; airway pressure is ambient. Application of CPAP (B) increases the airway pressure, e.g., 10 cm H_2O, and thus increases/restores the expiratory lung volume to a normal physiological state. During spontaneous inhalation (C) the airway pressure decreases, e.g., 5 cm H_2O, while lung volume simultaneously increases. At end-expiration (D), the lung volume returns to FRC, regulated by an expiratory pressure valve.

resulting from a heightened fluid (and albumin) flux across the leaky pulmonary capillaries. The increased EVLW compromises the patency of small airways, especially in dependent lung regions, predisposing to absorption atelectasis (Fig. 6-5). If fluid continues to move unabated into the pulmonary interstitium, fluid "spills over" into the alveoli, disrupting surfactant and leads to peripheral, widespread atelectasis and a further reduction of FRC.

In ARDS the FRC is less than the critical closing volume during tidal ventilation. Critical closing volume is that lung volume at end-exhalation below which small airway closure and atelectasis begin to occur. It is as much a conceptual value as it is a discretely measured volume. When FRC decreases below critical closing volume, alveoli are predisposed to collapse, $\dot{V}_A/\dot{Q}$ worsens, and $\dot{Q}sp/\dot{Q}t$ increases. A decrease in Pa_{O_2} results. CPAP restores FRC toward normal and, more importantly, increases it above the critical closing volume (Fig. 6-6). Thus CPAP corrects a major mechanical abnormality and restores the lung to a more normal physiological state.

The applied level of CPAP is determined at the end of exhalation. Because this therapy increases expiratory lung volume, inspiratory and mean airway pressure do not reflect the total alveolar distending pressure at end-exhalation (Fig. 6-7).

Quite apart from variations in work of breathing, CPAP and PEEP produce other major respiratory and hemodynamic differences. CPAP increases mean airway pressure to a greater extent than an equal level of PEEP. Gherini et al.[28] demonstrated that significantly higher FRCs were maintained with CPAP than with PEEP at equal expiratory pressure. With respect to hemodynamic effects, the lower inspiratory airway pressure and Ppl during PEEP enhances venous return to the heart and increases $\dot{Q}t$.

Dead Space

Disorders that decrease or eliminate perfusion to ventilated alveoli increase alveolar dead space. Physiological, or total, dead space volume (V_D) (anatomical plus alveolar dead space) includes that portion of the conducting airways and alveoli not involved in gas exchange. Several factors predominate. Diffuse pulmonary emboli inhibit blood flow but affect ventilation minimally. Physiological dead space increases at the expense of available V_T.

Normally, V_D/V_T approximates 0.3 (i.e., 30 percent of the V_T is wasted and does not participate in gas exchange). In severe cases of ARDS the V_D/V_T may be two to three times above the normal value. With increased V_D total ventilation must increase in order to maintain oxygenation when patients breathe ambient air. CO_2 retention is rarely a problem initially, in contrast to oxygenation, and, as mentioned, Pa_{CO_2} is characteristically low.

Other causes of increased V_D/V_T are severe hemorrhage and hypotension. Under these circumstances, gravitational force and low pulmonary arterial pressure redistribute the blood volume and flow to the more dependent lung regions. The result is a greater number of nondependent, underperfused but still ventilated alveoli, i.e., areas of increased $\dot{V}_A/\dot{Q}$, which increase V_D. A precipitous drop in $\dot{Q}t$ may produce similar effects. Finally, as pointed out earlier, V_T decreases and respiratory rate in-

creases in ARDS. Therefore V_D represents a proportionally greater fraction of a given V_T as a result of this altered breathing pattern.

Positive-pressure therapy may also alter alveolar V_D.[19] The mechanical ventilator preferentially distributes inspired gas to areas of limited perfusion. In the supine, paralyzed individual a disproportionate amount of V_T is delivered anteriorly to nondependent lung regions with decreased perfusion.[20] Spontaneous ventilation, conversely, tends to promote more normal distribution of $\dot{V}_A/\dot{Q}$ and minimizes the ventilator-induced abnormalities (Figure 6-8). Some studies have demonstrated that V_D increases during mechanical ventilation with or without positive expiratory pressure.[18,49] Downs and Mitchell[18] showed that increases of V_D were related to the rate of mechanical cycling regardless of the ventilatory pattern and/or whether positive expiratory pressure was employed (Fig. 6-9).

Another cause of ventilated but nonperfused alveoli is the elevated mean airway pressure developed during mechanical ventilation with positive expiratory pressure. Excessive pressure in some alveoli may collapse pulmonary capillaries, eliminate perfusion, and increase V_D.[69] Such changes re-

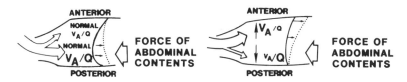

Fig. 6-8. Alteration in ventilation/perfusion ($\dot{V}_A/\dot{Q}$) matching as a result of therapy. Intermittent mandatory ventilation (IMV) tends to provide better $\dot{V}_A/\dot{Q}$ matching than controlled mechanical ventilation (CMV). With IMV (A), active contraction of the diaphragm during spontaneous inhalation facilitates the distribution of V_T to posterior areas of the lung. In the relatively low pressure pulmonary arterial system, blood flow also gravitates to the same areas. Thus in both posterior and anterior lung regions, normal physiological $\dot{V}_A/\dot{Q}$ matching results. CMV (B), however, tends to deliver a disproportionate amount of V_T anteriorly with passive diaphragmatic displacement. Thus the ventilator induces new $\dot{V}_A/\dot{Q}$ abnormalities: decreased $\dot{V}_A/\dot{Q}$ (relative shunt) in posterior perfusion-dependent areas and increased $\dot{V}_A/\dot{Q}$ (alveolar dead space) in anterior nondependent areas, or perhaps exacerbates existing abnormalities.

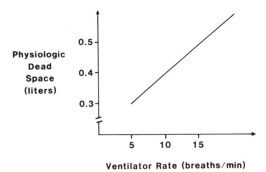

Physiologic Dead Space (liters)

Ventilator Rate (breaths/min)

Fig. 6-9. Physiological dead space (VD) and rate of mechanical ventilation. VD increases with increasing rates of mechanical ventilation with or without positive expiratory pressure. This effect is secondary to maldistribution of inspired gas during a mechanical breath and increased alveolar ventilation to nondependent areas of the lung. These effects increase the ventilation/perfusion ratio and therefore increase the VD. The combined effects of increased mechanical ventilation and loss of spontaneous ventilation precipitate increased VD (see Fig. 6-8). (Modified with permission from Downs JB, Mitchell LA: Pulmonary effects of ventilatory pattern following cardiopulmonary bypass. Crit Care Med 4:295, 1976.)

late to both the level of mean positive airway pressure and the pulmonary intravascular volume and pressure.

THERAPY IN ARDS

Raised Airway Pressure: PEEP/CPAP

Mechanical ventilation effects minimal improvement of oxygenation in patients with ARDS. Because alveolar ventilation is a primary goal of mechanical ventilation, one would suppose that the increase in airway pressure occurring with intermittent positive-pressure ventilation (IPPV) would expand areas of the lung which are poorly ventilated and perhaps open areas which are fluid-filled or atelectatic. Insofar as the events taking place during the inspiratory phase of each IPPV cycle are concerned, all of these considerations hold true. However,

at the end of each inspiration, airway pressure decreases to the normal, ambient level. Increased interstitial pressure, in combination with the instability of affected alveoli in ARDS, is sufficient to initiate significant alveolar volume loss and perhaps collapse during the expiratory phase. It is only when PEEP/CPAP are used to increase expiratory airway pressure that these abnormal changes can be at least partially offset. Under these circumstances, the mechanical breath delivers enough pressure to reexpand the involved areas, and PEEP or CPAP ensures continued expansion and gas exchange throughout the ventilatory cycle. The eventual level of expiratory pressure will be some value slightly above the mean alveolar closing pressure.

What is the optimal level of CPAP or PEEP? Although different therapeutic endpoints have been described, available evidence does not suggest the superiority of one or another. The most popular concept suggests that PEEP/CPAP be increased until the patient breathes less than toxic oxygen concentrations ($F_{IO_2} \leq 0.5$) and the hemoglobin is at least 90 percent saturated with oxygen ($Pa_{O_2} = 60$–70 mm Hg at normal pH). If the initial F_{IO_2} is greater than 0.5, as Pa_{O_2} improves the F_{IO_2} is progressively decreased to 0.5 or less as long as hemoglobin saturation remains equal to or greater than 90 percent.

High levels of PEEP and CPAP have been alleged to produce cardiovascular depression and pulmonary barotrauma. Consequently, most authorities have recommended some arbitrary limit to the level of PEEP or CPAP used, usually less than 15 cm H_2O. However, as Kirby et al.[42] pointed out, some patients require much higher levels before gas exchange improves. Arbitrary limitation of therapy to preselected maximal values may prevent attainment of designated therapeutic endpoints. Only by observing the individual response can we expect, in each particular case, to correct the problem.

Another approach to ascertain the acceptable limits of CPAP or PEEP correlates raised airway pressure to maximal combined thoracic and lung compliance (C_{LT}).[65] Because C_L decreases in ARDS, PEEP/CPAP may be expected to improve C_{LT} as alveolar reexpansion occurs and FRC improves. Studies have demonstrated that the "best" C_{LT} obtained with PEEP or CPAP does not always correlate with the best Pao_2 or lowest $\dot{Q}sp/\dot{Q}t$.[65,66] The level of PEEP/CPAP that optimizes C_{LT} is often considerably less than the level that which maximizes gas exchange. Because therapy in ARDS is usually initiated to improve alveolar gas exchange and arterial oxygenation, we advocate treating patients with PEEP or CPAP until $\dot{Q}sp/\dot{Q}t$ is restored to and maintained at 0.15 (15 percent or less).[25,26] The original definition of ARDS[2] stipulated an alveolar-arterial oxygen tension gradient greater than 300–350 mm Hg as one of the diagnostic criteria ($Fio_2 = 1.0$). This value results when $\dot{Q}sp/\dot{Q}t$ is 0.15 if $\dot{Q}t$ and $\dot{V}o_2$ are normal. Hence it is reasonably incorporated as a major endpoint of therapy. Calculation of $\dot{Q}sp/\dot{Q}t$ requires a mixed venous blood sample from a pulmonary artery catheter to determine mixed venous oxygen content ($C\bar{v}o_2$). In those patients with stable hemodynamic and metabolic function and without pulmonary artery catheters, we calculate the Pao_2/Fio_2 ratio. If that value exceeds 300, we assume venous admixture of less than 0.15. This method has been used successfully to treat over 300 cases without any serious errors in diagnosis and therapy.

Although it is unclear which therapeutic endpoint—adequate arterial hemoglobin saturation, best compliance, or shunt reduction to 0.15—is most advantageous, some conclusions may be evident. Overall mortality in ARDS seems to be similar in major medical centers regardless of the selected endpoints of treatment; mortality presumably is not a useful discriminant. On the other hand, information such as the duration of ventilatory support, types and numbers of complications, or the need for adjunctive cardiovascular support might provide insight into which method to use, if indeed differences exist.

Use of the same endpoint in all patients might provide other useful information. For example, if the level of CPAP or PEEP necessary to reduce $\dot{Q}sp/\dot{Q}t$ to 0.15 is 25 cm H_2O in one patient and only 10 cm H_2O in another, the relative severity of the pulmonary lesion may be estimated. Whether such information ultimately has any clinical value, as in the prediction of outcome, remains to be seen.

Once the desired therapeutic endpoint has been reached, how long should that level of PEEP or CPAP be maintained? Currently, there are no definitive answers. When increased airway pressure is applied, changes in oxygenation are readily apparent. Most improvements in Pao_2 and decreases in $\dot{Q}sp/\dot{Q}t$ occur within 10 minutes. When little or no change occurs after increasing PEEP or CPAP, one assumes that either lung function is deteriorating further or the level of therapy is inadequate (a third possibility is that lung function did improve but cardiovascular function was depressed). The "response curve" remains variable and often unpredictable for each patient. Whereas most individuals respond quickly to moderate levels of PEEP/CPAP, others may require much more aggressive treatment before oxygenation improves.

Some clinicians have noted an increase in pulmonary barotrauma when patients with ARDS improve after $\dot{Q}sp/\dot{Q}t$ has been reduced to 0.15. Perhaps this is related to an improvement in C_L and increased airway pressure transmission to the lung with resultant overdistention and possible alveolar rupture. Because both peak inflation pressure (PIP) and V_T are associated with barotrauma,[8] this consideration is plausible but not proved. PIP will be increased at higher PEEP/CPAP. For these reasons, we advocate limiting the duration of the optimal level of CPAP or PEEP to approximately 6 hours. Provided oxygenation does not deteriorate, we then reduce PEEP or CPAP by 3–5 cm H_2O decrements every 2–3 hours. The more time required to initially reduce $\dot{Q}sp/\dot{Q}t$ to 0.15, or the greater the level of PEEP or CPAP, the more slowly and cautiously we reduce therapy. We believe it reasonable to assume that the more diseased the lung is initially, as evidenced by the level of PEEP or CPAP required, the slower the resolution. No objective data have been published to show that this is necessarily true.

Weaning from PEEP or CPAP is independent of other ventilatory modalities. In our experience, patients who require PEEP or CPAP of more than 15 cm H_2O rarely can be weaned in 24 hours to a baseline PEEP of 5 cm H_2O or less. Normally we attempt to reduce the level of support by no more than half over each 24-hour period. Exceptions to this rule include near-drowning and pulmonary edema secondary to congestive heart failure. Both of these problems are usually resolved within 24 hours. Blood gas determinations are made within 10–15 minutes of each ventilator adjustment. The Pao_2 of patients with chronic, proliferative changes of ARDS may deteriorate when PEEP or CPAP drops below 5–10 cm H_2O. Then either the new level of therapy is inadequate or the low value represents the baseline condition of the patient and further improvement in the long-term status of the patient is unlikely. Parenthetically, we have noted that the oxygenation of some patients with acute exacerbation of chronic lung disease, but without ARDS, improves markedly when they are exposed to *low* levels of PEEP or CPAP. This observation contradicts the conventional teaching that PEEP/CPAP is contraindicated in COPD.

Mean Airway Pressure

Thus far we have discussed PEEP and CPAP and their effects on oxygenation but have ignored an aspect of positive-pressure therapy which many clinicians believe may be equally important. Recent work with neonates and adults has focused on reversal of the inspiratory:expiratory (I:E) ratio in ventilator therapy. In reality, this term is something of a misnomer if prolongation of the inspiratory time with a pressure plateau is actually what takes place.[57] The ratio refers specifically to the duration of the mechanical ventilator's inspiratory and expiratory times but does not take into account the postexpiratory pause before the next cycle.

When mechanical inspiration is prolonged, mean airway pressure increases. Both PEEP and CPAP also contribute to the elevation of mean airway pressure. In our studies of patients with severe ARDS requiring high levels of CPAP to maintain a $\dot{Q}sp/\dot{Q}t$ of 0.15, a 50 percent reduction of CPAP was accompanied by a fall in mean airway pressure and, as expected, an increase of $\dot{Q}sp/\dot{Q}t$. We then increased the duration of the ventilator's inspiratory time from 1.5 seconds up to as much as 5 seconds while limiting the PIP with a "pop-off" valve. $\dot{Q}sp/\dot{Q}t$ began to decrease and returned to its original value when the patients had been treated with high CPAP.[23] Mean airway pressure in both situations was the same, but when inspiratory prolongation was employed the CPAP requirement was only 50 percent of its original value to achieve identical Pao_2. These data seem to indicate that mean airway pressure is an important determinant of oxygenation, regardless of the particular modality of support used. Similar findings have been reported in neonates with RDS and in experimental studies with high-frequency oscillatory ventilation. PEEP/CPAP do not seem to be the therapeutic sine qua non for maintaining arterial oxygenation.

Mechanical Ventilation

Mechanical ventilation is required if spontaneous ventilation is inadequate (or absent) and a normal Pa_{CO_2} and pHa cannot be maintained. Current modes of mechanical ventilation include controlled mechanical ventilation (CMV), CMV with end-expiratory pressure (continuous positive-pressure ventilation; CPPV), assisted mechanical ventilation (AMV), and assist-control ventilation. These forms of positive-pressure ventilation do not allow normal spontaneous breathing and may require sedation, neuromuscular paralysis, or both to blunt spontaneous attempts to breathe. Intermittent mandatory ventilation (IMV) combined with PEEP or CPAP permits spontaneous and controlled ventilation. Synchronized IMV (SIMV) is a special form of IMV.[41]

In addition to ensuring adequate alveolar ventilation, other goals for ventilatory support for ARDS are essential (see section on Raised Airway Pressure: PEEP/CPAP).

Controlled Mechanical Ventilation. CMV delivers a preselected ventilatory rate that is independent of spontaneous effort on the part of the patient (Fig. 6-10A). The PIP generated mechanically varies inversely with C_{LT} and directly with airway resistance (if the ventilator is volume- or time-cycled). Indications for CMV include apnea secondary to central nervous system depression (brain or spinal cord trauma or both), drug overdose, neuromuscular paralysis (either drug-induced or the result of pathology, e.g., Guillain-Barré syndrome, myasthenia gravis, poliomyelitis).

CPPV delivers a positive-pressure breath followed by a fall in airway pressure to the previously selected positive-pressure plateau; airway pressure never returns to zero (Fig. 6-10B). CPPV was popularized by Ashbaugh et al.[2] as a treatment for ARDS to prevent alveolar collapse during the ventilator's expiratory phase and thereby improve and maintain overall $\dot{V}_A/\dot{Q}$ relationships.

Because many patients treated with CMV are sedated, paralyzed, or hyperventilated below their apneic threshold, accidental

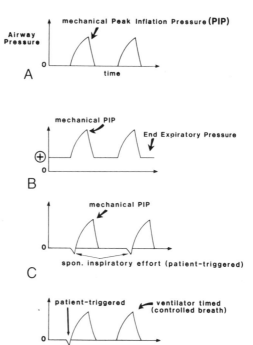

Fig. 6-10. (A) Mechanical ventilatory airway pressure patterns. Controlled mechanical ventilation (CMV). Mechanical ventilator rate and tidal volume (V_T) are preset and cannot be affected by the patient's respiratory efforts. (B) CMV with end-expiratory pressure or continuous positive-pressure ventilation (CPPV). When mechanical inhalation ends, pressure drops to a set positive-pressure plateau, i.e., the end-expiratory pressure level. (C) Assisted mechanical ventilation (AMV). Patient-triggered mechanical inhalation; V_T is preset and cannot be affected by the patient. If the patient does not initiate inhalation, the ventilator does not switch on. (D) Assist-control ventilation. The ventilator may be triggered to mechanical inhalation by the patient's inspiratory efforts or by a timing device, whichever comes first. The patient may trigger the ventilator as often as desired, and the timing device determines the minimum ventilator cycling rate.

disconnection or a mechanical malfunction represents a life-threatening situation. A "disconnect" or "failure-to-cycle" alarm must be provided.

Assisted Mechanical Ventilation. AMV is more appropriately termed "patient-trig-

Table 6-1. Physiological Effects of Respiratory Alkalemia (Hypocapnia)

Decreased
  Cardiac output
  Cerebral blood flow
  Coronary blood flow
  Lung compliance
  P_{50} (leftward shift O_2-hemoglobin dissociation curve—decreased oxygen availability)
  Serum ionized calcium
  Serum potassium
Increased
  Airway resistance
  Oxygen consumption

gered'' mechanical positive-pressure ventilation (Fig. 6-10C). If the patient does not initiate a spontaneous breathing effort, the ventilator *will not* deliver a mechanical breath. Thus apnea can be fatal with this mode of ventilation. AMV has been employed as intermittent positive-pressure breathing (IPPB) for short-term delivery of gases and therapeutic aerosols to patients with pulmonary parenchymal or airway disease. It is also used (infrequently now) for support of patients with acute or chronic respiratory failure. Some practitioners also use AMV to wean patients from CMV and to promote spontaneous breathing.

AMV was more popular during the 1960s than now because it was thought to be more "physiological" than CMV. The prevalent idea at that time—that AMV enhances maintenance of respiratory muscle tone, augmentation of venous return, and more normal pHa and Pa_{CO_2}—has not proved to be significant in severe ARDS. Patients treated with AMV tend to develop respiratory alkalemia, the deleterious effects of which are listed in Table 6-1, to the same extent as those managed with CMV.

The greatest operational difficulty with AMV is that many of the assist mechanisms, which trigger the inspiratory phase, are unreliable.[41] Response sensitivity must be preset, and as the patient's condition changes his capability to generate an appropriate signal (usually a decrease in circuit pressure associated with spontaneous inspiratory effort) varies. The ventilator sensitivity may then be too great (resulting in repetitive cycles or autocycling) or too slight, so that the ventilator fails to cycle.

Assist-Control Ventilation. This technique combines AMV and CMV; the ventilator may be triggered by the patient's spontaneous inspiratory efforts or by a timing device, whichever comes first (Fig. 6-10D). The patient may trigger the ventilator at any time, but the timer determines a minimal preselected rate. Hence CMV acts as a backup should the patient become apneic or attempt to breathe at a lower rate than that set by the timer.

All the aforementioned modes of mechanical ventilation predispose the patient to ventilator-induced $\dot{V}_A/\dot{Q}$ abnormalities. This untoward effect is related to the maldistribution of ventilation to nondependent lung regions, as described earlier (Figs. 6-8 and 6-9).

Intermittent Mandatory Ventilation. IMV allows the patient to breathe spontaneously; however, at preset intervals a mechanical inflation is provided (Fig. 6-11A). IMV per se is the mechanical ventilatory rate and, like CMV, cannot be influenced by the patient. Between sequential mechanical breaths, an unrestricted flow of gas equal to or greater than the patient's peak spontaneous inspiratory demand must be provided.

IMV was introduced initially as a method to wean patients from mechanical ventilation[16,44,45] by permitting a smooth transition from mechanical ventilation to spontaneous breathing as the rate of cycling was gradually decreased and spontaneous effort increased. As clinical experience has been accumulated, IMV has evolved as a primary ventilatory technique.

Several physiological advantages have been proposed for IMV. Spontaneous breathing, with its attendant lower inspiratory Ppl, and a decreased rate of me-

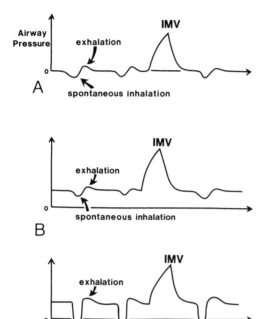

Fig. 6-11. (A) IMV airway pressure patterns. With IMV, the patient is allowed to breathe spontaneously as desired; however, at set intervals a mechanical inflation is provided (the ventilator rate is the IMV rate). IMV tidal volume is set and cannot be affected by the patient. (B) With IMV and CPAP, the patient breathes spontaneously as desired with CPAP (Fig. 6-3A) between IMV breaths. (C) With IMV and PEEP, the patient is allowed to breathe spontaneously as desired with PEEP (Fig. 6-3B) between IMV breaths.

chanical cycling combine to lower mean Ppl below that associated with CMV and AMV. Thus right heart filling pressure and cardiovascular function may be better preserved with IMV than with CMV.[42,43] Moreover, when IMV is combined with CPAP or PEEP (Figs. 6-11B,C) and contrasted with CPPV, the cardiopulmonary effects differ substantially (Fig. 6-12). IMV seems to allow the use of higher PEEP with fewer deleterious effects on venous return and $\dot{Q}t$ than does CPPV.[42,43] Also, spontaneous breathing with IMV promotes more normal $\dot{V}_A/\dot{Q}$ than CMV or AMV (Figs. 6-8 and 6-9).

The IMV rate should be titrated to deliver only that support which, in conjunction with spontaneous breathing, maintains normal alveolar ventilation and Pa_{CO_2}. When used in patients with antecedent pulmonary disease (emphysema, chronic bronchitis), IMV is extremely useful in regulating Pa_{CO_2} and pHa compared with either CMV or AMV.

Synchronized IMV (SIMV), like IMV, allows the patient to breathe spontaneously between mechanical breaths. At regular intervals, the mandatory breath is synchronized to begin with the next spontaneous inhalation (Fig. 6-13) in a manner analogous to AMV. This technique, also termed intermittent assisted ventilation or intermittent demand ventilation, was introduced because of concern that a mechanical breath might be superimposed on a spontaneous breath ("breath stacking"), which might predispose to increases of peak inflation mean airway, and mean intrapleural pressures. Similar fears were expressed if the mechanically delivered volume was added at the peak of spontaneous exhalation.[61]

Subsequently, investigations were conducted to examine the clinical efficacy of SIMV. Shapiro et al.[61] noted that mean Ppl measured with an esophageal balloon was substantially lower with SIMV than with IMV in normal volunteers. However, Hasten et al.[34] compared SIMV with IMV in 25 critically ill patients and found that, although PIP was greater with IMV than with SIMV, cardiovascular variables (blood pressure, $\dot{Q}t$, stroke index, central venous pressure, and pulmonary artery pressure) in the two groups did not differ significantly.

In another study Heenan et al.[35] obtained baseline data from spontaneously breathing, anesthetized dogs which were subsequently near-drowned and ventilated with IMV or SIMV. Again, no differences between the two modes were noted with re-

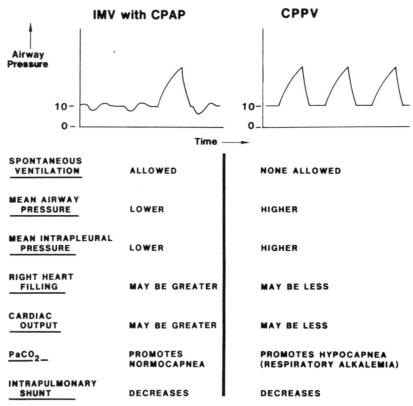

	IMV with CPAP	CPPV
SPONTANEOUS VENTILATION	ALLOWED	NONE ALLOWED
MEAN AIRWAY PRESSURE	LOWER	HIGHER
MEAN INTRAPLEURAL PRESSURE	LOWER	HIGHER
RIGHT HEART FILLING	MAY BE GREATER	MAY BE LESS
CARDIAC OUTPUT	MAY BE GREATER	MAY BE LESS
$PaCO_2$	PROMOTES NORMOCAPNEA	PROMOTES HYPOCAPNEA (RESPIRATORY ALKALEMIA)
INTRAPULMONARY SHUNT	DECREASES	DECREASES

Fig. 6-12. Comparison of the physiological effects of IMV with CPAP, and controlled mechanical ventilation with end-expiratory pressure, or CPPV. (The rate of IMV is assumed to be 1–4 breaths/minute compared with the CMV rate of 10–16 breaths/minute; both have the same end-expiratory pressure.)

spect to $\dot{Q}t$, stroke volume, Ppl, and $\dot{Q}sp/\dot{Q}t$. Peak inflation and mean airway pressures were significantly increased with IMV, and breath stacking occurred but without demonstrable adverse effects. Based on these data, SIMV does not seem to offer any physiological advantage compared with IMV and may be thought of as an expensive solution to a problem that has not been shown to exist.

Weaning from Ventilatory Support

Several considerations apply during the weaning process. Once treatment is begun, we prefer to keep FIO_2 constant between 0.3 and 0.5.[13] With this approach, some fall in PaO_2 may result. Physiological changes are noted rapidly when the same FIO_2 is maintained, an important consideration when more than one person is caring for a patient. Attempts to continually wean the patient to a lower FIO_2 require more work and blood gas analyses without necessarily effecting a therapeutic improvement.

Before extubation, the patient should be capable of breathing spontaneously with minimal PEEP or CPAP (5 cm H_2O or less). A PaO_2 greater than 55 mm Hg is adequate under these conditions, provided all other parameters are acceptable. Patients so treated are usually in no danger of acute hypoxemia if for some reason they do not

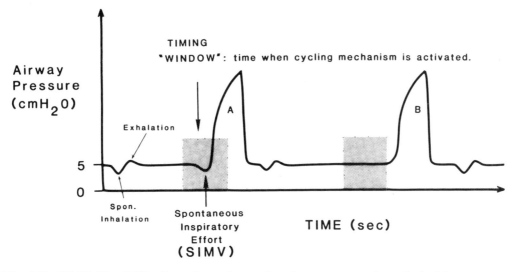

Fig. 6-13. SIMV, like IMV, allows the patient to breathe spontaneously as desired between ventilator breaths. At set intervals, the ventilator's electrical rate-timing circuit becomes activated and a timing "window" appears. If the patient initiates a breath in the timing "window," the mandatory breath is delivered, as shown in A. Thus IMV is synchronized to occur with the patient's spontaneous inspiratory effort. If no spontaneous inspiratory effort registers during the timing "window," the ventilator delivers the mandatory breath at the end of the timing sequence, as in B. This tracing shows a combination of SIMV with 5 cm H_2O CPAP.

receive supplemental oxygen after extubation.

We have previously discussed weaning from PEEP or CPAP. The goal of weaning is adequate gas exchange at 5 cm H_2O or less of expiratory pressure. Reduction of the IMV rate should occur independently of any changes in FIO_2 or positive expiratory pressure. Initial IMV seldom exceeds 6–8 breaths/minute. In weaning, decreases of 1–2 breaths/minute are acceptable as long as the pHa is maintained at or slightly above 7.30 and the spontaneous breathing rate is 30 breaths/minute or less. pH, rather than $PaCO_2$, is used as the primary guide to the adequacy of ventilation as knowledge of many patients' previous ventilatory status—i.e., if they are eucapnic or hypercapnic—may not be available.

Spontaneous respiration above 30 breaths/minute indicates markedly increased respiratory work. Above this level, exhalation changes from passive to active,

significantly increasing $\dot{V}O_2$ and causing fatigue.

We attempt to maintain a minimal IMV rate of 2 breaths/minute. Studies have indicated that patients who breathe spontaneously for a prolonged time often sustain a fall in PaO_2, even with PEEP or CPAP.[21] Almost without exception, IMV at 2 breaths/minute corrects this problem. Apparently, some unstable alveoli begin to collapse with time. The addition of positive-pressure breaths recruits and reexpands these units and does not require additional expiratory pressure.

Occasionally, elderly patients with chronic lung disease or those requiring prolonged mechanical ventilatory support may be difficult to wean. They become exquisitely sensitive to any changes in the rate of ventilation. Any usual decrease of IMV results in an increase in $PaCO_2$ and their spontaneous breathing rate, and weaning may be protracted over several days. After an IMV rate of 2 breaths/minute is achieved, the interval between mandated breaths may increase in 3- to 5-second increments, i.e., an IMV breath every 33–35 seconds and so on, until weaning is complete. Why such subtle changes have such a profound effect is unclear, but these are consistent observations.

Removing the endotracheal tube is predicated not only on F_{IO_2}, arterial blood gas tensions, pH, IMV rate, and PEEP or CPAP values but also on the patient's ability to maintain a patent airway with intact pharyngeal and laryngeal reflexes. Other criteria for extubation include absence of residual paralysis, the ability to cough and mobilize secretions, and cardiovascular stability.

The increased use of enteral feeding must be considered before extubation. Nasal feeding tubes are intended to be placed in the duodenum. However, because of gastric atony, many never enter the duodenum. Despite the presence of bowel sounds, the stomach can fail to empty. Under these conditions, and despite the presence of a cuffed endotracheal tube, feedings can be aspirated. This possibility is increased during the period immediately following tracheal extubation.

COMPLICATIONS OF VENTILATORY CARE

Aspiration

Chemical pneumonitis from aspiration of stomach contents poses a serious threat and contributes to significant pulmonary morbidity and mortality. Johanson and Harris[40] described the effects of aspiration of gastric contents which depend on the pH of the material, the presence or absence of particles (e.g., food), and the presence or absence of bacteria. Acidic fluid is widely disseminated in the lung and rapidly produces diffuse hemorrhage and pulmonary edema.

The severity of the lesion depends on the pH of the aspirate: a pH less than 2.5 damages the lung severely.[71] Large aspirated particles may obstruct the airway acutely and result in an "asthma-like" illness or atelectasis.

Irregularities in the endotracheal tube cuff, an improperly inflated cuff, a faulty valve on the inflation lumen of the pilot balloon, negligence (e.g., failure to reinflate the cuff after deflation), and rupture of the cuff from mechanical stress or accidental overinflation can all permit aspiration. Additionally, if the cuff is positioned inadvertently between the vocal cords, it cannot adequately protect against aspiration.

After diagnosis of aspiration, vigorous suctioning, saline lavage, and on occasion fiberoptic bronchoscopy may be indicated if particulate matter has been aspirated. Aspiration decreases Pa_{O_2}, lung compliance, and FRC and is an indication for immediate CPAP.

Pathogenic organisms may be introduced by the aspiration of oropharyngeal matter. The normal human pharynx contains enormous numbers of gram-positive and gram-negative aerobic and anaerobic cocci and rods. Represented in this bacterial population are staphylococci, streptococci, diphtheroids, neisseriae, and the more pathogenic pneumococci, group A beta-hemolytic streptococci, *Cornynebacterium diphtheriae*, and *Hemophilus influenzae*. The aspiration of even minute quantities of oropharyngeal secretions presents an enormous bacterial challenge to the lung. For example, 0.01 ml of aspirated secretions contains about 10^5 aerobic and 10^6 anaerobic bacteria.[40]

Cardiovascular Complications

$\dot{V}_A/\dot{Q}$ Impairments. Perhaps the most frequent major complication of mechanical ventilation is cardiovascular impairment. The application of raised airway pressure can greatly increase Ppl from its usual value of −5 mm Hg. Increased pressure impedes venous return to the right heart and reduces stroke volume; this induces a relative hypovolemia which, however, can usually be rectified by fluid administration. Although not well-documented, experimental data suggest that humoral factors are released from the distended lung during PEEP or CPAP therapy[52] and may directly impair myocardial contractility.

Increased airway pressure may also interfere with right ventricular performance. Overdistention of the alveoli compresses the pulmonary vascular bed, which increases pulmonary vascular resistance and right ventricular afterload. In response, particularly in patients with compromised ventricular function, the right ventricle dilates until it is restricted by the surrounding pericardium. At this point, with further dilatation impossible, pressures within the ventricle increase significantly, which causes the interventricular septum to bulge into the left ventricular outflow tract and, thus, impede left ventricular output.[39]

When fluid therapy fails to correct low $\dot{Q}t$, inotropic support is usually indicated. If increased pulmonary vascular resistance results from mechanical ventilation, vasodilator therapy is inappropriate as mechanical forces, not vasoconstriction, are the source of the problem.

Cardiac output can play a substantial role in arterial oxygenation. Failure to recognize this fact can lead to a misinterpretation of the cause of low Pao_2 and eventually to inappropriate therapy. The amount of oxygen extraction depends on tissue metabolism. Higher metabolic rates are associated with increased oxygen uptake. Trauma, sepsis, burns, and major surgery all increase $\dot{V}o_2$ and may necessitate increased delivery of oxygen to the tissues. An increase of the major oxygen carrier, hemoglobin, and a rightward shift of the oxyhemoglobin dissociation curve present more readily extractable oxygen to the tissues. When these mechanisms are insufficient to meet metabolic demands, cardiac output ($\dot{Q}t$) must increase. The relationship between cardiac output, oxygen uptake, and arterial and venous oxygen contents is expressed by the Fick equation:

Cardiac output (L/minute)

$$= \frac{\dot{V}o_2 \text{ (ml/minute)}}{Cao_2 - C\bar{v}o_2 \text{ (ml/L)}} \quad (4)$$

where Cao_2 is the arterial oxygen content, and $C\bar{v}o_2$ is the mixed venous oxygen content. $\dot{V}o_2$ may be seen to equal the product of $\dot{Q}t$ and ($Cao_2 - C\bar{v}o_2$). When $\dot{Q}t$ and Cao_2 are maximal but still insufficient to meet metabolic demands, an increase of oxygen extraction must take place from arterial blood and the numerical value of $Cao_2 - C\bar{v}o_2$ must increase beyond the normal value of 3.5–5.5 ml/dl.

In patients with ARDS, arterial blood is not maximally oxygenated at any given FIo_2 because of increased $\dot{Q}sp/\dot{Q}t$. Depending on the degree of pulmonary impairment, only limited amounts of oxygen may be transferred into the blood perfusing the alveoli. When $\dot{Q}t$ is inadequate, increased tissue extraction of oxygen must occur, and the oxygen content of mixed venous blood returning to the lungs is decreased. That blood which passes through perfused but non-ventilated (shunt) areas of the lungs does not have a "step-up" in oxygen content. When this blood reaches the left ventricle, it is mixed with blood which passed through "normal" $\dot{V}a/\dot{Q}$ areas and is oxygenated. The net result is a reduction of overall Cao_2, the magnitude of which is dependent on both the degree of shunting and the $C\bar{v}o_2$. In other words, if venous blood entering the lungs has a low $C\bar{v}o_2$ and a portion passes through pulmonary shunt areas, the resulting Cao_2 and Pao_2 are lower than would be caused by the shunt alone. If the clinician incorrectly assumes that the decrease in Pao_2 is related only to pulmonary dysfunction, when in actuality cardiac impairment is also present, therapy will be inappropriate and potentially harmful. The application of PEEP/CPAP might further decrease cardiac output and cause an additional decline in Pa_{O_2}. For this reason, the calculation of $\dot{Q}sp/\dot{Q}t$ with values of Ca_{O_2} and $C\bar{v}_{O_2}$ for blood obtained from arterial and pulmonary arterial catheters is a more reliable indicator of respiratory function than is Pa_{O_2} alone.

Pulmonary Barotrauma

A major complicaton of mechanical ventilatory support is pulmonary barotrauma, including pneumothorax, interstitial emphysema, pneumomediastinum, subcutaneous emphysema, pneumopericardium, and pneumoperitoneum. The initiating problem is rupture of alveoli into adjacent perivascular sheaths and dissection along these sheaths to the mediastinum where free rupture may occur into the pleural cavity (pneumothorax) or further dissection takes place into the mediastinum along the aortic sheath or into the fascial planes of the head and neck.

Barotrauma has been blamed on high levels of PEEP or CPAP. However, it is more likely associated with the large V_T and PIP of mechanical ventilation. Studies of the early 1970s showed that the incidence of pneumothorax was the same during mechanical ventilation with or without PEEP. IMV may protect the lung because of the decreased number of mechanical breaths and spontaneous breathing, both of which combine to reduce mean airway pressure. Furthermore, the fewer mechanical breaths with IMV minimize the time of airway exposure to high PIP.

There is no good evidence to support the prophylactic placement of chest tubes into patients treated with high levels of PEEP or CPAP. The cause-effect relationship between PEEP and barotrauma is tenuous at best. Prophylactic tubes can become inoperative before they are needed and do not really prevent pneumothoraces. Patients with severe ARDS may have adherence of the visceral and parietal pleura which prevents the lung from collapsing completely if a pneumothorax develops. However, numerous small, loculated pneumothoraces can form; prophylactic chest tubes provide little or no benefit under these circumstances unless they are located at the site(s) of the air leak. Obstruction of the chest tube by lung parenchyma, fibrin, or hemorrhagic clot can all interrupt the function of the tube.

The best defense against barotrauma, especially tension pneumothorax, remains a high index of suspicion. Patients with severe ARDS are at high risk, especially after blunt trauma.[27] Clinical assessment indicates that barotrauma often develops after the patient's condition has improved, the $\dot{Q}sp/\dot{Q}t$ is regressing, and the C_L is returning to normal. It is at this time that pressure transmission is maximal and the tendency for alveolar rupture greatest.

Infection

In spite of good respiratory care, pulmonary infection develops frequently in patients receiving mechanical ventilation. This problem may present as tracheitis, bronchitis, or pneumonia. Sputum cultures often show abundant gram-negative rods, commonly *Pseudomonas aeruginosa*, *Klebsiella pneumoniae*, and *Bacillus proteus*. Infectious processes involving the airway are often manifested by bronchial secretions. Pneumonia results in edema of the alveolar septae and intraalveolar exudates. Early hyperemia is followed by vascular sludging and diminished capillary blood flow. The products of inflammation drained by the lymphatics overflow into the venous circulation and produce bacteremia.

Bacteria colonize the tracheobronchial tree soon after placement of an endotracheal tube and initiation of mechanical ventilation. Intubation bypasses the primary respiratory tract defense mechanisms including the nasal and pharyngeal passages. In addition, cough and mucociliary function are blunted. Tracheal intubation decreases the patient's ability to eliminate secretions, and suctioning may introduce pathogenic bacteria into the tracheobronchial tree. Consequently, such care requires strict adherence to aseptic technique and the use of sterile suction catheters and gloves. A trap attached to the catheter can be used to collect secretions for gram stain and culture. This technique gains importance if any change in the quality of sputum occurs. Antibiotic therapy administered without knowledge of offending organisms or sensitivities may predispose the patient to superinfection, or resistant bacterial strains may develop.

Respiratory infection is a serious complication, particularly in patients with COPD. An exacerbation of bronchitis or newly acquired respiratory infection in such patients frequently provokes acute respiratory decompensation. Increased secretions and bronchospasm substantially increase airway resistance and the work of breathing. Finally, the chronically reduced $\dot{V}_A/\dot{Q}$ areas may be extended acutely, which results in severe hypoxemia and hypercapnia.

Humidifiers and nebulizers are easily contaminated with organisms, e.g., *Pseudomonas aeruginosa*, and the effluent from these devices may cause pulmonary infection. This problem can be avoided or at least minimized by replacing all equipment with sterile units every 24–48 hours. More frequent changes have not been shown to reduce the incidence of respiratory infection.

Other factors implicated in the spread of pulmonary infections include contaminated respirometers, improper suctioning techniques, and improperly stored and packaged supplies. A major problem in the spread of nosocomial infection is the result of improper hand-washing techniques.

Table 6-2. Measures to Prevent Pulmonary Infection

1. Atraumatic placement of aseptic endotracheal and tracheostomy tubes
2. Meticulous removal of secretions and suctioning
3. Frequent changing of ventilatory equipment (every 24–48 hours) with sterilization of tubing, humidifiers, nebulizers, valves, and any other devices
4. Use of sterile water (never tap water) in humidifiers and nebulizers
5. Prevention of cross infection by the use of isolation facilities
6. Maintenance of maximal host resistance to infection by ensuring adequate hydration, nutrition, blood volume, tissue perfusion, and tissue oxygenation
7. Prevention and immediate treatment of air space collapse, i.e., CPAP

Many hospital staff members go from patient to patient to perform tracheal suctioning, change bedclothes, turn patients, remove dressings, place and irrigate urinary catheters, empty bed pans, care for tracheostomies, and provide mouth care. Handwashing, the simplest measure to control infection, becomes of paramount importance in minimizing infections of highly susceptible patients. Methods to prevent pulmonary infection are listed in Table 6-2.

Nutrition

Many critically ill patients receive some form of parenteral nutrition. Often intravenous hyperalimentation relies almost exclusively on glucose as a source of calories. Metabolism of excessive amounts of exogenously administered glucose produces up to two to three times the normal amount of carbon dioxide. Normally minute ventilation increases to accommodate the increased load. However, the patient with acute or chronic lung disease may not be able to handle this extra burden, and CO_2 retention develops. One solution to this problem is to increase the rate and/or V_T of the mechanical ventilator. An alternative solution is to decrease the caloric load or to replace up to 50 percent of the glucose calories with intravenously administered lipid solutions. Because most enteral formulas include substantial fat, carbon dioxide production does not usually increase when the gastrointestinal tract is used for feeding.[3]

Oxygen Toxicity and Related Problems

Oxygen therapy can be either beneficial or harmful. Pulmonary oxygen toxicity in humans apparently occurs only at an F_{IO_2} greater than 0.5. Important factors include the duration and interval of exposure and the atmospheric pressure. At an F_{IO_2} of 0.6, several days may pass before clinical changes become apparent. However, 100 percent oxygen produces changes in pulmonary function within 6–12 hours.

The exact mechanisms involved in pulmonary oxygen toxicity are not clearly delineated.[70] Major effects seem to be related to toxic oxygen radicals, which seem to act on capillary endothelium. Initial symptoms include burning and retrosternal pain (tracheitis?), which is associated with a decreased vital capacity. Nonspecific changes ascribed to oxygen toxicity include atelectasis, increased capillary permeability, interstitial edema, alveolar septal thickening, alveolar hemorrhage, inflammation, fibrin deposition, and hyaline membrane formation. Destruction of surfactant and a decrease in type II alveolar cells are common. The final pathophysiological changes are not dissimilar to those occurring from ARDS. Because many patients with ARDS require a high F_{IO_2} for long periods of time, the relative contributions of the disease process and oxygen are impossible to delineate.

The morphological alterations seem to develop from tissue interaction with various oxygen radicals. Hydrogen peroxide, superoxide, hydroxyl radicals, and singlet oxygen have been implicated as causative agents. Oxygen toxicity presumably develops when normal defenses, e.g., catalase, perioxidases, and superoxide dismutase, have been overwhelmed and/or inactivated.

Other pulmonary abnormalities induced by oxygen are not reflections of oxygen toxicity per se. Douglas et al. described a "response curve" for $\dot{Q}sp/\dot{Q}t$ in patients with significant venous admixture.[13] Increasing the F_{IO_2} from 0.21 to 0.35 reduced the $\dot{Q}sp/\dot{Q}t$, presumably because alveoli with minimal but nevertheless finite ventilation ("hypoventilated" alveoli) at the higher F_{IO_2} contained more oxygen for exchange across the alveolar-capillary membranes. From an F_{IO_2} of 0.6 to 1.0, $\dot{Q}sp/\dot{Q}t$ increased linearly. One possible explanation for these observations is the phenomenon of resorption (absorption) atelectasis.[68] This model presumes increased pulmonary interstitial pressure and minimal but finitely ventilated alveoli. When the F_{IO_2} is less than 1.0, the alveolar gas mixture is composed primarily of nitrogen and oxygen molecules. Equal amounts of nitrogen enter and leave the alveoli so that P_{AN_2} remains constant. In contrast, oxygen may be taken up by pulmonary capillary blood flow more rapidly than it is replaced in those alveoli with reduced ventilation. Because nitrogen is still present, however, the alveoli do not collapse. As the F_{IO_2} is increased and nitrogen is washed out of the lung, it no longer can "splint" the alveoli. As oxygen is taken up more rapidly than it is supplied, alveolar volume decreases until eventual collapse occurs (the interstitial pressure increase is no longer opposed by gas within the vulnerable alveoli). The result is a progressive increase in $\dot{Q}sp/\dot{Q}t$, that reaches a maximum at an F_{IO_2} of 1.0. One troublesome aspect of this explanation is that the expected decrease in FRC that should accompany the increase in $\dot{Q}sp/\dot{Q}t$ at high F_{IO_2} has not been demonstrated.[66]

A second possible explanation for the increased $\dot{Q}sp/\dot{Q}t$ involves hypoxic pulmonary vasoconstriction. When localized pulmonary parenchymal hypoxia develops as a result of decreased $\dot{V}_A$, the regional pulmonary vascular bed reflexly constricts. As a result, $\dot{V}_A/\dot{Q}$ relationships in that area tend to remain normal, and pulmonary blood flow is shunted to other areas of the lung where ventilation is not so affected. When the F_{IO_2} increases, localized hypoxia decreases with a subsequent decrease of hypoxic pulmonary vasoconstriction. The resultant increase in blood flow exceeds any increase in ventilation and the result is a decreased $\dot{V}_A/\dot{Q}$ and an increased $\dot{Q}_{sp}/\dot{Q}_t$. Because FRC changes minimally, this explanation for changes in $\dot{Q}_{sp}/\dot{Q}_t$ with increasing F_{IO_2} may be more plausible than the mechanism of absorption atelectasis.

PROBLEMS IN MONITORING

Pulmonary Capillary Wedge Pressure

Problems exist in interpreting the pulmonary capillary wedge pressure (PCWP) during positive-pressure therapy. The pressure, which is measured through a pulmonary artery catheter, reflects both intravascular and transmitted airway pressure, and the cardiovascular implications of a given value are often unclear. Some clinicians have suggested measuring the wedge pressure with the patient connected to and then disconnected from the ventilator. The difference presumably represents the airway pressure component, which can then be subtracted from subsequent readings. A large discrepancy between readings "on" and "off" the ventilator may indicate significant hypovolemia, excessive PEEP or CPAP, or both. Others have suggested always disconnecting the patient from the ventilator system during pressure measurements. However, the relationship of measurements obtained without the ventilator artifact to those which are present the majority of the time while mechanical ventilation is occurring is unclear. One doubts that any clinically useful assumptions can be made.

At least one study demonstrated a discrepancy between transmural wedge pressure (PCWP$_{TM}$) (PCWP minus Ppl) measurements and simultaneous direct measurements of left ventricular end-diastolic pressure (LVEDP).[15] This difference was pronounced during CPPV. Increased Ppl does not seem to affect all intrathoracic structures equally. In the study mentioned, PCWP was always higher than LVEDP. Clinically, PCWP might be interpreted as adequate when, in fact, LVEDP is low, reflecting absolute or relative hypovolemia. The low $\dot{Q}_t$ observed during positive-pressure ventilation may also reflect hypovolemia rather than mechanical ventilation-induced cardiovascular depression.

Cardiac Output

Cardiac output frequently must be monitored for several hours or days to provide a complete hemodynamic assessment of critically ill patients receiving mechanical positive-pressure support. Conventional methods to measure $\dot{Q}_t$ include thermodilution and dye dilution techniques and variations based on the Fick principle. A newer noninvasive, computer-assisted, transcutaneous ultrasonic technique is also used.[10,22,38]

In recent years the easiest and most clinically reliable technique has been the thermodilution variant of the Stewart-Hamilton method. A balloon-tipped, flow-directed pulmonary artery catheter with a thermistor for sensing changes in blood temperature mounted on its distal end is required. The catheter is inserted percutaneously into a peripheral vein and advanced until the tip is positioned in the pulmonary artery. If a known volume of indicator (D_5W) at known temperature (usually 0°C) is injected into the right atrium, the thermistor senses the resulting decrease in blood temperature as it passes the tip. An analog computer attached to the thermistor lumen of the catheter first records the area under the curve described by the temperature-time signal and then provides a digital readout of the calculated cardiac output, which is inversely proportional to this area (Fig. 6-14):

$$\dot{Q}t = \frac{(indicator)(K)}{\int \Delta Tdt} \qquad (5)$$

where: $\dot{Q}t$ is the cardiac output (L·minute^{-1}); (indicator) is the 10 ml of 0°C solution (usually D$_5$W); K is the combined computation constant (taking into account pulmonary artery catheter dead space, heat change in transit, injection rate, and density factors of injectate and blood); and $\int \Delta Tdt$ is the change in blood temperature with time. If $\dot{Q}t$ is low, the reduced flow past the thermistor produces a longer time when cooler blood is detected. The result is a large temperature-time integral indicating a reduced Qt.

Mechanical ventilation can interfere with thermodilution determination of $\dot{Q}t$. Because gases moving into the lungs are often less than body temperature, the thermistor recording may be altered and, as a result, the computed $\dot{Q}t$ erroneous. When mechanical ventilation transiently reduces venous inflow, a determination made just before or during a mechanical breath may be inaccurate. Most experts recommend determining $\dot{Q}t$ at the same point in each respiratory cycle.[1] However, recent work has demonstrated that there are cyclic variations in $\dot{Q}t$ regardless of the mechanical ventilation interval during which it is measured.[63]

ALTERNATIVES TO TRACHEAL INTUBATION AND VENTILATION

CPAP Mask

For patients with respiratory distress who can breathe spontaneously, the administra-

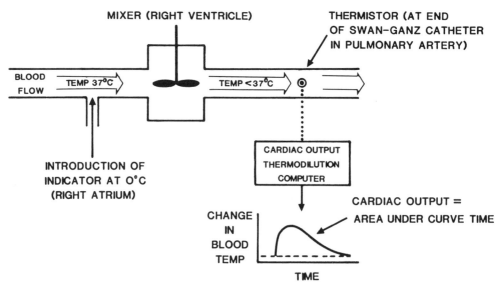

Fig. 6-14. Thermodilution principle for measuring cardiac output. In this model a change in the heat content of the blood is induced at one point in the circulation (right atrium) by the injection of a 10-ml bolus indicator (usually D$_5$W at 0°C), the resultant change in blood temperature being detected by a thermistor at a point downstream. As the thermodiluted (temperature reduced) blood flows by the thermistor, a transient change in blood temperature with respect to time at the thermistor is detected by a computer, which generates an appropriate curve. The area under this curve is the cardiac output as determined by the Stewart-Hamilton dilution equation (Eq. 5).

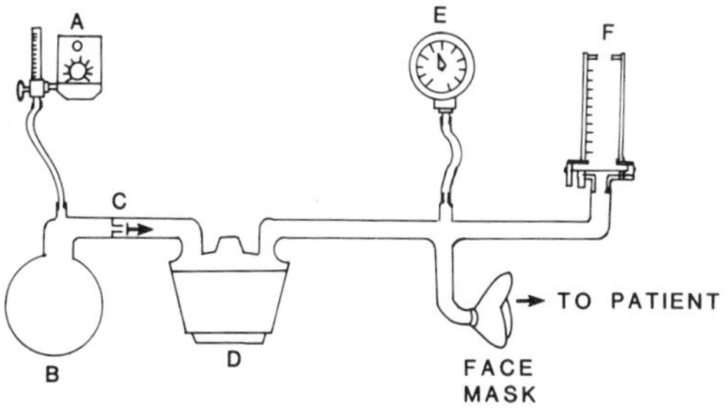

Fig. 6-15. Face mask CPAP system. (A) Air/O_2 blender. (B) Five-liter reservoir bag. (C) Unidirectional valve. (D) Humidifier or nebulizer. (E) Pressure manometer. (F) Threshold resistor expiratory pressure valve.

tion of CPAP through a face mask rather than an endotracheal tube may be possible. The CPAP mask is a soft, cushioned, form-fitting translucent mask for easy application and comfort. Other required circuit components are shown in Figure 6-15. Avoidance of tracheal intubation, with its potential to increase the risk of nosocomial infection and tracheal injury (erosion and stenosis), are among the compelling reasons to use face-mask CPAP.

The application of CPAP by face mask is not a new technique. Barach et al.[4] used this form of positive pressure to treat patients with acute pulmonary edema during the 1930s. During the same decade, Bullowa[7] described its use to manage pneumonia. In both reports the technique proved effective. During subsequent years, Gregory et al.[32] and later Sugarman et al.[64] successfully applied CPAP by using a plastic head chamber rather than a mask. In recently published reports, face-mask CPAP has been used for adults with respiratory distress. Greenbaum et al. described its use in 14 patients,[30] Smith et al. in 44 patients,[62] and Covelli et al. in 35 patients.[11] In all subjects the administration of face-mask CPAP rapidly reduced $\dot{Q}sp/\dot{Q}t$ and enhanced arterial oxygenation.

The decision to administer face-mask CPAP can be made when arterial oxygenation deteriorates progressively despite oxygen therapy, coughing, deep breathing,

and chest physiotherapy. Specific indications for face-mask CPAP have been proposed[62] and include: (1) an awake, cooperative patient; (2) the ability to breathe spontaneously; (3) normo- or hypocapnea; (4) $Pa_{O_2}/F_{I_{O_2}}$ less than 300; and (5) stable cardiovascular status. The technique is also useful for the treatment of postoperative atelectasis. Paul and Downs[53] described the responses of such patients to intermittent positive-pressure breathing (IPPB), incentive spirometry, and face-mask CPAP. Unlike IPPB and incentive spirometry, which required a great deal of effort and cooperation by the patient, face-mask CPAP was simple, effective, and required little effort.

Nevertheless, face-mask CPAP is not innocuous and may be associated with some problems. CPAP by mask or endotracheal tube may decrease $\dot{Q}t$ by decreasing ventricular filling pressure (preload) and increasing pulmonary vascular resistance (right ventricular afterload). Another potential complication is vomiting and aspiration of gastric contents. This problem can be minimized if the technique is used only for patients who are awake and alert and have no illness that predisposes them to nausea and vomiting. In some patients the risks of gastric distention and air swallowing may be reduced by placement of a nasogastric tube. A translucent face mask is recommended for early detection of vomitus or accumulated secretions.

Some reports suggested that carbon dioxide retention limits the use of face-mask CPAP,[5,30] whereas others have demonstrated that hypercapnea is not a significant problem.[11,62] More than likely the circuitry and methodology used, rather than the mask, are responsible for the differences reported. In our experience, hypercapnia has not been a clinical problem. Other complications are skin ulceration and facial trauma, especially when the mask is left in one position for a long period. These problems occur more frequently when opaque, black rubber anesthesia masks are used. Smith et al.[62] reported that the use of soft, silicone elastomer masks resolved such difficulties. Eye trauma may also result if the mask compresses the eye. Corneal lacerations have been reported as has obstruction of retinal venous return which produced hemorrhage and blindness.[31] Finally, taut head straps to maintain a tight seal may be poorly accepted by patients. The prescribed level of CPAP can be maintained even with slight air leaks around the mask if a self-sealing mask is used in combination with high flow rates.

MECHANICAL VENTILATION DURING TRANSPORT

Maintenance of life support during intra- and interhospital transport is a critical aspect of adult ventilatory therapy.[48] Demands for intrahospital transport arise daily; for simpler cases, self-inflating bags suffice for transferring the intubated, postoperative patient from the operating room to the intensive care unit (ICU) or recovery room. Often a patient needs to be moved from the ICU for computerized axial tomography (CAT) scans or other diagnostic tests. Frequently these patients require supplemental oxygen therapy, PEEP/CPAP, or mechanical ventilation to be continued during this time.

Interhospital transportation of the critically ill may involve aircraft as well as ground vehicles. Adequate pneumatic and electrical power as well as emergency airway equipment are required for the patient who is mechanically ventilated.

Transport Ventilators

Ventilation of patients during transport is often accomplished with a manual, self-inflating bag, flow-inflating (Mapleson D) system, or oxygen-powered breathing device (i.e., Elder demand valve). Because the V_T, PIP, and FIO_2 that these manually operated devices deliver may vary from breath to breath, a portable ventilator is a superior alternative. Such a device should be time-cycled with IMV; deliver CPAP (up to 45 cm H_2O) and a constant V_T (100–2000 ml); have controls to adjust the rate (2–45 breaths/minute), FIO_2, and airway humidification; and be capable of a high PIP ($\geq$150 cm H_2O) and high inspiratory flow rate (>100 L/minute). The ventilator must be light enough for one person to carry and compact enough to be stored in a locker or on a bed. A transport ventilator must also be reliable and adaptable to adults and children. Additionally, the controls of such a ventilator must be easily identifiable. Finally, it should be pneumatically powered to facilitate mobility. A new transport ventilator that incorporates a demand-flow valve CPAP system and satisfies the aforementioned criteria has been introduced.[17]

Gas Supply

A self-contained gas supply for pneumatic transport ventilators can be provided in two ways. Because the duration of intrahospital transport rarely exceeds 15 minutes, a small "E" size oxygen cylinder with a 660-L capacity is usually sufficient. If additional gas consumption is anticipated, two E-cylinders can be yoked together. A gas supply for interhospital transport (and sometimes intrahospital as well) requires a large "H" size oxygen cylinder with a capacity of approximately 6660 L. On occasion, two to three such large cylinders may be necessary. The disadvantage of the H-cylinder is its height (5 ft) and weight (approximately 150 lb).

A more efficient alternative is a liquid oxygen reservoir, which provides 860 cu ft of gaseous oxygen from 1 cu ft of liquid oxygen. One unit (Linde PCU 500) has a capacity of 13,200 L of gaseous oxygen, equivalent to two large H-cylinders. It is approximately 3 ft high, weighs only 70 lb when full, and occupies 0.25 sq M of floor space. Another advantage of liquid oxygen is that it can provide pneumatic power for two ventilators, if necessary, simply by placing a Y-connector on the reservoir outflow connection. Thus the transfer of up to two patients is easier without the cumbersome necessity of using multiple H-cylinders.

When properly used, the liquid oxygen reservoir complies with U.S. Federal Aviation Administration regulations for airborne ambulance use.[33] The full reservoir provides enough oxygen to power a ventilator for approximately 7 hours at 30 L/minute. The unit has a standard oxygen connector which supplies 50 psig for ventilator operation. In the ambulance, a 20-ft length of high-pressure oxygen hose between the reservoir and the ventilator allows the patient to be moved into and out of the vehicle without disconnection from the ventilator.

Manual Ventilation

As in the ICU, an alternative means of ventilation with a manually operated bag that provides CPAP is essential. A 100 percent oxygen, flow-inflating Mapleson D system is preferable to the conventional self-inflating "ambu" type bag[6] (Fig. 6-16). Advantages of the Mapleson D system include: the F_{IO_2} can be maintained at 1.0; the patient can breathe spontaneously with CPAP; and "IMV" can be provided manually by squeezing the bag. We have used this particular flow-inflating manual ventilation system successfully for transporting adults and children with respiratory failure. The major disadvantage is the gas consumption; a continuous, high rate of inflow up to 20–25 L/minute must be provided. However, use of a liquid oxygen system minimizes this disadvantage.

Other Medical Equipment

In addition to portable mechanical ventilators and manual resuscitators, other respiratory transport equipment is required. A kit containing airway management paraphernalia is essential (Table 6-3). The necessity to change an endotracheal tube rapidly to maintain ventilation after a cuff ruptures or to place a McSwain dart or Heimlich valve to treat a pneumothorax are examples of lifesaving interventions possible with equipment from such a kit. This equipment should be given the same care as the transport ventilator.

Equally important is suction equipment. Portable or fixed suction equipment must have an adjustable vacuum up to 300 mm Hg subatmospheric pressure. It should be fitted with large-bore, nonkinking tubing with a rigid suction tip. There should also be sterile catheters of various sizes for suctioning through an endotracheal or tracheostomy tube. A nonbreakable collection bottle and a supply of water for rinsing the tubes must be provided. The suction force must be easily adjustable, especially for use with children.

One must consider the problem of electromagnetic interference. No medical device should be used that interferes with aircraft navigation or communications equipment. Medical equipment should be tested before use to ensure this compatibility.

Altitude-Related Problems

Altitude-related problems are always a threat to patients in aircraft with unpressurized cabins. Gas expands with increasing altitude, which presents several problems. At sea level the average cabin pressure is 760 mm Hg, or 29.92 inches Hg (14.7 psig). At 8000 ft the barometric pressure decreases to 564.6 mm Hg (11.9 psig), and gas in a closed space within the body expands by approximately 26 percent. Personnel must be aware of this hazard as it relates to volume changes in the gut, thorax, lungs, central nervous system, and other

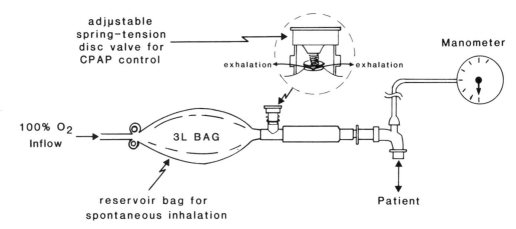

Fig. 6-16. Mapleson, flow-inflating, manual ventilation device. The manometer allows measurement of CPAP and peak inflation pressure. IMV breaths are provided by squeezing the bag at set intervals (see text).

body spaces. A nonfunctioning thoracostomy tube can be fatal in a patient with a pneumothorax. Gastric distention must be relieved before transport, and the pressure in endotracheal tube cuffs and pneumatic splints may have to be decreased during ascent. Intravenous fluids packaged in glass containers are impractical during flight; plastic bags with pressure administration cuffs are used instead.

Changes in atmospheric pressure alter the partial pressure of inhaled oxygen (P_{IO_2}). Although the proportion of oxygen in air remains the same (21 percent) at all altitudes, total barometric pressure varies inversely with ascent to altitude, which causes the P_{IO_2} to decrease. The P_{IO_2} at any altitude is calculated by multiplying the barometric pressure at that altitude by the constant 0.21. At sea level the P_{IO_2} is 160 mm Hg, the partial pressure of alveolar oxygen (P_{AO_2}) is about 105 mm Hg, and the Pa_{O_2} is about 95 mm Hg. At 8000 ft, the P_{IO_2} is 116 mm Hg, the P_{AO_2} about 70 mm Hg, and the Pa_{O_2} about 60 mm Hg in a healthy person with normal cardiac and pulmonary function. In a patient with impaired oxygenation a decreased P_{IO_2} at an increased altitude can be life-threatening. Supplemental oxygen should be provided for such patients, i.e.,

those with COPD, a history of myocardial infarction, or anemia (hemoglobin <7 g/dl) who are transported in unpressurized aircraft.

SPECIALIZED TECHNIQUES

Body Positioning

On occasion, pulmonary parenchymal involvement may be confined to one lung or one lobe. Atelectasis, aspiration pneumonia, or contusion are common examples (Fig. 6-17). Attempts to use conventional techniques of CPAP or mechanical ventilation to restore lung volume and improve oxygenation may fail. Instead, more specialized methods are needed.

Simple altering of body position can directly influence blood gas exchange. In the upright position dependent alveoli are maximally compressed at end-exhalation compared with those in the nondependent portions of the lung. However, the dependent alveoli receive a greater proportion of total gas flow during inspiration. The majority of pulmonary blood flow is also partitioned to the dependent lung areas and thereby maximizes the optimal $\dot{V}_A/\dot{Q}$.

Table 6-3. Airway Management Kit for Ventilation During Emergency Transport

1. Laryngoscope with curved and straight blades in various sizes with spare batteries and bulbs
2. Endotracheal tubes of various sizes
3. Adaptors for attaching endotracheal tubes to ventilators and gas sources
4. Forceps
5. Magill forceps
6. Oral and nasal airways
7. Esophageal obturator airway with gastric suction capability
8. McSwain dart or Heimlich valve
9. Syringes (10 and 50 cc)
10. Cetacaine
11. Surgical lubricant (water-soluble)
12. Adhesive tape (1 and 2 inches)
13. Suction catheters (various sizes)

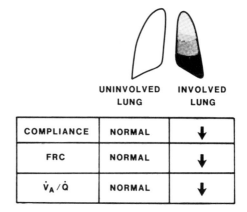

	UNINVOLVED LUNG	INVOLVED LUNG
COMPLIANCE	NORMAL	↓
FRC	NORMAL	↓
$\dot{V}_A/\dot{Q}$	NORMAL	↓

Fig. 6-17. Unilateral pathophysiology: atelectasis, pneumonia, aspiration, or contusion occurring in only one lung. Compliance, FRC, and ventilation/perfusion matching ($\dot{V}_A/\dot{Q}$) are decreased only in the involved lung.

In cases of unilateral lung involvement, when the goal is to improve gas exchange, the patient should be moved into the lateral decubitus position. This maneuver can be simplified by using a special bed.[60] With the uninvolved lung down, inspired gas and blood are preferentially distributed to that side during spontaneous breathing. Confirmation that this position is optimal can be elicited by turning the patient 180 degrees and placing the involved lung down. Blood gases should deteriorate.

Independent Lung Ventilation

Unfortunately, positioning does not always substantially improve oxygenation, and lung volume may need to be increased. Application of CPAP and mechanical ventilation can actually cause further deterioration. Compliance of the diseased lung is decreased so that positive airway pressure preferentially influences the healthy lung, and produces overdistention and an abnormally high $\dot{V}_A/\dot{Q}$. Not only are these alveoli now overdistended, but the resulting increase in pressure shifts blood away from the normal lung to diseased areas with a de-

crease of $\dot{V}_A/\dot{Q}$ (Fig. 6-18). In such circumstances, if 15 cm H_2O of CPAP does not restore appropriate function, we initiate independent lung ventilation to prevent the

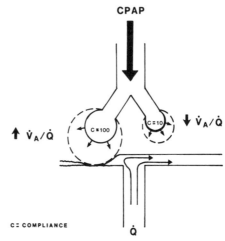

Fig. 6-18. Ventilation maldistribution with conventional application of CPAP to lungs with differential compliance (C). Grossly overdistended healthy lung with a C = 100 compresses pulmonary capillaries and directs perfusion to low compliant involved lung, predisposing to severe alveolar ventilation perfusion ($\dot{V}_A/\dot{Q}$) mismatching. Thus conventionally applied CPAP is inappropriate for treating unilateral pathophysiology.

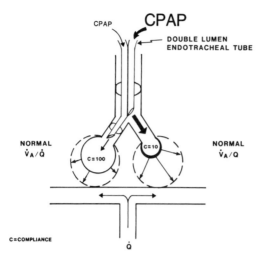

Fig. 6-19. Independent lung ventilation. Lung fields are isolated with a double-lumen endotracheal tube, and a greater level of CPAP is applied only to the involved lung. Thus overall normal alveolar ventilation/perfusion ($\dot{V}_A/\dot{Q}$) matching is maximized. FRC is restored to the involved lung (see text).

previously described problems of $\dot{V}_A/\dot{Q}$ mismatch.

Normally, the right lung receives 60 percent of the V_T. We attempt to maintain that ratio during independent lung ventilation. However, if high PIP becomes necessary in order to recruit atelectatic lung segments, we can modify ventilation accordingly. Devices are currently available for independent lung ventilation.[9,24,56,59] All provide complete control and isolation of V_T and CPAP to each lung field by timer synchronizers attached to separate ventilators or circuits. These synchronizers may not be necessary so long as inspiration to each lung is not more than 90 degrees out of phase.

A double-lumen endotracheal tube permits isolation of each lung and allows independent lung therapy. CPAP or mechanical ventilation can then be directed only where needed to provide the appropriate support necessary to restore function to each lung (Fig. 6-19). This tube should be treated with great care. The narrow lumen on each side means more difficulty during suctioning and a greater likelihood of obstruction by mucous plugs. Correct placement can be confirmed by clamping one side of the special adapter, which is attached to a conventional self-inflating bag. Breath sounds should stop in the lung on the side that is clamped but continue on the other side. Cuffs on some double-lumen tubes are not specific for high-volume/low-pressure applications. Therefore care must be taken to select a proper size and not to overinflate the cuff. Once the level of required CPAP is again below 15 cm H_2O, we prefer to substitute a single-lumen tube and to begin conventional ventilation.

ACKNOWLEDGMENTS

Ms. Lynn M. Carroll gave editorial assistance, and Ms. Joy Kuck provided the graphics with the assistance of Ms. Heidi Hengstenberg.

REFERENCES

1. Armengol J, Man GCW, Balsys AJ, et al: Effects of the respiratory cycle on cardiac output measurements: reproducibility of data enhanced by timing the thermodilution injections in dogs. Crit Care Med 9:852, 1981
2. Ashbaugh D, Bigelow D, Petty T, et al: Acute respiratory distress in adults. Lancet 2:319, 1967
3. Askanazi J, Nordenstrom J, Rosenbaum SH, et al: Nutrition for the patient with respiratory failure: glucose vs. fat. Anesthesiology 54:373, 1981
4. Barach AL, Martin J, Eckman M: Positive pressure respiration and its application to the treatment of acute pulmonary edema. Ann Intern Med 12:754, 1938
5. Belenky DA, Orr RJ, Woodrum DE, et al: Is continuous transpulmonary pressure better than conventional respiratory management of hyaline membrane disease? A controlled study. Pediatrics 58:800, 1976
6. Berninger GT, Forrette MJ: Adult manual resuscitators. Curr Rev Respir Ther 1:115, 1979

7. Bullowa JGH: The Management of Pneumonias. p. 192. Oxford University Press, New York, 1936

8. Caldwell EJ, Powell RD, Mullooly JP: Interstitial emphysema: a study of physiologic factors involved in experimental induction of the lesion. Am Rev Respir Dis 102:516, 1970

9. Carlon CG, Ray C, Klein R: Criteria for selective positive end-expiratory pressure and independent synchronized ventilation of each lung. Chest 74:501, 1978

10. Colocousis JS, Huntsman LL, Curreri PW: Estimation of stroke volume changes by ultrasonic doppler. Circulation 56:914, 1977

11. Covelli HD, Weled BJ, Beekman JF: Efficacy of continuous positive airway pressure administered by face mask. Chest 81:147, 1982

12. Douglas M, Downs JB: Special correspondence. Anesth Analg 57:347, 1978

13. Douglas ME, Downs JB, Dannemiller FJ, et al: Changes in pulmonary venous admixture with varying inspired oxygen. Anesth Analg 55:688, 1976

14. Downs JB: Mechanical ventilatory support. Part II. Curr Rev Respir Ther 3:82, 1981

15. Downs JB, Douglas ME: Assessment of cardiac filling pressure during continuous positive pressure ventilation. Crit Care Med 8:285, 1980

16. Downs JB, Klein EF, Desautels D, et al: Intermittent mandatory ventilation: a new approach to weaning patients from mechanical ventilators. Chest 64:331, 1973

17. Downs JB, Marston A: A new transport ventilator: an evaluation. Crit Care Med 5:113, 1977

18. Downs JB, Mitchell LA: Pulmonary effects of ventilatory pattern following cardiopulmonary bypass. Crit Care Med 4:295, 1976

19. Dueck R, Wagner PD, West JB: Effects of positive end-expiratory pressure on gas exchange in dogs with normal and edematous lungs. Anesthesiology 47:359, 1977

20. Froese AB, Bryan AC: Effects of anesthesia and paralysis on diaphragmatic mechanics in man. Anesthesiology 41:242, 1974

21. Gallagher TJ: Effect of positive pressure ventilation on oxygenation. Crit Care Med 6:119, 1978

22. Gallagher TJ, Banner MJ: Cardiac output measured noninvasively by continuous-wave ultrasonic doppler computer. Anesth Analg 62:261, 1983

23. Gallagher TJ, Banner MJ: Mean airway pressure as a determinant of oxygenation. Crit Care Med 8:244, 1980

24. Gallagher TJ, Banner MJ, Smith RA: A simplified method of independent lung ventilation. Crit Care Med 8:396, 1980

25. Gallagher TJ, Civetta JM: Goal-directed therapy of acute respiratory failure. Anesth Analg 59:831, 1980

26. Gallagher TJ, Civetta JM, Kirby RR: Terminology update: optimal PEEP. Crit Care Med 6:323, 1978

27. Gallagher TJ, Civetta JM, Kirby RR, et al: Post-traumatic pulmonary insufficiency: a treatable disease. South Med J 70:1308, 1977

28. Gherini S, Peters RM, Virgilio RW: Mechanical work on the lungs and work of breathing with positive end-expiratory pressure and continuous positive airway pressure. Chest 76:251, 1979

29. Gibbs CP, Schwartz DJ, Wynne JW, et al: Antacid pulmonary aspiration in the dog. Anesthesiology 51:380, 1979

30. Greenbaum DM, Millen JE, Eross B, et al: Continuous positive airway pressure without tracheal intubation in spontaneously breathing patients. Chest 69:615, 1976

31. Gregory GA: Devices for applying continuous positive airway pressure. In Thibeault DW, Gregory GA (eds): Neonatal Pulmonary Care. p. 183. Addison-Wesley, Reading, MA, 1979

32. Gregory GA, Kitterman JA, Phibbs RH, et al: Treatment of the idiopathic respiratory distress syndrome with continuous positive airway pressure. N Engl J Med 284:1333, 1971

33. Harless KW, Morris AH, Cengiz M, et al: Civilian ground and air transport of adults with acute respiratory failure. JAMA 240:361, 1978

34. Hasten RW, Downs JB, Heenan TJ: A comparison of synchronized and nonsynchronized intermittent mandatory ventilation. Respir Care 25:554, 1980

35. Heenan TJ, Downs JB, Douglas ME, et al: Intermittent mandatory ventilation—is synchronization important? Chest 77:598, 1980

36. Henning RJ, Shubin H, Weil MH: The measurement of the work of breathing for the

clinical assessment of ventilator dependence. Crit Care Med 5:264, 1977

37. Hobelmann CF Jr, Smith DE, Virgilio RW, et al: Mechanics of ventilation with positive end-expiratory pressure. Ann Thorac Surg 24:68, 1977

38. Huntsman LL, Gams E, Johnson CC, et al: Transcutaneous determination of aortic blood flow velocities in man. Am Heart J 89:605, 1975

39. Jardin F, Farcot JC, Boisante L, et al: Influence of positive end-expiratory pressure on left ventricular performance. N Engl J Med 304:387, 1981

40. Johanson WG Jr, Harris GD: Aspiration pneumonia, anaerobic infections and lung abscess. Med Clin North Am 54:385, 1980

41. Kirby RR: Mechanical ventilation in acute respiratory failure: facts, fictions and fallacies. In: Gallagher TJ. Advances in Anesthesia Year Book Medical Publishers, Chicago pp 51–88, 1984

42. Kirby RR, Downs JB, Civetta JM, et al: High level positive end-expiratory pressure (PEEP) in acute respiratory insufficiency. Chest 67:156, 1975

43. Kirby RR, Perry JC, Calderwood HW, et al: Cardiorespiratory effects of high positive end-expiratory pressure. Anesthesiology 43:533, 1975

44. Kirby RR, Robison EJ, Schulz J, et al: A new pediatric volume ventilator. Anesth Analg 50:533, 1971

45. Kirby RR, Robison E, Schulz J, et al: Continuous flow ventilation as an alternative to assisted or controlled ventilation in infants. Anesth Analg 51:871, 1972

46. Mendelson CL: The aspiration of stomach contents into the lungs during obstetric anesthesia. Am J Obstet Gynecol 52:191, 1946

47. Modell JH: The Pathophysiology and Treatment of Drowning and Near Drowning. Charles C Thomas, Springfield, IL, 1971

48. Murphy EJ, Desautels DA, Modell JH: A compact headboard and ventilator transport system. Crit Care Med 6:387, 1978

49. Murphy EJ, Downs JB: Ventilator induced ventilation-perfusion mismatching. In: Abstracts of Scientific Papers. 1976 ASA Annual Meeting. p. 345. American Society of Anesthesiologists, Park Ridge, IL, 1976

50. Nixon JR, Brock-Utne JG: Free fatty acid and arterial oxygen changes following major injury: a correlation between hypoxemia and increased free fatty acid levels. J Trauma 18:23, 1978

51. Otis AB: The work of breathing. In: Fenn WO, Rahn H (eds): Handbook of Physiology: A Critical, Comprehensive Presentation of Physiological Knowledge and Concepts. Section 3: Respiration. Vol I. pp. 463–476. American Physiological Society, Washington, DC, 1964

52. Patten MT, Liebman PR, Hechtman HB: Humorally mediated decreases in cardiac output associated with positive end-expiratory pressure. Microvasc Res 13:137, 1977

53. Paul WL, Downs JB: Postoperative atelectasis: intermittent positive pressure breathing, incentive spirometry, and face-mask positive end-expiratory pressure. Arch Surg 116:861, 1981

54. Peters RM, Hilberman M: Respiratory insufficiency: diagnosis and control of therapy. Surgery 70:280, 1970

55. Proctor HJ, Woolson R: Prediction of respiratory muscle fatigue by measurements of the work of breathing. Surg Gynecol Obstet 136:367, 1973

56. Ray C, Carlon CG, Miodownik S: A method of synchronizing two MA-1 ventilators for independent lung ventilation. Crit Care Med 6:71, 1978

57. Reynolds EOR: Effect of alterations in mechanical ventilator settings on pulmonary gas exchange in hyaline membrane disease. Arch Dis Child 46:152, 1971

58. Robin ED, Cross CE, Zelis R: Pulmonary edema. N Engl J Med 288:239, 1973

59. Sayer DM, Jung RC, Koons R: A unilateral lung ventilator. Respir Ther 3:41, 1973

60. Schimmel L, Civetta JM, Kirby RR: A new mechanical method to influence pulmonary perfusion in critically ill patients. Crit Care Med 5:277, 1977

61. Shapiro BA, Harrison RA, Walton JR, et al: Intermittent demand ventilation (IDV): a new technique for supporting ventilation in critically ill patients. Respir Care 21:521, 1976

62. Smith RA, Kirby RR, Gooding JM, et al: Continuous positive airway pressure (CPAP) by face mask. Crit Care Med 8:43, 1980

63. Snyder JV, Powner DJ: Effects of mechanical ventilation on the measurement of cardiac output by thermodilution. Crit Care Med 10:677, 1982

64. Sugarman HJ, Rogers RM, Miller LD: Positive end-expiratory pressure (PEEP); indications and physiologic considerations. Chest 62:86S, 1972

65. Suter PM, Fairley HB, Isenberg MD: Optimum end-expiratory airway pressure in patients with acute pulmonary failure. N Engl J Med 292:284, 1975

66. Suter PM, Fairley HB, Schlobohm RM: Shunt, lung volume and perfusion during short periods of ventilation with oxygen. Anesthesiology 43:617, 1975

67. Teplitz C: The core pathobiology and integrated medical science of adult acute respiratory insufficiency. Surg Clin North Am 56:1091, 1976

68. Turaids T, Nobrega FT, Gallagher TJ: Absorptional atelectasis breathing oxygen at simulated altitude: prevention using inert gas. Aerospace Med 38:189, 1967

69. West JB: Pulmonary Pathophysiology—The Essentials. p. 193. Williams & Wilkins, Baltimore, 1977

70. Winter PM, Smith G: The toxicity of oxygen. Anesthesiology 37:210, 1972

71. Wynne JW, Modell JH: Respiratory aspiration of stomach contents. Ann Intern Med 87:466, 1977

7

Neonatal Respiratory Support

Eduardo Bancalari
Esther Eisler

Babies are not just small adults.
Neonatologists' Credo

Respiratory failure is one of the most common problems of the newborn period, especially in the premature infant. The reasons for this are several, but most are related to the incomplete structural and biochemical development of the respiratory system.[58]

CHARACTERISTICS OF RESPIRATORY FUNCTION IN THE NEWBORN

Lung Development and Maturation

Between 17 and 24 weeks of gestation, the development of the lung is in a canalicular stage characterized by elongation of the subdivisions of the airways and appearance of cuboidal cells in the epithelium. The mesoderm becomes thinner, and toward the end of this stage a proliferation of capillaries comes close to the air spaces for the first time. The terminal sac period begins at 24 weeks' and lasts until 40 weeks' gestation. This stage of development is characterized by approximation of the blood capillaries to the respiratory epithelium and differentiation of the epithelial cells into their mature forms. At 24 weeks, it is already possible to identify type I and type II cells lining the air spaces. This is the earliest stage at which gas exchange can occur in the lung, but the thickness of the tissue between the air spaces and capillaries is two to three times that of the adult. By 30–32 weeks, the terminal bronchioli divide into four generations of respiratory bronchioli which eventually give origin to several elongated saccules. These continue to subdivide until term and give origin to alveolar sacs. Between 24 and 32 weeks' gestation, the lung gradually increases its functional surface and capacity for gas exchange. The production of surfactant also begins at 23–24 weeks' gestation, first appearing at the same time osmiophilic bodies are seen in the type II cells. However, it is only after 28–30 weeks that surfactant appears in sufficient quantities to be detected in the amniotic fluid.[47] At this time, the risk for developing hyaline membrane disease (HMD) decreases rapidly.[33]

Both the structural and biochemical development of the lung can be accelerated by corticosteroids.[26,70] Steroid levels in the fetus can be increased by administration to the mother or by conditions that produce fetal stress, e.g., placental insufficiency, prolonged rupture of membranes, or active labor.[9,82] Other substances, e.g., aminophylline and thyroid hormone, also accelerate fetal lung maturation.[51,90]

Cardiopulmonary Adaptation at Birth

Oxygen uptake and carbon dioxide elimination by the fetus in utero is accomplished in the placenta where gas exchange between the fetal and maternal circulation occurs. The fetal circulation has several adaptive mechanisms that allow adequate oxygenation despite the low P_{O_2} of blood returning from the placenta through the umbilical vein and the fact that this blood enters the fetal venous system. The most important characteristics are: (1) low pulmonary blood flow due to high pulmonary vascular resistance; and (2) right-to-left shunting through the foramen ovale and the ductus arteriosus. Hence perfusion by blood with a higher oxygen content is maintained to the coronary and central nervous system (CNS) circulations.

At birth, gas transfer across the placenta is suddenly interrupted and the newborn must establish effective pulmonary gas exchange within seconds if he is to survive intact. In order to accomplish this transition, several drastic changes must occur rapidly and in a given sequence. The most important alterations are triggered by the initiation of breathing followed by a rapid decrease in pulmonary vascular resistance and an increase in blood flow through the lungs. This is, in turn, followed by an increase in left atrial and systemic blood pressure which eliminates the right-to-left

shunting through the foramen ovale and the ductus arteriosus. Later, functional and anatomical closure of the ductus occurs. The drop in pressure in the pulmonary circulation is also an important factor in the reabsorption of fluid that fills the air spaces at birth. The most important cardiopulmonary changes that occur after birth are summarized in Figure 7-1.

All these events normally occur within a few minutes after birth and allow the infant to achieve arterial O_2 and CO_2 tensions similar to those of the adult during the first 12–24 hours of life. A number of pathological conditions can interfere with these changes, sometimes culminating in severe respiratory failure. Furthermore, most of these adaptive changes are reversible, and under conditions of hypoxia, acidosis, or cold stress an increase in pulmonary vascular resistance and pressure may recur with development of a right-to-left shunt and severe hypoxemia.

Respiratory Function in the Newborn

A number of characteristics in the respiratory function of the newborn render this group particularly susceptible to the development of respiratory failure.

Control of Breathing. The neonate, particularly if preterm, has frequent episodes of periodic breathing and short-duration apnea. These episodes are more common during sleep, and in the premature they may be accompanied by bradycardia. In such instances, stimulation is often required to induce a resumption of spontaneous breathing. Ventilatory response to CO_2 is decreased in the premature and is even lower in those presenting with frequent apnea.[45,93]

One of the most important differences in the neonatal control of breathing is a *decreased* ventilatory response to hypoxemia. Full-term infants during the first few days of life and premature infants for a longer

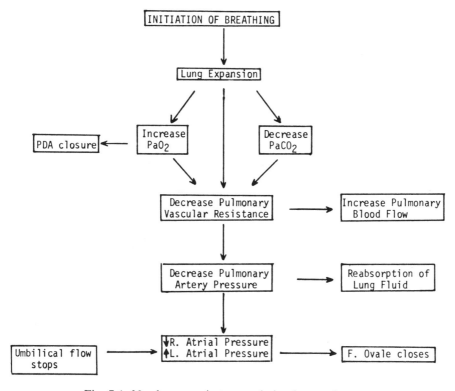

Fig. 7-1. Newborn respiratory and circulatory changes.

period of time may respond with a decrease in ventilation or apnea when their Pa_{O_2} falls below 30–40 mm Hg.[16,92] The mechanism for this respiratory depression by hypoxemia is not clear but most likely is due to CNS depression as peripheral chemoreceptors are active in the neonate.

Newborns seem to have an active inflation reflex which, in contrast to the adult, may play a role in the control of the tidal volume. Whereas the premature of more than 32 weeks' gestation responds with an increased inspiratory effort to respiratory loads (e.g., airway obstruction), infants below this gestational age frequently become apneic when they are stressed by an increased work of breathing.[19,43]

Because of increased oxygen consumption, minute ventilation in proportion to body weight is higher in the newborn than in the adult. The increase is achieved with a high respiratory rate of 30–50/minute and a tidal volume of only 5–7 ml/kg. A high dead space/tidal volume ratio results, especially in small preterm infants.

Mechanics of Breathing. In absolute terms, lung compliance in the newborn is very low, but if corrected for lung volume the value is similar to that in the adult (60 ml/cm H_2O/L functional residual capacity). The same considerations apply to airway resistance, but because of the very small airway size obstruction occurs more easily in the newborn than in the adult.

Another disadvantage of prematurity is high chest wall compliance.[42] This factor, coupled with a decreased lung compliance, results in a lower functional residual capacity (FRC) and a tendency for airway closure and low ventilation/perfusion ratios ($\dot{V}_A/\dot{Q}$) to develop.

Gas Exchange. In the premature infant, gas exchange can be limited because of incomplete vascularization of the air spaces.

Diffusion may also be decreased because of the increased alveolocapillary membrane thickness. Finally, the predisposition for air space closure and decreased lung volume frequently produces a decrease in $\dot{V}_A/\dot{Q}$ with resultant increased pulmonary shunting and hypoxemia.

RESPIRATORY FAILURE IN THE NEWBORN

Causes and Pathophysiology

Hypoventilation. Alveolar hypoventilation in the neonate may occur at birth as a result of respiratory center depression due to perinatal asphyxia or analgesic drugs administered to the mother during labor. Central depression also occurs frequently in infants with intracranial hemorrhage and meningitis. In preterm infants apnea is seen without a pathological substrate and is known as apnea of prematurity. It is probably due to structural and functional immaturity of the respiratory control system.

In cases of traumatic delivery, damage to the phrenic nerve may occur, resulting in diaphragmatic paralysis and hypoventilation. This complication is seen infrequently nowadays.

Still another mechanism leading frequently to hypoventilation in the newborn is increased work of breathing, which can be secondary to airway obstruction or decreased lung compliance. Airway obstruction results from aspiration of meconium, blood, or mucus; mucosal edema due to trauma; inflammation or heart failure; or retained secretions. Obstruction is also associated with congenital anomalies, e.g., tumors, webs, or vascular rings which occupy the lumen of the airway or produce extrinsic compression of the tracheobronchial tree.

Decreased lung compliance is one of the most common functional changes in neonatal pulmonary diseases. It may be secondary to decreased surfactant in HMD, increased pulmonary interstitial fluid associated with heart failure, or pulmonary inflammation due to infection or aspiration of substances that produce chemical injury. Decreased compliance is also present in infants with chronic lung disease and interstitial fibrosis, e.g., bronchopulmonary dysplasia. As in the adult, hypoventilation by the newborn results in hypercapnia and hypoxemia. Because of immature control of breathing and respiratory mechanics, the preterm infant is more prone to develop hypoventilation than the full-term infant.

Venous Admixture. Venous admixture is the most common cause of hypoxemia in the neonate. Right-to-left shunting of blood can occur in the lung parenchyma or in the cardiovascular system. Venous admixture in the lung is usually the result of a low $\dot{V}_A/\dot{Q}$ ratio resulting from diffuse alveolar collapse as occurs in HMD, alveolar exudate in pneumonia, or segmental or lobar atelectasis associated with localized airway obstruction. Lung collapse also occurs with pneumothorax, accumulation of pleural fluid, or other space-occupying lesions, e.g., diaphragmatic hernia or cardiomegaly.

Extrapulmonary shunting results from lesions associated with congenital malformations of the heart but more frequently is secondary to pulmonary hypertension and right-to-left shunting through the foramen ovale or a patent ductus arteriosus. This condition is known as persistent fetal circulation (PFC), persistent transitional circulation, or persistent pulmonary hypertension (PPH). It is usually associated with perinatal asphyxia or respiratory failure due to meconium aspiration, bacterial pneumonia, or other causes of pulmonary insufficiency. Such shunting increases the hypoxemia caused by the primary problem.

Although few studies have measured diffusing capacity in newborns with respiratory failure, most pathological conditions are characterized by increased interstitial fluid and, in chronic lesions, fibrous tissue. These abnormalities, coupled with the fact that the distance between air spaces and capillaries in the immature lung is already increased, make it likely that many of these patients also have a decreased diffusing capacity.

Diagnosis

Clinical Diagnosis. The diagnosis of respiratory failure is usually based on signs of increased work of breathing. Clinical manifestations include nasal flaring and intercostal, subcostal, and sternal retractions. The latter are due primarily to the increasingly subambient intrathoracic pressure required to maintain normal ventilation and to the high elasticity of the chest wall in the newborn. Most infants also have an increased respiratory rate, and those with conditions characterized by decreased lung volume frequently demonstrate expiratory grunting. Cyanosis may be evident in cases with severe hypoxemia but is a late sign because of the increased oxygen affinity of fetal hemoglobin.

All these signs are nonspecific and are of little help in defining the etiology of the respiratory failure. In cases of airway obstruction, inspiratory stridor may be audible if the obstruction is in the upper airway, or wheezing with prolonged expiration may be detectable if it is lower airway. HMD is characterized by severe retraction with poor breath sounds, whereas infants with penumonia may have abundant rales and, in most cases, other signs of systemic infection.

Infants with meconium aspiration have coarse and diffuse bronchial sounds and frequently have an overexpanded chest. They also may show meconium staining of the skin, nails, and umbilical cord.

Blood Gases. The definition and/or diagnosis of respiratory failure commonly includes abnormal arterial blood gas tensions. In the newborn, however, normal values vary depending on the gestational and postnatal age of the infant. Although a Pao_2 of 65 mm Hg is in the normal range for a 28-week gestational age premature, it is below normal for a full-term infant. The same considerations apply to the $Paco_2$, which tends to be higher in small premature infants. In general, one should consider a Pao_2 below 65 mm Hg abnormal in an infant under 37 weeks' gestation and under 75 mm Hg in a full-term infant (air-breathing under stable conditions).[68] Samples collected while the infant is crying are unreliable because the Pao_2 and $Paco_2$ may change significantly. The upper normal limits for $Paco_2$ are 40 mm Hg for the full-term and 50 mm Hg for the premature infant.[83] During the first hours of life, most infants have some degree of hypoxemia and hypercapnia, both of which become normal by 6–12 hours of age.

Although specific arterial blood gas tensions are not pathognomonic of specific disease states, the response of the Pao_2 to certain forms of treatment may help to define the mechanism underlying the respiratory failure. Infants with HMD characteristically respond with a rapid increase in Pao_2 when treated with continuous or intermittent positive pressure. This response is less clear in infants with pneumonia or meconium aspiration. In patients with extrapulmonary right-to-left shunting, Pao_2 does not increase significantly with increasing Fio_2 or high transpulmonary pressures. In fact, deterioration in Pao_2 may be evident when high airway pressure is applied because of the resultant increase in pulmonary vascular resistance. Patients with persistent pulmonary hypertension may have a higher Pao_2 in the blood "above" (right radial artery) than below (descending aorta) the ductus arteriosus. They also have wide spontaneous fluctuation in Pao_2 with values that are below what would be expected in relation to the severity of their lung disease.

Radiography, Angiography, and Radionucleotide Imaging. Chest radiographs are a valuable tool for the differential diagnosis of pulmonary diseases in the newborn.

248 • *Mechanical Ventilation*

HMD is characterized by diffuse increased lung density, a fine granular appearance, and loss of lung volume reflected by elevated diaphragms and air bronchograms. In bacterial pneumonia, the radiographic appearance may be similar to that of HMD, but in most cases the infiltrates are coarser, less symmetrical, and sometimes accompanied by evidence of pleural effusion. In meconium aspiration, coarse infiltrates are present, usually bilaterally, and later in the course of the disease the lungs may be hyperinflated.

Angiography is helpful when congenital malformation of the pulmonary or systemic circulation is suspected.

Radionucleotide scanning is used to define the distribution of ventilation and perfusion, either by rebreathing of xenon or by injection of the same gas into a vein. In the latter case, imaging of pulmonary perfusion is obtained initially, followed subsequently by elimination of the gas through ventilation.

Pulmonary Function Testing. The use of pulmonary function tests as a diagnostic tool is limited in the newborn because of the technical difficulties encountered. When available, the measurement of FRC, lung compliance, pulmonary resistance, and alveolar arterial gradients may be helpful to establish a diagnosis, follow the progression of the disease, and evaluate the response to therapy. Lung mechanics can be measured in infants breathing spontaneously or during mechanical ventilation. Tidal volume is measured using a pneumotachograph and integrating the flow signal to obtain volume. Esophageal pressure can be measured with a water-filled feeding tube, and airway pressure is determined by connecting the ventilator circuit to a pressure transducer.

Evaluation of respiratory control functions may also be helpful in cases of apnea or central hypoventilation. The most common tests of respiratory control are ventilatory response to CO_2, high and low O_2, and airway occlusion. Such tests can be performed on the full-term or premature infant by measuring ventilation with a pneumotachograph.

MANAGEMENT OF RESPIRATORY FAILURE IN THE NEWBORN

Management of the neonate with respiratory failure has improved considerably over the last 10–15 years, resulting in a significant increase in survival and a reduction in neurological sequelae due to severe hypoxia. Oxygen therapy was the only treatment available until modern techniques of mechanical respiratory assistance were introduced into the care of the newborn. These methods have not only improved the outcome of infants with respiratory failure but have also stimulated the development of other areas of neonatal intensive care, drastically changing the approach to the critically ill neonate.[46]

The care of any newborn with respiratory failure involves at least three considerations: The first is specific treatment of the condition causing respiratory failure, e.g., the use of antibiotics in pneumonia or the administration of methylxanthines to a premature with apnea. This aspect is not discussed here. The second consideration is the general management of a critically ill neonate, and the final area of concern is correction of respiratory failure, independent of the cause, to ensure adequate oxygenation and avoid acute hypercapnia and acidosis. This goal may be accomplished by increasing the inspired oxygen concentration using continuous distending airway pressure or by mechanical ventilation with intermittent positive pressure.

General Management

Introduction of sophisticated techniques of intensive care have resulted in a tendency to forget some of the basic principles of neonatal support, with occasionally disastrous consequences. Today, most infant deaths from respiratory failure are not related directly to the primary disease but are more often due to complications of treatment. For this reason, basic principles of neonatal care must continue to be stressed.

Temperature Control. This area is of essential importance, especially in the premature infant. Ambient temperature below the neutral thermal environment increases oxygen consumption, favors hypoglycemia and metabolic acidosis, and can increase pulmonary artery pressure with resultant increases of right-to-left extrapulmonary shunting. The ambient temperature must be kept between 32° and 35°C to maintain the body temperature between 36.5° and 36.8°C. For this purpose, incubators or radiant warmers equipped with a servo control system may be used effectively. Because heat loss can occur within a few minutes in small prematures, it is critical to keep these patients in the same thermal environment during diagnostic or therapeutic procedures.

Fluids and Electrolytes. Adjustment of fluid and electrolyte intake to maintain a normal balance is often difficult in the sick newborn because of the large surface area, increased skin permeability, and limited renal function. Dehydration may cause arterial hypotension, hypernatremia and renal failure, and excessive fluid intake in the small premature is associated with an increased incidence of symptomatic patent ductus arteriosis (PDA), necrotizing enterocolitis, and bronchopulmonary dysplasia.[10,11,17] Fluid requirements range widely depending on gestational age, postnatal age, environmental temperature and humidity, and the clinical condition of the infant. The administration of fluids must be based on these factors and on accurate and repeated determination of body weight, urine output, and urine and serum osmolarity. Normal water requirements range from 80 to 160 ml/kg/24 hours, sodium and potassium needs are 2–4 mEq/kg/24 hours, and calcium needs are 0.5–2 mEq/kg/day.

Nutrition. Adequate caloric intake is also essential for the survival of sick infants, but these infants are usually unable to receive oral feedings. A solution of 10 percent dextrose at a volume of 150 ml/kg/day provides the basic caloric requirements during the first few days of life. If oral feedings cannot be started after the first 3–5 days of life, total parenteral nutrition must be initiated, adding amino acids and lipids to the intravenous solution. We do not recommend the use of oral feedings in infants with acute respiratory failure who are receiving mechanical respiratory support as they may cause complications, e.g., aspiration pneumonitis or necrotizing enterocolitis. We do consider oral alimentation in infants who require intermittent positive-pressure ventilation (IPPV) because of chronic respiratory failure.

Infection Control. The large number of invasive procedures utilized during neonatal respiratory support considerably increases the risk of infection in these patients. Infection may be localized to the skin or airway but frequently spreads to the bloodstream, resulting in sepsis. Infections acquired through respiratory equipment are usually produced by gram-negative bacteria; however, *Staphyloccoccus aureus* or beta-hemolytic *Streptococcus* group B can also be acquired through contaminated hands or equipment. Therefore strict rules must be enforced for aseptic technique in all sick neonates, especially small prematures or those requiring respiratory assistance. The prophylactic use of antibiotics in these patients has not proved to be effective and in fact may increase the risk of colonization with resistant bacteria.

Blood Gas Monitoring

Proper management of respiratory failure in the newborn requires a 24-hour availa-

Table 7-1. Intermittent and Continuous Neonatal Blood Gas Monitoring

Arterial blood gases
  Umbilical catheter
  Peripheral percutaneous arterial catheter
  Arterial punctures

Capillary blood gases

Transcutaneous
  Oxygen
  Carbon dioxide

Continuous oxygen saturation with indwelling fiberoptic catheter

Continuous oxygen with indwelling polarographic electrode

bility of accurate arterial blood gas analysis. Blood gas measurements provide the physiological data necessary for appropriate clinical evaluation of the effectiveness of respiratory care and are the key determinants for modifications in this support. Values obtained reflect overall function of the cardiorespiratory system, including the adequacy of oxygenation, ventilation, acid-base homeostasis, pulmonary and peripheral perfusion, and the severity of respiratory or cardiac compromise. Measurements may also give early indications that complications, e.g., pneumothorax or endotracheal tube displacement, have occurred. Results can be accurately interpreted only when the clinical status of the patient is known, including such information as vital signs, oxygen concentrations, ventilator settings, and the site of blood sampling. In addition to intermittent blood sampling, recent advances have provided the technology to allow continuous invasive and transcutaneous monitoring techniques. Some of the most common clinically useful blood gas and continuous monitoring techniques for neonatal application are listed in Table 7-1. These are discussed in this section.

Arterial Catheters. Umbilical artery catheters are usually placed in the newborn who requires oxygen therapy or ventilatory support. In addition to blood sampling for arterial blood gas determinations, the umbilical line establishes a route for continu-ous infusion of fluids and medications, blood sampling for other laboratory tests, and direct blood pressure measurements. Frequent sampling is possible without repeated needle punctures, an important consideration as an agitated infant who is crying or holding his breath generally lowers his Pa_{O_2}, changes his Pa_{CO_2}, and adversely affects assessment of the efficacy of his respiratory support. When medications such as sodium bicarbonate are given through umbilical lines, care must be taken to flush the line to prevent contamination of a subsequent blood sample, which would result in false values for measured pH and Pa_{CO_2} and for calculated bicarbonate and base excess or deficit.

The advantage of an indwelling catheter which permits the sampling of arterial blood as needed must be weighed against possible complications. Blanching or cyanosis of the leg or toes may occur, indicating vascular spasm or obstruction to flow. Warming the nonischemic limb to initiate reflex contralateral vasodilation and improvement in color or pulse has occasionally been recommended. Otherwise the catheter should be removed. Thrombosis around the catheter tip occurs frequently. Major complications occur when there is embolization to the kidneys or intestines. Bacterial colonization of the umbilical catheters may be as high as 57 percent, but less than 5 percent of patients develop catheter-related bacteremia.[59] However, sterile techniques must be used in manipulating the catheter. Blood loss from loose connections or vascular perforation may also occur. Finally, one additional clinically relevant problem must be taken into consideration. When a right-to-left shunt causing venous admixture occurs through a PDA and the umbilical catheter tip is below the ductus, the oxygen tension measurement from this blood does not represent the oxygen tension in the preductal blood perfusing the eyes, heart, and brain. However, preductal blood gas tensions from the temporal, right radial, or right brachial arteries or transcutaneous oxygen measurements from the right upper chest may be compared to postductal blood values from the descending aorta in order to determine if a substantial ductal right-to-left shunt exists.

Peripheral percutaneous lines or surgical cutdowns may be necessary when an umbilical line cannot be placed or must be removed because of complications. The radial artery is the most common site for percutaneous line placement. The adequacy of collateral circulation in the ulnar artery should be determined before placement of the line. The temporal artery may also be catheterized; however, indwelling catheters in this portion of the circulation have been associated with cortical tissue infarction secondary to cerebral emboli.[97]

Arterial Punctures. Once the arterial line is removed and less frequent sampling is required, arterial punctures may be performed. The radial artery is the most common site, followed by the brachial, temporal, dorsal pedal, and posterior tibial arteries. Femoral arterial punctures are usually avoided because of potential injury to the legs caused by damage to the contiguous nerves, bones, or vasculature during the puncture. Complications of radial artery puncture should be minimal if peripheral circulation through the ulnar artery is ensured and good technique is used. The brachial artery is larger than the radial artery but is more difficult to puncture because it lies deeper and is less well fixed than the radial. A 13 percent incidence of median nerve damage caused by brachial punctures has been described in a group of infants weighing less than 1500 g.[84] Other possible complications include infection, blood loss, arterial laceration, hematoma formation, and spasm of the artery, causing loss of blood flow to the limb.

The puncture should be performed with a 1-ml heparinized tuberculin syringe and either a 25-gauge needle or a butterfly scalp vein needle. The needle should have a clear hub so that when the artery has been entered blood flashback is easily identified. Heparin should be used only to coat the barrel of the syringe. All air and heparin should be eliminated from the syringe. After location of the arterial pulse, the site should be cleaned with an antiseptic and the needle then inserted at a 45 degree angle to the point of strongest pulsation. A transillumination device can be used to assist in locating the artery, but care must be taken to avoid thermal burns.[104] The needle is inserted against the direction of blood flow. Slight "negative" pressure is developed by gentle traction on the syringe plunger. After successful penetration, blood should gradually flow into the syringe without additional force on the plunger. Once the blood is obtained, pressure must be applied to the site for at least 5 minutes to avoid hemorrhage and hematoma formation.

Capillary Blood Gases. Determination of capillary blood gases is useful in assessing pH and carbon dioxide levels because these values generally correlate well with those measured in arterial blood. However, their usefulness for evaluating arterial oxygenation is not as reliable. If proper technique is employed, good correlation may be present when arterial oxygen tension is 40–70 mm Hg. Simultaneously obtained capillary blood Pao_2 is usually 5–15 mm Hg less than arterial Pao_2 because of some venous admixture. However, when Pao_2 is greater than 70 mm Hg, capillary samples often do not reflect the higher value.

Proper collection of a capillary blood sample from the infant's heel requires warming to cause vasodilatation and local hyperemia. The heel should then be wiped with an antiseptic and punctured anterolaterally. The medial aspect of the heel must be avoided because of the proximate location of the posterior tibial artery and the potential for excessive bleeding. The site should be wiped with dry gauze and the blood allowed to flow freely into the heparinized capillary tube. Exposing the blood to air or allowing air bubbles to form within the tube affects the results. If the heel is squeezed at all, causing venous admixture, results are not accurate. Complications include blood loss, lacerations, and chronic scarring. Aseptic technique should be used as superficial infections sometimes lead to osteomyelitis of the heel and foot.[71] Repeated punctures of the same site should be avoided.

Capillary blood gases should not be used during the first 24 hours of life or any time when peripheral circulation is poor. If the infant has arterial hypotension or badly bruised heels, the results may be inaccurate. In any event, the validity of capillary samples is directly related to the appropriateness of the technique used. Strict quality control in obtaining capillary samples must be maintained in order to provide meaningful results.

Technical Problems. Because blood gas results are used to modify respiratory support, several technical problems need special attention. Modern blood gas analyzers are very accurate provided qualified technicians are operating the equipment. Most errors result from poor technique in collection of the samples. Samples should be capped and stored in ice when the blood is not analyzed immediately. Such technical considerations apply to adult samples and analysis as well.

The effect of heparin dilution has specific impact on neonatal blood sampling as 0.3 ml or less is often used. Small amounts of blood should be withdrawn to minimize the hemodynamic impact of repeated sampling, and the blood should be replaced. Several authors have shown that the amount of heparin left in the dead space of a syringe and needle is sufficient to alter the Pa_{CO_2} of a small blood sample 15–17 percent. Heparin dilution does not affect the pH but does decrease the Pa_{CO_2} and alter the calculated bicarbonate and base excess or deficit calculations in direct proportion to the amount of dilution.[15,32,48,52] Inappropriate thera-

Table 7-2. Advantages of Continuous Monitoring

Prevents acute hypoxia, hyperoxia, hypocapnea, or hypercapnea

Allows faster weaning from oxygen and ventilator

Allows determination of optimal ventilator assistance

Reduces blood sampling, avoids trauma and transfusion

peutic interventions with ventilatory support and alkali administration may result from these inaccuracies. This excess heparin must be removed from the barrel and dead space of the syringe.

Continuous Monitoring Techniques. Continuous transcutaneous (Tc) monitoring of oxygen and carbon dioxide tensions is now available. Indwelling catheters which continuously monitor arterial oxygen saturation by fiberoptic techniques and arterial oxygen tension by polarographic electrodes are also available. Continuous monitoring has provided increased knowledge of the neonate's cardiorespiratory function which intermittent sampling was unable to supply. The variability of transcutaneous oxygen tracing has shown the unreliability of a single Pa_{O_2} measurement. These monitoring devices have been especially helpful in determining the effect of routine procedures on the neonate's oxygenation and have demonstrated that conventional intermittent sampling identifies, on the average, only 5 percent of the total time that infants are hypoxic or hyperoxic. Continuous monitoring also reveals that 75 percent of hypoxia ($TcP_{O_2} < 40$ mm Hg) and hyperoxia ($TcP_{O_2} > 100$ mm Hg) result from interventions by nursing personnel and can be reduced by modifying intensive care unit (ICU) procedures.[72] The advantages of such monitoring are summarized in Table 7-2.

The transcutaneous oxygen sensor is composed of two basic parts: (1) a miniaturized Clark-type polarographic electrode consisting of a low oxygen consumption platinum cathode, silver anode, electrolyte, and an oxygen-permeable membrane; and

(2) a heating section and a precision thermistor for measuring and controlling the oxygen sensor temperature.

The sensor heats the skin surface directly under it to 43–44°C, causing local vasodilation of cutaneous vessels and hyperemia. Oxygen diffuses through the skin and the membrane and initiates current flow between the cathode and anode. An amplifier measures the amount of current flow and converts it into a value proportional to the oxygen tension at the electrode-membrane interface. This information is then displayed on a digital meter or strip chart recorder. Pao_2 and $TcPo_2$ are not identical, but correlation is good and of definite clinical significance.[60,85,103] The equipment is noninvasive, safe, and easy to use.

Transcutaneous oxygen measurements have been shown to be lower than arterial oxygen tensions during infusions of tolazoline (vascular vasodilator) and when the mean arterial blood pressure is more than 2.5 standard deviations below predicted normal values.[85] In shock states when perfusion is poor, transcutaneous monitoring may not provide an accurate indication of arterial oxygenation.

Although the transcutaneous monitor may not be helpful in assessing the severely asphyxiated, peripherally vasoconstricted infant in shock, an indwelling fiberoptic catheter which continuously monitors oxygen saturation or a catheter which incorporates a polarographic electrode for continuous arterial oxygen tension monitoring may be very useful. Each has shown good correlation with conventional blood gas measurements, and neither is affected by hypotension.[27,87,106] The fiberoptic catheter utilizes reflected light to illuminate blood inside the vascular space. Light is reflected back to a photodetector in the optical module, converted to an electrical signal, transmitted to the processor, and displayed as a saturation measurement. The umbilical catheter polarographic electrode measures oxygen tensions directly and displays this

information as a digital reading. The electrode functions similarly to the Clark transcutaneous electrode. Both of these catheter methods have the same disadvantages of a conventional indwelling umbilical catheter but do not seem to increase the risks of such monitoring.

The transcutaneous carbon dioxide electrode is a more recent development. The sensor utilizes a pH electrode based on the Stow-Severinghaus principle and is composed of two parts: (1) a carbon dioxide electrode consisting of a pH electrode, a reference electrode, and an electrolyte- and carbon dioxide-permeable membrane; and (2) a heating section and thermistor. The sensor heats the skin, causing vasodilatation and hyperemia. Carbon dioxide which has diffused through the skin passes through the permeable membrane and reacts with the electrolyte. The pH of the electrolyte solution is altered, changing the voltage across the pH and reference electrodes. An amplifier measures the voltage and converts it into a value corresponding to the carbon dioxide tension. Several authors have reported clinical usefulness of this method.[12,53,76] $TcPco_2$ values are higher than $Paco_2$ values because: (1) the sensor measures skin Pco_2, which must be greater than $Paco_2$; (2) the heated sensor increases local cellular metabolism, which increases the production of carbon dioxide; and (3) excess carbon dioxide is not consumed so it may accumulate in the sensor. The transcutaneous carbon dioxide value must be divided by a correction factor (anaerobic temperature coefficient) in order to estimate the arterial value. Hypoxia and acidosis, which affect peripheral circulation and tissue metabolism, may decrease the correlation between $Paco_2$ and $TcPco_2$.[12] However, the correlation seems to remain good, even with severe hypotension, until the systolic blood pressure falls below 15–20 mm Hg.[18,53] Transcutaneous carbon dioxide monitoring may prove to be very helpful in managing neonates who are mechanically ventilated. Because of the small size of the neonate, optimal future sensors should have the capability to monitor both oxygen and carbon dioxide tensions and pH with one sensor.

Clinical Guidelines. Any infant in the acute phase of respiratory failure requires frequent measurements of blood gases and pH or continuous monitoring. Arterial blood gases should be determined as soon as possible after initiation of respiratory support. Subsequent measurements should be obtained within 15–30 minutes after any change in respiratory support. More frequent samplings at shorter intervals are often indicated. Transcutaneous monitoring or continuous monitoring by indwelling catheter may be used instead of intermittent arterial blood gas measurements when available. Repeated sampling should be done at least every 4–6 hours even when no changes in respiratory support have been made.

An infant in the chronic phase of his respiratory disorder requires less frequent blood gas sampling. Blood gases or transcutaneous monitoring should be obtained at least every 24 hours in infants less than 1500 g who are receiving oxygen therapy. Chronically oxygen-dependent infants weighing more than 1500 g should have blood gas sampling or transcutaneous monitoring done at least every 3 days. When these larger infants have required oxygen for a month or more, even less frequent sampling may be acceptable. However, any change in respiratory support during the chronic phase still requires blood sampling or transcutaneous monitoring within 15–30 minutes.

Oxygen Therapy

Basic Principles. Most neonates with cardiopulmonary problems present with hypoxemia requiring oxygen therapy. The goal of such therapy is to minimize the ef-

Table 7-3. Basic Principles of Oxygen Therapy

Maintain Pao_2 at 50–70 mm Hg

Control FIo_2

Monitor airway FIo_2 at least every 2 hours

Warm and humidify gas

Allow sufficient gas flow to avoid rebreathing

Practice strict infection control

fects of continued hypoxemia and tissue hypoxia, which may produce diffuse metabolic and functional changes. It must be carefully administered in order to prevent the damaging effects of hyperoxia on various organ systems. Hence rational oxygen therapy must be based on the monitoring of arterial oxygen tensions, whether by blood gas analysis or transcutaneous or indwelling methods. Clinical observation is not sufficient because peripheral cyanosis may be present despite normal or above-normal arterial oxygen tensions, and hypoxemia may not be accompanied by cyanosis in cases of severe anemia.

Oxygen most commonly is administered to the neonate through a plastic oxygen hood, although it may be provided directly to an incubator, face mask, T-tube, or nasal catheter. The basic principles of oxygen therapy which apply to all methods are outlined in Table 7-3. An arterial oxygen tension of 50–70 mm Hg should provide adequate tissue oxygenation while avoiding the problems of hyperoxygenation.

Methods and Equipment. Oxygen may be delivered directly to the incubator through an oxygen inlet. Establishing precise and consistent concentrations is difficult as opening of the port holes during routine nursing care causes frequent fluctuations.

Plastic oxygen hoods provide a more efficient method for precise oxygen administration. A ''bubble'' encloses the infant's head with a neck opening to vent excess gas flow and exhaled gas; it has additional ports as well for the gas inlet, thermometer, and intravenous tubing. The concentration of oxygen actually delivered to the hood may have to be slightly higher than that desired because of dilution by ambient gas through the neck opening and access ports. Precise oxygen concentration can be delivered most accurately with a high-pressure oxygen/air blender which provides accurate oxygen concentration from 21 to 100 percent irrespective of external factors. If a nebulizer which incorporates a venturi device is used to provide specific concentrations, care must be taken to avoid changes in resistance and back-pressure within the tubing (e.g., occurs when water condensate is allowed to accumulate. Increasing the back-pressure causes an increase in F_{IO_2} because less air is entrained by the venturi device.

An accurate oxygen analyzer, which is calibrated a minimum of once a day to both low and high gas mixtures, must be used at least every 2 hours and whenever changes are made. Accurate analysis is important for correct interpretation of arterial blood gases and assessment of the infant's clinical status. Continuous anlyzers which sound an alarm at preset low and high limits are desirable but the humidity within the hood may shorten the life of the electrode and reduce its accuracy. Gas should be analyzed as close to the baby's airway as possible because the F_{IO_2} may vary from one location to another within the hood (the density of oxygen is higher than that of nitrogen). In addition, when all measurements are performed at the same location, variability from one analysis to the next is decreased. Reporting of oxygen levels in terms of liters per minute flow delivery is not sufficient as concentrations may vary, making clinical status difficult to evaluate.

All gas delivered to the hood must be warmed and humidified. Neonates, especially when premature, are very sensitive to heat and water loss. Temperature of the delivered gas becomes more critical at lower weights and gestational ages. If the gas is not warmed, oxygen consumption is increased and apnea may ensue. If the gas is too warm, apnea and hyperthermia may occur. Hood temperature should be kept at approximately the same temperature as the neutral thermal environment of the incubator and should be monitored as frequently as the oxygen concentration. In the very small premature, a servo-controlled, heated humidifier may be needed to more precisely control the temperature of the delivered gas. Humidification is necessary to prevent inspissation of secretions and to assist in their removal, to maintain an adequate moisture content of the mucous membranes, and to minimize the insensible water loss which occurs during normal breathing through evaporation from the mucosal surface. Infants who are tachypneic are at increased risk for such water loss.

Gas flows must be sufficient to flush exhaled carbon dioxide from the hood. Carbon dioxide levels above 1 percent have been measured in the hood when gas flows were inadequate.[40] An increase of this magnitude may be detrimental to a tachypneic infant. Adequate flushing of the hood to avoid carbon dioxide rebreathing occurs with gas flows of 3–7 L/minute.

Because any water reservoir is a potential source of bacterial contamination, sterile water should be used in the humidifier or nebulizer, and equipment used for oxygen therapy should be changed at a minimum of every 24 hours. The risk of pulmonary infection is always present in systems colonized with gram-negative bacteria. In addition, when venturi systems are used for nebulization and room air is entrained, airborne organisms become potential sources of contamination.

Face masks also may be used to provide therapy, but most infants do not tolerate the masks and dislodge them. Masks are best used for emergencies, transport, and stabilization, or during procedures when the infant must be removed from the hood. Hence they may be useful while the baby is being weighed, x-rayed, or having a lumbar puncture performed. At such times, even brief periods of hypoxia may cause an immediate change in the infant's clinical status or have long-term neurological effects. Venturi adaptors which provide precise concentrations may be used with masks for brief periods. Oxygen may also be delivered by a hood or a T-piece adaptor to an endotracheal tube. The oxygen tubing should be carefully positioned to prevent accidental extubation.

Nasal catheters are not employed routinely but seem to be acceptable for chronically oxygen-dependent infants.[50] Mobility is thereby improved as the infant no longer must be confined in a hood or mist tent, and the development of normal mental and motor skills is encouraged. Nasal catheters with oxygen flow rates of 0.25–0.75 L/minute provide concentrations less than 30 percent. Unfortunately, some infants may not tolerate the catheter because of excessive nasal discharge, inflammation of the nasal mucosa, and catheter dislodgement.

Complications. Oxygen is an important drug in the treatment of the neonatal patient, but, as is true with most other drugs, deleterious side effects may occur. Pulmonary oxygen toxicity, eye damage (retrolental fibroplasia; RLF), infection, and hearing impairment have been described.

Infants weighing less than 1500 g are at greatest risk for developing RLF. The incidence of RLF is inversely proportional to birth weight and/or gestational age and seems to be directly related to the duration of oxygen therapy. No effective treatment exists for this condition which, in its most severe form, leads to blindness. Because high Pao_2 has been shown to cause retinal artery vasoconstriction in the neonate, the hypothesis has been advanced that arterial oxygen tensions greater than 90–100 mm Hg may predispose the susceptible premature to eye damage.[2] However, a national collaborative study did not show a direct correlation between arterial oxygen tension and RLF.[63] Continuous oxygen monitoring

may help to reduce the incidence of RLF yet ensure oxygenation sufficient to prevent neurological damage. Further research is necessary to pinpoint the specific factors which predispose to the development of RLF. In the interim, efforts should be made to maintain arterial oxygenation within the physiologically adequate 50–70 mm Hg range.

Pulmonary oxygen toxicity is related to the inspired oxygen concentration and the length of therapy. Lung tissue changes, including interstitial edema, fibrosis, and metaplasia of the bronchial epithelium, have been associated with administration of high oxygen concentrations for more than 2–3 days.[89] High oxygen concentrations may also be a contributing factor to the development of bronchopulmonary dysplasia (BPD) in infants who have been mechanically ventilated. High Fio_2 also increases the tendency for alveolar collapse due to the rapid reabsorption of alveolar oxygen in areas of the lung which are poorly ventilated. Oxygen decreases the ciliary movement of airway epithelial cells, preventing mucous and bacterial clearance. In newborn animals, high concentrations of oxygen interfere with cell multiplication and lung growth.[20,80,94]

The risk of infection has already been described but must be emphasized again because the defense mechanisms of neonates receiving oxygen usually are already compromised. Strict infection control policies must be established and followed to prevent acquired nosocomial infections.

One final complication must be mentioned. Measured incubator noise levels frequently exceed recommended upper limits for adults. Oxygen delivery systems are potential sources for excessive noise because of high gas flow rates and the reverberation of water condensation within the oxygen or ventilator tubing.[13] Because no one is certain what levels may be damaging to the infant ear, more investigation is needed so that guidelines may be established.

Continuous Distending Airway Pressure

Continuous distending airway passure, another method of respiratory support, is used primarily in infants with HMD. Approximately one-third of all infants with HMD improve after a few days of oxygen therapy without requiring more aggressive types of respiratory assistance. Another one-third includes infants with more severe forms of the disease who require continuous distending airway pressure (CDAP); the remainder are very small prematures or infants with severe respiratory failure who require IPPV to maintain their ventilation and oxygenation.

Basic Principles. The volume of air remaining in the lungs at the end of each expiration is determined primarily by the balance of two forces acting in opposite directions. Retractive forces, which tend to promote lung collapse, result from the elastic tissue and surface tension of the alveoli. Opposing collapse, and thereby tending to increase lung volume, is the outward directed elasticity of the chest wall. In prematures with HMD, increased surface tension tends to collapse the alveoli. Compliance of the chest wall is very high and therefore cannot counterbalance the high collapsing forces of the lungs.[42] The result is a decrease in lung volume and a tendency for alveolar closure at the end of each expiration, resulting in increased pulmonary shunt and hypoxemia. When CDAP is applied, increased transpulmonary pressure at the end of each expiration tends to produce lung distention and avoid alveolar closure. Such pressure can be generated either by applying CPAP or by using continuous "negative" pressure (CNP) around the chest. The result with either technique is an increased FRC and a reduction of the pulmonary shunt resulting in a rapid improvement of the arterial Po_2.[6]

We have also observed in some patients with small airway obstruction (meconium pneumonitis, PDA, or BPD) that CDAP can distend the small airways, decrease airway resistance, and improve minute ventilation.[44]

Indications. Prime indications for CDAP are conditions associated with decreased $\dot{V}a/\dot{Q}$ or pulmonary shunt related to alveolar collapse. The best results are obtained in infants with HMD when CDAP is used early in the course of the disease. If CDAP is used before the oxygen requirement is above an Fio_2 of 0.7, to maintain a Pao_2 of at least 50 mm Hg, patients require less exposure to high oxygen concentrations and require IPPV less frequently.[41,75] CDAP should not be delayed until an infant with HMD is in severe respiratory failure. In very small premature infants, the results with CDAP are less favorable, and most infants with birth weights under 1200 g who have moderate or severe HMD develop hypoventilation and require IPPV. In such cases, it may be advisable to initiate IPPV without trying CDAP if severe respiratory failure develops.

Because application of CDAP may decrease lung compliance and increase the work of breathing,[6] it should be used with caution in infants with CO_2 retention unless the latter is related to small airway obstruction. In these cases, the use of a low CDAP (2–4 cm H_2O) may improve minute ventilation, reduce $Paco_2$, and increase Pao_2. In infants with PDA and increased pulmonary blood flow, CDAP may exert a beneficial effect by increasing pulmonary vascular resistance and decreasing pulmonary blood flow and left ventricular overload.

CDAP has also been used in infants with apnea of prematurity.[62] Here, CDAP decreases the incidence of apnea presumably by modifying pulmonary and chest wall reflex activity. Because these infants have normal lung compliance, low pressures (below 4 cm H_2O) should be used to avoid adverse side effects. One of the limitations of this treatment in infants with apnea is that oral feedings must be interrupted because nasal CDAP produces gastric distention. It is also difficult to keep the nasal tubes (prongs) in place for long periods in infants who are active.

Methods. The first system to apply CDAP in the newborn was described by Gregory et al.[49] It consists of a continuous gas flow system ending in an anesthesia bag and connected to a pressure manometer and an underwater pressure relief valve. The apparatus is connected to the patient's endotracheal or nasal tube and the pressure adjusted by changing the resistance at the outlet of the bag or by changing the gas flow. This system is effective, simple to assemble, and economical. Because of the many component parts required, it may be easier to use commercial products which, although more expensive, are more compact and practical. Most neonatal ventilators also have a mode to provide CPAP.

To avoid the need for the endotracheal tube, a plastic box was developed to deliver pressure over the entire head. This system requires a tight seal around the neck that can increase venous and CNS pressure. It also makes access to the airway for suctioning difficult and may expose the infant to high noise levels. A variation of this method is a chamber which fits over the face, but this has proved to be impractical and is seldom used. CDAP has also been applied by using a tight face mask; however, this method requires continuous attention to avoid aspiration of gastric contents or excessive leaks. Facial and even CNS damage can occur because of excessive pressure from head straps used to secure the mask.

The most common method used today to apply CDAP in infants with effective spontaneous ventilation is the nasal route. Because the newborn breathes preferentially through the nose, one can connect any of the systems to the nasal orifice using a small nasal prong or a shortened endotracheal tube passed into the nasopharynx. This method is safe and simple but has the disadvantage that some pressure loss may occur through the mouth. Also, when the infant cries and inspires through his mouth, he decreases the FIO_2. This problem can be solved by placing an oxygen hood over the patient's head so that the ambient FIO_2 can be adjusted to match that delivered by the nasal route.

Transpulmonary pressure can be increased by applying positive pressure to the airway or by decreasing the pressure around the chest wall while the airway remains exposed to atmospheric pressure. The effect in terms of increasing FRC and reducing pulmonary shunt is similar with positive airway pressure or "negative" pressure around the chest.[6] Negative pressure is advantageous as the apparatus does not require attachment to the airway and/or tracheal intubation. Deleterious effects on systemic and pulmonary circulation are minimal if the negative pressure is applied only over the chest. Problems associated with this method include high equipment costs, poor access to the patient, and difficulties with temperature control due to leaks through the seals of the negative-pressure chamber. In spite of these difficulties, when nursing personnel are familiar with the system continuous negative pressure is an effective and simple mode of treatment for infants that weigh more than 1200 g.

One of the difficulties when CDAP is used is to determine the level of pressure necessary to obtain optimal results with minimum side effects and complications. Pressure requirements vary from one patient to another and may change in the same patient as the disease evolves. When CDAP is applied, continuous monitoring of the appropriateness of clinical response is mandatory. The pressure requirement usually varies between 2 and 8 cm H_2O. In particularly severe cases, higher pressure is required to stabilize air spaces and the problem of deleterious side effects is reduced because of decreased pressure transmission beyond the lungs. The simplest method for determining the proper amount of CDAP is to increase the pressure in 2 cm H_2O increments with measurement of arterial blood or transcutaneous gases after each change until the best results are obtained. Persistence of sternal retraction and grunting respiration usually indicates the need for higher pressure. On the other hand, a fall in Pao_2, an increase in $Paco_2$, or active expiration evidenced by contraction of the abdominal muscles are findings that suggest excessive CDAP. The chest radiograph may also be helpful in this regard, showing pulmonary overdistention with depressed diaphragms. Excessive pressure may also reduce cardiac output, resulting in poor peripheral perfusion, arterial hypotension, and metabolic acidosis.

The suggestion has been advanced that pressure transmission from the airway to the esophagus can be used to determine the best level of CDAP. These measurements are difficult to evaluate because esophageal pressure is influenced by active expiratory efforts made by the infant as CDAP is increased.

Another method used in adults to determine the best CDAP is serial measurement of lung compliance at different pressure levels. In the newborn, this determination is not possible because compliance decreases with a progressive increase in CDAP in most infants with HMD.[6]

Weaning from CDAP is accomplished by a gradual decrease of pressure over a period of hours to days. Arterial or transcutaneous blood gas values must be followed closely after each change in pressure because in some patients a rapid decrease in CDAP may result in sudden deterioration of respiratory function. Decreases in pressure should be alternated with decreases in Fio_2 so that excessive pressure is avoided in infants in whom lung function is improving. A simple way of preventing this problem is to use pressures that are one-tenth or less the percent of inspired oxygen. For example, an infant requiring 40 percent oxygen

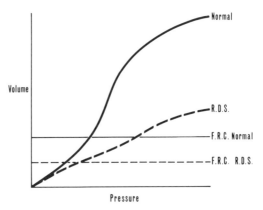

Fig. 7-2. Pressure-volume curves from normal and respiratory distress syndrome (RDS) lungs. Note the difference in FRC and the decrease in slope as volume increases and the lungs become "stiffer."

should not receive CDAP higher than 4 cm H_2O. When an infant tolerates a CDAP of 2–3 cm H_2O while breathing 40 percent oxygen or less, the endotracheal or nasal tube should be removed. The endotracheal tube should not be left in place without CDAP because a loss of lung volume and decrease in Pao_2 frequently result.[37]

Complications. Several problems related to the specific method of application of CDAP were mentioned earlier. Increased transpulmonary pressure can also have serious adverse effects when used in cases where it is not indicated or when the amount of pressure applied is excessive in relation to the degree of lung compromise, independently of the system used. These side effects are manifested mainly by changes in the mechanics of breathing and cardiovascular function.

Mechanics of Breathing. CDAP stabilizes alveoli that tend to collapse but may simultaneously overdistend those with better compliance. This overdistention produces a shift of these units to the flatter portion of their pressure-volume curve, reducing their distensibility[6] (Fig. 7-2). An increased risk of alveolar rupture and pneumothorax and an increased work of breathing results. Subsequent fatigue frequently leads to hypoventilation and CO_2 retention; therefore hypercapnia is one sign that may indicate the use of excessive end-expiratory pressure.

In some infants with airway obstruction and increased resistance, CDAP increases lung volume and airway diameter and reduces airway resistance[25,44] (Fig. 7-3). Because these patients may have normal lung compliance compared to those with HMD, one must avoid high pressures to minimize pulmonary overdistention and cardiovascular side effects.

Cardiovascular Effects. Pressure applied to the airways is partially transmitted to the pleural space and cardiovascular structures within the chest. The amount so transmitted is directly proportional to the compliance of the lungs and inversely related to the compliance of the chest wall. This relationship suggests that transmission

is lower in sicker infants in whom lung compliance is very low and higher in infants with relatively normal lungs[42] (Fig. 7-4). It is also less in premature infants who have a very high chest wall compliance (Fig. 7-5). Hemodynamic consequences include interference with venous return to the right heart and reduction of cardiac output, increased pulmonary vascular resistance, and decreased pulmonary blood flow. Increased pulmonary artery pressure can exacerbate arterial hypoxemia by increasing an already existing right-to-left shunt through the foramen ovale or ductus arteriosus.[79] A falling Pao_2 therefore is another indication that CDAP may be excessive and that transpulmonary pressure should be reduced.

Results. CDAP improves oxygenation in infants with HMD, reducing the requirement for oxygen therapy. Evidence for the influence of CDAP on the course of the disease and mortality is less certain.

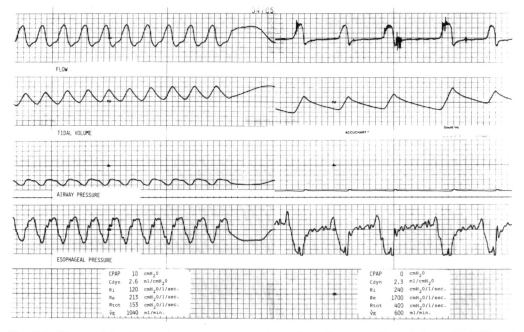

Fig. 7-3. Flow, tidal volume, airway pressure, and esophageal pressure in an infant with BPD and airway obstruction. Left portion obtained with CPAP of 10 cm H_2O, right with zero CPAP. At zero CPAP the pulmonary resistance increased, resulting in prolongation of expiration, increased esophageal pressure fluctuations with each breath, and a decrease in minute ventilation.

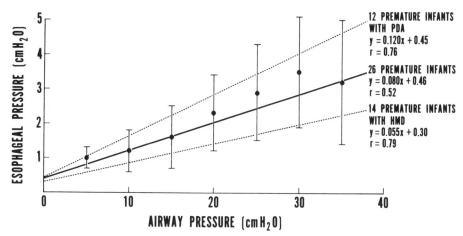

Fig. 7-4. Airway pressure transmission to the esophagus during IPPV in 26 preterm infants (heavy line). The upper dotted line reflects pressure transmission in infants with a PDA, and the lower dotted line represents transmission in infants with HMD. Transmission is lower in infants with HMD because of their lower lung compliance. (Reprinted with permission from: Gerhardt T, Bancalari E: Chest wall compliance in full-term and premature infants. Acta Paediatr Scand 69:359, 1980.)

A few controlled studies with small numbers of patients suggest that CDAP reduces the severity of HMD and shortens the course of the disease. They also suggest that CDAP reduces the number of infants who require IPPV and therefore reduces the complications associated with this mode of therapy.[41,75] Overall results obviously depend on the type of patients treated. When CDAP is used in infants with birth weights over 1200 g early in the course of the disease, results are excellent, with a survival close to 100 percent and no need for IPPV. Results are less satisfactory in infants below 1200 g or those in whom CDAP is delayed to a point until they require 70 percent or more oxygen. Most of these patients deteriorate until they require IPPV. Thus CDAP should be initiated before the infants are in critical condition or require a very high F_{IO_2}.

Most clinicians prefer to use IPPV in prematures under 1200 g without attempting the use of CDAP because of the infants' increased tendency to develop respiratory acidosis. Chronic pulmonary damage, e.g.,

BPD, is extremely uncommon in infants treated with CDAP alone. Although this fact may be used as evidence favoring the safety of this procedure, the observation may simply be related to the fact that infants with more severe HMD usually require IPPV.

Intermittent Postive-Pressure Ventilation

Mechanical ventilation has been widely used in the treatment of respiratory failure of the newborn for more than 20 years. Initially, the machines and methods were similar to those used in adults, and complications and mortality were very high. As a result, ventilator therapy often was restricted to patients in whom the mortality was near 100 percent without IPPV. In the last 10 years techniques for IPPV have improved considerably and the indications for ventilator support have been liberalized. Today, more than 50 percent of infants ad-

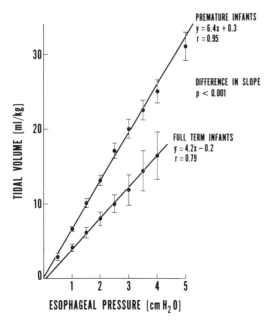

PREMATURE INFANTS
$y = 6.4x + 0.3$
$r = 0.95$

DIFFERENCE IN SLOPE
$p < 0.001$

FULL TERM INFANTS
$y = 4.2x - 0.2$
$r = 0.79$

Fig. 7-5. Esophageal pressure change during IPPV with different tidal volumes in premature and full-term infants. With the same tidal volume the pressure change is larger in full-term infants because of their decreased chest wall compliance. (Reprinted with permission from: Gerhardt T, Bancalari E: Chest wall compliance in full-term and premature infants. Acta Paediatr Scand 69:359, 1980.)

mitted to neonatal ICUs receive some type of mechanical respiratory assistance.

The basic rationale for IPPV is to replace the patient's inspiratory muscle activity with a system that generates a tidal volume by intermittent delivery of pressurized gas to the airway (Fig. 7-6). Exhalation, in most cases, occurs passively as the airway pressure drops to the expiratory level and the combined elastic recoil of the lungs and chest wall decreases the thoracic gas volume to FRC. The primary goal of mechanical ventilation is to maintain adequate minute ventilation and Pa_{CO_2}. In pathological conditions such as HMD, in which air space collapse is a prominent feature, a combination of IPPV and positive end-expiratory pressure (PEEP) favors opening of the air space and prevention of further collapse of unstable units. A significant reduction in

pulmonary shunt and increase in arterial Po_2 often results. IPPV also reduces or abolishes the work of breathing and decreases oxygen consumption of the respiratory muscles.

Indications. Mechanical ventilation is indicated in cases of severe acute respiratory failure not responding to other modes of treatment including oxygen therapy, respiratory stimulation, or CDAP. Two specific indications for IPPV may be considered. The first is hypoventilation and hypercapnia due to CNS depression caused by asphyxia, drugs, hemorrhage, or infection, to apnea of prematurity, or to increased work of breathing. The latter may be associated with airway obstruction and/or decreased lung compliance. The second indication is severe hypoxemia caused by pulmonary shunting.

Frequently more than one abnormality indicates the need for IPPV in the newborn. For example, a small preterm infant may initially require ventilation at birth because of respiratory depression due to asphyxia but may later develop progressive pulmonary failure due to HMD or pneumonia. Then, while improving from his pulmonary disease, a large left-to-right shunt through a PDA may become evident, producing additional deterioration in pulmonary function. Subsequently, the same infant may require prolonged ventilation because of chronic lung disease or central depression due to brain hemorrhage. This sequence of events is very common in infants less than 28–30 weeks' gestation.

In many cases the decision as to the most appropriate time to initiate IPPV is difficult. The criteria used most commonly are based on certain minimum values of arterial blood gases. Such indications are useful, especially in emergency situations or when personnel with limited experience in neonatal respiratory care have to make the decision. Nevertheless, this approach has important limitations. When IPPV is considered, clinicians must weigh the benefits that this mode of treatment offers to a particular in-

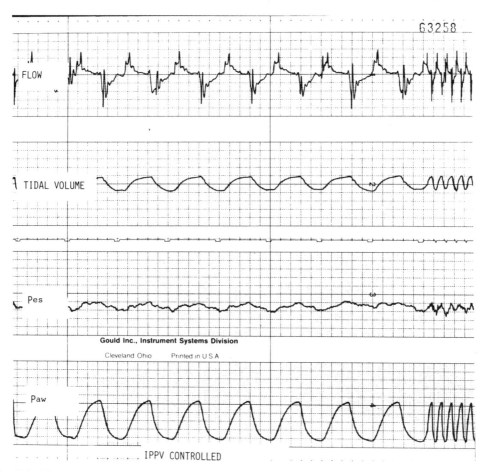

Fig. 7-6. Flow, tidal volume, and esophageal and airway pressures in an infant receiving controlled IPPV. Each ventilator cycle produces an increase in airway pressure that results in a tidal volume of approximately 9 ml. The change in airway pressure is partially transmitted to the esophagus.

fant against the possible complications. The incidence of these complications varies in different units depending on experience, staffing patterns, available equipment, and type of patient ventilated. Standard criteria to initiate IPPV are difficult to establish. Instead, criteria must be developed in each unit based on its results and experience. As specific unit care becomes more sophisticated, the incidence of certain complications decreases, and the indications for IPPV may be liberalized. On the other hand, IPPV should be used only as a last resort in units with limited experience.

Because each patient presents specific clinical problems, an experienced clinician often makes individual treatment decisions based on factors other than simple evaluation of blood gas values alone. Hence the latter should be used only as general guidelines and must be applied with flexibility in each unit and for each patient. They include:

1. Requirement of F_{IO_2} greater than 0.7 to maintain Pa_{O_2} above 50 mm Hg. If the infant has HMD and weighs more than 1200 g, this indication applies only after CDAP has failed.
2. Pa_{CO_2} above 60 mm Hg with a pH below 7.2 in two consecutive blood gas determinations.

3. Respiratory arrest not reversed by ventilation with a mask and high oxygen concentrations.

In perinatal centers with a large high-risk population, many infants require ventilation from the first minute of life because of perinatal asphyxia and central depression; one often does not have the chance to measure arterial blood gases before tracheal intubation and therapy are implemented.

Indications for IPPV are important in determining the eventual outcome of each patient. The morbidity and mortality of infants treated with IPPV in a given unit are closely related to the categories of patients who are ventilated. In order to compare figures from different centers, the indications for IPPV must be clearly defined.

Characteristics of the "Ideal" Neonatal Ventilator. The ideal neonatal ventilator must be capable of safely ventilating infants with varying degrees of abnormal lung compliance, airway resistance, dead space, and ventilation/perfusion abnormalities. It should be simple, easy to operate, and reliable. Because no agreement has been reached concerning the optimal techniques of neonatal ventilation, the perfect ventilator has not yet been designed. Respiratory care practitioners must weigh the relative advantages and disadvantages of each machine for operation within a particular clinical setting. Important characteristics to consider are listed in Table 7-4. Several points need to be emphasized.

Safety features must be incorporated into any ventilator. Because barotrauma is a potential complication of positive-pressure ventilation, all neonatal ventilators must include both pressure- and inspiratory-time-limiting devices. If alarms are not included as an integral part of the ventilator, a separate alarm system must be used. It should incorporate a low-pressure component to indicate patient disconnection or a circuit leak. As neonatal tidal volumes are small, any leaks must be identified to maintain adequate ventilation.

Table 7-4. Desired Characteristics for Neonatal Ventilators

General characteristics
 Designed specifically for neonatal use
 Reliable and easy to operate
 Simple, inexpensive, and readily accessible calibration and repair
 100% Relative humidity of inspired gas
 Minimal dead space
 Minimal internal compressible and distensible volume; nondistensible ventilator circuit tubing
 Minimal noise
 Low cost

Functional characteristics
 Precisely controlled F_{IO_2}
 Cycling rate 0–200/minute
 Continuous flow system for IMV
 Tidal volumes, 5–100 ml
 CPAP or PEEP, 0–15 cm H_2O (independent of flow, peak inspiratory pressures, or rate)
 Independently adjusted inspiratory and expiratory times (inspiratory time 0.2–1.5 seconds)
 Adjustable inspiratory flow rate 0–20 L/minute
 Manual cycling device
 Adjustable inspiratory time-limiting device
 Adjustable pressure-limiting valve
 Failsafe valve in case of ventilator malfunction

Alarms
 Visual, audible, adjustable, and battery-powered
 High and low pressure for PEEP and peak inspiratory pressure (based on proximal airway pressure)
 High and low rate
 High and low F_{IO_2}
 Prolonged inspiratory time
 Inspired gas temperature
 Electrical or pneumatic power failure

Monitoring capability
 F_{IO_2}
 Inspiratory and expiratory time
 I:E ratio
 Proximal airway pressure
 Duration of positive pressure
 Respiratory rate
 Mean airway pressure

Compressible volume represents the amount of gas not delivered to the patient during inspiration because of compression within the internal components of the ventilator, ventilator circuit, and humidifier. Compliance loss includes that volume of gas which does not reach the patient because of expansion of the tubing. Both are normally expressed in milliliters per centimeter of H_2O. In a volume- or time-cycled ventilator which is not pressure-limited, increases in peak inspiratory pressures are associated with corresponding increases of compressible volume and the volume loss due to the system's compliance. If compressible volume and system compliance are high, further increase in peak inspiratory pressure, necessitated by decreasing patient compliance, may provide a minimal increase in alveolar ventilation.

Compressible volume and compliance losses are kept to a minimum through the use of ventilators specifically designed for neonates with noncompliant circuits for the patient/ventilator interface and by reducing the volume added to the circuit by water traps and airway connectors. In both volume- and time-cycled ventilators, variations in alveolar ventilation are also influenced by the amount of water in the humidifier. Humidifier systems that have a small, constant compressible volume (0.2 ml/cm H_2O) and utilize a continuous feed and float system (Bird 3M humidifier), maintain constant volume levels in the humidifier and minimize the compressible volume. This feature is particularly important in neonatal ventilation because of the small tidal volume.

As previously described, the neonate is especially sensitive to heat and water loss, particularly when intubated and mechanically ventilated. Because the endotracheal tube completely eliminates upper airway humidification and warming, delivered gas must be externally warmed and humidified. Inspired gas temperature must be monitored close to the airway. A temperature gradient exists between the humidifier and patient which varies directly with the length of tubing and inversely with the temperature of the room. Cooling of the delivered gas and water condensation in the tubing occurs unless the ventilator circuit is heated.

In addition to interfering with adequate temperature and humidity control, condensation results in water accumulation in the circuit which may flood the endotracheal

tube, causing excess hydration and fluid overload. The water may also cause pressure fluctuations and a turbulent flow pattern. Water traps should be used to drain excess water and prevent accumulation in the ventilator circuit. Heating elements for the ventilator circuit have been recommended.[78] As much of the circuit as possible should be kept under the radiant warmer or within the incubator to minimize condensation. Future improvements in design will probably incorporate improved methods of maintaining the desired temperature through servo-controlled humidifiers and heating wires within the circuit itself.[3,69]

Some authors have suggested that in the future computers will be incorporated which are programmed to make changes in ventilator settings automatically based on continuous monitoring and laboratory data.[46,88] For example, air/oxygen blenders will be adjusted automatically to vary the F_{IO_2} as necessary to maintain transcutaneous oxygen levels within certain preset limits, and ventilator rates will be adjusted to maintain a given range of Pa_{CO_2}. Experience will be necessary to determine if this type of approach is either feasible or appropriate within the neonatal ICU setting.

Modes of Ventilation. Most neonatal ventilators in use today are time-cycled. They have the advantage of being able to deliver a relatively constant volume with precise control of the maximal inspiratory pressure. The duration of inspiration and expiration, as well as the inspiratory flow rate, are adjusted independently. During the expiratory phase, a continuous flow of gas through the system allows spontaneous ventilation and the use of intermittent mandatory ventilation (IMV) and PEEP. Most time-cycled ventilators are equipped with a gas mixer to adjust the F_{IO_2}, are relatively simple to operate, and are inexpensive when compared with comparable volume-cycled ventilators.

Modern ventilators offer a wide variety of possible settings to optimize gas exchange. The limitations today are not so much in the performance of the machines but in our knowledge of how to use them in the most effective and safe way. Various modes of IPPV have been suggested for the neonate, but little clinical or experimental evidence is available to support many of these recommendations. Several reports are based on retrospective reviews, comparing results with previous experience but not taking into account that many other changes in patient care have occurred simultaneously and may account, at least partially, for the difference in results. For this reason, definitive guidelines concerning techniques to ventilate sick neonates are difficult to establish. Until more information is available, one should select those modes of ventilation which minimize complications related to the use of IPPV.

The following discussion outlines some basic principles and techniques which allow safe operation of a neonatal ventilator. To date, no single type of mechanical ventilation is superior in all infants. Some techniques of IPPV are more effective in certain conditions than in others, and in some patients a given mode may be indicated at one point in the evolution of the disease but may be deleterious at a later stage. For example, a prolonged inspiratory time may improve oxygenation in a patient with severe HMD but cause deterioration of the Pa_{O_2} in an infant with persistent pulmonary hypertension or pneumonia, or even in the same infant with HMD during the recovery phase.

Controlled IPPV. In this mode the patient's respiratory effort is suppressed by slight hyperventilation, sedation, or muscle relaxation. Minute ventilation is entirely dependent on the mechanical ventilator. Advantages of controlled IPPV include elimination of the work of breathing performed by the patient and a potentially decreased risk of pneumothorax, as, if it is used appropriately, spontaneous efforts to breathe are absent and "stacking" of ventilator generated tidal volume on top of spontaneous breaths is eliminated. It also avoids excessive increase in intrathoracic pressure and hypoventilation by eliminating active spontaneous expiratory efforts which may occur during the inspiratory cycle of the ventilator. In this manner, deleterious effects on venous return and the risk of intracranial hemorrhage in very small infants may be reduced.

Some of the disadvantages of controlled IPPV include inactivity of the respiratory muscles and a loss of "fitness," or tone, which may delay the weaning process. If the ventilator malfunctions or is accidentally disconnected, the infant may not resume voluntary respiration until severe hypoxia has occurred. The chance for mechanical hyper- or hypoventilation is increased because the patient's ventilatory effort is lost as an indicator of respiratory drive and Pa_{CO_2}. Finally, the beneficial effect on venous return of the "negative" intrathoracic pressure from spontaneous inspiration is lost.

In many cases the suppression of spontaneous breathing is difficult to achieve by hyperventilation, and sedation or muscle relaxation must be employed. Muscle relaxants in the small preterm infant may effect an increase in Pa_{O_2} but do not seem to reduce the incidence of pneumothorax.[7] Because of the possibility that muscle relaxation may increase the risk of CNS hemorrhage, we do not recommend its use in small prematures.[7] In full-term infants significant side effects of muscle relaxants are less likely, and their use frequently results in improved oxygenation. This relationship is especially true in infants with pulmonary hypertension and right-to-left shunting associated with meconium aspiration in whom a sudden improvement in Pa_{O_2} is frequently observed after muscle relaxation.

Assisted IPPV. Each inspiratory cycle from the machine is triggered by the patient's spontaneous inspiratory effort. This mode is not available in modern neonatal ventilators, having been replaced by IMV.

Intermittent Mandatory Ventilation. This technique requires the work of breathing to be divided between the patient and the ventilator. The infant breathes from a continuous flow of gas which can be delivered at a constant positive pressure, and the ventilator cycles intermittently, providing mandatory tidal breaths at a preset frequency and pressure wave characteristic[64,65] (Fig. 7-7).

The alleged advantages of IMV are many. Because the patient's own breathing is maintained, IMV reduces intrathoracic pressure, thereby partially offsetting the adverse effects on venous return induced by the positive-pressure cycles. It also facili-

tates weaning by gradually reducing the number of breaths supplied by the ventilator and allowing a slow resumption of the infant's level of spontaneous breathing. In the case of ventilator malfunction or disconnection, the patient's own respiratory effort ensures some minute ventilation and gas exchange

Possible disadvantages of IMV are that it increases the work of breathing and oxygen consumption from the respiratory muscles. Some spontaneous respiratory efforts may occur in synchrony with those from the ventilator, increasing transpulmonary pressure and tidal volume with the consequent risks of pneumothorax (Fig. 7-8). Alternatively,

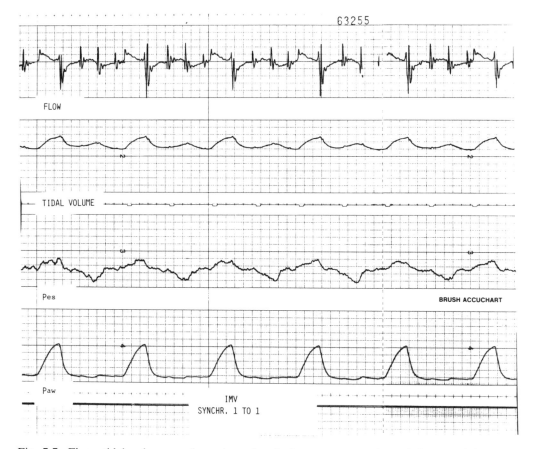

Fig. 7-7. Flow, tidal volume, and esophageal and airway pressures in an infant receiving IMV. After each ventilator cycle, a small tidal volume generated by the infant's spontaneous respiratory effort is reflected by a decrease in esophageal pressure.

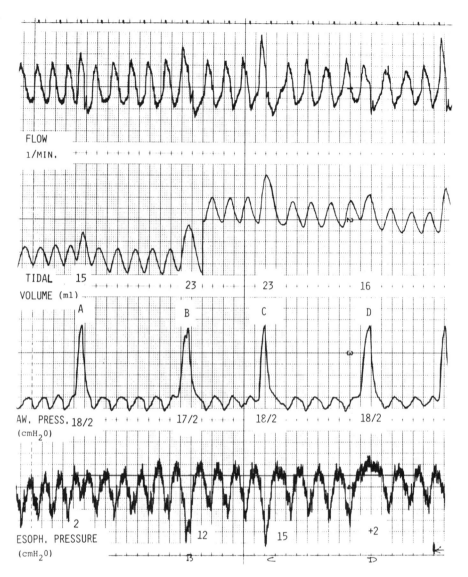

Fig. 7-8. Flow, tidal volume, and airway and esophageal pressures in an infant ventilated with IMV. Note the higher flows and tidal volumes in cycles B and C with summation of the ventilator cycle and the infant's spontaneous breath in comparison to cycles A and D with no spontaneous effort. The infant's inspiratory effort is reflected by the larger "negative" esophageal pressure in cycles B and C.

when the patient's own breath is out of synchrony with the mandatory breath, the active spontaneous expiration may occur during the ventilator's inspiration, increasing both airway and intrathoracic pressure with a consequent deleterious effect on venous return and cardiac output (Fig. 7-9). Finally, if a significant portion of total ventilation is spontaneous and the infant then becomes apneic, he may become hypoxemic and hypercapnic because the low ventilator rate is not sufficient to maintain normal minute ventilation.

Based on these considerations, we recommend the use of controlled ventilation in newborns with severe respiratory failure

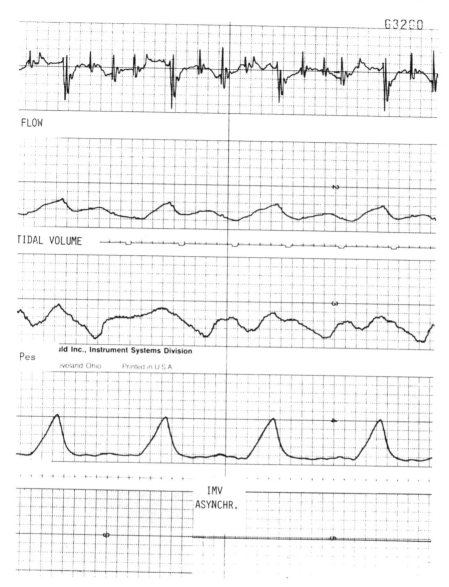

Fig. 7-9. Flow, tidal volume, and esophageal and airway pressures in an infant receiving IMV. The infant's spontaneous respiratory efforts occur in total asynchrony with the ventilator cycles, and most spontaneous inspirations begin before the previous expiration is completed.

who require an F_{IO_2} of more than 0.7. In small prematures, control can be accomplished by slight hyperventilation. This method abolishes spontaneous respiratory effort, reduces oxygen consumption, and maintains more stable Pa_{O_2} and Pa_{CO_2}. In larger infants with severe respiratory failure, sedation with phenobarbital, morphine, or chloral hydrate, or muscle relaxation, may be necessary. As they improve and are able to maintain strong respiratory efforts, the ventilator rate can be reduced gradually, converting the control mode to IMV as the F_{IO_2} requirement decreases from 0.7.

Ventilator Settings. Most neonatal ventilators available today offer a wide flexibility in the settings that can be used. In addition to the usual variables of respiratory rate, airway pressures, and F_{IO_2}, one may also alter the pressure waveform by manipulation of gas flow, inspiratory time, and the pressure-limiting valve.

The following general principles can be used to adjust ventilator settings according to arterial blood gas levels. These principles apply to the majority of patients with pulmonary failure; however, exceptions occur which make it necessary to evaluate each patient's response carefully and individually. Low Pa_{O_2} in most neonates results from a decreased ventilation/perfusion ratio due to alveolar fluid or terminal airway and alveolar collapse. This abnormality usually can be improved by increasing the mean airway pressure by one or more of the following steps: (1) increasing peak inspiratory pressure (PIP); (2) prolonging inspiratory time; (3) increasing positive end-expiratory pressure; and (4) changing the shape of the pressure wave from a "fin" to a "square."

The latter can be accomplished by increasing the inspiratory flow rate (Fig. 7-10). Selection between these four alternatives is not simple, and one must take into consideration the type and stage of the disease-producing respiratory failure.

Peak Inspiratory Pressures. In a time-cycled ventilator, increases in PIP can be achieved by increasing the flow rate or the inspiratory time if the peak pressure is not limited or by increasing the PIP limit if a relief valve is used to control the peak pressure. An increase in PIP increases tidal volume and minute ventilation and may recruit areas of the lung that are collapsed or poorly ventilated. The result in most cases is an increase in Pa_{O_2} and a decrease in Pa_{CO_2}. The increase in Pa_{O_2} is usually more than what can be expected by improved ventilation alone and reflects the reduction in pulmonary shunt.

High pressures increase the risk of alveolar rupture, leading to pulmonary inter-

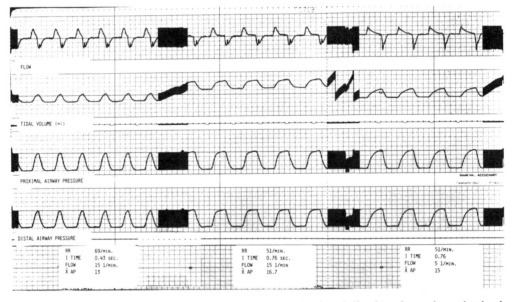

Fig. 7-10. Flow, tidal volume, and airway pressure proximal and distal to the endotracheal tube during IPPV in a neonatal lung model. The four cycles in the center of the figure have a longer inspiratory time than those to the left, resulting in a higher mean airway pressure. The four cycles to the right have a lower inspiratory flow rate, producing a decreased slope of the pressure and tidal volume curves and a slightly lower mean airway pressure.

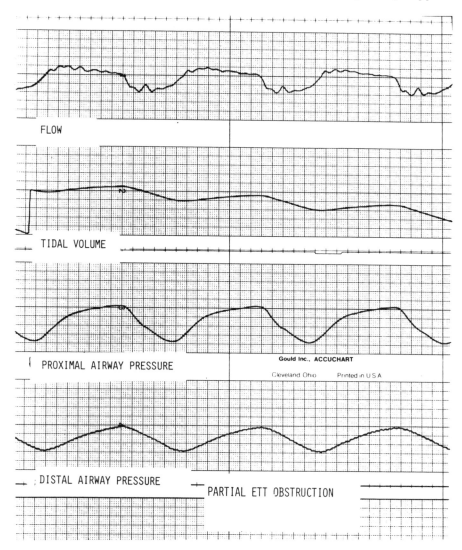

FLOW

TIDAL VOLUME

PROXIMAL AIRWAY PRESSURE

Gould Inc., ACCUCHART

Cleveland Ohio   Printed in U.S.A

DISTAL AIRWAY PRESSURE

PARTIAL ETT OBSTRUCTION

Fig. 7-11. Flow, tidal volume, and airway pressure proximal and distal to a partially obstructed endotracheal tube during IPPV in a neonatal lung model. Note the difference between the two pressure traces, with a dampening of the slope and peak inspiratory and end-expiratory pressures distal to the obstruction.

stitial emphysema (PIE) and pneumothorax, and may also impair pulmonary and systemic circulation. These risks are less in patients with severe disease and low lung compliance; however, high pressures may exacerbate extrapulmonary right-to-left shunting in patients with pulmonary hypertension. The lowest PIP necessary to main-

tain adequate minute ventilation and oxygenation should be used.

As lung compliance improves during the recovery phase of the disease, PIP must be gradually reduced to avoid hyperventilation and other complications related to high airway pressure. A significant pressure drop occurs between the proximal airway, where

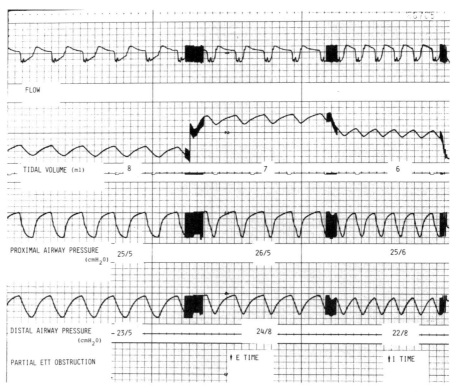

FLOW

TIDAL VOLUME (ml)   8   7   6

PROXIMAL AIRWAY PRESSURE   25/5   26/5   25/6
(cmH₂0)

DISTAL AIRWAY PRESSURE   - 23/5   24/8   22/8
(cmH₂0)

PARTIAL ETT OBSTRUCTION   ↑ E TIME   ↑↑ TIME

Fig. 7-12. Flow, tidal volume, and airway pressures proximal and distal to a partially obstructed endotracheal tube during IPPV in a neonatal lung model. Shortening of expiratory time in the four cycles in the center of the figure results in higher end-expiratory pressure distal to the tube (inadvertent PEEP) and a decrease in tidal volume. A decrease in inspiratory time in the five cycles to the right decreases the peak inspiratory pressure distal to the tube and further reduces the tidal volume.

PIP is measured, and the distal airways. It results from the resistance to flow offered by the endotracheal tube and airways and is more significant in cases of airway obstruction or during ventilation with high flows and/or short inspiratory times (Fig. 7-11).

Inspiratory Time. In most neonatal ventilators inspiratory time (IT) can be adjusted independently from the other parameters. Inspiratory time, or duration of inspiration, is frequently confused with the duration of positive pressure. Expiratory gas flow is associated with a decrease in airway pressure, but the airway pressure remains positive for some time because of flow retardation through the ventilator exhalation valve.

Hence the duration of positive pressure is longer than the duration of inspiration. A longer inspiration (the termination of which is defined by the onset of expiratory flow) may result in a larger tidal volume because PIP increases or because more time permits increased filling of slowly ventilated areas (Fig. 7-12). The longer duration of positive pressure also decreases alveolar collapse and/or increases alveolar recruitment, thereby reducing pulmonary shunt. Because longer inspirations increase tidal volume and allow greater pressure transmission to the distal airways, the risk of barotrauma and cardiovascular effects is probably increased.[5,56] For these reasons, an IT over 0.7 second is usually not advisable. In most cases, improved oxygenation and ventilation result from an IT of 0.3–0.5 second.

Positive End-Expiratory Pressure. The stated goal of PEEP therapy is to increase lung volume and avoid alveolar collapse during expiration. It is indicated in conditions such as HMD which are characterized by decreased alveolar stability. PEEP, like CDAP, can decrease flow resistance in patients with small airway obstruction.

Side effects are related mainly to the reduction of pulmonary blood flow and cardiac output. Excessive PEEP may increase and aggravate hypoxemia in infants with extrapulmonary shunts.[79] Because tidal volume is proportional to the difference between end-expiratory pressure and peak inspiratory pressure, an increase of expiratory pressure produces a decrease in tidal volume and minute ventilation if pressure-limited ventilation is employed (Fig. 7-13). PEEP can also produce overdistention of some alveoli and reduce lung compliance, leading to hypoventilation and CO_2 retention. During IPPV at rapid rates with short expiratory times, pressure in the distal airways may remain higher than the value recorded in the proximal airway at end-expiration. This condition is known as inadvertent PEEP and is more likely to occur in cases of increased airway resistance or endotracheal tube obstruction (Fig. 7-12). The possibility of this complication must also be considered when the appropriate level of PEEP is sought for a given patient.

Pressure Waveform. Little is known about the effects of various waveforms on pulmonary function and resultant complications in neonates with respiratory failure. In theory, lower inspiratory gas flow rates should be beneficial in infants with evidence of airway obstruction or poor distribution of ventilation. Such flow should favor improved distribution of inspired gas to areas with prolonged time constants (slow-filling areas). High flow rates, on the other hand, increase the rate of rise of inspiratory pressure, resulting in increased turbulence and higher mean airway pressure (Fig. 7-10).

Respiratory Rate. Increased Pa_{CO_2} is the result of alveolar hypoventilation and can often be corrected by increasing the respiratory rate or tidal volume. An increase in respiratory rate is achieved by shortening inspiration, expiration, or both. Very short inspirations reduce tidal volume and mean airway pressure and may produce a fall in Pa_{O_2} (Fig. 7-10). Shortening of expiration (below 0.3 second) may produce air trapping, especially if small airway obstruction is present[96] (Fig. 7-12). It may also interfere with venous return and reduce cardiac output. High respiratory rates are used in some cases of persistent pulmonary hypertension with right-to-left shunting in order to induce respiratory alkalemia and reduce pulmonary vascular resistance. They may also be used in infants with pulmonary interstitial emphysema in conjunction with low tidal volumes.

Tidal volume can be augmented by increasing PIP and/or decreasing PEEP. Excessive PEEP overdistends normal alveoli, reducing their compliance, and larger transpulmonary pressures are required to generate a normal tidal volume. Therefore too high a level of PEEP must be ruled out as the cause of CO_2 retention before any other change in ventilator settings is made.

Mean Airway Pressure. In recent years the effectiveness and complications of IPPV have been related to mean airway pressure (area under the pressure curve of each respiratory cycle).[14,23,57,98] This attempt to simplify matters tended to obscure the importance of the variables during IPPV. Although it is true that an increase in mean airway pressure, within certain limits, results in a better Pa_{O_2}, patients respond quite differently to the same mean airway pressure, depending on the ventilatory pattern used to achieve this pressure.[98] Thus an infant ventilated at 10 cm H_2O PEEP and a PIP of 20 cm H_2O has a high mean airway

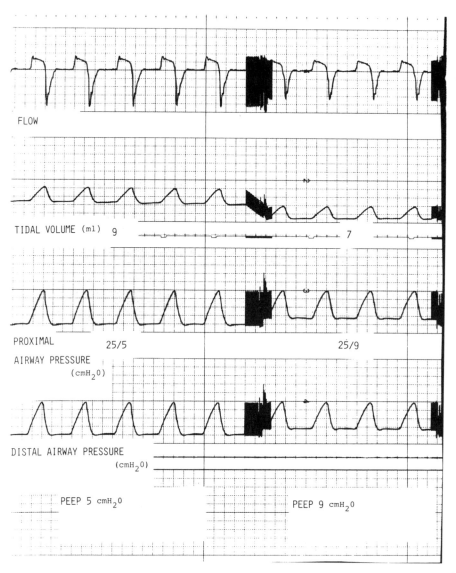

FLOW

TIDAL VOLUME (ml) 9   7

PROXIMAL   25/5   25/9
AIRWAY PRESSURE
(cmH$_2$0)

DISTAL AIRWAY PRESSURE
(cmH$_2$0)

PEEP 5 cmH$_2$0   PEEP 9 cmH$_2$0

Fig. 7-13. Flow, tidal volume, and airway pressure proximal and distal to the endotracheal tube during IPPV in a neonatal lung model. An increase in PEEP in the four cycles to the right of the figure results in a reduction in transpulmonary pressure and a smaller tidal volume.

pressure but may well be severely hypoxic and hypercapnic because of alveolar hypoventilation. If the mean airway pressure is decreased by lowering the PEEP to 4 cm H$_2$O, the Pao$_2$ and Paco$_2$ are likely to improve. Mean airway pressure lumps together PIP, PEEP, duration of positive pressure, and the shape of the pressure curve, all of which produce different effects on ventilation, distribution of inspired gas, changes in FRC, and the dynamics of the pulmonary and systemic circulation. Mean airway pressure is probably more important in the evaluation of the effects of positive pressure on pulmonary and systemic circulation.

Combinations. Recommendations have ranged from those of Reynolds and Taghizadeh,[91] who suggested that very low rates with prolonged inspiration and low PIP may reduce the incidence of chronic lung disease, to the more recent attempts to use very high frequencies to reduce pulmonary barotrauma.[38] This wide range of clinical application reflects how little is known and how empirical is the basis for mechanical ventilation of the newborn. Although the incidence of barotrauma may be reduced by using low PIP, the resulting increased FIO_2 requirement increases the risk of oxygen toxicity. Because the relative risk of these two factors is not established, we recommend reduction of both PIP and FIO_2 until "safe" levels are achieved (PIP < 30 cm H_2O, FIO_2 < 0.7, respectively).

In a prospective controlled study of 111 infants, we found that long IT (1–1.4 seconds) and low PIP (< 25 cm H_2O) did not reduce the incidence of chronic lung disease but did increase the incidence of barotrauma.[5] Based on these results, we recommend the use of IT under 0.7 second in infants with severe HMD and under 0.5 second when the FIO_2 requirement is below 0.7. PEEP between 2 and 8 cm H_2O produces generally satisfactory results according to the severity of the disease.

Infants with pneumonia usually have better lung compliance than infants with HMD and can be ventilated with lower PIP; however, their response to specific ventilator settings is more unpredictable. In cases of severe pulmonary involvement, very high PIP may be necessary to achieve a normal PaO_2. A frequent complication which makes the management of such infants even more difficult is the development of pulmonary hypertension and systemic hypotension with right-to-left shunting through the foramen ovale or ductus arteriosus. If evidence of alveolar rupture and PIE or pneumothorax is present, the lowest possible PIP with short IT and high rates should be employed.

Newborns with severe meconium aspiration are very difficult to ventilate. They frequently retain CO_2, requiring the use of high PIP and rapid rates but also manifest increased airway resistance with air trapping and a high incidence of pneumothorax. Extrapulmonary shunts may also be exacerbated by high airway pressures.

Infants who require IPPV because of apnea but have normal lungs should be ventilated with PIP under 20 cm H_2O, PEEP of 2 cm H_2O, and a low rate to maintain $PaCO_2$ between 35 and 45 mm Hg.

High-Frequency Ventilation. Recently, much speculation has focused on the possible use of high-frequency ventilation (HFV) in adults and infants with various forms of respiratory failure. Possible advantages of this technique of positive-pressure ventilation includes improvement of ventilation and oxygenation at lower tidal volumes and lower mean airway pressures, thereby reducing the risk of barotrauma and cardiovascular depression.

Although the principle is not new, much controversy exists concerning the mechanism(s) by which tidal volume, often considerably less than physiological dead space, can maintain normal gas exchange. Enhancement of diffusion and coaxial, bidirectional gas flows are but two theories which seek to explain this observation.[39] Only a few reports concerning the use of HFV in neonates are available in the literature. One group reported improvement in gas exchange and a decrease in the radiographic evidence of pulmonary interstitial emphysema in five infants ventilated with frequencies of 8–12 Hz (480–720 cycles/minute) for approximately 48 hours.[38] In a separate study, eight neonates were ventilated with frequencies ranging from 8 to 20 Hz (480–1200 cycles/minute) and showed some improvement in PaO_2.[73] Mean airway pressure was measured in only three patients and was higher during HFV than during conventional IPPV, making the interpretation of these results difficult. More experience is required before this mode of

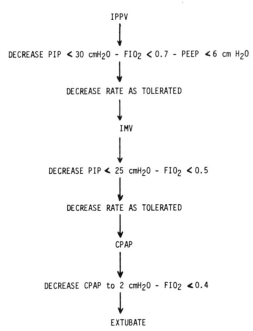

IPPV
↓
DECREASE PIP < 30 cmH$_2$O - FIO$_2$ < 0.7 - PEEP < 6 cm H$_2$O
↓
DECREASE RATE AS TOLERATED
↓
IMV
↓
DECREASE PIP < 25 cmH$_2$O - FIO$_2$ < 0.5
↓
DECREASE RATE AS TOLERATED
↓
CPAP
↓
DECREASE CPAP to 2 cmH$_2$O - FIO$_2$ < 0.4
↓
EXTUBATE

Fig. 7-14. General guidelines for weaning infants with acute respiratory failure from IPPV. At each step, try to maintain PaO$_2$ between 50–70 mm Hg, PaCO$_2$ between 35–45 mm Hg. If possible, make only one change at a time.

IPPV can be recommended for the newborn.

Weaning. Because of the number of complications associated with IPPV in small infants, the duration of this therapy should be kept to a minimum. As soon as arterial blood gases begin to improve, ventilator support should gradually be reduced. The order in which support modalities are reduced varies with each case, but in general those responsible for the highest incidence of complications (PIP > 30 cm H$_2$O, IT > 0.7 second, and FIO$_2$ > 0.7) deserve special attention. Figure 7-14 provides a guideline for weaning from IPPV. Gradual changes performed individually are recommended so the clinician can evaluate patient response to the decrement of each variable. Arterial or transcutaneous readings of PO$_2$ and PCO$_2$ must be obtained after each change. Successful reduction of ventilator rate is determined by observation of the infant's respiratory effort and PaCO$_2$. Lowering of PIP, PEEP, and FIO$_2$ depends on the results of measurement of both PaO$_2$ and PaCO$_2$.

In small prematures a point is often reached at which acceptable blood gases are obtained with a very slow ventilator rate but not with spontaneous breathing and CDAP. In spite of this finding, some of these infants are able to maintain acceptable gas exchange after tracheal extubation, perhaps through elimination of both increased resistance by the endotracheal tube and partial airway obstruction from secretions.

In most cases, extubation can be attempted after the infant has breathed an FIO$_2$ lower than 0.4 at a CDAP of 2 cm H$_2$O and has maintained acceptable blood gas levels for at least 4 hours. Weaning can be delayed by complications which alter pulmonary function (PDA, atelectasis due to airway damage and/or retained secretions, residual pulmonary disease, pulmonary infection, and CNS depression due to CNS hemorrhage, meningitis, or drugs). These problems should be corrected before completing ventilator weaning. Whenever possible, patients developing chronic lung disease should be weaned from IPPV to avoid further pulmonary damage produced by the ventilator even if they are not able to maintain normal arterial blood gas values. In small prematures, secretions are commonly retained after extubation, producing airway obstruction and deterioration of respiratory status and often leading to reintubation and additional IPPV. In many cases this scenario can be avoided by chest physiotherapy and repeated airway suction under direct laryngoscopy as often as necessary during the hours after extubation. In very small infants, CDAP or IPPV through a nasal tube or periodic ventilation with a bag and mask may stabilize the lungs, avoiding progressive alveolar collapse and the need for reintubation. The use of aminophylline as a respiratory stimulant sometimes facilitates the weaning of infants with weak respiratory effort.

Table 7-5. Endotracheal Tube Complications
Tracheal dislodgement—accidental extubation
Bronchial intubation
Kinking
Plugging (mucus, blood)
Suctioning
Hypoxia and atelectasis
Airway trauma—pneumothorax
Infection
Nasal, laryngeal, and tracheal trauma
Upper airway obstruction, subglottic stenosis
Damage to palate and teeth

Table 7-6. Supplies for Securing Neonatal Endotracheal Tube
Appropriate size endotracheal tube
Smallest size safety pin available (stainless)
Clear tape 0.5 inch (Johnson & Johnson)
Reston self-adhering foam pads (3M Company)
Tincture of benzoin
Cotton swabs

Complications. Complications occur frequently in infants treated with IPPV. Often it is difficult to determine whether the complications are produced directly by IPPV or are related to the primary disease. Most common complications are related to ventilator malfunction, the use of endotracheal tubes, high inspired oxygen concentration, infection, and barotrauma. Most of these problems were discussed earlier.

Ventilator. Proper ventilator operation must be ensured by utilizing a checkout procedure appropriate to that particular device before connecting it to an infant. Whenever a mechanically ventilated neonate experiences sudden deterioration, the possibility of ventilator malfunction must be considered immediately. Alarms should notify nursery personnel of any deviation in preselected pressures, rate, or F_{IO_2}. The infant should be examined carefully and manually ventilated while the ventilator is checked for problems. Because tidal volumes are small, slight leaks in the system caused by loose connections significantly affect ventilation. Proper operation of the blender and accuracy of oxygen concentration should also be checked. Electrical or pneumatic power sources should be ensured and valves examined for proper assembly to make sure there are no tears or holes in the material. All tubing must be assembled in the proper configuration. Gaskets and O-rings on humidifiers and water traps should be in place and properly sealed.

Airway. Complications associated with tracheal intubation are listed in Table 7-5. The tube must be well secured in order to prevent accidental extubation or inadvertent right mainstem bronchial intubation. Various methods have been described.[36,67,95] We have used the technique illustrated in Figure 7-15 for the past 10 years and find it to be simple and reliable when used with the supplies listed in Table 7-6. After intubation a safety pin is inserted through the wall of the endotracheal tube at the level of the patient's lip. The pin should barely pass into the lumen of the tube as suctioning is difficult if it is too close to the center. After the pin is in place, tincture of benzoin is applied to the face, the Reston square is inserted underneath the pin, and two diagonal strips of tape with an opening in the center are placed over the tube to secure it. If a chest x-ray shows the tip of the endotracheal tube to be improperly positioned, it can easily be readjusted by repeating the above procedure.

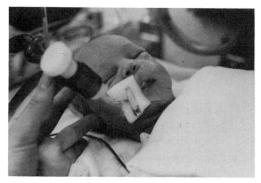

Fig. 7-15. Well-secured endotracheal tube using the method described in the text.

If the ventilator tubing pulls or twists the endotracheal tube, it may kink and the infant is thus not ventilated. A mucous plug which totally occludes the tube produces the same effect. Adequate humidification and good suctioning technique should help to prevent the latter complication. Local trauma to the nose, larynx, and trachea may occur if the tube fits too tightly. It should be as large as possible but still allow a small circumferential leak. One recent study showed that the newborn larynx tolerates long periods of intubation with uniform diameter polyvinyl chloride endotracheal tubes without serious clinical problems. This finding was surprising because autopsy of infants who died revealed that the majority had ulcerations within the highly resilient cricoid cartilage.[55] Upper airway obstruction or subglottic stenosis may be seen in patients requiring long-term or repeated intubations.

Additional reports have shown damage to the developing teeth in as many as 18 percent of intubated survivors. Because most of the problems occurred on the right side, trauma from laryngoscopy was considered to be the aggravating factor.[77] Palatal grooves caused dentition defects in another series of patients. These too were primarily right-sided, presumably because the endotracheal tubes were usually secured at the right side of the mouth, and prolonged trauma resulted from the pull and drag of the ventilator tubing.[105]

Endotracheal tubes must be suctioned to maintain patency. Suctioning may cause bradycardia, hypoxia secondary to atelectasis, and mucosal damage. Several authors have recommended the use of an endotracheal tube adaptor with side hole ports to allow maintenance of mechanical ventilation and oxygen administration while suctioning is performed.[21,107] The transcutaneous oxygen monitor is helpful for monitoring the adequacy of oxygenation during suctioning. Because each infant responds differently, variations in the procedure may be employed while following the readings.[8]

Several authors have described pneumothoraces caused by suction catheters which perforated the airway when they were passed beyond the carina.[1,102] Care should be taken to gently advance the suction catheter only until a slight resistance is felt.

Suctioning must be performed using sterile technique to prevent bacterial colonization of the respiratory tract. The risk for development of systemic infection after airway colonization is high in the compromised premature because the endotracheal tube provides direct access to the lower respiratory tract.[99] In addition, natural filtration of the nose and upper airway is bypassed. The endotracheal tube causes mucosal damage which establishes sites for bacterial growth. The infant's nutritional status is frequently poor, providing lowered resistance, and drug therapy for other infections predisposes to secondary infections with antibiotic-resistant bacteria. Sources for infection include contaminated gas cylinders, pipelines, or the atmosphere, as well as the nebulizer (more commonly) or humidifier (rarely) water reservoirs which support growth of bacteria. These reservoirs may initially be inoculated with bacteria traced back from the patient to the ventilator.[100] All respiratory circuits should be changed at least every 24 hours. More frequent changes have not been clearly demonstrated to reduce the incidence of infection. Sterile water should be used to fill humidifiers, and closed continuous water feed systems are preferable to prevent handling and contamination of the humidifier.

Cardiovascular Effects. The cardiovascular effects of positive airway pressure, e.g., the decrease in cardiac output and the increase in pulmonary vascular resistance, were discussed before with the use of CPAP. They are increased significantly with IPPV, with or without PEEP.

Pulmonary Effects. One of the major acute complications associated with IPPV is alveolar rupture, leading to PIE, pneumomediastinum, pneumothorax, or pneumopericardium.[66] Pneumothorax occurs in 15–30 percent of infants with severe HMD who require IPPV[5] and is associated with a significant increase in morbidity and mortality. It usually occurs during the more severe stages of the disease and in most cases produces a marked deterioration in the patient's condition which requires emergency treatment and adjustments in the ventilator settings. The cause of alveolar rupture is most likely overdistention of some areas of the lung produced by the positive pressure and/or prolonged inspiratory time. Initial gas dissection occurs around small vessels and airways, causing interstitial emphysema and, from here, continues to the mediastinum, pleural spaces, pericardium, retroperitoneal area, and fascial planes of the head and neck.

A significant number of infants who require IPPV survive with abnormal lung function that may persist for years.[35] Whether this damage is due to the initial disease, the use of intermittent positive pressure with high inspired oxygen concentration, or both is unknown.[30,81] The most severe form is known as bronchopulmonary dysplasia (BPD), stage IV, and occurs in 5–15 percent of all HMD survivors who require IPPV for more than 3 days.[4] It is characterized by chronic respiratory failure aggravated by infection or heart failure.

The pathogenesis of this process is not fully understood but most likely is the result of multiple factors, including incomplete development of the lung, initial damage produced by HMD, persistence of a ductus arteriosus, oxygen toxicity, and airway damage caused by positive pressure. Many IPPV treatment survivors who do not have such a severe alteration in their lung structure may nevertheless have milder changes that predispose them to respiratory illness later in life.

Outcome. As we have mentioned, the survival of infants treated with IPPV is closely related to the indications used to initiate mechanical ventilation and to the experience and skills of the personnel providing this therapy. When IPPV is used in infants with HMD and severe respiratory failure after other modes of therapy have failed, the mortality is around 30 percent.[56] In contrast, when IPPV is applied more liberally, the mortality is probably lower. Survival is closely related to the gestational age and birth weight in prematures. The direct cause of death or sequelae in the majority of very small infants is not respiratory failure but a massive intracerebral hemorrhage.[34,35] The role of IPPV in the pathogenesis of CNS hemorrhage is not known; however, high airway pressures, increased $Paco_2$, low Pao_2, and pneumothorax are factors which may increase the incidence of this complication.[29]

The long-term outcome of survivors from IPPV also vary according to the severity of the disease and incidence of complications. Recent reports indicate that 70–80 percent of the survivors from IPPV have normal physical and mental development.[34,54,61]

In summary, IPPV is a method of treatment used very frequently in ill neonates and is one of the major factors responsible for the improved outcome of infants with severe respiratory failure during the last decade. Although IPPV is an effective method of treatment, it is also associated with a significant risk of complications. It should be used only with clear indications and when experienced personnel and proper facilities are available.

Respiratory Support During Resuscitation

Whenever neonatal resuscitation is required, the first step should be to establish a patent airway and provide assisted ventilation as needed. Whether this step occurs in the delivery room or the nursery, appropriate equipment must be readily accessible and organized, and the personnel involved must be ready to initiate action immediately.

Following is the equipment that should be available in any setting where neonatal resuscitation may be required.

Resuscitator Bags. Two types of resuscitator bags are available: self-inflating manual resuscitators and nonrebreathing modifications of the Jackson-Reese anesthesia system. Several points concerning this equipment deserve emphasis. Self-inflating bags reinflate automatically after each manual compression and may be used without a high-pressure gas source. Addition of oxygen and reservoir tubing increases the FIO_2 of delivered gas. Other factors of importance in determining the final FIO_2 include the rate of ventilation, volume delivered, refill time, reservoir size, and oxygen flow rate. A precisely controlled FIO_2 is usually difficult to obtain. The neonatal breathing valve should be lightweight, offer minimal dead space and resistance, and be a nonrebreathing type. A relief valve, inserted for safety and to prevent pulmonary barotrauma, may prevent adequate ventilation when lung compliance is poor because it opens at too low an inflation pressure. Adjustment or override of the relief valve should be possible when necessary.

The anesthesia bag requires a compressed gas source for inflation and to provide ventilation. For neonatal support, a 0.5-L bag is used. The delivery of precise oxygen concentrations is possible when an oxygen/air blender is used as the gas source. The flow rate should be adjusted as necessary to provide various tidal volumes, pressures, breathing rates, and PEEP levels. Spontaneous ventilation is possible from the continuous flow of gas. This resuscitator requires greater familiarity to provide safe ventilation than does the self-inflating bag.

Both resuscitator bags should be used in conjunction with an airway pressure monitor to prevent excessive pressure side effects. Only enough pressure to provide chest excursion should be used. High pressures may be harmful but in some cases are necessary to achieve adequate ventilation.

During neonatal resuscitation, manual ventilation should be continued at a rate of one breath for every three cardiac compressions. Adequate compressions require a rate of 100–120/minute; hence ventilation should be performed at a rate of 30–40/minute without pause.

Because an infant may initially generate a pressure of -80 cm H_2O (first gasp) to expand his lungs, manual ventilation with high pressure may be necessary for the first few breaths in the delivery room. Various methods have been suggested to establish the infant's FRC. Some clinicians have recommended prolonged inspiratory times, but because of the increased risk of barotrauma we prefer the following method: An initial breath of 20–30 cm H_2O for 1–2 seconds should be followed by a shorter inspiratory time of 0.25–0.50 second at a rate of 40–60/minute. Pressure should be just enough to expand the upper chest. This pattern should then be repeated three or four times during the first 2 minutes. The heart rate should increase and the onset of regular spontaneous respiration follow.[86]

If continued ventilation is necessary, a resuscitator bag and mask may be used initially. The airway should be suctioned with a bulb syringe, a deLee suction trap, or gentle wall suction. Care must be taken as stimulation of the larynx and trachea may elicit vagal responses and blind nasopharyngeal suctioning may cause cardiac dysrhythmias or apnea.[28] A rolled diaper may be placed under the infant's shoulders to extend the neck slightly in order to maintain a patent airway. The mask should be held tightly enough to provide a seal; however care must be taken to avoid nasal obstruction. An additional problem associated with

Table 7-7. Neonatal Endotracheal Tube Size

Weight (g)	Tube Size (mm)
≤1199	2.5
1200–1999	3.0
2000–2999	3.5
≥3000	4.0

bag and mask ventilation is insufflation of gas into the stomach and gastrointestinal tract. A nasogastric tube should be inserted and the stomach emptied to prevent pulmonary aspiration of stomach contents.

When the cardiopulmonary response to ventilation with a mask is inadequate, tracheal intubation may be necessary. During intubation the heart rate should be monitored, and attempts at intubation should be stopped when the heart rate falls. Proper placement of the tube may be determined by equal chest expansion, improvement in color and heart rate, and auscultation of bilateral breath sounds. A chest x-ray film should be obtained for confirmation.

Appropriate neonatal endotracheal tube size is based on body weight (Table 7-7). The "tip-to-lip" rule of "7-8-9"[101] may be used as a guideline for determining the length of the endotracheal tube from the tip of the tube to the fixation site at the lip:

1 kg infant = 7 cm insertion
2 kg infant = 8 cm insertion
3 kg infant = 9 cm insertion

The tube should then be secured as previously described.

Whenever possible, arterial blood samples should be obtained for gas analysis to determine the adequacy of ventilation. If Pa_{CO_2} is still high, more rapid rates or high pressure may be necessary to increase minute ventilation. A low or high Pa_{O_2} requires adjustments in the delivered oxygen concentration, either by varying the reservoir size on a self-inflating bag or adjusting the blended gas source to the anesthesia bag. When perfusion is adequate, transcutaneous Pa_{O_2} measurements may also be help-

ful. If the infant has been hyperventilated during resuscitation, he may remain apneic when manual inflation stops. Manual support should be gradually discontinued to allow the return of spontaneous ventilation.

Respiratory Support During Transport

The regionalization of neonatal intensive care requires the transport of critically ill infants to hospitals where they may receive specialized treatment. Neonatologists generally agree that such transportation must be well controlled with the utilization of personnel trained in assessment and supportive care of the newborn. Transport teams may include various combinations of neonatologists, nurses, respiratory therapists, pediatric house staff physicians, anesthesiologists, and emergency medical technicians. The small infant weighing less than 1500 g who is transported by well trained and skilled personnel, has a better chance for survival than the infant transported by inexperienced staff. This may be due to the trained team's ability to deliver an infant to the newborn, ICU in better thermal, cardiopulmonary and metabolic condition.[22]

Transportation of sick newborns requires careful organization and perfectly functioning equipment. Meticulous attention must be paid to each detail as the only resources available are those brought by the team. Nothing must be left to chance.

Most transported neonates require some form of respiratory support. In some cases, clearance of the airway and administration of oxygen suffices. Other sicker infants, however, require insertion of an artificial airway and application of CDAP or positive-pressure ventilation. Support for these infants also requires maintenance of a neutral thermal environment, adequate glucose levels, adequate circulating blood volume, and relatively normal acid-base status. The same guidelines which apply to long-dis-

Table 7-8. Assessment of Respiratory Status for Transport

Respiratory rate
Heart rate
F_{IO_2}
Ventilator settings
Blood gas and pH values
X-ray findings
Verification of endotracheal tube placement
Auscultatory findings
Feeding status
Umbilical artery catheter placement
Temperature
Serum glucose (Dextrostix)
Blood pressure
Hematocrit

tance transport should be adapted for those within the hospital, i.e., for computed axial tomography (CAT) scans, cardiac catheterization, or surgery.

Organization. Any transport begins with the initial communication from the referring hospital. At this time, all pertinent information regarding the respiratory status of the patient must be obtained in order to plan for transport and to give advice for stabilization before the team's arrival (Table 7-8). The necessary team members must be assembled, arrangements made for activation of the transport vehicles, and the presence and function of equipment and supplies verified. A careful checking of equipment is mandatory. An increase of problems and iatrogenic complications during transport results if this procedure is omitted or done in anything less than a thorough manner. Improvisation does not offset the absence of a laryngoscope handle or the presence of an empty oxygen cylinder.

A checkout list should be developed so that all supplies and equipment are known to be present before departure and are restocked after the transport is completed. All supplies may be included in a large fishing tackle box, or respiratory support items may be maintained in a separate carrier. A large camera accessory bag with a shoulder strap and zippered pouch makes a convenient carrying case. When both a nurse and respiratory therapist are on the transport, separate supply cases make access to needed supplies easier. The equipment listed in Table 7-9 represents only that needed for respiratory stabilization of the neonate. It should not be considered all-inclusive as additional medications and nursing supplies often must be taken along.

Most required items are small and can be assembled in the carrier bag. The list is long but everything needed must be readily available as team members cannot count on

Table 7-9. Respiratory Support Equipment

Carrier bag
  Laryngoscope handles, 2
  Extra batteries and bulbs
  Straight Miller laryngoscope blades, 2—size 0
  Straight Miller laryngoscope blade, 1—size 1
  Endotracheal tubes with adaptor, 8 (2 each of size 2.5, 3.0, 3.5, 4.0)
  Magill forceps, 1
  Endotracheal tube stylets, 2
  Supplies for endotracheal tube fixation—scissors
  Anesthesia bag
  Manual self-inflating bag with reservoir tubing
  Pressure manometer
  Anesthesia masks, 1 newborn and 1 premature
  Bulb syringe
  DeLee suction with trap
  Suction catheters, 9 (3 each of size 5, 6.5, 8 Fr)
  Saline for lavage
  Disposable newborn oxygen mask and oxygen connect tubing, 1
  Oxygen cylinder wrench
  Blood gas syringes, heparin, and syringe caps
  Stethoscope
Transport system components
  Ventilator
  Oxygen/air blender
  Oxygen analyzer
  Suction machine
  Oxygen hood
  Heated nebulizer or humidifier and bottle sterile water
  Oxygen cylinder with regulator or liquid oxygen vessel
  Compressed air cylinder (or air compressor) with regulator
  Transcutaneous oxygen and carbon dioxide monitor and electrodes
  Chest tube tray
  Umbilical artery catheter tray
  Heart rate monitor and respiratory rate monitor

additional supplies at the referral hospital. If the team is using their hospital's self-contained neonatal transport vehicle, all supplies should be routinely stored in the vehicle. However, additional portable supplies must be prepared for use in the referral nursery and in the move between the nursery and transport vehicle. Larger components are either part of the commercial transport system or should be mounted on or attached to the basic infant transport incubator. Individuals who design a transport system must balance the advantages of adding more equipment against the disadvantages of increased weight and lack of portability. The system must be sufficiently portable to be lifted into ambulances, helicopters, or airplanes.

Equipment. Adequate oxygen is necessary for successful transport. Oxygen may be supplied either in gaseous form in high-pressure cylinders or in liquid form in a portable carrying case. Liquid oxygen has the advantage of being much lighter in weight than an equal amount of cylinder gas. In a van specifically designed for neonatal transport, a large H-cylinder of oxygen or a large liquid reservoir (the equivalent of two H-cylinders) may be used while in transit. The smaller, portable E-cylinders, or a portable liquid oxygen supply, must be mounted directly adjacent to the transport incubator. A 10-lb liquid carrying case holds the equivalent of 1.5 E-cylinders but weighs less than half as much. Because pressure gauges cannot be used with liquid oxygen, a portable scale must be used to determine the amount remaining. Each pound of liquid oxygen equals approximately 342 L of gaseous oxygen. After weight is converted to liters, the duration of gas flow at a specific flow rate is (Table 7-10):

Duration of flow (minutes)
$$= \frac{\text{liters remaining in case}}{\text{liter flow/minute}}$$

The portable case should be filled as close to the start of transport as possible as liquid oxygen evaporates even when not in use. Evaporation of a carrying case holding 3 lb of liquid oxygen occurs at approximately 10 L/hour.

Calculation for measuring the length of time a cylinder of oxygen will last are based on the following formula (Table 7-10):

Duration of flow (minutes)
$$= \frac{\text{gauge pressure (psi)} \times \text{factor}}{\text{liter flow/minute}}$$

The factor for an E-cylinder is 0.28 and for the H-cylinder 3.14.[31]

Members of the team must be able to assess the oxygen requirements for transport, usually based on the anticipated duration of the transport; 1.5 to 2 times this amount should be taken to provide for unusual or unexpected circumstances. Tanks must be well secured because they will be used in a moving vehicle.

An oxygen/air blender is necessary to provide precise oxygen concentrations when an oxygen hood, ventilator, or anesthesia type bag is used. Several commercial transport systems utilize an internal miniature air compressor; otherwise a compressed air cylinder is needed. The length of time an air cylinder will last can be calculated by the same formula and factor used to calculate the duration of oxygen flow. If compressed air is not available, a nebulizer with a venturi dilution device can be used for varying oxygen concentrations within the hood. Whichever method is selected, the F_{IO_2} of the gas mixture must be analyzed frequently during transport. In addition, the gas should be warmed and humidified. Even for short trips, cold, dry gas may affect the infant's thermoregulation.

Suction may be needed during the transport. Portable units are available which are powered by either their own battery source or compressed gas. They are relatively inexpensive and simple to operate.

Until recently, one of the most difficult factors to assess during transport was the

Table 7-10. Weights and Capacities of Oxygen Cylinders and Liquid Vessels

Parameter	E-Cylinder	H-Cylinder	Typical Portable Liquid Carrying Case	Typical Liquid Oxygen Reservoir
Weight: gas and container (lb)	15	130	10 (3 lb 02)	68 (40.4 lb 02)
Volume (L)	600	6,900	1,026	13,800
Duration factor	0.28	3.14	—	—
Weight/liter conversion	—	—	1 lb 02 = 342 L	1 lb 02 = 342 L

arterial oxygen tension. Lighting in most transport vehicles is less than ideal, and the baby's color, or that of the arterial blood, are poor indicators of Pa_{O_2}. Some self-contained ground vehicles include blood gas machines; however, maintenance is expensive and operation difficult while moving; thus they are rarely found on air ambulances. A satisfactory alternative may be the portable transcutaneous oxygen monitor. Two recent evaluations of the use of transcutaneous oxygen monitoring during transport have shown promising results.[24,74] Periods of hyperoxia or hypoxia may be limited by altering respiratory support as indicated by the monitor.

Clinical Assessment and Stabilization. Once the team arrives at the referring hospital, they must assess the infant's respiratory status (Table 7-8). Initial priorities include establishment and maintenance of the airway, oxygenation, and determination if CDAP or assisted ventilation is necessary. A nasogastric or orogastric tube should be placed and the stomach emptied to prevent aspiration while in transit. An umbilical artery catheter may be placed, and blood gas results should be evaluated in relation to the F_{IO_2}. If the infant was intubated by the referral hospital personnel, esophageal and bronchial placement should be ruled out and the presence of bilateral breath sounds confirmed. Once a chest x-ray confirms proper tube placement, the distance from the lip to the endotracheal tube adaptor should be measured so that during transport tube placement may be verified. If an en-

dotracheal tube is not in place, a decision should be reached before departure concerning the necessity of intubation. Tracheal intubation is difficult in a small vehicle and nearly impossible in a noisy vibrating aircraft that cannot pull over to the side of the road. Maximal stabilization at the referring hospital is essential before any attempt is made to transport.

Nasal CPAP may be started with an anesthesia bag system and a premixed gas source if a ventilator is not available. One hundred percent oxygen should not be given on the transport unless it is required to maintain the Pa_{O_2} between 50 and 70 mm Hg. If tracheal intubation and manual or mechanical ventilation are necessary, the tube should be well secured as the manipulation and movement inherent in the transport allow accidental extubations to occur easily. During movement to the transport vehicle, the endotracheal tube must be held and supported to provide additional fixation of the tube and to prevent kinking.

A mechanical ventilator is not essential during transport as an experienced team member can hand-ventilate the infant using either a self-inflating bag or an anesthesia bag with an attached manometer and a blended source of gas. However, hand ventilation is not as consistent as mechanical ventilation over an extended period in a moving vehicle. For this reason, we recommend that a well calibrated and maintained neonatal ventilator be included with the transport equipment. When a ventilator is used, the personnel must be thoroughly familiar with its operation. The high-stress environment during transport mitigates against on-the-job training in the mechanics of ventilator function. The ventilator should be monitored closely during transport. Tubing may disconnect or kink easily when the infant is moved or handled. Close observation is mandatory to detect any signs of distress.

Ventilator selection should be made according to availability, portability, ease of operation, and power source requirements. A pneumatic or fluidic ventilator should be capable of operating with low gas flow requirements as gas supplies are limited. An electronic ventilator should be adaptable to all sources of electrical current and should have fail-safe internal battery power in case of incubator or vehicular failure. Currently available neonatal ventilators are mainly time-cycled and pressure-limited and are described in Chapter 10.

Stabilization for respiratory support also includes maintenance of acceptable acid-base status, intravascular volumes, glucose level, and a neutral thermal environment. Hypoxia leads to increasing metabolic acidosis, which in turn aggravates hypoxemia if not corrected. Metabolic acidosis usually responds to improved cardiovascular and respiratory function and gradually resolves. Slow infusions of sodium bicarbonate may be necessary if acidosis is still severe. Tissue oxygenation is dependent on both circulating blood volume and local perfusion, so blood or fluid expanders should be given if hypovolemia is suggested.

Respiratory distress increases the body's demand for glucose, which is required by most tissues and is absolutely essential for cerebral metabolism. Measurement of blood glucose should be performed (Dextrostix) and glucose infusion started to maintain acceptable levels.

Finally, the increased oxygen consumption of a cold infant in respiratory distress exacerbates all existing problems. Unless body temperature is carefully controlled, stabilization of the respiratory status will be marginal at best.

Special Problems. Several neonatal problems require special consideration during stabilization and transport. An infant with a diaphragmatic hernia should have his head elevated and be placed with the affected side down. This position minimizes compression of the heart and allows expansion of the unaffected lung. A nasogastric tube should be inserted to prevent distention of the gastrointestinal tract. Bag and mask ventilation should be avoided as inadvertent inflation of the stomach (difficult to prevent) further compromises respiratory function. If the respiratory problem is severe, the newborn should be intubated before transport.

An infant with a tracheoesophageal fistula should be positioned with his head elevated. A feeding tube must be placed in the esophageal pouch and gently suctioned intermittently in an attempt to prevent reflux of gastric secretions. Nothing should be given by mouth, and oxygen should be administered as necessary.

Infants with choanal atresia or Pierre-Robin syndrome should be placed in the prone position to allow the tongue to move forward. An oropharyngeal airway should be placed to establish a patent airway. When an airway cannot be maintained, intubation is necessary.

Air Transport. Neonatal transport may involve the use of fixed-wing aircraft or helicopters as many regional centers are located more than 100 miles from the referring hospital. Common problems encountered in air transport include the small working area, difficulty with thermoregulation, noise and vibration, poor lighting, inability to stop en route for complicated procedures, and the possibility of expansion of free air within the thoracic or abdominal cavities because of decreased atmospheric pressure. If any free air is present before departure, a chest tube should be inserted and connected to an underwater seal or a Heimlich valve. During any transport, supplies must be available to relieve a tension pneumothorax. A butterfly needle, three-way stopcock, and 10-cc syringe can be used temporarily. Because a partially pressurized or unpressurized cabin aggravates existing hypoxia, the concentration of ambient oxygen must be increased to compensate for the decreased barometric pressure.

Successful transport results in the delivery of a stable infant to the receiving hospital. Vital signs, temperature, blood gases, and fluid volumes should be within normal limits. These results can be obtained consistently over a long period of time only through practice and experience by well trained and interested personnel.

Respiratory Therapist's Role in Neonatal Care

Respiratory therapists have an important role to fill in neonatal care and should be included as part of the team used to staff neonatal special care units. Actual practice differs from one unit to another, but therapists' education, training, and experience make them useful resources. They should be involved in a level I nursery because they are familiar with oxygen therapy equipment, oxygen analyzers, and blood gas analysis, all of which are essential for basic stabilization. Without the therapists' assistance, equipment is often used inappropriately by unskilled personnel. In addition, as members of an obstetrical stabilization team, they may assist during high-risk deliveries.

In level II and III nurseries, the therapists should be used to their fullest capabilities. As neonatal critical care becomes more complex in terms of both clinical management and technological advances, and as ventilators and continuous oxygen monitoring devices are employed almost routinely, it is unrealistic and inefficient to expect nursing and physician personnel to

provide the expertise necessary for proper selection, operation, and maintenance of mechanical ventilatory support. Skilled respiratory therapists are critical to the effective use of respiratory equipment. The most sophisticated ventilators are only as good in the successful management of respiratory problems as the personnel who operate them.

In many centers the neonatal respiratory therapy specialist is taking an additional active role in direct patient care by developing complementary and overlapping expertise and skills with the neonatologist and neonatal nurse specialist. The respiratory therapist's responsibilities within the neonatal ICU are categorized in Table 7-11.

For maximal operational efficiency, the respiratory therapy department must make a commitment to the establishment of a permanent, distinct support team for the level III neonatal ICU. A coordinator is needed to supervise and organize the team of therapists who volunteer to work in this area. A high level of involvement and input by the respiratory therapist in the neonatal ICU is related directly to the interest, motivation, competence, training, and availability of personnel, all of which are virtually impossible to accomplish unless a permanent assignment is made to the neonatal area.

Comprehensive orientation and training is essential because neonatal respiratory care is so specialized. Coordinators must train the staff to understand how the neonate's total clinical status influences their choice and application of respiratory therapy. Orientation must include didactic training in neonatal pathophysiology and disease processes, the indications for and hazards of respiratory therapy procedures, and clinical experience to develop the necessary practical skills. The importance of this training cannot be emphasized enough. Without it, the therapist is unable to deliver safe and effective respiratory support.

Coordinators must motivate therapists to work as a team with one goal in mind: the

Table 7-11. Responsibilities of Respiratory Therapist in the Neonatal ICU

Equipment
  Proper function
  Maintenance and calibration
  Minimize equipment misuse and downtime
  Sterilization and disinfection
  Infection control—random cultures
  Evaluation of new techniques and equipment
  Adaptation and/or development of equipment for new techniques

Direct patient care
  Continuous monitoring and evaluation of respiratory status
  Monitoring and management of oxygen
  Monitoring and management of CDAP and mechanical ventilation systems under physician direction
  Chest physical therapy and delivery of medication by aerosol
  Intubation and tube fixation
  Transportation (team)
  Member of perinatal stabilization team for high-risk deliveries
  Airway patency and suctioning
  Resuscitation
  Medical rounds and multidisciplinary clinical conferences

Diagnostic
  Arterial blood gas analysis and interpretation
  Arterial and capillary puncture
  Continuous transcutaneous oxygen and carbon dioxide monitoring
  Monitoring of indwelling oxygen saturation devices and polarographic electrodes
Bedside pulmonary function testing

Education and training
  Instruction of respiratory therapists, nurses, and physicians in proper usage and care of equipment, respiratory therapy techniques, blood gas interpretation, tracheal intubation, and application of mechanical ventilators and monitoring equipment

Research
  Investigations comparing effectiveness of respiratory support devices
  Investigations comparing effectiveness of techniques and applications of respiratory therapy

delivery of optimal respiratory care with continual efforts to reevaluate and improve the equipment and methods used to provide support. Qualified and well trained therapists can made a difference in the level of care patients receive. When equipment is well maintained and calibrated, infection control policies are adhered to strictly, and ventilator alarms and safety systems are carefully used, iatrogenic complications can be reduced.

If full utilization of the expertise and skill of the respiratory therapy team can be achieved to ensure optimal respiratory care, a foundation of mutual respect must be developed between the therapists, nurses, and physicians. All personnel must acknowledge the expertise, capabilities, and training of their colleagues. Communication between team members is the key to effective and efficient delivery of respiratory support. Multidisciplinary patient rounds, coordination of work schedules, and combined in-service education help to improve rapport. Scheduled meetings between the medical director, head nurse, administrative coordinator, and respiratory therapy team coordinator are important to maintain communication and to develop methods for continued improvement in the delivery of respiratory care.

REFERENCES

1. Anderson KD, Chandra R: Pneumothorax secondary to perforation of sequential bronchi by suction catheters. J Pediatr Surg 11:687, 1976
2. Aranda JV, Saheb N, Stern L, et al: Arterial oxygen tension and retinal vasoconstriction in newborn infants. Am J Dis Child 122:189, 1971
3. Baker JD, Wallace CT, Brown CS: Maintenance of body temperature in infants during surgery. Anesthesiol Rev 4:21, 1977
4. Bancalari E, Abdenour GE, Feller R, et al: Bronchopulmonary dysplasia: clinical presentation. J Pediatr 85:819, 1979
5. Bancalari E, Feller R, Gerhardt T: Prospective evaluation of IPPV settings in infants with RDS. Clin Res 28:879A, 1980
6. Bancalari E, Garcia OL, Jesse MJ: Effects of continuous negative pressure on lung mechanics in idiopathic respiratory distress syndrome. Pediatrics 51:486, 1973

7. Bancalari E, Gerhardt T, Feller R, et al: Muscle relaxation during IPPV in prematures with RDS. Pediatr Res 14:590, 1980

8. Barnes CA, Asonye UO, Vidyasagar D: Effects of bronchopulmonary hygiene on $Ptco_2$ values in critically ill neonates. Crit Care Med 9:819, 1981

9. Bauer CR, Stern L, Colle E: Prolonged rupture of membrane associated with a decreased incidence of respiratory distress syndrome. Pediatrics 53:7, 1974

10. Bell EF, Warburton D, Stonestreet BS, et al: Effect of fluid administration on the development of symptomatic patent ductus arteriosus and congestive heart failure in premature infants. N Engl J Med 302:598, 1980

11. Bell EF, Warburton D, Stonestreet BS, et al: High volume fluid intake predisposes premature infants to necrotizing enterocolitis. Lancet 2:90, 1979

12. Bhat R, Kim WD, Shukla A, et al: Simultaneous tissue pH and transcutaneous carbon dioxide monitoring in critically ill neonates. Crit Care Med 9:744, 1981

13. Blennow G, Svenningsen NW, Almquist B: Noise levels in infant incubators. Pediatrics 53:29, 1974

14. Boros SJ: Variations in inspiratory expiratory ratio and airway pressure wave form during mechanical ventilation: the significance of mean airway pressure. J Pediatr 94:114, 1979

15. Bradley JG: Errors in the measurement of blood Pco_2 due to the dilution of the sample with heparin solution. Br J Anaesth 44:231, 1972

16. Brady JP, Ceruti E: Chemoreceptor reflexes in the newborn infant: effect of varying degrees of hypoxia on heart rate and ventilation in a warm environment. J Physiol (Lond) 184:631, 1966

17. Brown ER, Stark A, Sosenko I, et al: Bronchopulmonary dysplasia: possible relationship to pulmonary edema. J Pediatr 92:982, 1978

18. Brunstler I, Enders A, Versmold HT: Skin surface Pco_2 monitoring in newborn infants in shock: effect of hypotension and electrode temperature. J Pediatr 100:454, 1982

19. Bryan AC, Bryan MH: Control of respiration in the newborn. In Thiebeault DW, Gregory G (ed): Neonatal Pulmonary Care. p. 2. Addison Wesley, Menlo Park, CA, 1979

20. Bucher JR, Roberts RJ: Development of the newborn rat lung in hyperoxia: a dose-response study of lung growth, maturation, and changes in antioxidant enzyme activities. Pediatr Res 15:999, 1981

21. Cabal L, Devashar S, Siassi B, et al: New endotracheal tube adaptor reducing cardiopulmonary effects on suctioning. Crit Care Med 7:552, 1979

22. Chance GW, Matthew JD, Gash J, et al: Neonatal transport: a controlled study of skilled assistance. J Pediatr 93:662, 1978

23. Ciszek TA, Modanlou HO, Owings D, et al: Mean airway pressure-significance during mechanical ventilation in neonates. J Pediatr 99:121, 1981

24. Clarke TA, Zmora E, Chen JH, et al: Transcutaneous oxygen monitoring during neonatal transport. Pediatrics 65:884, 1980

25. Cogswell JJ, Hatch DJ, Kerr A, et al: Effects of continuous positive airway pressure on lung mechanics of babies after operation for congenital heart disease. Arch Dis Child 50:799, 1975

26. Collaborative Group on Antenatal Steroid Therapy: Effect of antenatal dexamethasone administration on the prevention of respiratory distress syndrome. Am J Obstet Gynecol 141:276, 1981

27. Conway M, Durbin GM, Ingram D, et al: Continuous monitoring of arterial oxygen tension using a catheter tip polarographic electrode in infants. Pediatrics 57:244, 1976

28. Cordero L, Hon EH: Neonatal bradycardia following nasopharyngeal stimulation. J Pediatr 78:441, 1971

29. Dykes FD, Lazzara A, Ahmann P, et al: Intraventricular hemorrhage: a prospective evaluation of etiopathogenesis. Pediatrics 66:42, 1980

30. Edwards DK, Dyer WM, Northway WH: Twelve years' experience with bronchopulmonary dysplasia. Pediatrics 59:839, 1977

31. Egan DF: Fundamentals of Inhalation Therapy. Mosby, St. Louis, 1969

32. Fan LL, Dellinger KT, Mills AL, et al: Potential errors in neonatal blood gas measurements. J Pediatr 97:650, 1980

33. Farrell PM, Avery ME: Hyaline membrane disease. Am Rev Resp Dis 111:657, 1975

34. Fitzhardinge PM: Follow-up studies in infants treated by mechanical ventilation. Clin Perinatol 5:451, 1978

35. Fitzhardinge PM, Pape K, Arstikaitis M, et al: Mechanical ventilation of infants of less than 1,501 gm birth weight: health, growth, and neurologic sequelae. J Pediatr 88:531, 1976

36. Fletcher MA, Gluck L: Problems unique to the delivery of respiratory care in infants and children. In Burton GG, Gee GN, Hodgkin JE (eds): Respiratory Care: A Guide to Clinical Practice. p. 694. Lippincott, Philadelphia, 1977

37. Fox WW, Berman LS, Dinwiddie R, et al: Tracheal extubation of the neonate at 2–3 cm H_2O continuous positive airway pressure. Pediatrics 59:257, 1977

38. Frantz ID, Stark AR, Werthammer J: Improvement in pulmonary interstitial emphysema with high frequency ventilation. Pediatr Res 15:719, 1981

39. Fredberg JJ: Augmented diffusion in the airways can support pulmonary gas exchange. J Appl Physiol 49:232, 1980

40. Gale R, Redner-Carmi R, Gale J: Accumulation of carbon dioxide in oxygen hoods, infant cots and incubators. Pediatrics 60:453, 1977

41. Gerard P, Fox WW, Outerbridge EW, et al: Early versus late introduction of continuous negative pressure in the management of the idiopathic respiratory distress syndrome. J Pediatr 87:591, 1979

42. Gerhardt T, Bancalari E: Chest wall compliance in full-term and premature infants. Acta Paediatr Scand 69:359, 1980

43. Gerhardt T, Bancalari E: Components of effective elastance and their maturational changes in human newborns. J Appl Physiol 53:766, 1982

44. Gerhardt T, Bancalari E: Effect of CPAP on pulmonary mechanics in newborn with meconium aspiration. Pediatr Res 13:534, 1979

45. Gerhardt T, McCarthy J. Bancalari E: Effect of aminophylline on the respiratory center activity and metabolic rate in premature infants with idiopathic apnea. Pediatrics 63:537, 1979

46. Gluck L: Preventing obsolescence in the design of a perinatal unit. Clin Perinatol 3:349, 1976

47. Gluck L, Kulovich MB: Fetal lung development: current concepts. Pediatr Clin North Am 20:367, 1973

48. Goodwin NM, Schreiber MT: Effects of anticoagulants on acid-base and blood gas estimations. Crit Care Med 7:473, 1979

49. Gregory GA, Kitterman JA, Phibbs RH, et al: Treatment of the idiopathic respiratory distress syndrome with continuous positive airway pressure. N Engl J Med 284:1333, 1971

50. Guilfoile T, Dabe K: Nasal catheter oxygen therapy for infants. Resp Care 26:35, 1981

51. Hadjigeorgiou E, Kitsiou S, Psaroudakis A, et al: Antepartum aminophylline treatment for prevention of the respiratory distress syndrome in premature infants. Am J Obstet Gynecol 135:257, 1979

52. Hansen JE, Simmons DH: A systemic error in the determination of blood P_{CO_2}. Am Rev Resp Dis 115:1061, 1977

53. Hansen TN, Tooley WH: Skin surface carbon dioxide tension in sick infants. Pediatrics 64:942, 1979

54. Harrod JR, L'Heureux P, Wangensteen OD, et al: Long-term follow-up of severe respiratory distress syndrome treated with IPPB. J Pediatr 84:277, 1974

55. Hawkins DB: Hyaline membrane disease of the neonate, prolonged intubation in management: effects on the larynx. Laryngoscope 88:201, 1978

56. Heicher DA, Kasting DS, Harrod JR: Prospective clinical comparison of two methods for mechanical ventilation of neonates: rapid rate and short inspiratory time versus slow rate and long inspiratory time. J Pediatr 98:957, 1981

57. Herman S, Reynolds EOR: Methods for improving oxygenation in infants mechanically ventilated for severe hyaline membrane disease. Arch Dis Child 48:612, 1973

58. Hodson WA: Development of the lung. In: Lung Biology in Health and Disease. Vol. 6. Marcel Dekker, New York, 1977

59. Hodson WA, Belenky DA: Management of respiratory problems. In Avery GB (ed): Neonatology: Pathophysiology and Management of the Newborn. p. 265. Lippincott, Philadelphia, 1975

60. Huch A, Huch R: Transcutaneous noninvasive monitoring of P_{O_2}. Hosp Prac 11:43, 1976

61. Johnson JD, Malachowski NC, Grobstein R, et al: Prognosis of children surviving with the aid of mechanical ventilation in the newborn period. J Pediatr 84:272, 1974

62. Kattwinkel J: Neonatal apnea: pathogenesis and therapy. J Pediatr 90:342, 1977

63. Kinsey VE, Arnold HJ, Kalina RE, et al: Pa_{O_2} levels and retrolental fibroplasia: a report of the cooperative study. Pediatrics 60:655, 1977

64. Kirby RR, Robison EJ, Schulz J, et al: A new pediatric volume ventilator. Anesth Analg 50:533, 1971

65. Kirby RR, Robison EJ, Schulz J, et al: Continuous flow ventilation as an alternative to assisted or controlled ventilation in infants. Anesth Analg 51:871, 1972

66. Kirkpatrick BV, Felman AH, Eitzman DV: Complications of ventilator therapy in respiratory distress syndrome. Am J Dis Child 128:496, 1974

67. Klaus MH, Fanaroff AA: Care of the High Risk Neonate. Saunders, Philadelphia, 1973

68. Koch G, Wendel H: Adjustment of arterial blood gases and acid base balance in the normal newborn infant during the first week of life. Biol Neonate 12:136, 1968

69. Kopotic RJ: Role of humidifiers in regulation of neutral thermal environment. J Calif Perinatal Assoc 1:66, 1981

70. Liggins GC, Howie RN: A controlled trial of antepartum glucocorticoid treatment for prevention of the respiratory distress syndrome in premature infants. Pediatrics 50:515, 1972

71. Lilien LD, Harris VJ, Ramamurthy RS, et al: Neonatal osteomyelitis of the calcaneus: complication of heel punctures. J Pediatr 88:478, 1976

72. Long JG, Philip AGS, Lucey JF: Excessive handling as a cause of hypoxemia. Pediatrics 65:203, 1980

73. Marchak BE, Thompson WK, Diffty P, et al: Treatment of RDS by high frequency oscillatory ventilation: a preliminary report. J Pediatr 99:287, 1981

74. Miller C, Clymase RI, Roth RR, et al: Control of oxygenation during the transport of sick neonates. Pediatrics 66:117, 1980

75. Mockrin LD, Bancalari E: Early vs. delayed initiation of continuous negative pressure in infants with hyaline membrane disease. J Pediatr 87:596, 1975

76. Monaco F, McQuitty JC: Transcutaneous measurements of carbon dioxide partial pressure in sick neonates. Crit Care Med 9:756, 1981

77. Moylan FMB, Seldin EB, Shannon DC, et al: Defective primary dentition in survivors of neonatal mechanical ventilation. J Pediatr 96:106, 1980

78. Nelson D, McDonald JS: Heated humidification, temperature control, and "rainout" in neonatal ventilation. Resp Ther 7:41, 1977

79. Nelson RM, Egan EA, Eitzman DV: Increased hypoxemia in neonates secondary to the use of continuous positive airway pressure. J Pediatr 91:87, 1977

80. Northway WH, Petriceks R, Shahinian L: Quantitative aspects of oxygen toxicity in the newborn: inhibition of lung DNA synthesis in the mouse. Pediatrics 50:67, 1972

81. Northway WH, Rosan RC, Porter DY: Pulmonary disease following respirator therapy of hyaline membrane disease. N Engl J Med 276:357, 1967

82. Obladen M, Merritt TA, Gluck L: Acceleration of pulmonary surfactant maturation in stressed pregnancies: a study of neonatal lung effluent. Am J Obstet Gynecol 135:1079, 1979

83. Orzalesi MM, Mendicini M, Bucci G, et al: Arterial oxygen studies in premature newborns with and without mild respiratory disorders. Arch Dis Child 42:174, 1967

84. Pape KE, Armstrong DL, Fitzhardinge PM: Peripheral median nerve damage secondary to brachial arterial blood gas sampling. J Pediatr 93:852, 1978

85. Peabody JL, Willis MM, Gregory GA, et al: Clinical limitations and advantages of transcutaneous oxygen electrodes. Acta Anaesth Scand [Suppl] 68:76, 1978

86. Phibbs RH: Delivery room management of the newborn. In Avery GB (ed): Neonatology: Pathophysiology & Management of the Newborn. 2nd Ed. p. 190. Lippincott, Philadelphia, 1981

87. Pollitzer MJ, Soutter LP, Reynolds EO: Continuous monitoring of arterial oxygen

tension in infants: four years of experience with an intravascular oxygenation electrode. Pediatrics 66:31, 1980

88. Pomerance JJ: Neonatal intensive care unit: basic equipment needs. Clin Perinatol 3:353, 1976

89. Pratt PC: Pathology of pulmonary oxygen toxicity. Am Rev Resp Dis 110:51, 1974

90. Redding RA: Thyroid hormone influence upon lung surfactant metabolism. Science 175:994, 1971

91. Reynolds EOR, Taghizadeh A: Improved prognosis of infants mechanically ventilated for hyaline membrane disease. Arch Dis Child 49:505, 1974

92. Rigatto H, Brady JP, de la Torre Verduzco R: Chemoreceptor reflexes in preterm infants. I. The effect of gestational age and postnatal age on the ventilatory response to inhalation of 100% and 15% oxygen. Pediatrics 55:604, 1975

93. Rigatto H, Brady JP, de la Torre Verduzco R: Chemoreceptor reflexes in preterm infants. II. The effect of gestational age on the ventilatory response to inhaled CO_2. Pediatrics 55:614, 1975

94. Sackner MA, Landa J, Hirsch J, et al: Pulmonary effects of oxygen breathing: a 6-hour study in normal men. Ann Intern Med 82:40, 1975

95. Shannon DC: Respiratory care in newborn. Crit Care Med 5:10, 1977

96. Simbruner G, Gregory GA: Performance of neonatal ventilators: the effect of changes in resistance and compliance. Crit Care Med 9:509, 1981

97. Simmons MF, Levine RL, Lubchenco LG: Serious sequela of temporal artery catheters. J Pediatr 92:284, 1978

98. Stewart AR, Finer NN, Peters KL: Effects of alterations of inspiratory and expiratory pressures and inspiratory/expiratory ratios on mean airway pressure. Pediatrics 67:474, 1981

99. Storm W: Transient bacteremia following endotracheal suctioning in ventilated newborns. Pediatrics 65:487, 1980

100. Sykes MK: Sterilization of ventilators. Int Anesthesiol Clin 10:131, 1972

101. Tochen ML: Orotracheal intubation in the newborn infant: a method for determining length of tube insertion. Pediatrics 95:1050, 1979

102. Vaughan RS, Menke JA, Giacoia GP: Pneumothorax: a complication of endotracheal tube suctioning. J Pediatr 92:633, 1978

103. Vidyasagar D, Asonye UO: Practical aspects of transcutaneous oxygen monitoring. Crit Care Med 7:149, 1979

104. Wall PM, Kuhns LR: Percutaneous arterial sampling using transillumination. Pediatrics 59:1032, 1977

105. Wetzel RC: Defective dentition following mechanical ventilation. J Pediatr 97:334, 1980

106. Wilkinson AR, Phibbs RH, Gregory GA: Continuous measurement of oxygen saturation in sick newborn infants. J Pediatr 93:1016, 1978

107. Zmora E, Merritt TA: Use of side hole endotracheal tube adapter for tracheal aspiration. Am J Dis Child 134:250, 1980

8

Ethics, Law, and Medicine: Termination of Life Support and Mechanical Ventilation

Robert R. Kirby

Death is not the enemy, doctor, humanity is.[14]

In my youth, said the sage, I took to the law and argued each case with my wife. And the muscular strength that it gave to my jaw has lasted the rest of my life.
Lewis Carroll: *Through the Looking Glass*

Other chapters in this book are concerned primarily with the physics and physiology of mechanical ventilatory support, the operational characteristics of ventilators in general, and the application of therapy through the use of specific positive-pressure devices. Newer forms of treatment, e.g., high-frequency ventilation, are addressed, and adjunctive treatment, including airway management, positive end-expiratory pressure (PEEP), and continuous positive airway pressure (CPAP) are considered in some detail. Generally speaking, all of these topics may be considered to relate to the "mechanics" of ventilatory support—how to provide it and sometimes why. During the past decade, however, additional considerations have been thrust to the forefront of the decision-making pro-

cesses in mechanical ventilation. Arguments concerning the merits of PEEP/CPAP, intermittent mandatory ventilation (IMV), assist-control ventilation, and similar techniques of support pale to insignificance when compared to those involving the ethics, morality, and law pertaining to mechanical ventilation, the decision to initiate it, and, most importantly, when it should be stopped. Unfortunately, the answers to these questions and even the questions themselves are unclear and in a continual state of flux. Nevertheless, a significant body of information is available with which every respiratory care practitioner—physician, therapist, and nurse—should be familiar. It is likely that all individuals who treat critically ill patients requiring long-term ventilator support will have to deal with the ethical and medico-legal aspects of such treatment. Forwarned is forearmed!

HISTORICAL CONSIDERATIONS

The issues mentioned above constitute a relatively new area of concern in regard to mechanical ventilation. Tank respirators (iron lungs) were used primarily for subacute and chronic long-term support, and the problems of discontinuation were encountered much less frequently than today. Patients either had a resolution of their problem or required ventilation for the rest of their lives. Intensive care as we view it today was nonexistent, and monitoring, if it was even available, was crude and relatively ineffectual.

Subsequently, however, resuscitation and critical care medicine evolved almost explosively, and patients who previously would not have survived their initial illness or injury could be supported by artificial means for long periods of time. New developments in surgery were made possible because of improved capabilities to support the patient during the operative and perioperative period. Open heart and organ transplantation procedures are but a few of the examples that can be cited. Although many factors are identifiable as contributory to this enhanced capability, mechanical ventilation has to be close to the top of the list, not because the ventilator ever "cured" any dysfunction but because it provided a means for patient survival (not previously available) until definitive therapy could be implemented.

As is usually the case with major advances in medical care, a price was extracted. Patients could also be supported, sometimes indefinitely, who had little chance for any return to normal or even functional integrity.[18] For such individuals, long-term mechanical ventilation served only to extend the process of dying, usually at tremendous expense. Not so many years ago, a diagnosis of terminal illness was followed within a relatively short period by the patient's death. Now, however, an average of 30 months passes between the time of diagnosis and the time of death. Furthermore, 80 percent of patient deaths now occur in hospitals or chronic care facilities rather than at home, and during the final year of life an average of 80 days of hospitalization has been documented.[18] Dying, then, is no longer a private event involving the patient, family, a few friends, and the physician, but has become a process with tremendous socioeconomic, medicolegal, religious, and ethical overtones. The problems do not go away, cannot be ignored, and must be faced by all individuals who are involved.

THE ETHICS

Most health care providers have no special interest or training in ethics or ethical decisions and may feel uncomfortable discussing the ethical issues involved in matters of life and death. Although persons know in their minds what they mean by "ethics," probably few individuals can define the term specifically. Young[21] has pointed out that ethics may be descriptive, as a discipline in which morality is studied and in which the arguments, logic, presuppositions, and values underlying moral positions are scrutinized and analyzed. Normatively, however, ethics is the discipline concerned with what "ought" to be. In the latter regard, medical ethics go beyond mere description, instead weighing the pros and cons of moral issues and then proposing reasoned solutions of them.

Unfortunately, ethical principles may be as diversified as the number of individuals who enumerate them. What is "ethical" to one person (or group) may be "unethical" to another. Cassem[4] suggested that ethical decisions in an intensive care setting ultimately relate to the appropriateness of therapy for a given disease process and went on to enumerate certain general principles. If a form of therapy can reasonably be expected to restore health and recovery, it may be judged to be necessary and ethically justifiable. To deliberately withhold such treatment is unethical. An appropriate example is a patient with chronic peptic ulcer disease who develops a life-threatening gastrointestinal hemorrhage unresponsive to conservative therapy and blood replacement. Surgical intervention in this case may reasonably be expected to be life-saving and to restore health. Such treatment is therefore necessary and ethically justifiable. However, if this patient had a known unresectable, incurable brain tumor and was comatose, and subsequently developed the same gastrointestinal hemorrhage, the same operation would be unnecessary, inappropriate, and unethical. Even if the bleeding problem is corrected, no possibility exists that the patient's primary health problem (the brain tumor) can be reversed or that he can be restored to health.

Although these clinical examples are chosen to illustrate a specific point, one can easily construct a slightly different scenario which might change the course of events. Thus if the patient with the incurable brain tumor and gastrointestinal bleeding desired the abdominal surgery so as to have a few extra days or weeks to put his affairs in order, the operation might be justifiable, even if unnecessary and/or unethical by the strict interpretation of the terms as they were discussed earlier.

Apparently decisions not to *initiate* therapy do not trouble physicians nearly as much as do those involved with the *termination* of treatment, although the perceived differences in the decision-making process are not at all clear. Cassem[4] stated that stopping treatment is *no* different than starting it if certain guidelines are kept in mind. Therapeutic interventions are usually begun in hopes of establishing a cure or buying time until a diagnosis can be made. The latter circumstances are typified by a trauma victim with a potentially lethal closed head injury who is brought to a hospital emergency room. Until a comprehensive neurological assessment is made, possibly including neurosurgical exploration, a physician should by all means intubate the trachea, establish ventilatory support, and provide whatever therapy is necessary at the time. After completion of the assessment, however, it is appropriate *ethically* to discontinue support if on the basis of his best judgment and the extent of then current medical knowledge the condition is completely irreversible. Considerations as to whether one may *legally* take such steps have resulted during the past decade in the concept of "brain death" and legislative action in the majority of the United States.[1,7]

Many physicians, however, employ such an analysis reluctantly if at all. Reasons include objections based on religious belief (although many organized religions hold that "extraordinary" life support is *not* required in hopeless cases). Also, a large number of physicians fear medicolegal reprisal if they terminate life support in such cases. Available evidence suggests that such fears, although not groundless, are much overrated. Thus moral and ethical decisions become entangled with legal and financial ones, creating a morass of apparently incomprehensible and conflicting data with no clearly established guidelines to be followed.

In an attempt to bring some order out of this apparent chaos, various solutions have been proposed, including the establishment of hospital ethics or prognosis committees which are charged with evaluating individual cases impartially and objectively and with making nonbinding recommendations regarding further treatment. Such committees are advisory only, and the members, usually including physicians and lay persons (attorneys, clergymen, etc.), do not have anything to do directly with the care of the patients in question. Unfortunately, probably less than 5 percent of hospitals in this country have established groups such as these, so in most cases the attending physician is "on his own."

Improvement in diagnostic techniques (EEG, CAT scans, etc.) enable a more objective prognosis to be formed than was once possible. These tests, when combined with more conventional assessment, make it less likely that an error in diagnosis or interpretation will occur. Also, since 1970, legislative "definitions of death"[7] have been promulgated widely, and if adhered to properly they make the physician and other personnel less culpable in possible later malpractice actions. Factors which have contributed to the enactment of such legislation include the need to ensure a supply of donor organs for transplantation. Thus quite apart from ethical considerations, the practicalities of supply and demand also govern the way a terminally ill patient may be handled.

For reasons that are not altogether clear, mechanical ventilators have become the focal point when a question of the termination of life support arises. Physicians, it seems, do not perceive the discontinuation of any other instrument, e.g., an intraaortic balloon counterpulsation device, to present nearly the same degree of ethical difficulty. In this latter case, treatment is initiated for a period of time which is usually clearly defined. If the patient's condition has not improved sufficiently to allow survival independent from the machine when that period has elapsed, support is usually discontinued without fanfare.[4] Conversely, a decision to "pull the plug" when ventilator support is involved never seems to come so easily. Because discontinuation of either support mode results in death for the patient who is dependent on it, the differences in psychological impact on those caring for the patient are not easily explained.

The level of public consciousness regarding the ethical and legal issues of life sup-

port and its termination was elevated by the landmark case of Karen Ann Quinlan in 1975.[12] However, similar cases obviously had occurred on previous occasions, and one would be naive indeed to believe that decisions to continue or discontinue terminal care were not made. Indeed, the concept of "judicious neglect" was discussed by at least one expert witness in the Quinlan hearings in New Jersey, who pointed out that previously such decisions in the unconscious or incompetent patients had been handled quietly by the family, physician, and hospital administrators. The Quinlan case brought the issues into the open for the first time. From that time forward, the public became involved.

THE LAW

Since 1975 certain court decisions involving the care of terminally ill patients have been rendered and have had real or perceived major impact on the practice of medicine.[10–12,20] In some cases the actual significance of the decisions has been misinterpreted, and what physicians and other health care providers thought the courts meant was apparently not what the judges intended. Most individuals involved in critical care are familiar with the major cases, but an abbreviated review of a selected number of them is appropriate.

Karen Ann Quinlan

Karen Ann Quinlan[6,12,16] was a young woman who was comatose with irreversible brain damage but not brain death. No reasonable hope for recovery existed, and her family desired removal of the life support devices, including a mechanical ventilator. Accordingly, her father filed suit to discontinue ventilator support, being opposed at the time by the attending physicians, the local prosecutor, and the state attorney general. His request was granted by the New Jersey Supreme Court in April 1976 (a year after the suit was initiated). Gradual weaning took place during May 1976, and the patient resumed breathing. The court stated forcefully that decision-making in such cases should rest in the hands of the incompetent patient's guardian, in consultation with a hospital ethics committee, and that judicial review was to be discouraged[12]:

> We consider that a practice of applying to a court to confirm such decisions would generally be inappropriate, not only because that would be a gratuitous encroachment upon the medical profession's field of competence, but because it would be impossibly cumbersome.

Joseph Saikewicz

Joseph Saikewicz[5,16,17,20] was a 67-year-old, profoundly retarded man (mental age 2 years, IQ 10) who in April 1976 was diagnosed as suffering from acute myeloblastic monocytic leukemia. Chemotherapy was expected to provide at best a temporary remission and would be painful and associated with many undesirable side effects, none of which could be explained to the patient or understood by him. A guardian ad litem appointed by the Hampshire County (Massachusetts) Probate Court concurred with the physicians and recommended that therapy be withheld. The Probate court subsequently agreed and entered an order to that effect which was affirmed by the Supreme Judicial Court in July 1976. In November 1977 the Supreme Court issued its report, concurring with the medical ethical position that "extraordinary means should not be employed to maintain life in cases where there is no hope for recovery." However, they disagreed with the New Jersey Supreme Court in Quinlan, stating that they took[12]:

> . . . a dim view of any attempt to shift the ultimate decision-making responsibility away from the duly established courts of

proper jurisdiction to any committee, panel or group, adhoc or permanent. . . . Rather, such questions of life and death seem to us to require the process of detached but passionate investigation and decision that forms the ideal on which the judicial branch of government was created. Achieving this ideal is our responsibility . . . and is not to be entrusted to any other group purporting to represent "the morality and conscience of our society," no matter how highly motivated or impressively constituted.

Thus in Massachusetts in 1977 the decision to withdraw or to withhold life support measures from terminally ill, incompetent patients apparently could be made only by appropriate courts of law.

Shirley Dinnerstein

Shortly after Saikewicz, another Massachusetts case also caught the public eye. Shirley Dinnerstein[10,13] was a 67-year-old woman with terminal Alzheimer's disease and a life-threatening coronary artery condition complicated by stroke. Her attending physician, who diagnosed her case as hopeless and her life expectancy at less than a year, wished to enter a "no code" (do not resuscitate) order in her chart. Dinnerstein's adult children concurred. Because such an order was believed possibly to be addressed by the recent Saikewicz decision, the question of the need for judicial approval was presented to the Norfolk County Probate Court, which in turn presented findings of fact to the Massachusetts Court of Appeals. In June 1978 the Appellate Court held that judicial approval was not necessary to enter a do not resuscitate order in the medical record of an irreversibly, terminally ill 67-year-old severely demented person. They distinguished the need for judicial approval of withholding treatment in Saikewicz because the proposed treatment there might have brought about a substantial remission of symptoms. By contrast, in the event of resuscitation from a cardiac arrest, Dinnerstein's case would still be hopeless.

Brother Joseph Fox

During a herniorrhaphy Brother Joseph Fox[11,15] sustained a cardiac arrest and, although resuscitated, never regained consciousness. Subsequently, he required ventilator support for the maintenance of respiration. When neurological consultants agreed that he was in a "permanent vegetative state" with a hopeless prognosis, his guardian requested the ventilator be discontinued. However, the attending physician, neurosurgical consultant, and hospital administration refused. To complicate matters, the Naussau County (New York) District Attorney had stated that anyone who disconnected life support apparatus could be prosecuted for homicide. Eventually, a ruling was obtained from the New York Supreme Court that treatment could be stopped, but the decision was appealed. In March 1980 the Appelate Division of the New York Supreme Court issued its ruling in which it restated "the right of the terminally ill to refuse treatment and to allow the natural process of death to run its course," and that these rights applied to both competent and incompetent patients. However, the court held that incompetent patients had to be terminally ill, in a vegetative coma characterized as chronic or irreversible, lacking cognitive brain function, and with an extremely remote possibility of recovery. The reasoning which was behind approval for the removal of life support devices from such patients was that:

> As a matter of established fact, such a patient has no health and, in the true sense, no life for the State to protect. . . . Indeed, with Roe [abortion opinion] in mind, it is appropriate to note that the State's interest in preservation of the life of the fetus would appear greater than any possible interest the State may have in maintaining the life of a terminally ill comatose patient . . . [whose] claim to personhood is certainly no greater than that of a fetus.

In other words, a chronically vegetative patient was decreed to be dead. However, an elaborate judicial process was directed which, at a minimum, would require four to six physicians, five attorneys, and a judge before a ventilator would be withdrawn from a terminally ill, chronically vegetative patient.[15] The results of such litigation in the words of Father Philip Eichner, who as guardian for Fox sought to have ventilator support discontinued, is "a lawyer's paradise not to mention a doctor's bonanza."

Comment

As is clear from a comparison of the preceding four cases, no consensus exists concerning the procedures for termination of life support for incompetent, terminally ill patients. However, the picture may not be as black as is often portrayed. For example, Justice Paul J. Liacos, author of the Saikewicz decision, pointed out that the Massachusetts Attorney General's Office argued both for the protection of the patient's life through the administration of chemotherapy and, through its civil rights division, for the right of the patient, competent or incompetent, to refuse such treatment. Hence the civil rights division recognized the duty of the state to ensure the exercise of this choice in the face of what it construed to be less substantial state interests. In the final analysis, the court rejected the traditional parens patriae doctrine that the interests of the state with respect to the preservation of life always prevails against the interest of individuals to make their own choice concerning their bodies and fate.

Liacos also stated that questions of life, death, morality, ethics, and individual rights have been traditional concerns of the judiciary in a wide variety of human endeavors. That the medical profession should be exempted from court scrutiny would deny the very principles on which our society was founded.[2] The judiciary is the only institution charged with protecting individual rights and the rights of the State in an impartial fashion.[13]

Finally, he suggested that Dinnerstein should never have been litigated and that in Saikewicz it was never the court's intention that a "do not resuscitate" order could not be written or that a terminally ill patient had to be resuscitated time after time in the absence of a court order to the contrary. He stated that such an interpretation represented poor legal advice given to both physicians and hospitals and that most of the controversy in Saikewicz was the result of misinterpretation and misinformation by lawyers who should know better.[13]

Returning to the definition of ethics mentioned earlier, we may ask what "ought" to be done in circumstances similar to those of Quinlan, Saikewicz, Dinnerstein, and Fox. Paris addressed this problem eloquently, referring to John Rawls Theory of Justice, and suggested that at the least[15]:

> . . . one would insist on a procedure that would not be unreasonably dragged out, that would not distress one's family, and that—as much as the human condition of fallibility allows—would not fail to safeguard the right to decide to struggle for yet another morning or slip gently into the night.

He further stated that such individuals would not wish a full adversarial hearing and the unwelcome, costly, and cumbersome arena of litigation. Technological advancements have made death more dramatic, but the questions of life and death are not new. They have been determined within families and with physician guidance since the dawn of history.[15]

LEGISLATION

Another problem closely related to those already discussed is the determination of death. Classic pronouncement, which considers only cessation of cardiopulmonary function, has long been regarded as inadequate in selected cases in which technologically advanced life support measures are capable of maintaining vegetative existence long after higher cerebral function has ceased. Early attempts to define irreversible loss of cerebral function or brain death either were too restrictive or were generally not accepted by the medical community.

Brain Death Statutes (Definitions of Death)

Since 1970 the majority of states have enacted legislation based on either the American Bar Association's proposed definition of death[7] or the Capron-Kass[3] models. Although the wording differs to some extent, as does the interpretation from one state to another, the following is more or less representative:

> A person will be considered dead if in the opinion of a physician, based on ordinary standards of approved medical practice, the person has experienced an irreversible cessation of spontaneous respiratory and circulatory function. In the event that artificial means of support preclude a determination that these functions have ceased, a person will be considered dead if in the announced opinion of a physician, based upon ordinary standards of approved medical practice, the person has experienced an irreversible cessation of brain function. Death will have occurred at the time when the relevant functions ceased. In any case, when organs are to be used in a transplant, an additional physician, not a member of the transplant team, must make the pronouncement of death.

Many reasons can be cited which led to the enactment of such legislation, including a desire to reduce the cost of care of hopeless cases, the need to free intensive care beds for other patients with a reasonable chance of survival, and the maintenance of the supply of transplant organs. Although such legislation has been generally regarded as enlightened, objections have been raised. The problem, according to Byrne et al.,[1] is the equating of loss of brain function with death of the brain or of the person. They suggest that legislative attempts to "define" death are misguided.

> Death is the word we use to name a certain empirically given state of affairs, a state difficult to describe in full generality, yet one with which we are all too familiar as a situation of fact. Someone we have known ceases to breathe, sags wherever not supported; we find no pulse; there is no sign of inner activity or of reaction; all is silent, inert then cold; the body grows rigid, later becomes flaccid and begins to putrify, decomposing until only bones remain. Most importantly, from a certain moment on—"the moment of death"—whatever happens, whether it involves putrescence, mummification, incineration, or nuclear vaporization, is entirely describable in terms of disintegration, dissolution, destruction of the unity of the single organism that was formerly present: a human being has, so far as this world can tell, simply ceased to be.

Legislative definitions of death actually refer to criteria by which death may be inferred to have taken place, not to death itself. In the past, general criteria (cessation of cardiopulmonary function) were intended to prevent the possibility that someone who was alive would be mistakenly treated as dead. Newer "definitions of death" may be construed to prevent someone who is "dead" from being treated as alive. Byrne et al. suggested that our ability to determine that brain death (destruction of the brain) has occurred is imperfect and our methods are in a continual state of flux. Historically, cessation of spontaneous ventilation, and later of cardiac function, were considered to be diagnostic of death. Yet nowadays such events are commonly treated, not only by medical personnel but also by lay people. They are, in fact, often

reasons for admission to an intensive care unit. Current diagnostic tests, though technically more advanced, may be similarly criticized at some time in the future.

Although such arguments have a logical appeal, they are not practical. Should a physician be required to biopsy the brain to determine that putrescence is actually present? Would a single sample from a specific location be necessarily representative of the entire brain? Carried to their logical conclusion, such arguments might preclude the declaration of death of a terminally ill, apneic patient with no detectable cardiac or brain function who is maintained for days, weeks, or (in the future) months by extracorporeal circulation. Such a state of affairs seems neither necessary or desirable. As Byrne et al. pointed out, once rigor mortis is observed, we can certainly conclude that death has occurred.[1] That we should wait for this event seems unrealistic at best.

Natural Death Statutes

At least 14 states (Alabama, Arkansas, California, Delaware, Idaho, Kansas, Nevada, New Mexico, North Carolin, Oregon, Texas, Vermont, Virginia, and Washington) as well as the District of Columbia have enacted legislation which establishes a way for patients, while competent, to direct that at the end of their lives, if they become incompetent, treatment will not include artificial interventions which prolong dying.[6] Such statutes proscribe the formalities which must be observed in the establishment of such a directive, exclusions, revocation, the duration or term of the directive, duties of physicians to patients who have chosen this means of overseeing their final days, and in some cases penalties to be assessed against those who do not comply. Certain precautionary clauses also are incorporated, including the fact that any individual who initiates such a directive is *not* committing suicide. Physicians who comply with the directive, so long as they act in good faith and are not negligent, are immune from civil and criminal prosecution.

Although these statutes are well conceived, they do not help many of the problems they were designed to eliminate. For example, the California natural death act (the first in the nation) provides that a terminally ill patient must wait 14 days after being told of his/her illness before signing a directive.[21] Yet a study by California physicians 1 year after the law was enacted found that only one-half the patient's diagnosed as terminally ill (death being imminent regardless of the life-sustaining procedures used) were still conscious by 14 days.[6] Furthermore, patients such as Karen Quinlan, who in part was the inspiration for such acts, would not be helped by them because their deaths would not be imminent. Indeed, the total number of such patients to whom such legislation applies constitutes a relatively small percentage of all such patients from whom decisions about life-sustaining equipment must be made.

Durable Power of Attorney Statutes

A durable power of attorney is a document by which an individual (principal) legally authorizes another person to perform certain acts on his behalf, including decisions about health care matters if the principal becomes incompetent.[6] Unlike common-law powers of attorney, a durable one allows the agent to act even when the principal is incapacitated. At least 42 states have such laws. Although durable power of attorney statutes were not specifically developed for health care decision-making, they are easily accommodated to such purposes. However, because little experience has been gained in this regard, further study of their applicability is warranted. One obvious problem is the possibility that the individual on whom the durable power of attorney is conferred may have a vested interest in the outcome (debtor, creditor, heir, etc.).

PROBLEMS OF DECISION-MAKING

Withdrawal (or withholding) of life support is for the most part exclusively a problem involving unconscious or incompetent patients.[8] At the very least, physicians must be as certain as they can about the condition of the patients in question. A determination of unconsciousness generally is based on evidence that an individual has no response to the internal or external environment (except unmodulated reflexes), engages in no purposeful activity, and gives no evidence of mental activity. The condition must also be permanent, so far as the current state of medical knowledge and past experience allow one to make such an inference.[17,21]

If one sifts through the massive amount of material relating to terminal care and its withdrawal, he cannot help but be suspicious that the useless continuation of life support in a permanently unconscious or completely incompetent patient is based on fear of a possible malpractice action at a later date or of civil or criminal prosecution. This is not to say that many people are not guided by moral or religious principles which prevent them from accepting any form of "enthanasia," active or passive. To them, the withholding or withdrawing of life support violates the basic principles which guide their entire lives. No criticism should be levied against them. At most, such individuals should be encouraged to transfer the care of patients who fall into the above described categories to other physicians not constrained by the same factors. No doubt some physicians do not become actively involved in such decisions because for them it is easier to continue support than to engage in frank and meaningful discussions with the family about discontinuation.

However, the number of such individuals must be very small.

With respect to euthanasia, the distinction made by Young[21] is useful between "benemortasia"—a good death accomplished by simply allowing the disease to take its course while providing palliative treatment for pain—and "euthanasia"—a good death caused by withdrawal of one or more forms of treatment without which the patient cannot survive. The distinction between the two involves the difference between actions and omissions that lead to death. Although these differences on occasion are obscure, such is not usually the case. Just as no *ethical* difference can be established between not starting a form of therapy (omission) and withdrawing it once started (action),[4] so also nothing in law makes stopping a treatment more serious than not starting it.[17] In fact, *not* starting treatment which may be in the patient's best interest may be held more serious in a civil or criminal court than withdrawing it once it is found to be of no benefit.

Although the question of euthanasia is not yet resolved, that of mercy killing is. In all states, mercy killing is forbidden by law, and a prohibition against it is contained in all the natural death statutes which have been enacted.[6,20]

> Nothing in this chapter shall be construed to condone, authorize, or approve mercy killing, or to permit any affirmative or deliberate act or omission to end life other than to permit the internal process of dying as provided in this chapter.

Even here, however, the courts have been extremely lenient, even compassionate, in the few cases on record for both physicians and lay persons. To some extent, it seems that how harshly an individual is dealt with depends on the motivation which was present, i.e., was "mercy" really involved?[21] Thus the continuous administration of morphine to control intolerable pain but also to depress respiration and ulti-

mately result in death would probably be viewed more leniently than would strangulation. Of interest is the fact that until recently only two American physicians were ever tried for mercy killing, and both were acquitted by juries.[6] For the most part, prosecutors are often reluctant to pursue such issues either because they have empathy for the individuals involved or because of the historical difficulty in obtaining a conviction. In one well known case the court stated that:

> . . . it is reported that apparently no prosecutor has proceeded to trial in a case where a physician chose to terminate life-preserving treatment or omit emergency treatment in a hopeless case. [In re Spring, 405 N.E.2d 115, 121 (Mass, 1980)]

More recently, however, two physicians were indicted on criminal liability charges of murder and conspiracy to commit murder involving deliberate omissions of care. The indictments were dismissed after a preliminary hearing.[6] For the foreseeable future, society seems disposed to maintain the statutory prohibition against mercy killing but to deal compassionately with individuals, physicians and nonphysicians alike, who take the law into their own hands to end the suffering of terminally ill patients.[6,21]

Baby Doe I and II

The rapid growth of the neonatal intensive care field and the significant improvement in survival of premature infants have created new problems. Despite the reduction in mortality, significant numbers of babies still die during the neonatal period. As in the case in adult intensive care, costs have skyrocketed ($1.5 billion in 1978), and legal and ethical problems have kept pace.

In a now "famous" case[19,21] the parents of a newborn child with Down's syndrome, tracheoesophageal atresia, and possible other anomalies elected to forego treatment. Child welfare authorities brought suit to prevent this decision, but a trial court sustained the parents' position. In the wake of this decision, however, the Department of Health and Human Services (DHHS) published a proposed rule, "Discrimination Against the Handicapped by Withholding Treatment or Nourishment: Notice to Health Care Providers" (from the Office of the Secretary, Department of Health and Human Services, 47 Federal Regulation 26, 027, 16 June 1982). Although the initial rule was struck down in federal court, a second was recently published. In essence, it states that it is unlawful for a recipient of federal financial assistance to withhold from a handicapped infant nutritional sustenance or medical or surgical treatment required to correct a life-threatening condition if: (1) the withholding is based on the fact that the infant is handicapped; and (2) the handicap does not render the treatment or nutritional sustenance medically contraindicated. Notices to be placed in hospitals include a toll-free DHHS "hotline" number to enable anyone suspecting that such events are taking place the opportunity to report them. In response, a "Special Assignment Baby Doe Squad" is to be dispatched immediately to investigate the complaint.

Quite apart from the legality of such proceedings, the question which has been raised is whether the federal government can effectively dictate and enforce a standard of medical decision-making to apply to every critically ill infant in every hospital without, in the process, jeopardizing the health of the subjects it is allegedly trying to protect.[19] Furthermore, the implications of such a process, should it in the future be applied to the incompetent adult patient, are staggering.

TERMINAL WEANING

Although much has been written about the legal and ethical aspects of withdrawing life-sustaining measures, almost nothing has been detailed about the mechanics. Once a patient has been determined to be in a persistently vegetative state and the decision has been made to stop all but hygienic and comfort care, how does one go about discontinuing ventilator support? As Grenvik pointed out in a recent editorial,[9] abrupt termination may be viewed as an act committed with intent to kill. To forestall this impression, a "terminal weaning" protocol has been developed at the University of Pittsburgh.

The major difference between regular and terminal weaning is that the latter proceeds despite deterioration in vital signs and arterial blood gas and pH measurements. In addition, the process continues over a period of hours rather than days, and many patients die in this phase. As was the case with Karen Quinlan, an occasional patient tolerates weaning and extubation. Should gasping or other signs of "distress" appear, incremental doses of morphine, 1–2 mg, are given intravenously. Such treatment, of course, has no effect on the patient insofar as awareness or suffering are concerned because by definition these are nonexistent, but it may benefit the family members and intensive care unit personnel who will be upset by signs of suffering.

Although one may be able to generate a philosophical debate as to whether there is really any difference between abrupt discontinuation or more gradual terminal weaning over a period of hours, it seems that the method suggested by Grenvik has a great deal in favor of it with respect to the family's response. It is at least one measure which can be employed to prevent prolongation of dying.

CONCLUSIONS

In one chapter it is impossible to do more than skim the surface of the complex medicolegal and ethical considerations of terminally ill patients and their care. That this is so, however, is a reflection of just how far we have come during the past decade. Ten years ago this chapter probably could not have been written because the subject matter was largely taboo. During the intervening period, physicians, attorneys, judges, philosophers, ethicists, legislators, and others too numerous to count have become increasingly concerned about the issues which must be dealt with.

Many physicians in the past considered the loss of each patient as a personal defeat and felt obligated to carry on therapy regardless of the hopelessness in a given case. Human beings, at least so far as their earthly existence is concerned, are not immortal, and a time comes when it should be relatively clear to all concerned that to continue therapy and resuscitation serves no useful purpose. A final point written by a long-suffering patient before he turned off his ventilator expressed this most poignantly: "Death is not the enemy, doctor, humanity is."[14] Public awareness, with respect to the problems and possible solutions which have been proposed, is at an all time high. Although court decisions and legislative actions may not always be either enlightened or correct (and who is to say?), the fact that they exist at all is testimony to the interest and concern which are inherent in their formulation. Physicians and respiratory therapists, nurses, and all others charged with the responsibility to care for the terminally ill owe it to themselves and their patients to become familiar with the problems and to participate in finding the solutions.

REFERENCES

1. Byrne PA, O'Reilly S, Quay PM: Brain death—an opposing viewpoint. JAMA 242:1985, 1979

2. Callahan D: Shattuck lecture—contemporary biomedical ethics. N Engl J Med 302:1228, 1980

3. Capron AM, Kass LR: A statutory definition for the standards for determining human death: an appraisal and a proposal. Univ PA Law Rev 121:87, 1972

4. Cassem NH: Ethical considerations in critical care: Refresher Courses Anesthesiol 5:13, 1977

5. Curran WJ: Law-medicine notes: the Saikewicz decision. N Engl J Med 298:499, 1978

6. Deciding to Forego Life-Sustaining Treatment: Ethical, Medical and Legal Issues in Treatment Decisions. President's Commission for the Study of Ethical Problems in Medicine and Biomedical and Behaviorial Research. US Government Printing Office, Washington, DC, 1983

7. Dornette WHL: How does your state define death? Leg Aspects Med Pract 8:11, 1980

8. Dunn LJ Jr: Who "pulls the plug": the practical aspect of the Saikewicz decision. Med Malpract Cost Contain J 1:161, 1979

9. Grenivk A: "Terminal weaning": discontinuation of life-support therapy in the terminally ill patient. Crit Care Med 11:394, 1983

10. In re Dinnerstein, 380 N.E. 2d 134 (Mass App Ct 1978)

11. In re Eichner, AD2d, 637 E, March 28, 1980, Supreme Court: Appellate Division Second Department

12. In re Quinlan, 70 N.J. 10, 355 A.2d 647, act denied, 429 U.S. 922 (1976)

13. Liacos PJ: Dilemmas of dying. Medicoleg News 7:4, 1979

14. Opp M: Pulling the plug. Med World News 29 May 1978

15. Paris JJ: Court intervention and the diminution of patients' rights: the case of Brother Joseph Fox. N Engl J Med 303:876, 1980

16. Savage D: After Quinlan and Saikewicz: death, life, and God committees. Crit Care Med 8:87, 1980

17. Schram RB, Kane JC Jr, Roble DT: "No code" orders: clarification in the aftermath of Saikewicz. N Engl J Med 299:875, 1978

18. Snider GL: Thirty years of mechanical ventilation: changing implications. Arch Intern Med 143:745, 1983

19. Strain E: The American Academy of Pediatrics comments on the "Baby Doe II" regulations. N Engl J Med 309:443, 1983

20. Superintendent of Belechertown State School vs Saikewicz, Massachusetts Supreme Judicial Court NO. 5JC-711, 1977

21. Young EWD: Euthanasia: a new civil right? In: Civil Rights: A Staff Report of the Subcommittee on Constitutional Rights of the Committee on the Judiciary. United States Senate, 94th Congress, Second Session, 1976, pp. 277–300

9

High-Frequency Ventilation: History, Theory, and Practice

Neel B. Ackerman, Jr.
Donald M. Null, Jr.
Robert A. deLemos

> New things are usually feared and re-
> jected: rejected because of a belief that they
> would not work; feared because of a suspi-
> cion that they might.
>
> A.R. Feinstein, M.D.
> West Haven, Conn.

Techniques of high-frequency ventilation (HFV) have been viewed as a new and innovative respiratory approach, although in fact the underlying theory was described almost 70 years ago.[69] Since their redis-covery by Sjöstrand, Bryan, and others,[14,18,27,31,44,56,60,81,132] they have re-ceived great attention as tools for better un-derstanding of respiratory gas exchange and as a group of techniques theoretically ca-pable of providing respiratory support with a decreased risk of airway injury. The pur-poses of this chapter are to define the ter-minology, history, physiology, and clinical application of HFV.

DEFINITIONS

No unanimity of opinion exists as to what constitutes HFV. The problem occurs be-cause different species and different ages of animals breathe at different rates; therefore what may be a supraphysiological respira-tory rate in one setting is normal in another. In this discussion, we consider HFV to be ventilation with a rate at least twice the rest-ing respiratory rate and a tidal volume close to or less than the anatomical dead space.

High-frequency techniques are usually categorized in three groups: (1) high-fre-quency positive-pressure ventilation (HFPPV); (2) high-frequency jet ventilation (HFJV) or high-frequency flow interrup-tion (HFFI); and (3) high-frequency oscil-latory ventilation (HFOV). HFPPV refers to the use of a low-compliance ventilator to deliver small volumes through a small air-way at frequencies of 1–2 Hz (one Hz = 60 cycles/minute). HFJV and HFFI describe systems which deliver small volumes at high velocities through a narrow orifice. A high-pressure source is interrupted intermittently to produce pulsatile gas flow, and additional gas is usually entrained to augment volume delivery. Rates vary from 1 to 20 Hz depending on the system and clinical model. As can be seen from the definitions, some ventilators can be placed in either group 1 or 2, and as such the categorical assignments may be somewhat arbitrary. HFOV uses a piston or diaphragm oscillator in line with the patient's airway. With HFOV, no net displacement of gas occurs in and of itself, so a source of bias gas flow must be provided into the ventilator circuit. Oscillators have been shown to function at frequencies of 50 Hz or higher.

The method by which HFV is delivered and the pulmonary pathology of the subject affects the physiology of gas transport, the optimum frequency, and the clinical response. Therefore one high-frequency technique may prove to be best suited to a selected set of circumstances whereas others fail.

HISTORICAL PERSPECTIVE

In 1915 Henderson et al.,[69] observing rapid, shallow breathing in dogs during heat "polypnea," commented: "There may easily be a gaseous exchange sufficient to support life even when tidal volume is considerably less than the dead space." As an integral part of their observations, they performed experiments which still form the basis for our incomplete understanding of how gas exchange is accomplished during HFV. Brisco et al.[25] confirmed Henderson et al.'s observations and demonstrated that with tidal volumes as small as 60 ml (in a patient with a dead space of 170 ml), alveolar gas exchange occurred.

By the late 1950s Emerson suggested that the application of high-frequency oscillations during ventilation with a conventional positive-pressure ventilator improved pulmonary gas mixing. In 1959 he patented a device which "vibrated" gas in the airway and asserted that "vibrating the column of gas undoubtedly causes the gas to diffuse more rapidly within the airway and, therefore, aids in the breathing function by circulating the gas more thoroughly."[136] This device, although probably the first true high-frequency ventilator, was never fully applied or adequately tested. Scotter et al.[130] demonstrated enhanced dispersion of gases into porous materials by using either sinusoidal gas flows or oscillations; and Lunkenheimer et al.,[95,96] during studies on cardiac impedance in dogs, fortuitously discovered that eucapnia could be maintained while oscillating the animal's airway at rates of 23–40 Hz after placing a loudspeaker diaphragm at the orifice of an endotracheal tube. These investigations were the first to report *conclusively* that effective ventilation of animals could be accomplished with tidal volumes that were less than the dead space volume. Other investigators have confirmed and expanded these results during the past several years.

Insufflation techniques similar to those now used in HFJV were described during the early 1900s.[101,113] Their use was short-lived, however, because of the introduction of the McGill endotracheal tube. This form of ventilation was not reevaluated with respect to patient application until 1956 by Jacoby et al.[77] They used an 18-gauge needle inserted transtracheally with oxygen flow at 4–6 L/minute and demonstrated that adequate oxygenation was possible; within 30 minutes, however, ventilation proved inadequate. Sanders[122] described a technique for ventilating patients during bronchoscopy. He used a 50-psi oxygen source connected to a small cannula. Adequate oxygenation and ventilation were obtained by intermittently opening and occluding the jet of oxygen. He also noted that flow and volume were enhanced by gas entrainment. Spoerel et al.[140] and Jacobs[76] obtained effective ventilation through small transtra-

$$\text{ALVEOLAR VENTILATION} = \left[\text{TIDAL VOLUME} - \text{DEAD SPACE VOLUME}\right] \times \text{VENTILATORY FREQUENCY}$$

Fig. 9-1. The classic relationship between alveolar ventilation, tidal volume, and dead space volume. If applied to HFV when the tidal volume is less than the dead space volume, alveolar ventilation is predicted to be zero. Thus gas exchange during HFV must occur via alternative mechanisms.

cheal catheters. Spoerel used a Bird Mark 2 pressure-limited, time-cycled ventilator at rates of 12–16 breaths/minute and 50 psi driving pressure. Jacobs used 60 psi driving pressure and similar low rates. Klain et al.,[87] using a 14-gauge angiocath placed transtracheally and connected to a fluidic ventilator, obtained adequate gaseous exchange at rates of 20–200 breaths/minute. They coined the term high-frequency jet ventilation.

During the early 1970s Sjöstrand and associates described positive-pressure ventilation with low compressibility ventilators at rates of 60–100/minute. They used a small insufflation catheter or endotracheal tube and a pneumatic valve connected to a time-cycled volume-controlled ventilator.[80,81,131] By the mid 1970s, HFPPV was used clinically for bronchoscopy, laryngoscopy, pediatric anesthesia, and neonatal artificial ventilation.

PHYSIOLOGY

Classic pulmonary physiology presumes that alveolar ventilation is determined by respiratory frequency and alveolar volume (Fig. 9-1).[41] It has also been assumed that alveolar ventilation is impossible when dead space volume exceeds tidal volume. However, in HFV the tidal volume is often considerably less than the anatomical dead space, yet adequate alveolar ventilation has been demonstrated using a wide variety of

techniques. A number of theories have been advanced to explain these observations, but none can explain all facets of the observed phenomenon.[40,46,50,61,62,74,75,83,93,94,105,107, 118,120,121,123,124,126, 135, 137, 138]

In normal spontaneous breathing, air is transported in the large proximal airways primarily by convective mechanisms. Wilson and Lin[150] estimated that pure convective forms of transport dominate until the eighth bronchial generation. When the airways narrow and convective velocities decrease, radial diffusion becomes an additional transport mode,[22] whereas molecular and axial diffusion seem to be major factors in the most distal air spaces.[150] During HFV, gas dispersion is enhanced so that less of the airway is involved in bulk convective flow and other less well defined, dispersive mechanisms predominate (Fig. 9-2). Most investigators have developed their hypotheses as extensions of a model suggested by Taylor to explain the dispersion of gases in areas of turbulent flow.[144] Fredberg proposed that augmented diffusion in the large airways combined with molecular diffusion at the periphery of the lung can explain most of the gas transport during HFV.[61,137] It is interesting that Fredberg's concept predicts an optimum frequency not based entirely on the diffusive mechanisms themselves but also on the pressure, flow, size, and tensile strength characteristics of the airway. Scherer and Haselton[125] believed that a longitudinal convective transport mechanism may exist in the airway. They measured the effective axial diffusivity of gas as it passed through a bronchial tree model and noted that axial *diffusivity* was 4000 times greater tham molecular diffusion when the velocity of flow was 100 cm/second.[125] The mechanism allegedly depends on differences in the shapes that exist between the inspiratory and expiratory waveform velocity profiles during both laminar and turbulent flow in airways and not on bulk flow itself (similar to the observation by Henderson et al. in 1915[69]); Fig. 9-3). The importance of crit-

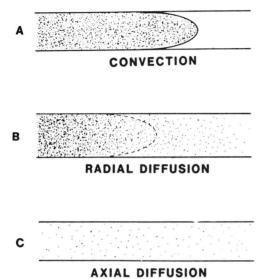

CONVECTION

RADIAL DIFFUSION

AXIAL DIFFUSION

Fig. 9-2. (A) Convective or bulk flow predominate in large airways. In these airways, convection is so rapid that no appreciable time is available for diffusion. (B) When the airways decrease in caliber and the relative cross-sectional area increases, convective velocities decrease and radial diffusion, which smooths out concentration differences along the radius of the tube, become a prominent transport mode. (C) Beyond the 12th generation, axial gas velocity is so slow that no radial diffusion occurs and thus transport occurs by convective block flow and axial diffusion.[15]

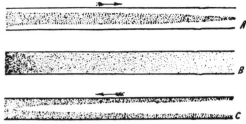

Fig. 9-3. The Henderson "spike." (A) If smoke is blown into one end of a long glass tube, it does not immediately fill the tube but, instead, passes to the other end as a thin spike. Although the volume of smoke is less than that of the tube, it nevertheless is able to traverse the entire length. The quicker the puff, the thinner and sharper the spike. (B) If as the tip of the spike reaches the distal end the proximal end is occluded by the tongue, the spike instantaneously breaks up and fills the tube. (C) When an inspiration occurs, a thin spike of clean air passes through the smoke-filled tube from the distal end back to the smoker's mouth. (Reproduced from Henderson Y, Chillingworth FP, Whitney JL: et al: The respiratory dead space. Am J Physiol 38:1, 1915.)

erate simultaneously, convection generally predominating in the upper airways where gas velocities are high and diffusion predominating in the lower and peripheral airways where gas velocities are low (Fig. 9-4). More exact information regarding mech-

ical inspiratory flows and flow velocities is supported by observations made during continuous-flow apneic ventilation and HFJV.

Investigators have noted that the position of the airway catheter is extremely critical, with 1–2 cm difference in positioning the tip causing marked changes in ventilation.[10,84,92] Slutsky et al.[138] have shown that the most important factor in CO_2 elimination during HFV is the magnitude of the inspiratory flow.

It seems that lower ranges of HFV primarily act through enhanced convection whereas the higher-frequency ranges result in augmented diffusive exchange. However, in most circumstances both modes op-

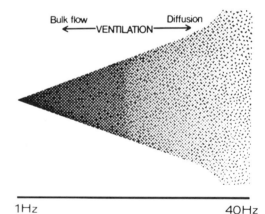

Fig. 9-4. A spectrum of gas exchange from pure convection to pure diffusion occurs as ventilatory frequency increases.

anisms of gas transport is not available because of the geometrical complexity of the bronchial tree. Further elucidation awaits the development of improved mathematical and physical models or more refined and innovative animal experiments to better define the complex parameters involved in gas exchange.

During HFV, oxygenation is closely related to the mean airway pressure, as it is during conventional ventilation.[20,23,60,90,99,102,147] This relationship is best shown when the underlying pulmonary condition involves diffuse alveolar injury. HFV has also been shown to improve the distribution of gas during ventilation, thus "homogenizing" the ventilation/perfusion ($\dot{V}/\dot{Q}$) ratio.[27,49,54] The observation of Calkins et al.[30] that airway diameter changes uniformly during inspiration tends to confirm the observation made regarding homogeneous gas distribution. In situations where oxygenation is altered by a $\dot{V}/\dot{Q}$ mismatch (chronic obstructive pulmonary disease; COPD), a significant reduction in intrapulmonary shunt has been demonstrated during HFOV, presumably as a result of the improvement of gas distribution.[27]

The pressure relationships seen within airways are of great interest to many investigators. At slow ventilatory rates the pressure distribution is such that peak pressures reached in the proximal and distal airways are approximately equal.[119] On a theoretical basis, distal peak airway pressures should be lower at higher respiratory frequencies. If the airways responded similarly to a series of rigid tubes of decreasing diameter, a predictable pressure modulation would occur as frequency increases.[115,119] However, attempts to measure airway pressures directly have led to the preliminary conclusion that such theoretical predictions may not be valid under all circumstances. In fact, some investigators have measured distal peak pressures higher than those in the proximal airway.[3,5] The mechanisms involved in the production of

the higher pressures are not fully defined but are more likely to occur when the inspiratory/expiratory (I:E) ratio is greater than 50 percent and/or distal lung compliance is low. The higher distal pressures are most likely related to high expiratory resistance ("air trapping") and the elastic recoil of the airways themselves. Thus one cannot assume that HFV is uniformly associated with lower peak pressures in the distal airways.

Estimation of alveolar pressures after transient clamp occlusion of the proximal airway during HFV has also produced unexpected results.[3,55] The equilibration pressure distal to the clamp is an approximation of alveolar pressure in an unobstructed system. Alveolar pressures measured in this manner have also been higher than proximal airway pressures under some circumstances. As with peak airway pressures, the paradoxical results seem to occur most frequently in situations where lung compliance is poor and the I:E ratio long. Because of these data, no predictions can be made regarding the role of HFV in the prevention of pulmonary baroinjury. Because the circumstances (poor lung compliance) where baroinjury is most likely are similar to those where paradoxical pressure relationships have been observed, the widespread use of HFV for *prevention* of pulmonary baroinjury needs to be delayed until realistic theoretical models or carefully designed animal and human trials have been performed.

A great deal of interest has been directed to a comparison between the effects of HFV and conventional ventilation (CV) on cardiovascular function. Conflicting data exist regarding the effects on cardiac output. Several studies have shown no statistically significant difference between cardiac parameters measured during comparable HFV and CV trials.[43,48,71,102,128,134,143,147] However, other studies have shown a decrease in cardiac output and/or an increase in pulmonary artery mean pressure in animals ventilated with HFV.[7,37,39,70,100,141]

Investigators have observed that healthy dogs with normal lungs can be ventilated with different HFV techniques at lower mean airway pressures while maintaining similar cardiac outputs compared to the same dogs ventilated with conventional techniques. However, if diffuse pulmonary injury is induced, similar or higher mean airway pressures may be required during HFV, and cardiac outputs are often lower than conventionally ventilated controls.[141] The cardiac variability seen during spontaneous respiration and conventional ventilation and the interdependence of lung inflation and left ventricular stroke output are not seen with HFV; however, no recognizable problems have been detected from their absence. Recent attempts by several groups to synchronize HFJV with the cardiac cycle have proved the feasibility of the technique. However, synchronization has not produced consistent augmentation of cardiac output or any other cardiovascular benefits.[33,34,112]

Problems have emerged when HFV is attempted in conditions associated with a left-to-right shunt. During positive- or negative-pressure ventilation, lung inflation exerts a mechanical effect on the pulmonary vascular bed, increasing resistance selectively in the pulmonary circuit.[65,145] This effect tends to decrease the magnitude of the left-to-right shunt. In a premature baboon model of respiratory distress syndrome, cardiovascular deterioration associated with patency of the ductus arteriosus is much more common during high-frequency ventilation than during conventional ventilation.[2] This observation, if confirmed in the human infant, might preclude the use of high-frequency techniques in infants with respiratory disease and a left-to-right vascular shunt. A number of studies with HFV have also revealed an unexplained metabolic acidosis after prolonged respiratory support.[2,95,96,117] More detailed studies of cardiovascular function, including measurements of tissue perfusion, are needed be-

fore we can say with certainty that these techniques have no adverse cardiovascular effects.[139]

Finally, some experimental and clinical data regarding the effect of HFV on the neural control of ventilation have become available. Several investigators have noted that in some animals and humans spontaneous respiration is ablated during HFV.[27,90,151] Thompson et al.[146] showed that bilateral vagotomy completely reversed this effect, suggesting an inhibitory mechanism on the respiratory center mediated by stretch receptors in the lung. This hypothesis has been confirmed by Man et al.,[98] who demonstrated the HFV increased discharge of pulmonary afferent fibers continuously and to a degree greater than that seen during static lung inflation. They postulated that the increased vagal activity seen during HFV probably caused inhibition of phrenic nerve activity through a central effect. The possibility of a central mechanism is further reinforced by observations made by Bryan,[26] who noted that during REM sleep patients who were apneic resumed respiratory efforts. The apneic effect of HFV is a matter of concern until the effects of HFV on other pulmonary receptor systems is established.

TECHNIQUES OF HFV

High-Frequency Positive-Pressure Ventilation

Sjöstrand et al.,[68,131,133,134] Bland et al.,[17] and others[19,21,47,67,80,81] have reported extensively on the use of either conventional ventilators or specially designed low-compliance systems which cycle at frequencies two to six times the normal physiological rate (Fig. 9-5). Premature infants with respiratory distress syndrome (RDS) have been successfully ventilated at rates up to 2.5 Hz using modified conventional ventilators and low tidal volumes.[17,67] The prev-

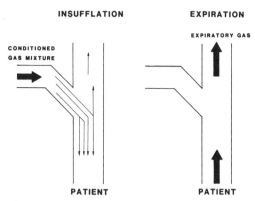

INSUFFLATION   **EXPIRATION**

Fig. 9-5. A "pneumatic valve" for use in HFPPV. (Modified and reproduced with permission from Sjöstrand U (ed): Experimental and clinical evaluation of high-frequency positive-pressure ventilation HFPPV. Acta Anaesthesiol Scand, Suppl 64, 1977, p. 15.)

alence of barotrauma may be somewhat reduced in infants treated in this manner, but the overall results are inconclusive. Mean airway pressures are similar or slightly higher than during conventional ventilation, but inflation pressures are lower at the proximal and presumably the distal airway.[17,67] Because gas exchange probably occurs by the same mechanisms as with conventional techniques, ventilator adjustment is similar. One major risk with this approach is the tendency to use ventilators with high internal and circuit compliance and with valve systems not designed to function effectively at the chosen frequency. This error may result in inadvertent air trapping, iatrogenic pulmonary hypertension, and air block syndrome.[20,21,57,114]

Sjöstrand and co-workers designed their system specifically to avoid these problems.[131–133] Gas is delivered through a small tube, and tidal volumes are slightly larger than the dead space volume. Gas egress occurs around the inflow catheter. This technique is particularly suited to laryngoscopy and microlaryngeal surgery.[19] It has also been applied in other surgical procedures where motion is undesirable. The relative

absence of cardiopulmonary interaction is said to be of potential benefit in cardiovascular surgery; however, this supposition remains unproved.

High-Frequency Jet Ventilation and High-Frequency Flow Interruption

Ventilators utilized for HFJV or HFFI deliver gas from a pressurized source through a valve to the patient. At preselected intervals, repetitive interruption of the gas source results in pulsatile flow (Fig. 9-6). The tidal volume thus depends on flow velocity and duration and the amount of entrainment that occurs because of the rapidly flowing stream of gas.[36]

Jet ventilators are simple to design and operate.[31,32,36,37] They have been shown to be effective over a wide range of patient sizes and in a variety of disease states.[28,29,31,37,42,127,128] The jet delivery port is placed in the airway, and exhalation occurs either around the tube or through an alternate lumen. The simplicity of the system, however, can cause serious problems. Movements of the tracheal catheter by only a few centimeters can result in ineffective ventilation.[10,84] Also because the technique relies on an open system for gas egress, obstruction of the exhalation limb can result in rapid and catastrophic lung overinflation. Even when the system is unobstructed, regulation of lung volume is difficult as it depends on many variables, including gas input, gas egress, lung compliance, and airway resistance.[32] Humidification repre-

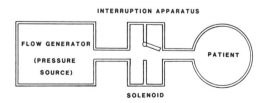

Fig. 9-6. A ventilator for HFJV or HFPI. The interruption apparatus may be a solenoid (as pictured), an eccentric cam, or a pneumatic valve.

sents a design problem with most jet ventilators.[32] The engineering tasks of humidifying a rapidly flowing gas stream are formidable,[116] and local drying probably accounts for some of the tracheal lesions seen during HFJV.[31] Other airway erosive lesions may occur, especially in neonates, from the "jackhammer" effect of a dry, high-pressure jet on tracheal mucosa.[109,110] Finally, the problems of making accurate distal pressure measurements are magnified owing to the high-velocity jet stream, producing a variety of measuring artifacts and inconsistencies.

In spite of these drawbacks, HFJV remains one of the only current available ventilatory systems capable of maintaining adequate oxygenation and ventilation in sick adult humans.[31,127,128] It has proved efficacious in surgery and in adult respiratory distress syndrome.[31,41,53] Because flow can be administered through a small cannula, it may also prove to be an effective emergency resuscitation technique when applied via a transtracheal cannula.[87–89] Most devices used for HFFI can be characterized as flow interrupters. As is the case with HFJV, a pressured source of gas is interrupted by a valve. In contrast, however, gas is delivered well back from the patient airway. Frequencies of 15–20 Hz can be obtained. By design, flow interrupters have a lower proximal airway velocity than do jets; however, the pressure fall-off within the patient's airway is less. As a result, the incidence of tracheal injury seems to be lower.[4] At higher frequencies and in larger animals, all HFFI ventilators require a source of bias or supplementary gas flow. The pressure waveform during HFFI varies from one instrument to another but is always positive relative to the baseline. Unlike jet ventilators, flow interrupters may have additional valves placed at the patient end of the circuit. When this configuration is employed, the same system can perform both low-frequency and high-frequency ventilation. Expiratory distending pressure (positive end-expiratory pressure/continuous positive airway pressure; PEEP/CPAP) is also easily controlled at the exhalation port. Tidal volume is determined by the pulsatile flow velocity, inspiratory cycle time, and entrained supplementary gas flow. Flow interrupters capable of effective ventilation in large and small animals and humans are currently being evaluated.[44,59,60,111,141] The gas flow rate results in an optimal frequency somewhat lower in the adult than in the infant. Clinical studies have shown these ventilators to be capable of maintaining adequate ventilation in selected cases where conventional techniques have been inadequate.[4,13,111]

High-Frequency Oscillatory Ventilation

Refinement of the observations of Lunkenheimer et al.[95,96] have led to the development of clinically effective oscillators. Two techniques for generating an oscillatory waveform have been employed: pistons and loudspeaker diaphragms (Fig. 9-7). An interesting, recently tested device (Texas Research, Inc., San Antonio, TX) employs a piston moving in a magnetic field, a technique which reduces the problems of mechanical fatigue in devices operating at extremely high frequencies.

As mentioned previously, an oscillator has both a positive- and negative-pressure waveform with equal forward and backward volume displacement. A system constructed in this fashion, by itself, delivers no volume to the patient. Hence an additional fresh gas source is supplied between the oscillator and the patient. This gas flow and the resistance to gas egress jointly determine the mean airway pressure (MAP). The oscillator merely displaces gas to and fro at pressures around this mean. Although oscillatory volumes are consistently less

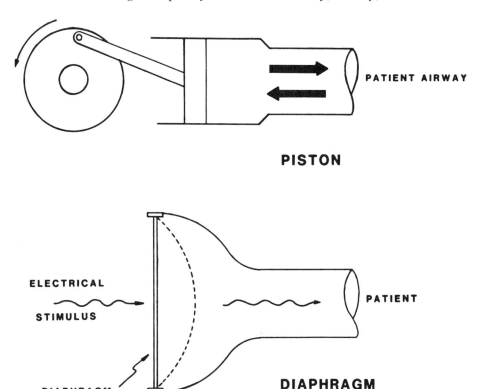

Fig. 9-7. The primary mechanisms by which oscillatory waveforms are generated. (Reprinted with permission from Gallagher TJ, Banner M, Desautels D: Presented as a scientific exhibit at the annual meeting of the American Society of Anesthesiologists, New Orleans, 1981.)

than the dead space volume, carbon dioxide elimination ($\dot{V}CO_2$) is primarily dependent on the oscillatory amplitude. At any frequency, $\dot{V}CO_2$ increases directly with the oscillatory amplitude whereas oxygenation, as with other forms of HFV, seems to be more closely related to the MAP.

Oscillators are capable of extremely high frequencies and of maintaining adequate gas exchange at rates greater than 50 Hz in small animals.[18] The ventilatory efficiency of an oscillator is critically dependent on the oscillatory volume, and all current available high-frequency oscillators are limited by the size of animal they can effectively ventilate. Although some oscillators achieve adequate $\dot{V}CO_2$ in large normal animals, none currently has sufficient capacity to ventilate a large subject with noncompliant lungs.

The relationship between frequency and $\dot{V}CO_2$ during oscillatory ventilation is still incompletely defined. Part of the difficulty lies in the increasing gas compression as higher frequencies and flow rates are used. Early investigators failed to take this fact into account and concluded that a single optimal frequency might exist. Recent studies suggest that a number of optimal and suboptimal frequencies may be defined in any given ventilator-lung system.[18,118] The frequency at which CO_2 is maximally eliminated may be dependent on the resonance of both the oscillator and the airways in question, with certain frequencies enhancing and others negating the delivered waveform. Mathematical models have been developed, but their applicability to various disease states is problematic. At present the available data suggest that, at constant oscillatory volumes, $\dot{V}_{CO_2}$ increases with increasing frequency up to 10–15 Hz. Above 20 Hz, the relationship between frequency and $\dot{V}_{CO_2}$ is not consistent.

Most oscillatory ventilators utilize an open circle with either a flow resistor or Starling resistor to provide expiratory resistance and thereby control volume loss through the exhalation port. Delivered oscillatory volume depends on the oscillatory amplitude and lung and expiratory resistance, and it is critically dependent on patency of the exhalation system. Entrainment of room air through the exhalation port is a recognized problem and is often dealt with by providing a low ambient flow at this point.

The strength of an oscillatory system is its ability to ventilate adequately with extremely small chest excursions. In theory, the very high frequencies possible with oscillators may give lower distal airway pressures and a lower risk of baroinjury, but as discussed earlier this speculation remains unsubstantiated. At the present time the effectiveness of oscillatory ventilation is limited by factors closely related to the size of the subject; therefore the development of equipment capable of ventilating adult diseased lungs may await proof of the efficacy of these very high frequencies. Because jets and pulse interrupters are simpler to design and use, and their main limitation is a lower maximal frequency, oscillators will probably be evaluated in small animals and children before being expanded for adults.

OTHER TECHNIQUES OF HFV

Several modifications of the previously mentioned techniques have been adapted for laboratory use. CO_2 scrubbers have been placed in line, reducing the requirement for large-amplitude oscillation.[106] External vibration has been shown to increase CO_2 elimination.[15,73,79,148] Combinations of loudspeaker diaphragms with conventional ventilators and interposition of conventional and high-frequency modes have also received interest.[23,66] None of these is sufficiently studied to be of clinical value at this time.

CLINICAL APPLICATIONS

Although a wealth of laboratory data exist, the proved clinical indications for HFV remain few at this time. In a real sense, HFV is a technique searching for a disease. It is probable that these various forms of HFV will ultimately find a place in the respiratory care armamentarium, but where this will be is not yet clear.

Low-compliance positive-pressure ventilators (e.g., the one designed by Sjöstrand) or high-frequency jet ventilators seem to have the most immediate clinical applicability. Extensive clinical work has been done on the use of HFPPV and HFJV in oropharyngeal, laryngeal, and tracheal surgery.[19] The techniques are simple and safe, and provide the surgeon with an unobstructed field. HFJV has also been used in ventilatory support during bronchoscopic and endoscopic procedures in infants, children, and adults.[19,38,41,53] It is reported to allow adequate ventilation and oxygenation despite the long, small cannula through which ventilation is accomplished.

The usefulness of HFV during other surgical procedures is not well established. Several investigators have used various high-frequency techniques during cardiovascular surgical procedures with apparently less detrimental effect on cardiac indices than occurs with conventional ventilator techniques.[43,97] The potential benefits of a relatively motionless thoracic operative field have not yet been fully explored. Similarly, HFV might be useful during certain microneurosurgical procedures where the effects of normal ventilation cause excessive movement of the operative site in the microscope's field of view. A reduction of intracranial pressure fluctuations may also be advantageous.[8,52,147] Hoff et al.[72] noted that dogs ventilated with HFV tolerated intravenous infusion of significantly more air with greater cardiovascular stability than dogs ventilated using conventional techniques. This observation suggests that HFV may add a safety factor during cardiovascular or neurosurgical procedures where air embolism is a potential complication.

Weaning from ventilation in patients with chronic lung disease is said to be facilitated by the use of HFV.[37,82,86] Patients interviewed after ventilation are reported to prefer HFJV compared to intermittent mandatory ventilation (IMV), although these data are purely subjective. Schwartz et al.[129] studied the psychiatric effects of ventilation and noted that the HFJV patient retains "respiratory autonomy," as spontaneous respiration is not eliminated using this method and the rapid jet rate is comfortably superimposed on the patient's own respiratory rhythm. Patients are reported to tolerate endotracheal suctioning better if HFJV is continued during the procedures.[64]

Klain et al.[89] and others have studied the usefulness of HFJV in a variety of emergency situations. They demonstrated that HFJV can provide excellent ventilatory support during cardiopulmonary resuscitation.[142] They produced convincing evidence that transtracheal HFJV is effective in preventing aspiration in nonintubated patients.[88] Limited experience with HFJV via a transtracheal catheter suggests that this technique may have an important place in emergency resuscitation by paramedical personnel unskilled in tracheal intubation or in emergency situations where the extent of injuries make intubation difficult or dangerous.[89] This supposition remains to be proved.

The usefulness of various HFV techniques to augment pulmonary toilet and mucous clearance in humans and experimental animals is not established. Studies of tracheal mucous clearance show decreased clearance during HFV compared to spontaneous respiration and conventional ventilation.[6,108] Clinical experience with several high-frequency ventilators has also demonstrated significant problems with bronchial mucous plugging after long-term ventilator support.[4,31] The mucous plugging may be secondary to inadequate humidification, disruption of mucociliary transport, or to other as yet unknown mechanisms. In contrast to these findings, a number of anecdotal reports in adults with chronic obstructive lung disease and in children with cystic fibrosis have demonstrated improvement in clinical, radiographic, and pulmonary function parameters in patients treated with a high-frequency intermittent positive-pressure ventilator.[12,13] This technique is used three or four times a day in a manner similar to that used with a conventional intermittent positive-pressure breathing (IPPB) device. It has been suggested that the high-frequency device vibrates secretions off the mucosa so that they can be effectively cleared by deep breathing and coughing. It is also possible that these devices can more effectively deliver water and medications to the distal airways than conventional IPPB machines because of the better overall distribution of gas which has been noted by some investigators.

In ventilated patients, as frequencies are increased downstream, peak pressures may fall, particularly when lung compliance is normal. In cases involving bronchopleural fistulas and other air leak syndromes, high-frequency techniques are said to reduce the volume of the air leak.[9,31,37,45,91,149] No controlled studies are available to support this contention, and laboratory experience suggests that improvement occurs only when it is possible to maintain adequate blood gas values at low airway pressures. If high pressures are required, air leaks persist.

Less clinical evidence is available for the more rapid high-frequency techniques. All have been tried in air leaks of various kinds. Improvement in pulmonary interstitial emphysema has been reported in approximately half of the patients treated with pulse interrupters.[17,60] Numerous reports have appeared concerning specific patients in terminal ventilatory failure. In most cases improved ventilation and/or oxygenation occurred when high-frequency techniques were employed after failure of conventional techniques.[16,31,35,48,111,128] However, the majority of patients died, and no controlled human data have shown HFV to be superior to conventional therapy. There are few long-term animal experiments,[138] and data with respect to potential toxicity are almost nonexistent.

Some of the strongest advocates of HFV point to its possible use in infants with RDS, particularly those under 1000 g where the incidence of bronchopulmonary dysplasia is highest.[17,78,99] Human and animal experience over short periods looks very promising, with oxygenation and ventilation at least equal to that obtained during conventional ventilation.[103] However, longer-term experience reveals the inability of HFOV alone to maintain alveolar volume early in the course of RDS, and the combined use of HFOV and an intermittent sigh can result in airway disruption identical to that seen with presently available techniques.[1,44] The development of an appropriate ventilatory strategy for the use of HFV in infants with RDS requires extensive laboratory and clinical investigation[11] before clinicians can even begin a trial to see if baroinjury is reduced. Until these studies are completed, there is no role for the *routine* clinical use of HFOV or HFPPV in this disease.

COMPLICATIONS AND SAFEGUARDS

HFV is not without potential serious complications. The inability to accurately measure distal airway pressures and distending volumes necessitates detailed and close monitoring of treated patients. Rapid changes may occur in Pao_2 and Pco_2, requiring frequent and accurate measurement of these values. If ventilator settings are changed, an assessment of arterial blood gases and pH should be made within a few minutes rather than 15–20 minutes, as has been advocated frequently with standard support.

Few guidelines are present to establish initial ventilatory settings. They may vary widely, depending on the patient's age, pulmonary problems, and type of high-frequency ventilator used. Blood gases and chest x-rays presently give the most information to help one decide the appropriateness of the therapy employed.

HFV has been heralded as a means of reducing the incidence of pulmonary barotrauma.[9,18,24,60] However, as noted previously, the assumption that distal pressures are always significantly lower than proximal pressures has been shown to be untrue,[3,5] particularly in disease states with low compliance. Also, the "position" of the patient's lungs on the pressure-volume curve when HFV is used may be crucial[26] (Fig. 9-8).

Mobilization and clearing of secretions in certain instances is said to be augmented by HFV.[12,13] However, we have observed two patients treated with continuous HFV for over 72 hours who developed severe problems with mucous plugging and inspissated secretions.[4] Improved humidification and/or more frequent suctioning than is used with standard ventilation may be necessary.

Gas flow rates with HFV are high. To prevent inadvertent pulmonary overdistention and/or rupture, the unobstructed venting of gas must be ensured. Circuits must incorporate pressure relief mechanisms. When using a jet ventilator, one must be certain that upper airway is free of obstruction.

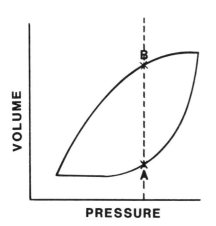

PRESSURE

Fig. 9-8. Representative pressure-volume curve. (A) Lung volume and compliance are low resulting in inefficient ventilation at high frequencies without further increases of pressure amplitude. (B) If lung volume is increased (PEEP/CPAP or a sigh), more effective gas exchange occurs during low-amplitude ventilation.

If alveolar distention does not occur during HFV, several problems may result. Ventilation without alveolar distention leads to a decrease in surfactant production.[51,63] Normal quantitative and qualitative surfactant function was noted in normal cats during HFV; however, in our baboon RDS model, we noted progressive alveolar collapse if sighs were not incorporated when HFV was used.[1,44] We have recently seen left-to-right ductal levels shunts—measured using a continuous wave doppler technique—decrease during peak inflation with standard mechanical ventilation. HFV did not produce a similar decrease to left-to-right shunting even at a mean pressure similar to that of the standard ventilator. This observation suggests that HFV may be of limited value in the treatment of congestive heart failure in patients with large left-to-right shunts. Although no major parenchymal changes have been noted in several short-term HFV experiments using normal animals,[58,85] severe interstitial air leaks have been noted in experiments using surfactant-deficient animals.[1,117]

CONCLUSIONS

The future of HFV is still clouded by conflicting data and results from many groups using different ventilators and ventilatory strategies. There are proved and potential benefits; however, well conceived and controlled animal and clinical studies must be accomplished before firm conclusions can be drawn and recommendations made regarding general clinical use. The development of safe, simple, and effective HFV systems, useful for the wide patient size and disease spectrum seen in clinical practices, is imperative before the techniques can be widely used. Much investigative work also remains to be done on unanswered questions regarding optimum frequency; I:E ratios; wave form, shape, and transmission; and pressure relationships between distal and proximal airways.

Even if HFV never reaches the level of clinical usefulness many have proposed, it probably will, at least, continue to stimulate the reevaluation of current ventilatory techniques and the physiological principles on which they are based. Perhaps this information will lead to a more complete understanding of the factors involved in normal and abnormal spontaneous respiration.

REFERENCES

1. Ackerman NB Jr, Coalson J, Kuehl RJ, et al: Pulmonary interstitial emphysema in the premature baboon with hyaline membrane disease. Crit Care Med 12:512, 1984
2. Ackerman NB Jr, Kuehl T, Mack J, et al: The premature baboon—a model for patent ductus arteriosus. Presented at the 10th Annual Meeting of Southern Perinatal Association, 27 January 1983
3. Ackerman NB Jr, Null DM, deLemos RA: Airway pressures during high frequency oscillatory ventilation. Pediatr Res 16:344A, 1982

4. Ackerman NB Jr, Null D, deLemos RA: Personal observations

5. Allen JL, Keefe DH, Fredberg JJ: Alveolar pressures and pulmonary impedance during high frequency oscillation in excised rabbit lungs. Pediatr Res 17:370A, 1983

6. Armengo JA, Man SFP, Logus JW, et al: Effects of high frequency oscillatory ventilation on canine tracheal mucous transport. Crit Care Med 9:192, 1981

7. Armengo JA, Wells A, Man GCW, et al: Hemodynamic and blood gas effects of high frequency oscillatory ventilation. Crit Care Med 9:192, 1981

8. Babinski MF, Albin M, Smith RB: Effect of high frequency ventilation in intracranial pressure. Crit Care Med 9:159, 1981

9. Baum M: Forced diffusion ventilation (FDV): mechanisms and applications. Anaesthetist 29:586, 1980

10. Baum M, Benzer H, Geyer A, et al: Gas exchange and flow properties during high frequency jet ventilation. Crit Care Med 9:159, 1981

11. Beardsmore CS, Stocks J, Silverman M: Problems in measurement of thoracic gas volume in infancy. J Appl Physiol 52:995, 1982

12. Bell R: Personal communication

13. Bird FM: Personal communication

14. Bird FM: The theoretical aspects of high frequency pulmonary ventilation. Flying Physician, Summer 1980, p. 12

15. Bitterman H, Kerem DH, Shabta Y, et al: Respiration maintained by externally applied vibration and tracheal insufflation in the cat. Anesth Analg 62:33, 1983

16. Bjerager K, Sjöstrand LL, Wattwil M: Long-term treatment of two patients with respiratory insufficiency. Acta Anesth Scand 64:55, 1977

17. Bland RD, Kim MH, Light MJH, et al: High frequency mechanical ventilation in severe hyaline membrane disease. Crit Care Med 8:275, 1980

18. Bohn DJ, Miyasaka K, Marehak BE, et al: Ventilation by high frequency oscillation. J Appl Physiol 48:710, 1980

19. Borg U, Eriksson I, Sjöstrand U: et al: High frequency positive pressure ventilation: a review based upon its use during bronchoscopy and for laryngoscopy and microlaryngeal surgery under general anesthesia. Anesth Analg 59:594, 1980

20. Boros SJ, Campbell K: A comparison of the effects of high-frequency low tidal volume and low-frequency high tidal volume mechanical ventilation. J Pediatr 97:108, 1980

21. Boros SJ, Mammel MC, Hagen E, et al: Infant ventilator performance: effects of altering frequency, peak inspiratory pressure, I : E ratio, and PEEP. Pediatr Res 17:372A, 1983

22. Bouhuys A: The Physiology of Breathing. pp. 48–49. Grune & Stratton, New York, 1977

23. Boynton BR, Friederichsen G, Kopotic R, et al: Combined high frequency oscillatory ventilation and conventional ventilation in neonates. Crit Care Med 11:223, 1983

24. Boysen PG: High frequency ventilation. Respir Ther Sept–Oct:105, 1982

25. Briscoe WR, Forster RE, Comroe J Jr: Alveolar ventilation at very low tidal volumes. Pediatr Res 7:27, 1954

26. Bryan C: Personal communication

27. Butler WJ, Bohn DJ, Bryan AC, et al: Ventilation by high frequency oscillation in humans. Anesth Analg 59:577, 1980

28. Calkins JM, Waterson CK, Hammeroff ST, et al: A simple fluidic high frequency ventilator. Anesth Analg 61:138, 1982

29. Calkins JM, Waterson CK, Hameroff SR, et al: Jet pulse characteristics for high frequency jet ventilation in dogs. Anesth Analg 61:293, 1982

30. Calkins JM, Quan SF, Conahan TJ, et al: Airway diameters in high frequency jet ventilation. Anesthesiology 55:A366, 1981

31. Carlon GC, Kahn RC, Howland WS, et al: Clinical experience with high frequency jet ventilation. Crit Care Med 9:1, 1981

32. Carlon GC, Miodownik S, Ray C Jr, et al: Technical aspects and clinical implications of high frequency jet ventilation with a solenoid valve. Crit Care Med 9:47, 1981

33. Carlon GC, Pierri MK, Groeger J, et al: Cardiac counterpulsation using high frequency jet ventilation. Crit Care Med 11:244, 1983

34. Carlon GC, Pierri MK, Ray C Jr, et al: Hemodynamic and respiratory variables with high frequency jet ventilation synchronized with heart rate. Crit Care Med 9:163, 1981

35. Carlon GC, Ray C Jr, Goetz WS, et al: High frequency jet ventilation in respiratory failure: influence of driving pressure and cannula size. Crit Care Med 9:159, 1981

36. Carlon GC, Ray C Jr, Griffin Jr, et al: Tidal volume and airway pressure on high frequency jet ventilation. Crit Care Med 11:83, 1983

37. Carlon GC, Ray C Jr, Pierri MK, et al: High frequency jet ventilation: theoretical considerations and clinical observations. Chest 81:350, 1982

38. Carlon GC, Turnbull AD, Alexander JD, et al: High frequency jet ventilation during tracheal surgery. Crit Care Med 9:163, 1981

39. Charkrabarti MK, Sukes MK: Cardiorespiratory effects of high frequency intermittent positive pressure ventilation in the dog. Br J Anaesth 52:475, 1980

40. Colgan FJ, Ten Eyck LG, Sawa T: Ventilation requirements during high frequency ventilation. Crit Care Med 11:173, 1983

41. Dalens B, Labbe A, Haberer JP: Respiratory assistance secured by jet ventilation during bronchofiberscopy in forty-nine infants. Anesthesiology 57:551, 1982

42. Davey AJ, Lay GR, Leigh JM: High frequency venturi jet ventilation. Anaesthesia 37:947, 1982

43. Dedhia HV, Schiebel F: Hemodynamic effect of high frequency ventilation in open heart surgery patients. Crit Care Med 9:158, 1981

44. deLemos RA, Kuehl T, Null D, et al: Ventilatory strategy for high frequency ventilation of baboons with hyaline membrane disease. Pediatr Res 17:310A, 1983

45. Derderian SS, Rajagopal KR, Abbrecht PH, et al: High frequency ventilation in bilateral bronchopleural fistulas. Am Rev Respir Dis 123:87, 1981

46. Dorkin HL, Jackson AC, Strieder DJ, et al: Interaction of oscillatory and unidirectional flows in straight tubes and an airway cast. J Appl Physiol 52:1097, 1982

47. Doyle JH, Fried JL: High frequency positive pressure ventilation with a Baby Bird ventilator and modified circuit. Crit Care Med 9:222, 1981

48. El-Baz N, Faber LP, Doolas A: Combined high frequency ventilation for management of terminal respiratory failure: a new technique. Anesth Analg 62:39, 1983

49. Eriksson I: Effects of high frequency positive pressure ventilation on intrapulmonary gas distribution. Anesth Analg 59:585, 1980

50. Eriksson I: The role of conducting airways in gas exchange during high frequency ventilation—a clinical and theoretical analysis. Anesth Analg 61:483, 1982

51. Faridy EE, Permutt S, Riley RL: Effect of ventilation on surface forces in excised dogs' lungs. J Appl Physiol 21:1453, 1966

52. Fein IA, Rackow EC, Winslow L: The effect of high frequency ventilation on intracranial pressure. Am Rev Respir Dis 123:85, 1981

53. Flatau E, Lewinsohn G, Konichezky S, et al: Mechanical ventilation in fiberoptic bronchoscopy: comparison between high frequency positive pressure ventilation and normal frequency positive pressure ventilation. Crit Care Med 10:733, 1982

54. Fletcher PR, Epstein RA: Constancy of physiologic dead space during high frequency ventilation. Respir Physiol 47:39, 1982

55. Fletcher PR, Epstein RA: Measurement of alveolar pressures during high frequency ventilation. Anesthesiology 65:A358, 1981

56. Fletcher PR, Epstein MA, Epstein RA: A new ventilator for physiologic studies during high frequency ventilation. Respir Physiol 47:21, 1982

57. Fontan JP, Heldt GP, Willis MM, et al: Changes in functional residual capacity and inadvertent positive end-expiratory pressure in rabbits ventilated at rapid rates. Pediatr Res 17:375A, 1983

58. Frantz ID, Stark AR, Davies P, et al: Frequency ventilation does not affect pulmonary surfactant, liquid, or morphologic features in normal cats. Am Rev Resp Dis 126:909, 1982

59. Frantz ID, Stark AR, Dorkin HL: Ventilation of infants at frequencies up to 1800/minute. Pediatr Res 14:642, 1980

60. Frantz ID, Werthammer J, Stark AR: High frequency ventilation in premature infants with lung disease: adequate gas exchange at low tracheal pressure. Pediatrics 71:483, 1983

61. Fredberg JA: Augmented diffusion in the airways can support pulmonary gas exchange. J Appl Physiol 49:232, 1980
62. Goldstein D, Slutsky AS, Ingram RH Jr, et al: CO_2 elimination by high frequency ventilation in normal subjects. Am Rev Respir Dis 123:251, 1981
63. Greenfield LJ, Ebert PA, Benson DW: Effect of positive pressure ventilation on surface tension properties of lung extracts. Anesthesiology 25:312, 1964
64. Guntupalli K, Klain M, Sladen A: High frequency jet ventilation with endotracheal suctioning. Crit Care Med 9:190, 1981
65. Hakim TS, Michel RP, Chang HK: Effect of lung inflation on pulmonary vascular resistance by arterial and venous occlusion. J Appl Physiol 53:1110, 1982
66. Hameroff SR, Calkins JM, Waterson CK, et al: High frequency alternating lung ventilation. Anesthesiology 54:237, 1981
67. Heicher DA, Kasting DS, Harrod JR: Prospective clinical comparison of two methods for mechanical ventilation of neonates: rapid rate and short inspiratory time versus slow rate and long inspiratory time. J Pediatr 98:957, 1981
68. Heijman K, Sjöstrand U: Treatment of the respiratory distress syndrome—a preliminary report. Opusc Med Bd 5:235, 1974
69. Henderson Y, Chillingworth FP, Whitney JL: The respiratory dead space. Am J Physiol 38:1, 1915
70. Hoff BH, Robotham JL, Smith RB, et al: Effects of high frequency ventilation (300–2400/min) on cardiovascular function and gas exchange in dogs. Am Rev Respir Dis 123:108, 1981
71. Hoff BH, Smith RB, Bunegin L, et al: High frequency ventilation in dogs with open chests. Crit Care Med 10:517, 1982
72. Hoff BH, Smith RB, Bunegin L, et al: Venous air embolism during high frequency ventilation and IPPV. Crit Care Med 9:164, 1981
73. Homma I, Nagai T, Ohashi M, et al: Effects of chest wall vibration on ventilation in patients with spinal cord lesion. J Appl Physiol 50:107, 1981
74. Horsefield K, Gabe I, Mills C, et al: Effect of heart rate and stroke volume on gas mixing in dog lung. J Appl Physiol 53:1603, 1982
75. Isabey D, Chang HK: Steady and unsteady pressure-flow relationships in central airways. J Appl Physiol 51:1338, 1981
76. Jacobs HB: Emergency percutaneous transtracheal catheter and ventilator. J Trauma 12:50, 1972
77. Jacoby JJ, Karmelburg W, Ziegler CH, et al: Transtracheal resuscitation. JAMA 162:625, 1956
78. James LS: High frequency ventilation for immature infants—special conference report. Pediatrics 71:280, 1983
79. Jammes Y, Mathiot MJ, Roll JP, et al: Ventilatory response to muscular vibrations in healthy humans. J Appl Physiol 51:262, 1981
80. Jonzon A, Oberg PA, Sedin G, et al: High frequency low tidal volume positive pressure ventilation. Acta Physiol Scand 80:21A, 1970
81. Jonzon A, Oberg PA, Sedin G, et al: High frequency positive pressure ventilation by endotracheal insufflation. Acta Anaesthesiol Scand [Suppl] 43:1, 1971
82. Kalla R, Wald M, Klain M: Weaning of ventilator dependent patients by high frequency jet ventilation. Crit Care Med 9:162, 1981
83. Kamm RD: Mechanisms of gas exchange in high frequency ventilation. Presented at AAMI, 10 May 1981 (Annual Meeting), Washington, DC
84. Keszler H, Klain M: Importance of position of jet orifice in high frequency jet ventilation. Crit Care Med 10:234, 1982
85. Keszler H, Klein R, McCellan L, et al: Effects of conventional and high frequency jet ventilation on lung parenchyma. Crit Care Med 10:514, 1982
86. Klain M, Kalla R, Sladen A, et al: Weaning from respiratory support by high frequency jet ventilation. Crit Care Med 9:190, 1981
87. Klain M, Keszler H, Brader E: High frequency jet ventilation in cardiopulmonary resuscitation. Crit Care Med 9:421, 1981
88. Klain M, Smith RB: High frequency percutaneous transtracheal jet ventilation. Crit Care Med 5:280, 1977
89. Klain M, Miller J, Kalla R: Emergency use of high frequency jet ventilation. Crit Care Med 9:160, 1981
90. Kolton M, Cattran CB, Kent G, et al: Oxygenation during high frequency ventila-

tion compared with conventional mechanical ventilation in two models of lung injury. Anesth Analg 61:232, 1982

91. Kuwik RJ, Glass D, Coombs DW: Evaluation of high frequency positive pressure ventilation for experimental bronchopleural fistula. Crit Care Med 9:164, 1981

92. Lehnert BE, Oberdorster G, Slutsky AS: Constant flow ventilation of apneic dogs. J Appl Physiol 53:483, 1982

93. Lehr J, Barkyoumb J, Drazen JM: Gas transport during high frequency ventilation. Fed Proc 40:384, 1981

94. Ludwig E: Gas mixing within the acinus. J Appl Physiol 54:609, 1983

95. Lunkenheimer PP, Frank F, Ising H, et al: Intrapulmonater goswechsel unter simulierter apnoe durch transtrachealer periodischen intrathorkalen Druckwechsel. Anaesthetist 22:232, 1972

96. Lunkenheimer PP, Rafflebeul W, Keller H, et al: Application of transtracheal pressure oscillations. Br J Anaesth 44:627, 1972

97. Malina JR, Nordström SG, Sjöstrand UH, et al: Clinical evaluation of high frequency positive pressure ventilation in patients scheduled for open chest surgery. Anesth Analg 60:324, 1981

98. Man GCW, Man SFP, Kappagoda CT: Effects of high frequency oscillatory ventilation on vagal and phrenic nerve activities. J Appl Physiol 54:502, 1983

99. Marchak BE, Thompson WK, Duffty P, et al: Treatment of RDS by high frequency oscillatory ventilation: a preliminary report. J Pediatr 99:287, 1981

100. McDonald JS, Reilley TE, Cook R, et al: Hemodynamic and pulmonary responses to volumetric diffusion respiration in the oleic acid canine model. Crit Care Med 9:197, 1981

101. Meltzer SJ, Auer J: Eine vergleichung der volhardschen methode derlkunstlichen atmung mit der von miltzer und auer in der kontinuierlichen respiration ohne respratorischen bewegungen verwendelen methode. Zentralbl Physiol 23:442, 1909

102. Meredith K, Walsh W, Ackerman N, et al: High frequency oscillatory ventilation as the initial ventilatory mode in diffuse alveolar disease. Pediatr Res 16:356A, 1982

103. Militzer HW, Quan SF, Calkins JM, et al: Effects of high frequency jet ventilation in a rabbit model of infant respiratory distress syndrome. Crit Care Med 11:222, 1983

104. Napolitano A, Doyle B, Duncan J, et al: Morphologic changes in the airway of dogs ventilated with high frequency jet ventilation compared to conventional ventilation. Pediatr Res 17:386A, 1983

105. Nilsestuen JO, Coon RL, Zuperku EJ, et al: Interrelationships among airway CO_2, airway pressure and breathing frequency. J Appl Physiol 52:190, 1982

106. Ngeow YK, Mitzner W: A new system for ventilating with high frequency oscillation. J Appl Physiol 53:1638, 1982

107. Ngeow YK, Mitzner W, Permutt S, et al: Carbon dioxide clearance during high frequency oscillation. Crit Care Med 9:164, 1981

108. Nordin U, Keszler H, Klain M: How does high frequency jet ventilation effect the mucociliary transport? Crit Care Med 9:160, 1981

109. Nordin U, Klain M, Keszler H: Electron-microscopic studies of tracheal mucosa after high frequency jet ventilation. Crit Care Med 10:211, 1982

110. Ophoven JP, Mammel MC, Gordon MJ, et al: High frequency jet ventilation: tracheobronchial histopathology. Pediatr Res 17:386A, 1983

111. O'Rourke PP, Crone RK: High frequency ventilation in 10 children with acute respiratory failure. Crit Care Med 11:222, 1983

112. Otto CW, Waterson CK, Conahan TJ, et al: Cardiovascular effects of ECG synchronized jet ventilation. Crit Care Med 9:160, 1981

113. Peck H: Intratracheal sufflation anaesthesia (Meltzer-Auer). JAMA 61:839, 1913

114. Pepe PE, Marini JJ: Occult positive end-expiratory pressure in mechanically ventilated patients with airflow obstruction. Am Rev Respir Dis 126:166, 1982

115. Poiseuille JLM: Recherches experimentales sur le mouvement des liquides dans les tubes de tres petits diametres. C R Acad Sci 11:961, 1041, 1840

116. Poulton TJ, Downs JB: Humidification of rapidly flowing gas. Crit Care Med 9:59, 1981

117. Raju T, Braverman B, Kim DW, et al: Some difficulties with high frequency os-

cillator and interruptor. Pediatr Res 16:360A, 1982

118. Robertson HT, Coffey RL, Standaert TA, Truog WE: Respiratory and inert gas exchange during high frequency ventilation. J Appl Physiol 52:683, 1982

119. Rohrer F: Der Stromung-Swiderstand in den menschlichen atemwegen und der einfluss der unregelmassign verzweigung des bronchialsystems auf den atmungsverlauf in verschiederen lungenbezirken. Pfluegers Arch 162:225, 1915

120. Rossing TH, Slutsky AS, Ingram RH, et al: CO_2 elimination by high frequency oscillations in dogs—effects of histamine infusion. J Appl Physiol 53:1256, 1982

121. Rossing TH, Slutsky AS, Lehr JL, et al: Tidal volume and frequency of carbon dioxide elimination by high frequency ventilation. N Engl J Med 305:1375, 1981

122. Sander RD: Two ventilating attachments for bronchoscopes. Del Med J 39:170, 1967

123. Scherer PW: Airway gas transport during high frequency ventilation. AMMI Annual Meeting, 10 May 1981, Washington, DC

124. Scherer PW, Haselton FR: Convective exchange in oscillatory flow through bronchial tree models. J Appl Physiol 53:1023, 1982

125. Scherer PW, Shendalman LH, Greene NM, et al: Measurement of axial diffusivities in a model of the bronchial airways. J Appl Physiol 38:719, 1975

126. Schmid ER, Knopp TJ, Rehder K: Intrapulmonary gas transport and perfusion during high frequency oscillations. J Appl Physiol 51:1507, 1981

127. Schuster DP, Klain M, Snyder JV: Comparison of high frequency jet ventilation to conventional ventilation during severe acute respiratory failure in humans. Crit Care Med 10:625, 1982

128. Schuster DP, Snyder JV, Klain M, et al: High frequency jet ventilation during the treatment of acute fulminant pulmonary edema. Chest 80:682, 1981

129. Schwartz L, Kala R, Klain M: Psychiatric response pattern to conventional ventilation compared with high frequency jet ventilation. Presented at the 9th Annual Scientific Meeting of the Society of Critical Care Medicine, 14 May 1980

130. Scotter DR, Thurtell GW, Raats PAC: Dispersion resulting from sinusoidal gas flow in porous materials. Soil Sci 104:306, 1967

131. Sjöstrand U: Experimental and clinical evaluation of high frequency positive pressure ventilation. Acta Anaesthesiol Scand [Suppl] 64:1, 1977

132. Sjöstrand U: High frequency positive pressure ventilation (HFPPV), a review. Crit Care Med 8:345, 1980

133. Sjöstrand U, Eriksson IA: High rates and low volumes in mechanical ventilation— not just a matter of ventilatory frequency. Anesth Analg 59:567, 1980

134. Sladen A, Guntapalli KK, Klain M, et al: High frequency jet ventilation and conventional ventilation: a comparison of cardiorespiratory parameters. Crit Care Med 10:212, 1982

135. Slutsky AS: Gas mixing by cardiogenic oscillations: a theoretical quantitative analysis. J Appl Physiol 51:1287, 1981

136. Slutsky AS, Brown R, Lehr J, et al: High frequency ventilation, a promising new approach to mechanical ventilation. Med Inst 15:229, 1981

137. Slutsky AS, Drazen JM, Ingram RH Jr, et al: Effective pulmonary ventilation with small volume oscillations at high frequency. Science 209:609, 1980

138. Slutsky AS, Kamm RD, Rossing TH, et al: Effects of frequency, tidal volume, and lung volume on CO_2 elimination in dogs by high frequency, low tidal volume ventilation. J Clin Invest 68:1475, 1981

139. Smith RB, Cutaia F, Hoff BH, et al: Long term transtracheal high frequency ventilation in dogs. Crit Care Med 9:311, 1981

140. Spoerel WE, Narayanan DS, Singh NP: Transtracheal ventilation. Br J Anaesth 43:932, 1971

141. Stoddard R, Minnick L, Ackerman N Jr, et al: A comparison between high frequency and conventional ventilation in dogs with oleic acid lung injury. Pediatr Res 16:362A, 1982

142. Swartzman S, Wilson MA, Hoff BH, et al: Percutaneous transtracheal jet ventilation for cardiopulmonary resuscitation. Crit Care Med 10:235, 1982

143. Szele G, Shahvari BC: Comparison of cardiovascular effects of high frequency ven-

tilation and intermittent positive pressure ventilation in hemorrhagic shock. Crit Care Med 4:161, 1981

144. Taylor G: The dispersion of matter in turbulent flow through a pipe. Proc R Soc Lond Ser 223:446, 1954

145. Thomas LJ Jr, Griffo ZJ, Roos A: Effect of negative lung pressure on pulmonary vascular resistance. J Appl Physiol 16:451, 1961

146. Thompson WK, Marchak BE, Bryan AC, et al: Vagotomy reverses apnea induced by high frequency oscillatory ventilation. J Appl Physiol 51:1484, 1981

147. Thompson WK, Marchak BE, Froese AB, et al: High frequency oscillation compared with standard ventilation in pulmonary injury model. J Appl Physiol 51:1484, 1981

148. Ward HE, Power JH, Nicholas TE: High frequency oscillations via the pleural surface: an alternative mode of ventilation? J Appl Physiol 54:427, 1983

149. Wilson EA, Hoff BH, Sjöstrand UH, et al: Conventional and high frequency ventilation in dogs with bronchopleural fistula. Crit Care Med 10:232, 1982

150. Wilson TA, Lin KH: Convection and diffusion in the airway and the design of the bronchial tree. In Bouhuys A (ed): Airway Dynamics; Physiology and Pharmacology. pp. 5–19. Charles C. Thomas, Springfield, IL, 1970

151. Zwart A, Jansen JRC, Versprilla A: Suppression of spontaneous breathing with high frequency ventilation. Crit Care Med 9:159, 1981

10

Mechanical Ventilators

Robert A. Smith
David Desautels
Robert R. Kirby

In some ways, we are as confused as ever;
but we believe we are confused on a higher
level and about more important things.

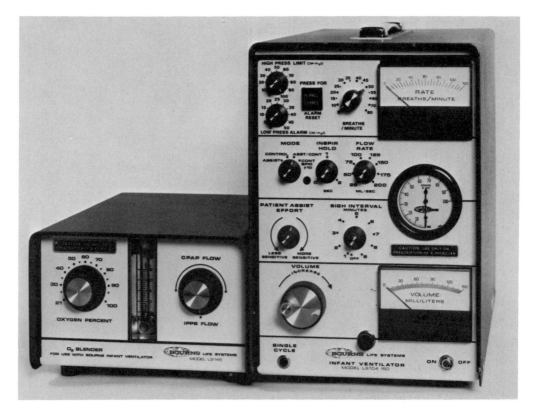

Fig 10-1. Bear LS 104–150 infant volume ventilator. (Courtesy of Bear Medical, Inc.)

During the past decade ventilator proliferation has occurred at an unprecented rate. Many advances have been a result of advances in computer technology, and the possible functions available to the clinician today are almost intimidating. Gone forever is the concept that the ventilator itself is relatively unimportant compared to the individual who uses it. Major differences in potential and actual capabilities are present, and understanding these differences often spells the difference between success and failure in the care of patients with acute and chronic respiratory insufficiency.

In the following pages we have selected representative ventilators to describe in detail, believing that our choices are used in well over 90 percent of all critical care units in the United States and in many other countries. In some cases the ventilators are no longer manufactured and/or available for purchase in this country. However, sufficient numbers are still in use, or have enough interesting features, to warrant inclusion. Others are so new that little information pertaining to their use or efficiency is available. Again, certain characteristics mandate their inclusion.

One exclusion deserves explanation. At the time of this writing the Food and Drug Administration (FDA) has limited commercially available high-frequency devices to a maximum rate of 150 cycles/minute. As a result of this constraint, we have elected not to include such ventilators in this chapter, feeling that they have minimal utilization potential. When this limit is removed in the future, high-frequency ventilation will as-

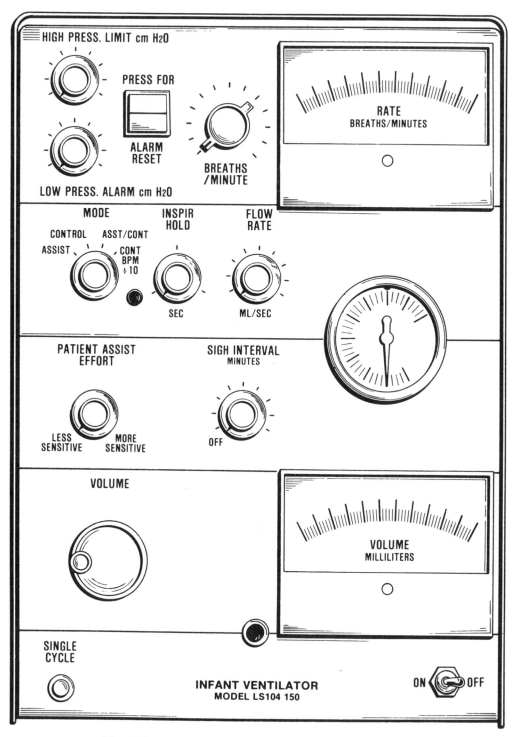

Fig. 10-2. Schematic of the Bear LS 104–150 control panel.

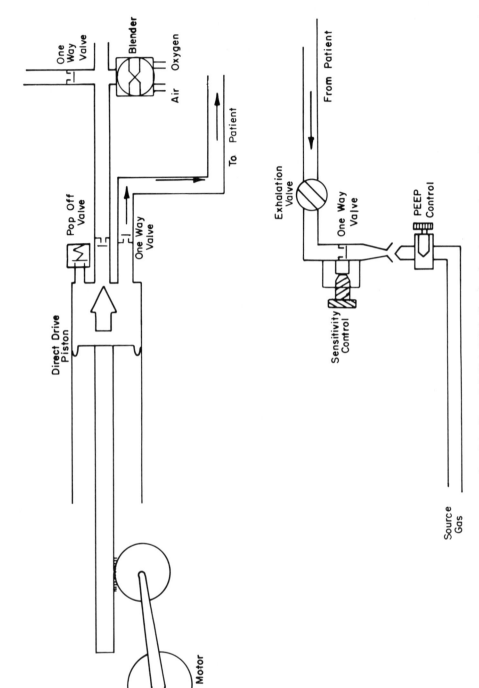

Fig. 10-3. Internal schematic of the Bear LS 104–150 indicating inspiratory phase gas flows.

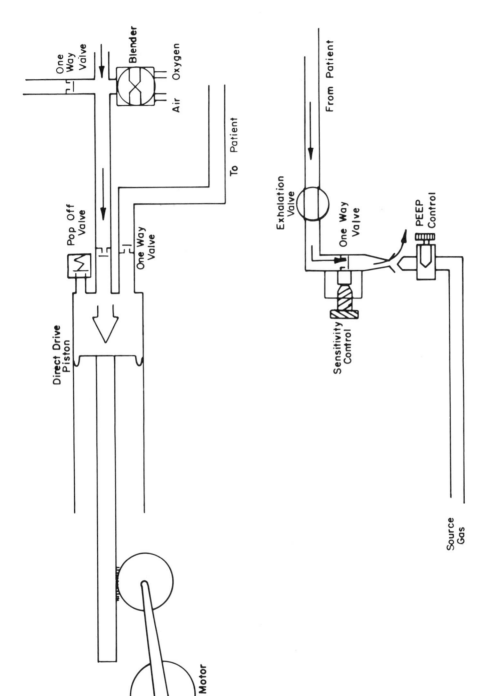

Fig. 10-4. Internal schematic of the Bear LS 104–150 indicating expiratory phase gas flows.

sume increasing importance and should naturally extend our capabilities in the field of respiratory care.

BEAR INFANT VOLUME VENTILATOR (LS 104–150)

The Bear LS 104–150 Ventilator (Fig. 10-1) is an electronically powered and controlled, volume-cycled, constant-flow generator. Inspiration may be extended by a postinflation hold (plateau). Controlled mechanical ventilation (CMV), assist, and intermittent mandatory ventilation (IMV) modes are available with or without positive end-expiratory pressure (PEEP).

Control and Surveillance

The electronic circuit is activated by a main power switch located on the control panel (Fig. 10-2). When ON, a pilot light is illuminated. Tidal volume (V_T) is adjusted by a hand crank with a range of 10–150 ml. The selected V_T is indicated on an analog meter. Ventilatory assist, control, assist-control, or CONT BPM ÷ 10 (control breaths·minute^{-1} divided by 10) modes are selected by a four-position rotary knob. The CMV rate is adjusted from 5 to 80 breaths·minute^{-1}. In the ASSIST mode (range 0–120 breaths·minute^{-1}), if patient-triggered breaths decrease to less than 60 percent of the selected CMV rate for 10–12 seconds, an audible apnea alarm sounds and CMV is activated for 7 seconds. After this CMV period, the ASSIST mode is automatically reestablished. The sequence is repeated if the assisted rate is less than 60 percent of the CMV rate. In the ASSIST-CONTROL mode, if patient-triggered breaths occur less frequently than the CMV rate, sufficient controlled breaths are provided to make up the disparity.

The effort necessary to initiate assisted mechanical breaths is adjustable from 0.1 to 1.0 cm H_2O. Low control rates, e.g., IMV, may be administered in the CONT. BPM ÷ 10 mode (range 0.5–8 breaths·minute^{-1}). Ventilator cycling frequency is displayed on an analog rate meter. In the CONT BPM ÷ 10 mode, this meter indicates the preselected CMV value.

The inspiratory flow rate is adjustable from 25 to 200 ml·second^{-1}. After inspiration, exhalation may be delayed up to 2 seconds with an inspiratory hold (plateau) control. In the assist mode, a single breath may be delivered by depressing a pushbutton. A sigh breath consisting of two consecutive piston compressions (stacked V_T) can be delivered at a preselected interval of 1–9 minutes.

Peak inspiratory pressure (PIP) is indicated on an anaeroid manometer and is adjustable from 0 to 100 cm H_2O. If the preset PIP is reached, inspiration is terminated and an audible and visual alarm engage. A minimal PIP may be selected (range 0–50 cm H_2O). If the minimal PIP is not reached, visual and audible low-pressure alarms activate, indicating a patient-ventilator interface leak or disconnection.

Ventilator rear panel controls (not illustrated) include a PEEP/CPAP (continuous positive airway pressure) regulator, a sensitivity/leak compensator, and a positive-pressure limit. PEEP/CPAP is adjustable from 0 to 15 cm H_2O when the oxygen source pressure is 50 psig. The sensitivity/leak compensator permits balancing of PEEP/CPAP in the presence of small circuit leaks by means of a retrograde circuit gas flow. Leak compensation is provided by oxygen; therefore if it exceeds the circuit leak the F_{IO_2} increases. Pressure developed by the piston compression stroke may be limited by a mechanical vent from less than 30 to more than 80 cm H_2O. This feature may be employed as a back-up to the PIP cycle control or as a means to provide a dynamic inspiratory pressure plateau. When activated it does not terminate the inspiratory phase.

The desired oxygen concentration for mechanical and/or spontaneous ventilation is provided by an air-oxygen blender. Blender outflow is either demand (intermittent positive pressure ventilation; IPPV) or continuous (CPAP) depending on the position of the control knob. An adjustable flowmeter range from zero to about 20 L·minute^{-1} regulates blender outflow in the continuous mode. When the ventilator is in ASSIST, CONTROL, or ASSIST-CONTROL modes, the blender control is set to demand (IPPV). In IMV or CPAP configuration the blender control is placed in the CPAP mode and the flow rate adjusted to the desired level.

Operation

Inspiratory (Fig. 10-3) and expiratory (Fig. 10-4) phase gas flows are illustrated. Unlike most piston ventilators, the Bear LS 104 delivers a square-wave flow pattern because its piston is directly gear-driven. The piston moves forward at variable speeds depending on the amount of voltage delivered to the direct current (DC) motor. During inspiration the exhalation valve solenoid closes, and forward piston motion occurs. As the piston completes its positive stroke, it makes contact with an electrical switch on the forward cylinder wall, signaling the end of inspiration. The piston then returns to its original position, which is determined by the adjusted tidal volume. This switch also deactivates (opens) the solenoid exhalation valve unless a postinflation hold (plateau) is employed. When a sigh breath is delivered, the initial switch contact is ignored, and a second piston stroke is completed before exhalation commences. As the piston returns to its exhalation position, it draws in fresh mixed gas from the air-oxygen blender. Check valves maintain proper flow direction of the piston and patient circuit. A pressure relief valve in the manifold system ensures that excessive pressure is not applied to the patient and piston rolling diaphragm, as too much pressure on the piston diaphragm can invert it.

PEEP is developed from the source gas, which powers a venturi device. Pressure generated by the venturi acts on a unidirectional leaf valve. A leak may be compensated by diverting PEEP venturi flow through a sensitivity control into the exhalation limb of the circuit. During spontaneous breathing the F_{IO_2} may be diluted by this flow.

Reference

Model LS 104/150 Instruction Manual No. 50000–10104. Bear Medical Systems, Inc., Riverside, CA.

BEAR BP-200 INFANT VENTILATOR

The Bear BP-200 infant ventilator (Fig. 10-5) is an electronically controlled, pneumatically and electronically powered, time-cycled, constant-flow generator. It may be employed in a CMV, IMV, or CPAP mode and is capable of providing an inspiratory pressure plateau. End-expiratory pressure is available in any mode.

Control and Surveillance

A compact control panel facilitates manipulation of ventilatory parameters (Fig. 10-6). A four-position rotary knob provides electrical power, alarm function testing, and mode selection (IPPB/IMV or CPAP). In any position but OFF, an amber light illuminates when the ventilator is connected to an appropriate electrical source. A buzzer sounds in the alarm test mode. To ascertain battery competence, one must disconnect the ventilator from the power source in the test mode; if the buzzer con-

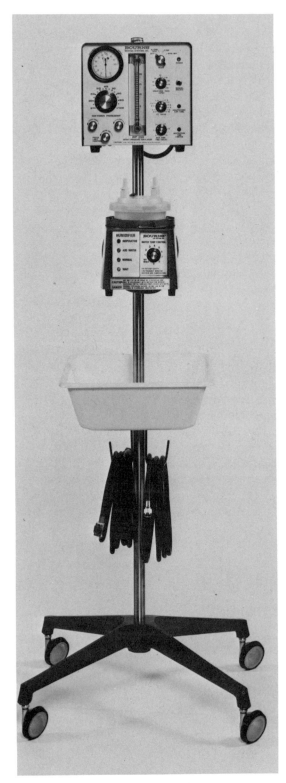

Fig. 10-5. Bear BP-200 infant ventilator. (Courtesy of Bear Medical, Inc.)

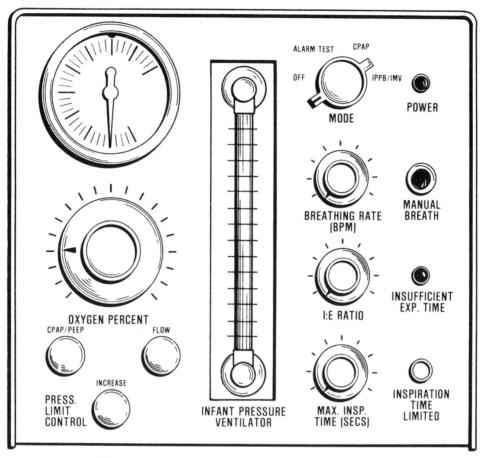

Fig. 10-6. Schematic of the Bear BP-200 control panel.

tinues to sound, battery function is adequate. When CPAP is selected, pneumatic and electronic alarm circuits are activated. If air or oxygen inlet pressures fall below 15 or 30 psig, respectively, or an electrical failure occurs, a battery-operated buzzer is activated. In the IPPB/IMV mode, time-cycled exhalation valve function and alarm system functions become operational.

Continuous gas flow at a given oxygen concentration (21–100 percent) is metered to the patient circuit via a calibrated Thorpe tube (0–20 L·minute^{-1}). In the CPAP mode, the infant breathes spontaneously from a continuous gas flow at either ambient or elevated baseline pressures. Baseline pressure is varied with a CPAP/PEEP control (0–20 cm H_2O). When positive-pressure

ventilation is desired, the mode selector is placed in the IPPB/IMV position. Mechanical V_T is determined by the cycling frequency (1–150 breaths·minute^{-1}), inspiratory:expiratory (I:E) ratio control (4:1 to 1:10), and continuous flow rate. At low IMV frequencies the maximum inspiratory time control (0.1–3.0 seconds) may be employed to override the I:E control, thereby preventing an excessively prolonged inspiratory time (T_I). When the maximum T_I limit is exceeded, a red lamp illuminates. An internal timer prevents mechanical exhalation from decreasing below 0.22–0.28 second. If this timer overrides the adjusted cycling parameters, the "insufficient expiratory time" lamp is illuminated. A "manual" breath may be administered by de-

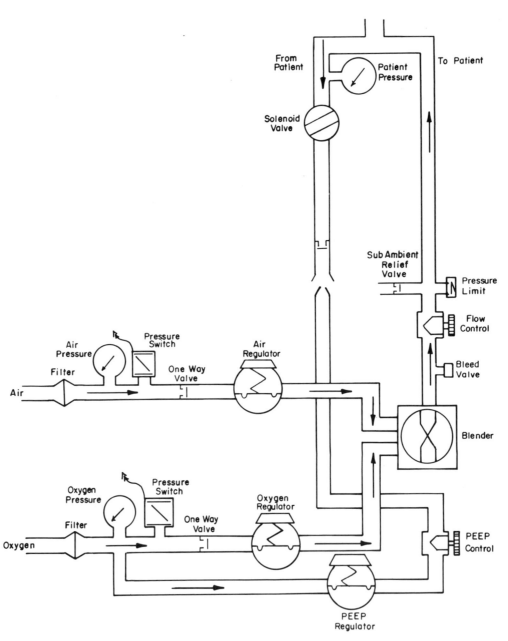

Fig. 10-7. Internal schematic of the Bear BP-200 indicating inspiratory phase gas flows.

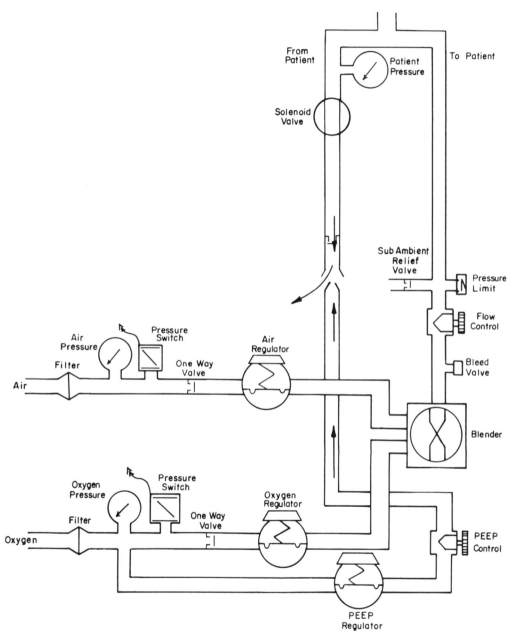

Fig. 10-8. Internal schematic of BP-200 indicating expiratory gas flows.

pressing a button when the ventilator is in the CPAP mode. The manual V_T is controlled identically to those provided during IPPB/IMV.

PIP is regulated by an uncalibrated control knob (12 cm H_2O at 2 L·minute^{-1} to > 80 cm H_2O at 20 L·minute^{-1}). The desired PIP is selected by observing an anaeroid manometer while adjusting the control knob during IPPB/IMV cycling against the occluded circuit outflow port. When the PIP is exceeded, the exhalation valve remains closed but all circuit flow is vented to ambient air. A pressure plateau is then established for the remaining T_I.

Operation

Inspiratory (Fig. 10-7) and expiratory (Fig. 10-8) phase gas flows are illustrated in pneumatic schematics of the BP 200. Air at 15–75 psig and oxygen at 30–75 psig are equilibrated to the lowest source pressure. A pressure switch monitors air and oxygen inlets to warn of low values, and anaeroid manometers indicate the pounds per square inch of each gas. Unidirectional valves are incorporated into each high-pressure system to ensure that retrograde flow does not occur.

Blended gas is directed through a needle valve into a calibrated Thorpe tube (not illustrated). Distal to the flowmeter system is a spring-loaded valve which limits outflow pressure. Should maximum pressure be attained, excess pressure is vented to ambient for the duration of inspiration. A subambient relief valve is available to allow spontaneous breathing of room air during pneumatic or electronic malfunctions.

Inspiration occurs when an electronic solenoid valve closes and diverts the continuous gas flow into the infant's lungs. This occlusion is abrupt, thereby creating a square-wave inspiratory flow pattern. At end-inspiration the solenoid valve opens to permit exhalation and venting of the con-

tinuous flow. End-expiratory pressure is developed by gas shunted from the oxygen source to a venturi jet, which pressurizes a unidirectional valve.

Reference

Model BP 200 Instruction Manual No. 50000–10200. Bear Medical Systems, Inc. Riverside, CA.

BEAR CUB INFANT VENTILATOR (BP-2001)

The Bear Cub infant ventilator (Fig. 10-9) is an electronically controlled, pneumatically and electronically powered, time-cycled, constant-flow generator. It may be used in CMV, IMV, or spontaneous ventilation modes with or without PEEP. Inspiratory pressure plateau may be provided.

Control and Surveillance

A four-position rotary knob, located on the control panel (Fig. 10-10), provides electrical power, alarm function testing, and mode selection (CPAP or CMV/IMV). In any position other than OFF, the power light is illuminated when the ventilator is connected to an appropriate electrical source. A buzzer activates, and all indicator lamps and LED displays are illuminated in the test mode. When the ventilator is disconnected from the electrical power source while in the test mode, a buzzer indicates adequate battery function.

Continuous circuit flow is adjusted with a rotary knob and indicated on a calibrated Thorpe tube (3–30 L·minute^{-1}). Continuous flow is usually adjusted at 1.5–2.0 times the estimated minute ventilation for spontaneous breathing or to minimize spontaneous inspiratory effort as indicated by the proximal airway pressure manometer. Oxygen concentration is continuously adjustable from 21 to 100 percent.

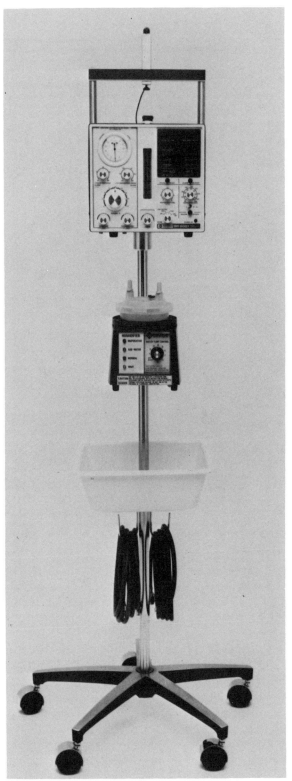

Fig. 10-9. Bear Cub infant ventilator. (Courtesy of Bear Medical, Inc.)

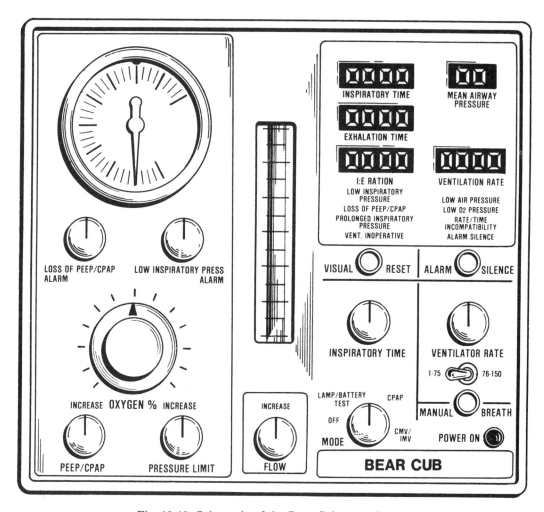

Fig. 10-10. Schematic of the Bear Cub control panel.

Mechanical ventilation is initiated by placing the mode selector in the CMV/IMV position. Tidal volume (VT) is primarily determined by the continuous flow rate, inspiratory time (TI) (range 0.1–3.0 seconds), and PIP limit control (0–72 cm H_2O). Once PIP limit occurs, circuit pressure is maintained for the duration of TI. Thus TI and PIP limit controls may be employed to establish an inspiratory pressure plateau (hold). Mechanical cycling frequency is adjustable either from 1 to 75 or 76 to 150 breaths·minute^{-1} depending on the position of the "rate range" toggle switch.

A manual inspiration (VT) at the programmed TI may be administered in the CPAP mode by depressing a pushbutton. End-expiratory pressure is continuously adjustable from −2 to 20 cm H_2O. Monitored ventilator and alarm functions are indicated in the upper right corner of the control panel. Inspiratory time, expiratory time, I : E ratio, ventilation rate, and mean airway pressure (P̄aw) are indicated on respective LED displays. "Loss of PEEP/CPAP" and "low inspiratory pressure" alarm controls are adjusted to levels slightly below selected PEEP/CPAP and observed PIP, respectively. A loss of PEEP/CPAP alarm may result from a circuit leak or a significant pressure decrease during spontaneous inspiration, indicating insufficient continuous circuit flow. A low inspiratory pressure alarm may indicate a circuit leak or exhalation valve dysfunction when PIP does not reach the preselected level.

A "prolonged inspiratory pressure" alarm activates when a pressure 10 cm H_2O higher than the loss of PEEP/CPAP alarm adjustment is sustained for longer than 3.5 seconds. A "ventilator inoperative" alarm engages when any of the following conditions occurs: failure to cycle, electrical power failure/disconnect, high/low T_I, panel control malfunction, and timing circuit failure. Low air and oxygen pressure alarms activate if inlet pressures fall below 22.5 psig. A "rate/time incompatibility" alarm activates when the selected frequency and T_I prevent an exhalation time (T_E) of at least 0.25 second. The ventilator then overrides the programmed T_I to provide the necessary T_E until the condition is corrected.

All alarm functions, except "rate/time incompatibility" and "alarm silence," must be reset by depressing a pushbutton after correction. Audible alarms may be silenced for 30 seconds by depressing another pushbutton.

Operation

Inspiratory (Fig. 10-11) and expiratory (Fig. 10-12) phase gas flows are illustrated. Air and oxygen at 15–75 and 30–75 psig, respectively, are regulated to within 2 cm H_2O of each other at the lowest inlet pressure before entering the blender. A pressure switch monitors each gas inlet to warn of low values, and anaeroid manometers indicate the respective pressures. Unidirectional valves are incorporated into each high-pressure system to prevent retrograde flow.

Once gas is blended, it passes through a flow control valve into a calibrated Thorpe tube (not illustrated). Distal to the flow meter system is a pressure relief valve which limits maximum circuit pressure. Should maximum pressure be attained before the inspiratory time has elapsed, excess flow (pressure) will vent to ambient. An internal overpressure relief valve is factory-adjusted to open at 87 ± 4 cm H_2O, decreasing the circuit pressire to 40 ± 15 cm H_2O. The resultant relief pressure depends on the adjusted flow. When pressure decreases to the lower relief level, the valve resets. If the problem causing excessive pressure is still present, the relief valve again opens at 87 ± 4 cm H_2O. Thus pressure rises and falls in the breathing circuit until the problem (e.g., obstruction or a circuit kink) is corrected. During any overpressure condition, the vented gas passes through a pneumatic whistle (alarm).

A subambient inspiratory relief valve permits spontaneous breathing from room air if ventilator malfunction occurs. An inspiratory effort of − 2 cm H_2O is required to open this valve.

During mechanical inspiration, a solenoid diverts gas from the pressure limit control through a metering valve to pressurize the exhalation valve. This valve occludes the exhalation port of the circuit and diverts the continuous flow to the infant. Exhalation valve pressure is equal to the selected pressure limit. Any excess circuit pressure generated during mechanical inspiration is bled (vented) past the exhalation valve. The metering valve modulates a pressure signal between the pressure limit control and the exhalation valve. At high continuous circuit flow, the metering valve facilitates rapid exhalation valve closure, thus creating a square-wave inspiratory flow pattern. Exhalation valve pressurization and closure is slower with low continuous flow, resulting in an exponential-wave contour. Proximal airway pressure is indicated on an anaeroid manometer and monitored by a transducer for electronic calculations. A 0.2

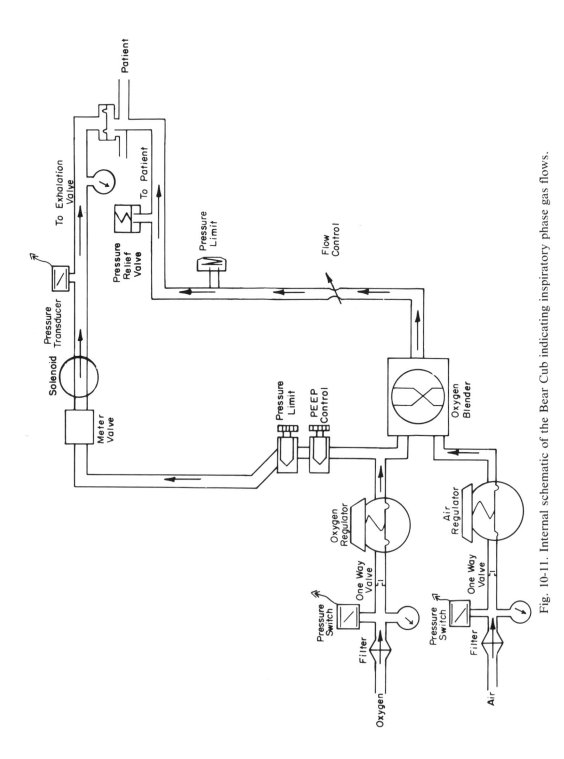

Fig. 10-11. Internal schematic of the Bear Cub indicating inspiratory phase gas flows.

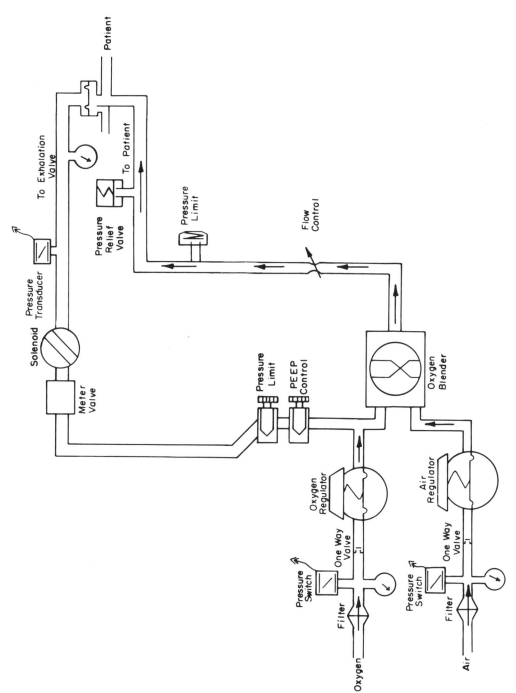

Fig. 10-12. Internal schematic of the Bear Cub indicating expiratory phase gas flows.

345

L·minute^{-1} flow of blended gas is purged through the proximal pressure line into the breathing circuit to prevent moisture contamination of the manometer and transducer.

During exhalation the signal from the pressure relief control is interrupted by a solenoid causing exhalation valve depressurization to ambient pressure (unless the PEEP control is activated). A PEEP control signal is directed through the solenoid to effect pressurization of the exhalation valve to the desired level during the expiratory phase. A fixed-flow jet venturi device (not illustrated) creates a subambient pressure in the exhalation valve assembly (0 to -2 cm H_2O depending on the resistance pressure developed by the continuous circuit flow. This mechanism helps to minimize circuit resistance to flow (back-pressure) and is balanced with the PEEP control to establish the desired expiratory pressure.

Reference

Model 2001 Instruction Manual No. 5000–10220 and Maintenance Manual No. 5000–12033. Bear Medical Systems, Inc., Riverside, CA

BEAR 1 ADULT VOLUME VENTILATOR

The Bear 1 adult volume ventilator (Fig. 10-13) is a pneumatically and electronically powered, electronically controlled, volume-cycled flow generator. Flow may be delivered with a constant or tapered waveform. It employs CMV, ASSIST-CONTROL, synchronized IMV (SIMV), and CPAP modes. Postinflation hold (plateau) and PEEP are available.

Control and Surveillance

Ventilatory controls and monitors are located on the main control panel (Fig. 10-14). Ventilation is programmed with the mode selector knob. Controls include: tidal volume (100–2000 ml) and cycling frequency (5–60 breaths·minute^{-1}). Not shown is a "rate ÷ 10" switch which provides 0.5–6 breaths·minute^{-1} and pressure cycle (0–100 cm H_2O). The ventilator may be placed in a standby mode. Controls and alarms (except "ventilator inoperative" and "low air pressure") are then inoperative, and the ventilator switches to the CPAP mode.

Single or multiple sigh breaths may be adjusted with a volume of 150–3000 ml delivered 2–60 times/hour. The sigh breath pressure limit is 0–100 cm H_2O.

When activated, a volume accumulator measures and displays minute volume (i.e., the sum of mechanical and spontaneous V_T over a minute). A "waveform" control regulates the ventilator driving pressure, providing flow taper capabilities. Maximum flow taper is achieved at the extreme counterclockwise setting and when circuit pressure exceeds 50 cm H_2O.

An assist control adjusts the inspiratory effort required to initiate a patient-triggered breath. A "ratio limit" control in the ON position terminates inspiration and activates audible and visual alarms if the inspiratory time exceeds the expiratory time.

F_{IO_2} control is continuously adjustable from 0.21 to 1.0. Mechanical V_T may be delivered at flows of 20–120 L·minute^{-1}. An end-inspiratory plateau control, when activated, delays exhalation valve opening for up to 2 seconds. The PEEP control range is 0–30 cm H_2O. No adjustment of the patient-triggering level is required when PEEP is changed.

A "low-pressure" alarm is adjustable from 0 to 50 cm H_2O and is activated (visually and audibly) when the inspiratory pressure does not exceed the set value (e.g., disconnection during IPPV). The exhaled volume alarm is adjustable from 0 to 2.0 L and activates (visually and audibly) when the exhaled V_T does not exceed the baseline value for three consecutive breaths. All audible alarms can be silenced for 60 seconds. A "PEEP/CPAP" alarm control activates

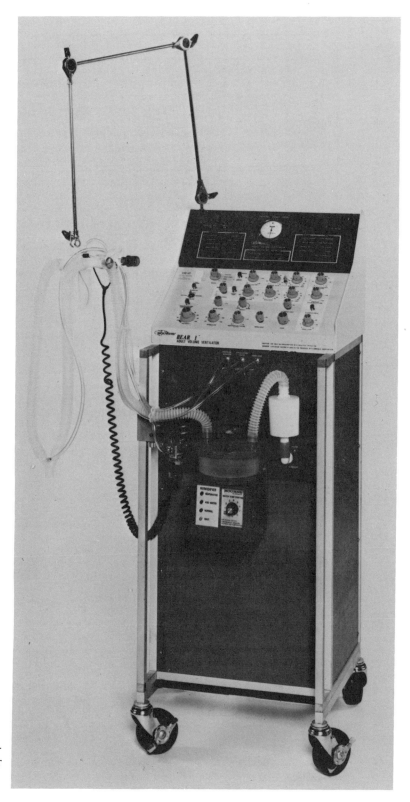

Fig. 10-13. Bear 1 ventilator. (Courtesy of Bear Medical, Inc.)

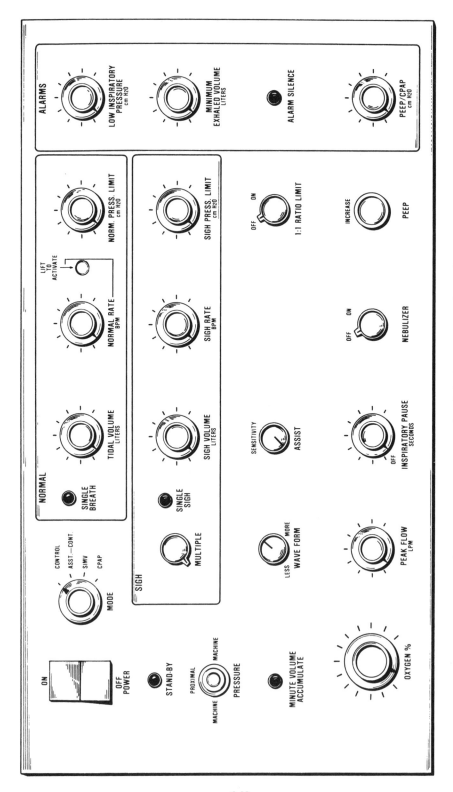

Fig. 10-14. Schematic of the Bear 1 control panel.

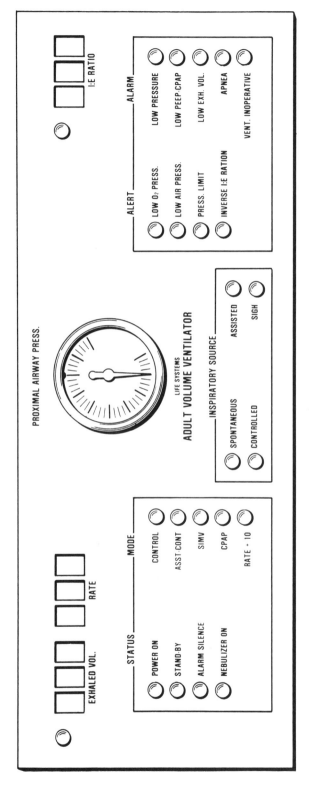

Fig. 10-15. Schematic of the Bear 1 mode/alarm panel.

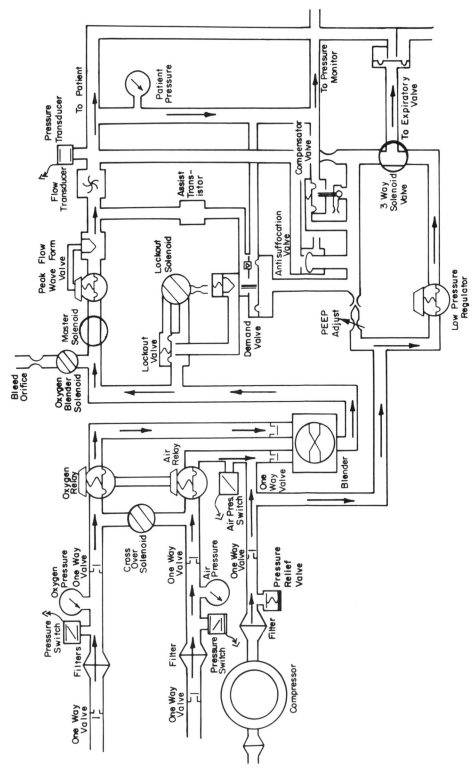

Fig. 10-16. Internal schematic of the Bear 1 indicating inspiratory phase gas flows.

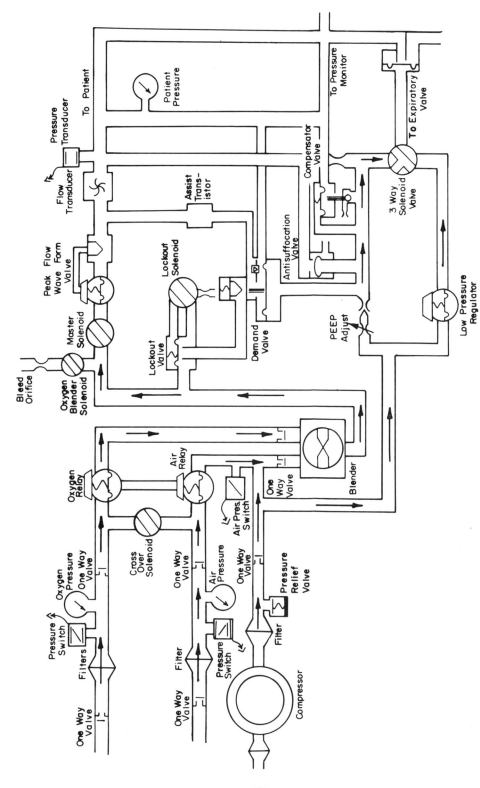

Fig. 10-17. Internal schematic of the Bear 1 indicating expiratory phase gas flows.

(visually and audibly) when expiratory pressure is less than the preselected value (e.g., disconnection in CPAP mode).

A vertical display panel contains the proximal airway pressure manometer and various function indicator and alarm lights (Fig. 10-15). The LED displays indicate exhaled volume, respiratory rate, and I:E ratio. "Status" indications include power on, stand-by, alarm silence, and nebulizer on. "Ventilator mode" indicates whether CONTROL, ASSIST-CONTROL, SIMV, CPAP, or RATE/10 is employed. Lamps under "inspiratory source" illuminate appropriately when spontaneous, controlled, assisted, or sigh breaths occur. "Alert" and "alarm" lights activate under the following conditions: low O_2 source pressure (<30 psig at FIO_2 > 0.21); low air pressure (<9.5 psig); circuit pressure limit; inspiratory exceeds expiratory time (I:E ratio); low circuit pressure; low PEEP/CPAP; apnea (20 seconds elapse between breaths); and ventilator inoperative (total gas, internal electronics, or AC power failure).

Operation

Inspiratory (Fig. 10-16). and expiratory (Fig. 10-17) phase gas flows are illustrated. Air and oxygen are delivered at 30–100 psig through sintered stainless steel filters which remove particles greater than 40 μm in size. Both pressures are regulated to approximately 11 psig and equilibrated ± 2 cm H_2O. Blended gas to ensure an accurate FIO_2 is available to the system at 11 psig if flow is 0 L·minute^{-1} but decreases to 5.5 psig when flow approaches 120 L·minute^{-1}. Should air pressure decrease below 27.5 psig, an internal air compressor is activated. No alarm is activated during this changeover as it may also be a normal mode of operation if external compressed air is unavailable. The compressor pressure is 9.5 psig. Should either gas decrease below operating pressure limits, a crossover solenoid opens to facilitate pneumatic power from the higher pressure source. If all gas pressure sources fail, an "antisuffocation valve" opens, permitting the patient to breathe ambient air.

The main solenoid valve determines tidal volume delivery in conjunction with the peak flow and waveform controls. It is electronically opened but closed by opposing spring tension. Inspiratory time, volume, and flow characteristics are integrated. Waveform contour is altered by manipulating the driving pressure prior to peak flow valve. It may be adjusted from 3.2 psig (225 cm H_2O) to 1.8 psig (125 cm H_2O) to generate constant (square-wave) or decelerating inspiratory flow patterns, respectively. With maximum flow taper, a 50 percent decrease in peak flow may occur toward the end of inspiration. The actual decrement depends on peak airway pressure; as the airway to driving pressure gradient narrows, flow deceleration is more pronounced.

Inspiratory flow is measured by a transducer utilizing a fixed vortex generator. Vortices created by flow through the transducer are sensed ultrasonically. By design, each vortex is equal to 1 ml of gas; thus inspiratory volume is measured. Outflow pressure (proximal to humidifier/circuit resistance) is transduced and signaled to the electronic logic unit. This pressure is *not* equal to the proximal airway pressure. Thus an alarm condition related to overpressurization caused by a kink in the ventilator outflow tubing proximal to the humidifier may not be detected by the anaeroid manometer connected to the proximal airway.

A demand system for spontaneous breathing capable of delivering up to 100 L·minute^{-1} is referenced to the PEEP/CPAP level by exposing both sides of the demand valve diaphragm to the baseline pressure. Demand flow is initiated when a 1 cm H_2O pressure gradient is developed across the diaphragm. Should the patient become disconnected from the ventilator while on PEEP/CPAP, a pressure differential equivalent to the PEEP/CPAP level is created across the diaphragm, and a maximal gas flow results. The pressure reference for this demand system is in the proximal airway connection; therefore any interruption of this line (even to measure pressure with a mercury manometer) is sensed as a patient disconnect. Demand flow comes directly from the blender, bypassing the main solenoid and peak flow control. A lockout valve prevents demand valve function during control mode. A 0.1 L·minute^{-1} retrograde flow through the proximal airway pressure line removes accumulated moisture.

PEEP/CPAP is adjusted by flow through a venturi device, which creates expiratory pressure with a three-way solenoid valve. During the expiratory phase the solenoid directs a residual pressure, determined by the PEEP/CPAP control, into the exhalation mushroom valve. It also maintains pressure in the exhalation valve during pause time (inspiratory plateau). A low-pressure regulator decreases the pneumatic driving pressure to the exhalation valve/PEEP circuitry. At end-inspiration (or after the plateau), exhalation valve gas is vented through a compensator valve, working in concert with the PEEP control.

Reference

Bear 1 Instruction Manual No. 50000–10500. Bear Medical Systems, Inc., Riverside, CA

BEAR 2 ADULT VOLUME VENTILATOR

The Bear 2 adult volume ventilator (Fig. 10-18) is a pneumatically and electronically powered, electronically controlled, volume-cycled, flow generator. Flow may be delivered with a constant or decelerating waveform. End-inspiratory pause and PEEP are available. It may be operated in CMV, ASSIST-CONTROL, SIMV, or CPAP modes.

Control and Surveillance

Power to the electrical circuitry is controlled by an ON/OFF switch (Fig. 10-19). The ventilatory mode is selected from a four-position rotary knob labeled CMV, ASSIST-CONTROL, SIMV, and CPAP.

Tidal volume (V_T) is continuously adjustable from 0.1 to 2.0 L at a cycling frequency of 0.5–60 breaths·minute^{-1}. PIP ranges up to 120 cm H_2O. When the selected PIP is exceeded, exhalation occurs immediately. A single breath equal to the programmed V_T may be administered 350 milliseconds or more into exhalation during any ventilatory mode. Deep breath or sigh volume is adjustable from 0.15 to 3.0 L at a rate of 2–60·hour^{-1}. The PIP cycle of a sigh is 0–120 cm H_2O and may be delivered in multiples of two or three. When the sigh function is activated, a single deep breath may be initiated by depressing a button any time 350 milliseconds or more into exhalation.

Tidal volume may be delivered with a continuous or decelerating inspiratory flow pattern. The desired waveform is selected with a two-position toggle switch. Constant or square-wave inspiratory flow is approximately equal to the adjusted peak flow (10–120 L·minute^{-1}). In the decelerating or tapered position, inspiratory flow initially is equivalent to peak flow, but as circuit pressure increases the outflow decreases. Maximum flow deceleration (approximately 50 percent of adjusted peak flow) occurs at 120 cm H_2O.

In ASSIST-CONTROL, SIMV, and CPAP modes, the effort required for patient-initiated breaths is regulated by an uncalibrated "assist" control. During mechanical V_T delivery, liquid in the circuit medication reservoir may be aerosolized by engaging the "nebulizer" control. The nebulizer control diverts a portion of the V_T to facilitate nebulization; thus F_{IO_2} and delivered V_T remain unaltered. Nebulization does *not* occur when peak flow is less than 30 L·minute^{-1}.

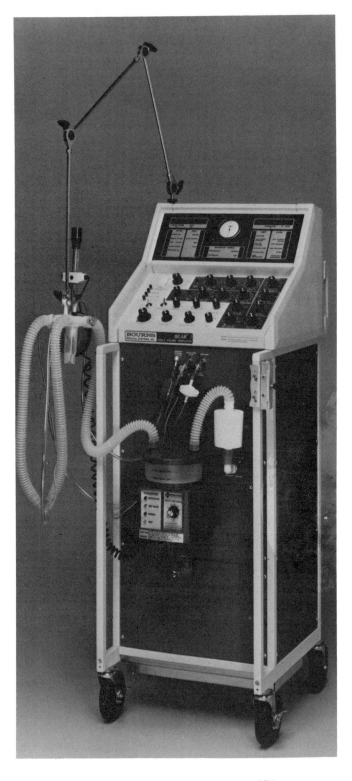

Fig. 10-18. Bear 2 adult ventilator. (Courtesy of Bear Medical, Inc.)

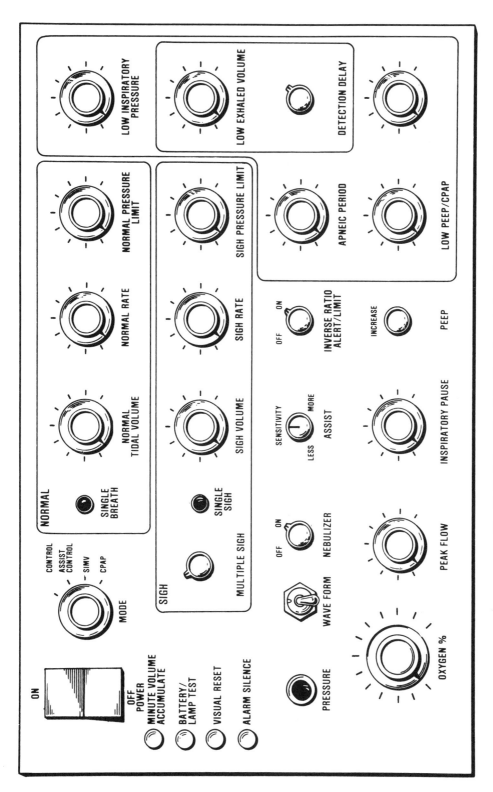

Fig. 10-19. Schematic of the Bear 2 control panel.

355

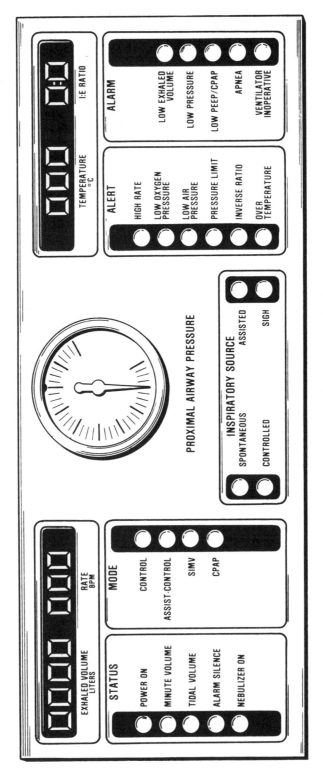

Fig. 10-20. Schematic of the Bear 2 mode/alarm panel.

Inspiration may be extended after V_T delivery by clockwise rotation of the inspiratory pause control which delays exhalation valve opening up to 2.0 seconds. If inspiratory time exceeds expiratory time, the ventilator automatically cycles to exhalation *unless* the inverse ratio alert/alarm is deactivated. PEEP is controlled by residual pressure in the exhalation valve regulated by an uncalibrated PEEP control (range 0–50 cm H_2O).

FIO_2 is regulated from 0.21 to 1.0. Machine-sensed circuit pressure is measured by leftward positioning of a self-returning toggle switch and is indicated on an aneroid manometer. At all other times the actual proximal airway pressure is indicated.

Ventilator and alarm functions are indicated on a display panel (Fig. 10-20). "Status," "mode," and "inspiratory source" lamps illuminate when the appropriate function activates. Proximal airway temperature is displayed in degrees centigrade. The I:E ratio is calculated and indicated. Alert/alarm conditions precipitate visual and audible indications of discrepancies. "High rate" alarms activate when the selected high rate control (10–80 breaths·minute^{-1}) is exceeded (mechanical plus spontaneous breathing). The alarm condition deactivates if the ventilatory rate subsequently decreases below the high rate setting. "Low oxygen pressure" alarms engage when the oxygen percentage control is set above 21 percent and the inlet pressure is below 27.5 ± 2.5 psig. A "low air pressure" alarm indicates a decreased external source and/or internal compressor pressure less than 27.5 ± 2.5 and 9.5 psig, respectively. When mechanical inspiration is pressure- or time-limited, audible and visual alarms activate. An activated "temperature" alarm is indicative of a proximal airway temperature ≥ 41°C.

Low exhaled volume is adjusted from 0.1 to 2.0 L. If monitored exhaled volume is less than the selected value for the number of consecutive breaths adjusted on the "detection delay" knob (2–5 breaths), alarms activate. Low inspiratory pressure is adjustable from 5 to 75 cm H_2O. If a CMV or SIMV breath is delivered with less PIP than the selected low inspiratory pressure, an alarm activates, usually indicating a circuit or airway leak. "Low PEEP/CPAP" alarm function is adjustable from OFF to 50 cm H_2O. Decrease of PEEP/CPAP below the selected level generally results either from a circuit/airway leak or an insufficient demand flow during spontaneous ventilation. If a mechanical or spontaneous breath fails to occur within the alloted time selected by the "apneic period" control (2–20 seconds), alarms are activated.

Mean ventilatory rate (mechanical and/or spontaneous) is calculated over 20 seconds and displayed in breaths·minute^{-1}. Breath-to-breath exhaled volume is indicated in liters. Accumulated minute volume is displayed for a 2-minute cycle when a pushbutton is depressed.

Internal rechargeable nickel cadmium battery function and control panel indicator lamps and LED displays are tested by depressing a pushbutton. Should external electrical power malfunction or disconnection occur, a battery-powered audible and visual alarm activate. Visual alarms may be reset by depressing the appropriate pushbutton after correcting the alarm condition. Audible alarms may be silenced for 60 seconds or can be manually reactivated by depressing a pushbutton.

Operation

Inspiratory (Fig. 10-21) and expiratory (Fig. 10-22) phase gas flows are illustrated. Air and oxygen are delivered at 30–100 psig through sintered stainless steel filters which remove particles greater than 40 μm in size. Gases are regulated to approximately 11 psig and equilibrated ± 2 cm H_2O. Blended gas to ensure accurate FIO_2 is available to the system at 11 psig if flow is 0 L·minute^{-1} but decreases to 5.5 psig when flow nears 120 L·minute^{-1}. Should air pressure decrease below 27.5 psig, an internal air com-

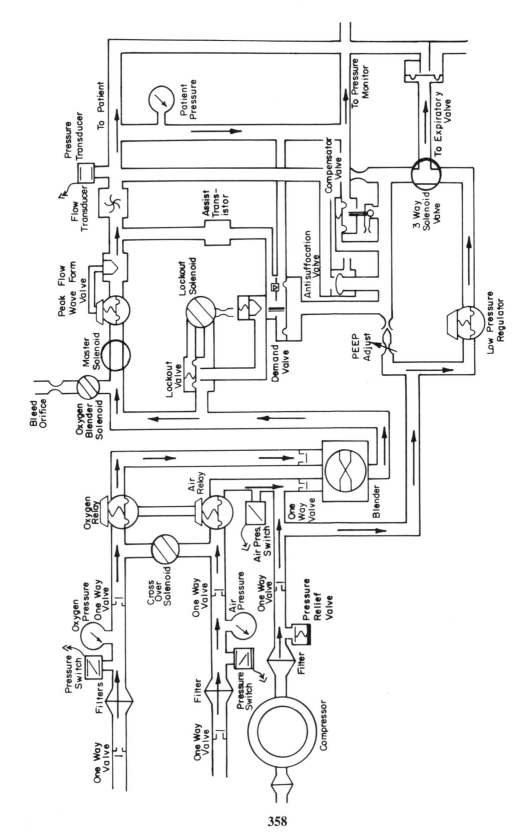

Fig. 10-21. Internal schematic of the Bear 2 indicating inspiratory phase gas flows.

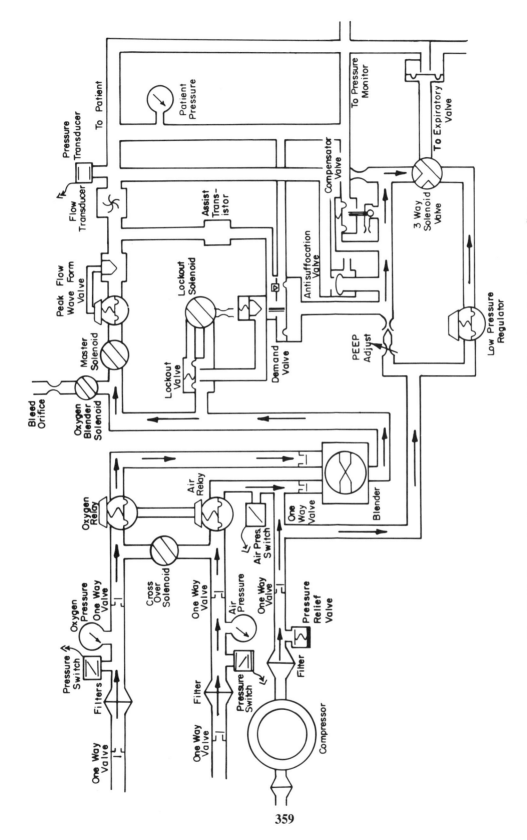

Fig. 10-22. Internal schematic of the Bear 2 indicating expiratory phase gas flows.

pressor automatically engages. No alarm sounds as this can be a normal mode of operation when external compressed air is unavailable. The compressor working pressure is 9.5 psig. When either compressed gas decreases below the minimal operating limit, a crossover solenoid opens to provide pneumatic power from the higher pressure source. If all gas pressure sources fail, an "antisuffocation valve" opens, permitting the patient to breathe ambient air spontaneously.

During mechanical inspiration, the main solenoid valve, working in tandem with the waveform and peak flow controls, determines not only inspiratory time but volume and flow characteristics as well. A constant or tapered inspiratory flow pattern is selected by a two-position toggle switch. In taper position, as much as a 50 percent decrease in peak flow may occur toward the end of inspiration, depending on the peak airway pressure; as the airway to driving pressure gradient narrows, flow deceleration is more pronounced.

Inspiratory flow is measured by a transducer utilizing a fixed vortex generator. Vortices created by flow through the transducer are sensed ultrasonically. By design, each vortex is equal to 1 ml of gas; thus inspiratory volume is measured. Outflow pressure proximal to the humidifier/circuit resistance is transduced and signaled to the electronic logic unit. This is outflow, not proximal airway pressure; therefore the machine may alarm, indicating an overpressure condition which is undetected by the proximal airway pressure gauge (anaeroid manometer).

A demand system capable of delivering 100 L·minute^{-1} is referenced to the PEEP/CPAP level by exposing both sides of the demand valve diaphragm to the baseline pressure. Demand flow is initiated by a 1 cm H_2O pressure gradient across the diaphragm. Should the patient become disconnected from the ventilator while on PEEP/CPAP, a pressure differential equivalent to PEEP/CPAP is created against the demand valve diaphragm, resulting in maximum flow. The pressure reference for this demand system is in the proximal airway connection. Any interruption of this line (even to measure pressure via a mercury manometer) is sensed as a patient disconnect. A 0.1 L·minute^{-1} retrograde gas flow through the proximal airway pressure line removes moisture. Demand flow comes directly from the blender, bypassing the main solenoid and peak flow control. A lockout valve prevents demand valve function during control mode.

PEEP/CPAP is adjusted by flow through a venturi device, which creates expiratory pressure with a three-way solenoid valve. The solenoid also maintains pressure in the exhalation mushroom valve during the postinflation pause (plateau). A low-pressure regulator decreases pneumatic driving pressure to the exhalation valve/PEEP circuitry. At end-inspiration exhalation valve gas is vented through a compensator valve, working in conjunction with the PEEP control.

Reference

Bear 2 Instruction Manual No. 50000–10530. Bear Medical Systems, Inc., Riverside, CA

BENNETT MA-1 VENTILATOR

The Bennett MA-1 ventilator (Fig. 10-23) is an electronically powered and controlled, volume-cycled, constant-flow generator. It may be used in CMV or ASSIST modes with optional PEEP and may be modified to provide IMV.

Control and Surveillance

Ventilator parameters are easily adjusted on a control panel (Fig. 10-24). A main switch controls all electrical circuitry. Nor-

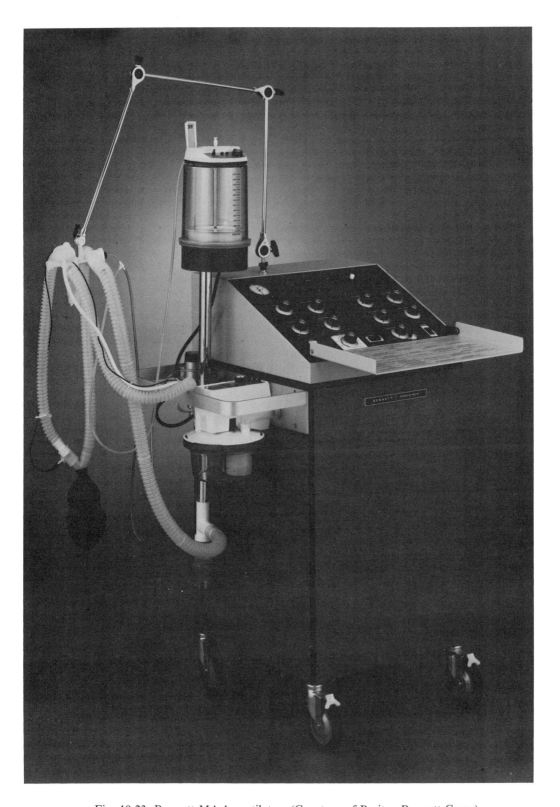

Fig. 10-23. Bennett MA-1 ventilator. (Courtesy of Puritan-Bennett Corp.)

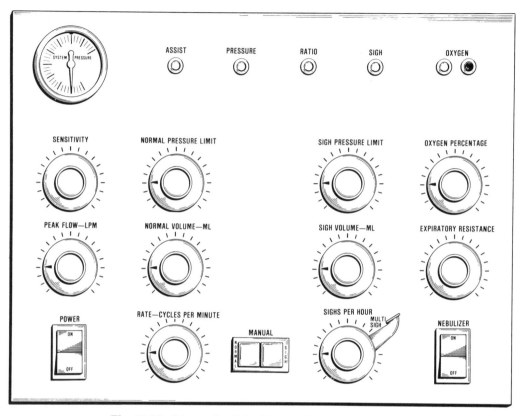

Fig. 10-24. Schematic of the Bennett MA-1 control panel.

mal tidal volume (V_T) is adjustable (0–2200 ml) at peak inflation pressure (20–80 cm H_2O). Peak flow is variable up to 100 L·minute^{-1}, and at any given setting is maximum at the onset of inspiration. As circuit pressure increases, this constant-flow-generating characteristic decreases. Ventilator cycling may be controlled from 1 to 60 breaths·minute^{-1} or the sensitivity adjusted to permit patient triggering. Deep breaths up to 2200 ml at 20–80 cm H_2O pressure may be administered by adjusting the sigh volume control for single breaths of 4, 6, 8, 10, or 15·hour^{-1} or multiples of two or three. A sigh is delivered in lieu of a controlled or assisted V_T at the programmed interval.

Manual delivery of a normal tidal volume or sigh is accomplished by depressing the appropriate pushbutton. Upon termination of the manual breath, the rate timer rephases to the programmed value. F_{IO_2} is regulated from 0.21 to 1.0 when the ventilator is connected appropriately to oxygen. An "expiratory resistance" control regulates the rate of the exhalation mushroom valve depressurization, thereby providing flow retardation. When this control is increased to maximum, a momentary delay in exhalation valve opening occurs, creating postinflation hold (plateau).

Aerosolized solutions may be administered via a small reservoir nebulizer in the patient circuit. When the nebulization button is placed in the ON position, a portion of the V_T or sigh volume is shunted to power the nebulizer jet. Aerosol therapy applied in this manner does not alter V_T or F_{IO_2}.

Circuit pressure is indicated by an aneroid manometer calibrated from -10 to 80 cm H_2O and connected proximal to the humidifier. Ventilator function monitoring utilizes a series of lights located in the upper portion of the panel. Proper illumination is ascertained by depressing the case enclosing each lamp. Monitoring includes an amber "assist" light, indicating a patient-initiated breath, and a red "pressure" light which illuminates when inspiration is pressure-cycled (an audible buzzer also sounds concomitantly). If the I:E ratio, which is dependent on V_T, peak flow, and controlled cycling frequency, exceeds 1:1, a red light illuminates. During each sigh breath, a white light is activated. The oxygen monitoring system is composed of a green and red light. When the F_{IO_2} is set above 0.21 while the ventilator is attached to *any* high-pressure gas source, the green light illuminates. The red light and an audible alarm are activated when the F_{IO_2} is set beyond 0.21 without a sufficiently high pressure gas source.

IMV Modification

IMV may be employed with the MA-1 after simple modification. Early production models provided a minimum rate of 6 breaths·minute^{-1}; however, factory-installed rate controllers down to 1 breath·minute^{-1} subsequently became available. An external source of fresh gas for spontaneous breathing must be interfaced with the circuit (see Fig. 2-32). When a continuous-flow system is used, the pressure gauge on the control panel registers a value higher than is actually present at the proximal airway. This "artifactual" back-pressure is derived from flow resistance produced by the cascade humidifier (tower assembly and water level). Another potential problem with this IMV modification is related to the delivered mechanical tidal volume. When a high continuous flow is delivered into the IMV circuit assembly and exceeds the flow delivered from the ventilator, the unidirectional valve does not completely close during mechanical inspiration. The continuous gas flow is then added to the programmed V_T, thereby increasing tidal volume. This condition occurs most frequently at low ventilator peak flows when the circuit pressure rises slowly and delays closure of the valve.

Operation

Inspiratory (Fig. 10-25) and expiratory (Fig. 10-26) phase gas flows are illustrated. Electrical (AC) power and compressed oxygen (for $F_{IO_2} > 0.21$) are necessary for operation. High-pressure oxygen is regulated to 40 ± 3 psig and then to 1.8–2.1 cm H_2O in the oxygen accumulator. When pressure in the accumulator decreases to 0.5–0.9 cm H_2O an alarm sounds. The oxygen is delivered to an oxygen percentage control, which adjusts gas flow to the stack valve electronically. This adjustment is made proportionately to filtered ambient air drawn into the stack valve assembly as the bellows descends during mechanical exhalation.

Bellows descent in the cannister to the designated tidal volume level is controlled by a pulley. Pulley displacement is selected by the volume control potentiometer. Once the bellows is in position, filtered ambient air from the compressor is delivered by the main solenoid to a venturi device, which boosts (via entrainment) total flow to 100 L·minute^{-1}. The resultant flow to the cannister is regulated by the "peak flow" control.

A portion of the venturi outflow is shunted to a "dump valve" to allow cannister pressurization. The peak flow determines the rate at which the bellows is compressed within the cannister or the time for tidal volume delivery. As the bellows ascends, gas passes through a unidirectional outlet valve system, then through a filter

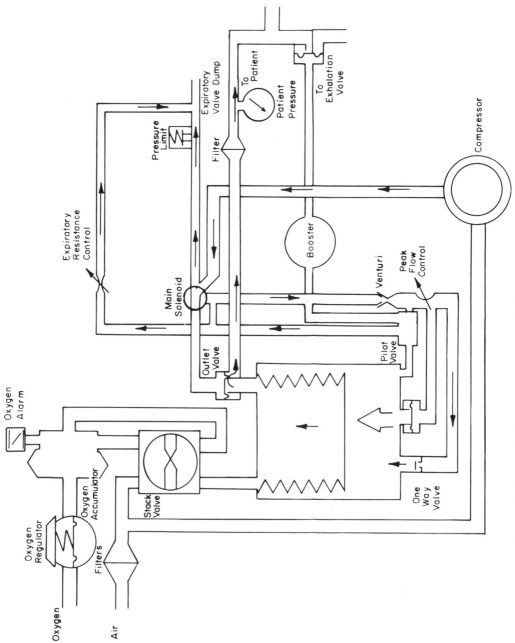

Fig. 10-25. Internal schematic of the Bennett MA-1 indicating inspiratory phase gas flows.

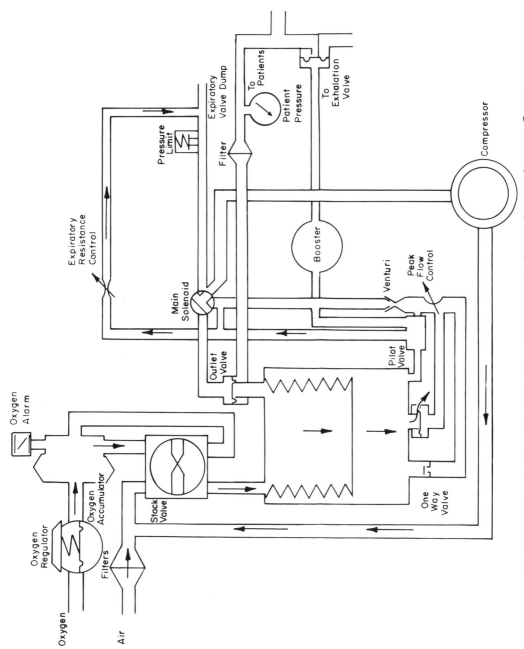

Fig. 10-26. Internal schematic of the Bennett MA-1 indicating expiratory phase gas flows.

365

and humidification system before entering the distal circuit and the patient's lungs. Simultaneously with the bellows compression, a secondary system closes the breathing circuit exhalation valve through a pilot valve which diverts gas into the exhalation valve system. Pressure from the pilot valve is regulated by a "PEEP" control which bleeds gas into the exhalation valve dump system. This control maintains pressure in the mushroom of the exhalation valve and controls the level of expiratory pressure in the breathing circuit. The control which cycles the ventilator to the exhalation phase when excessive peak inspiratory pressure is generated is also within this system. This same system must be pressurized during the expiratory phase to close the outlet valve so that the bellows refills only with gas from the stack valve.

Reference

Model MA-1 Operating Instructions No. 50300. Bennett Medical Equipment, Los Angeles, CA

BENNETT MA-2 VENTILATOR; BENNETT MA 2 + 2 VENTILATOR

The Bennett MA-2 ventilator (Fig. 10-27) is an electronically powered and controlled, volume-cycled, constant-flow generator at zero back-pressure. Mechanical inspiration is either continuous (CMV) or intermittent (IMV/CPAP) and may be extended by a postinflation hold (plateau). PEEP and SIMV are standard features.

Control and Surveillance

All electronic components (except the humidifier emersion heater) are activated by the power switch on the control panel (Fig. 10-28). The humidifier-heater is reg-

ulated independently by a temperature control. This feature permits heating of the water reservoir before anticipated use.

The desired ventilatory mode is engaged by depressing either IMV/CPAP or CMV buttons. In the former mode, the patient's minute ventilation (MV) may be augmented (IMV) or entirely spontaneous (IMV = 0 or CPAP). During CMV the entire minute ventilation is mechanical (by means of controlled or patient-triggered breaths).

Tidal volume for IMV and normal CMV breaths is adjustable up to 2200 ml at peak flow of 20–125 L·minute^{-1}. The selected peak flow is maximal during the initial phase of inspiration; as airway pressure rises, this value decreases. PIP during IMV and CMV ranges from 20 to 120 cm H_2O. A safety catch-pin is located at 80 cm H_2O and must be purposely depressed to permit greater PIP. When selected PIP is reached, the ventilator cycles to exhalation.

Independent cycling controls are provided for CMV (0 and 3–60 breaths·minute^{-1}) and IMV (0, 0.3–3, and 3–30 breaths·minute^{-1} in low and high ranges, respectively). The inspiratory effort threshold for patient-initiated CMV, IMV (SIMV), and demand flow (spontaneous breathing during IMV or CPAP) is adjustable from -10 cm H_2O to a maximum sensitivity level which results in autocycling. The programmed inspiratory effort required for a given ventilator response is not altered by subsequent adjustment of end-expiratory pressure. PEEP/CPAP (0–45 cm H_2O) is selected by an uncalibrated knob.

Inspiration may be extended (0–2.0 seconds) with the "plateau" control only in the CMV mode. When CMV inspiration is pressure-cycled, no plateau occurs. If inspiratory exceeds expiratory time (as determined by CMV rate selection), the plateau is terminated.

Manual inspiration equivalent to the CMV volume may be administered during the expiratory phase of IMV and CMV, or any time in the CPAP mode. After manual

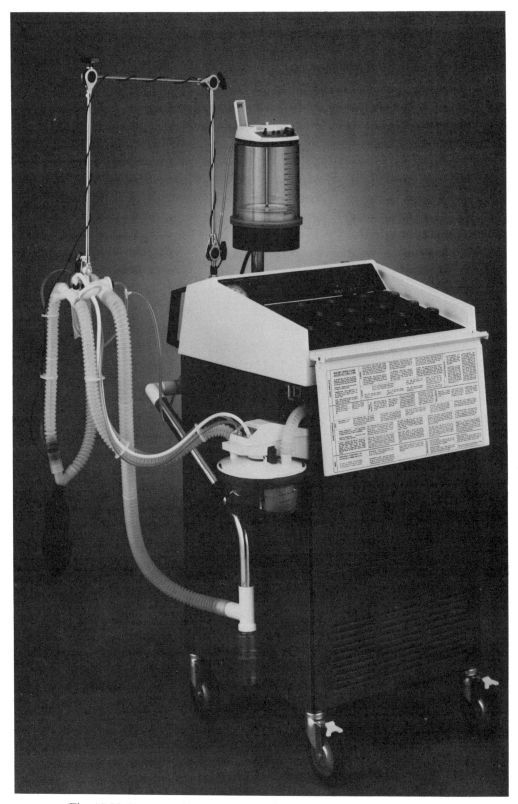

Fig. 10-27. Bennett MA-2 ventilator. (Courtesy of Puritan-Bennett Corp.)

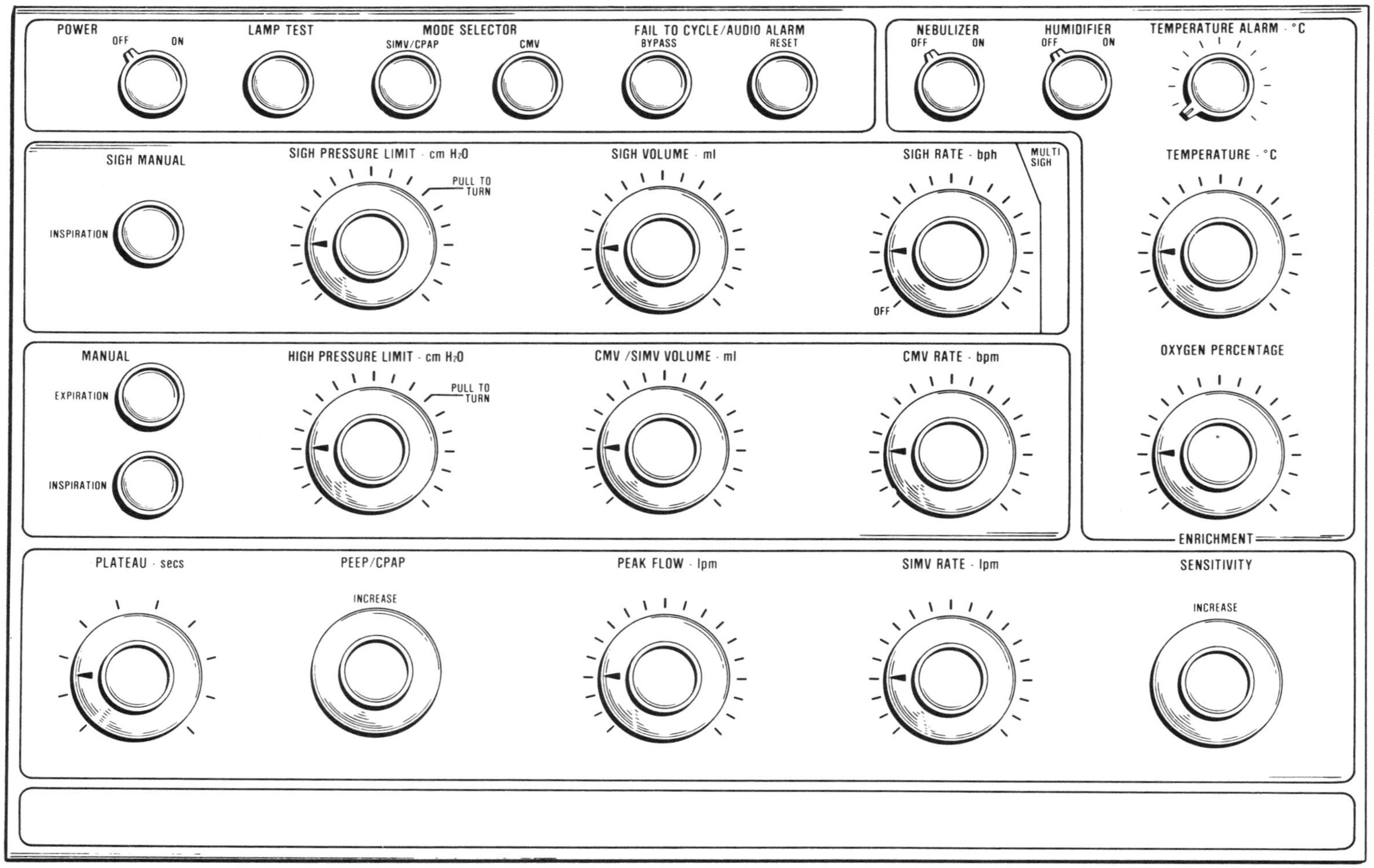

Fig. 10-28. Schematic of the Bennett MA-2 control panel.

inspiration, the rate timer resets to the established exhalation time. Mechanical exhalation may be initiated manually in any ventilator mode. This maneuver facilitates complete bellows refill, resetting the timer for the next CMV or IMV breath. The need for manual exhalation commonly arises during transient disruption in the patient-ventilator interface during IMV/CPAP. When the circuit pressure decreases as the patient is disconnected from the MA-2, the demand flow system rapidly exhausts the bellows volume (a functional sustained inspiration). To ensure availability of gas for subsequent demand, the manual exhalation is activated just before reestablishing the patient-ventilator interface.

When a deep breath is desired, adjustments must be made for: sigh pressure limit (20–120 cm H_2O), sigh volume (up to 2200 ml), and sigh rate (0–15 cycles·hour^{-1} either singly or in multiples of two or three consecutive breaths). A manual inspiration equivalent to the sigh volume may be delivered during the exhalation phase in any mode. After a manual sigh the rate timer resets to zero.

F_{IO_2} is adjustable from 0.21 to 1.0. Aerosol therapy in conjunction with mechanical inspiration may be employed by adding the desired solution to the circuit small reservoir cup and engaging the nebulizer control.

"Patient-ventilator interface" and "ventilator function" monitors and alarms are primarily located uppermost on the control panel (Fig. 10-29). LED displays (temperature, rate, and oxygen percent), "mode in use" lights (IMV, CPAP, CMV, oxygen, audioalarm bypass, sigh, and assist), and visual alarm indicators (fail-to-cycle, temperature, high pressure, low pressure, ratio, and oxygen) all illuminate when the "lamp test" button is depressed.

Proximal airway pressure (Paw) is indicated on an anaeroid manometer calibrated from − 10 to 120 cm H_2O. Paw may not correlate with the PIP cycle value. The indicated pressure is usually lower because the PIP cycle sensor is proximal to the humidifier and the inspiratory limb flow resistance of the breathing circuit.

Proximal airway temperature is measured by a thermister and displayed in degrees centigrade. Ventilatory rate (mechanical and spontaneous) is indicated and reassessed every four breaths. An optional polarographic oxygen sensor monitors and displays oxygen concentration. "High" and "low" oxygen percent limits may be selected, and if these are exceeded audible and visual alarms activate.

Each alarm condition evokes both visual and audible indicators. "Fail-to-cycle" alarm activation occurs when the main power is on, but 20 seconds elapse without a ventilator-"sensed" inspiration or expiration. It functions primarily as an apnea and back-up circuit disconnect alarm. The "temperature" alarm engages if proximal airway temperature exceeds a preselected value. "High pressure" illuminates when the PIP limit is exceeded and the ventilator cycles to exhalation. A "low-pressure" alarm condition exists when Paw relative to baseline either fails to increase at least 10 cm H_2O during mechanical V_T delivery or decreases 5 cm H_2O for more than 1 second. This alarm system is the primary mechanism for detecting disruption of the patient-ventilator interface (circuit leaks). The "ratio" alarm is activated when inspiration exceeds 50 percent of the total cycle time permitted by the CMV rate. During alarm conditions volume-cycling continues, but the plateau phase, if in use, is terminated. "Oxygen" illuminates when either low or high concentration limits are exceeded.

Audible alarms may be silenced for 2 minutes by depressing the bypass button (which also illuminates the "audio alarm bypass" indication). Audio alarms may be reset manually before the elapsed time. "Current ventilatory mode(s)" in progress (IMV, CPAP, CMV, OXYGEN, SIGH, ASSIST) is/are designated by respective illumination. A lighted oxygen indication occurs when the F_{IO_2} is greater than 0.21. Patient-

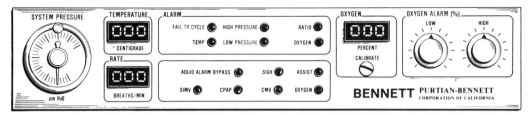

Fig. 10-29. Schematic of the Bennett MA-2 mode/alarm panel.

initiated ventilation, whether preset mechanical or demand breaths, illuminates the "assist" lamp.

Operation

Inspiratory (Fig. 10-30) and expiratory (Fig. 10-31) phase gas flows are illustrated. Electrical (AC) power and compressed oxygen (for an FIO_2 greater than 0.21) are necessary for operation. Compressed air may be employed in lieu of the internal AC-powered compressor. High-pressure oxygen is regulated to 40 ± 3 psig and then to 1.8–2.10 cm H_2O in the oxygen accumulator. When pressure in the accumulator decreases to 0.9–0.5 cm H_2O an alarm sounds. Oxygen is delivered to an oxygen percentage control which adjusts gas flow to the stack valve electronically. This adjustment is made proportionately to filtered ambient air drawn into the stack valve assembly as the bellows descends during exhalation.

Bellows descent in the cannister to the designated tidal volume level is controlled by a pulley. The pulley displacement is determined by signals from the volume control potentiometer. Once the bellows is in position, filtered ambient air from the compressed air source is delivered by the main solenoid to a venturi device, which boosts flow (via entrainment) to 125 L·minute^{-1}. The resultant flow to the cannister is regulated by the peak flow control.

A portion of the venturi outflow is shunted to a dump valve to allow cannister pressurization. Peak flow determines the rate at which the bellows is compressed within the cannister and the inspiratory time for tidal volume delivery. As the bellows ascends, gas passes through a unidirectional outlet valve system and filter and humidification system before entering the distal circuit and the patient's lungs. Simultaneously with bellows compression, a secondary system closes the breathing circuit exhalation valve. This is accomplished by a pilot valve which diverts gas into the exhalation valve system. Pressure from the pilot valve is regulated by a "PEEP" control which bleeds gas into the exhalation valve dump system. This "PEEP" control maintains pressure in the mushroom of the exhalation valve, thus regulating expiratory pressure in the breathing circuit. In this same system the IMV pilot valve and solenoid valve facilitate spontaneous breathing from gas in the bellows. If spontaneous ventilatory demand exceeds the bellows capacity, it may remain at the top of its stroke, interrupting further gas flow to the patient. The control which cycles the ventilator to exhalation should the upper pressure limit be exceeded is also here. The same system must be pressurized during exhalation to close the outlet valve so that bellows refill occurs only from the stack valve.

Bennett MA 2 + 2 Ventilator

Functionally the Bennett MA 2 + 2 ventilator is similar to the MA-2, with three modifications. The low inspiratory pressure alarm is adjustable from 2 to 80 cm H_2O

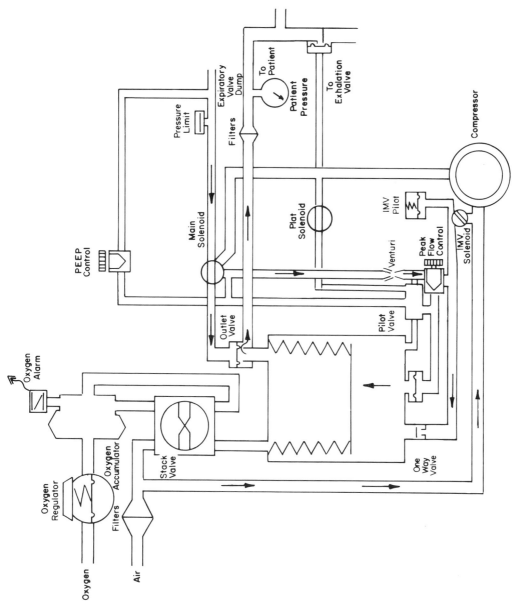

Fig. 10-30. Internal schematic of the Bennett MA-2 indicating inspiratory phase gas flows.

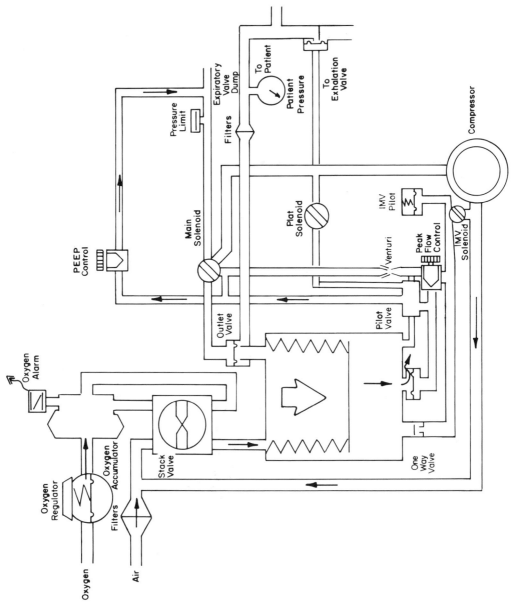

Fig. 10-31. Internal schematic of the Bennett MA-2 indicating expiratory phase gas flows.

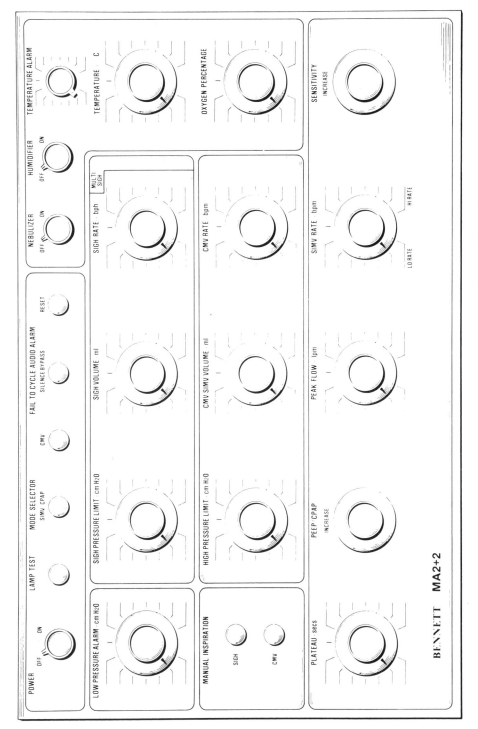

Fig. 10-32. Schematic of the Bennett MA 2 + 2 control panel.

rather than factory-set at 10 cm H_2O. A universal mount is provided to accommodate most commercially available heated humidifiers while retaining temperature display and adjustable alarms. The manual expiration pushbutton was deleted because an automatic bellows reset system was incorporated. This mechanism obviates the necessity for manual refilling of internal bellows in the face of exhaustive leaks on CPAP/PEEP or after transient disconnections. The most conspicuous change is the control panel (Fig. 10-32).

Reference

Model MA-2 Operating Instructions No. 11407A and MA-2+2 Operating Instructions No. 11040M. Bennett Medical Equipment, Los Angeles, CA

BENNETT 7200 MICROPROCESSOR VENTILATOR

The Bennett 7200 microprocessor ventilator (Fig. 10-33) is an electronically and pneumatically powered, microprocessor-controlled, volume-cycled, flow generator. It may be used in CMV, SIMV, or CPAP modes. Inspiratory flow is constant, is descending (tapered) or sine-wave in configuration, and may be extended by a postinflation pause (plateau). PEEP may be employed in any mode.

Control and Surveillance

The control panel (Fig. 10-34) is partitioned into three sections: ventilation settings, patient data, and ventilator status. All

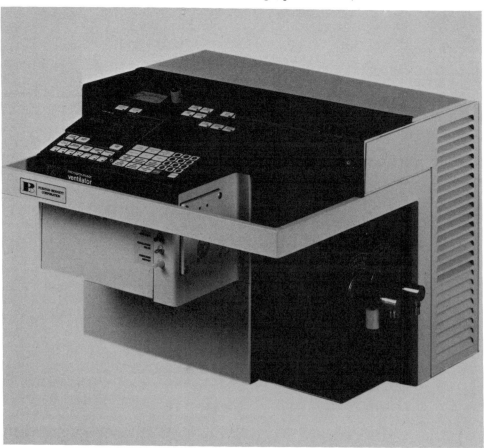

Fig. 10-33. Bennett 7200 microprocessor ventilator. (Courtesy of Puritan-Bennett Corp.)

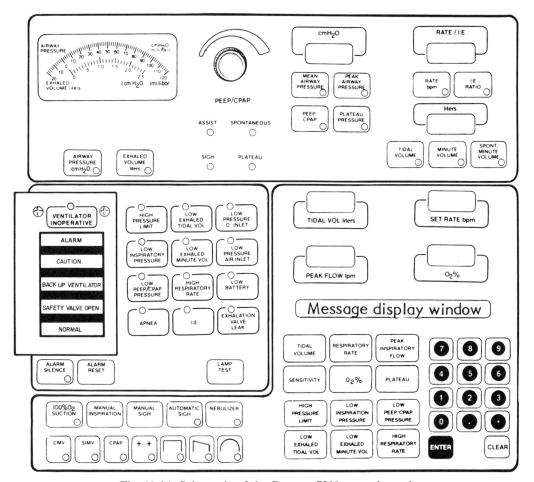

Fig. 10-34. Schematic of the Bennett 7200 control panel.

operations (except PEEP/CPAP) are actuated by depressing specific function and/or numerical keys. The microprocessor signifies a keyed selection with a single beep and displays it on a 20-character alpha-numerics (α-N) window. Displayed data are entered by depressing the ENTER key (on the numerical keyboard just below the α-N window) and are acknowledged by two beeps. If the selected value exceeds specifications, the microprocessor ignores the data, signifies the condition with four beeps, and displays an INVALID ENTRY in the α-N window. Depressing CLEAR redisplays the function to allow a corrected numerical entry compatible with the programmed specifications.

An extended self-test (EST) may be activated when the ventilator is not connected to a patient. The EST is initiated by depressing a pushbutton on the utility panel (not illustrated) on the left side of the ventilator chassis. The utility panel also contains the AC power inlet, main power ON/OFF switch, and audible alarm tone control. Once activated, the EST requires 2–3 minutes to assess the microprocessor electronic and pneumatic systems. The delivery circuit must be occluded at the patient connection before initiating EST. During EST all pressure transducers are automatically zero-referenced to ambient pressure, and circuit competence and compliance are determined to facilitate selected tidal volume

(V_T) delivery to the patient's airway. If any errors/malfunctions are detected during EST, mechanical ventilation cannot be initiated.

Microprocessor-entered mechanical V_T (0.1–2.5 L), selected respiratory rate (0.5–150 breaths·minute^{-1}), peak inspiratory flow ($\dot{V}_I$), and oxygen percent (21–100 percent) are displayed just above the α-N window. Sensitivity (20–0.5 cm H_2O) determines the inspiratory effort required for patient-initiated breaths. Mechanical inspiration may be extended by a plateau (0–2.0 seconds).

Ventilatory modes include CMV, SIMV, and CPAP. Submodes include: constant, descending, and sine-wave inspiratory flow patterns; and nebulizer, automatic sigh, and 100 percent O_2. When activated, a red lamp on the submode key is illuminated. The submode key designated + + is vacant.

During CMV all breaths are mechanical and may be initiated by the ventilator (controlled), patient (assisted), or operator (manually). In the SIMV mode breaths may be spontaneous, mechanical (either controlled or assisted) or operator (manually) initiated. During CPAP, breaths are spontaneous or operator (manually) initiated. With spontaneous ventilation (SV) in either SIMV or CPAP modes, $\dot{V}_I$ up to 180 L·minute^{-1} is available. Selected waveform submodes regulate $\dot{V}_I$ during mechanical/manual inspiration but not SV.

Nebulization may be activated to deliver medication during mechanical inspiration so long as $\dot{V}_I$ exceeds 20 L·minute^{-1}. Nebulizer function is automatically terminated 30 minutes after activation. When the automatic sigh is engaged, every 100th breath is twice the selected V_T. Transient delivery of 100 percent oxygen for up to 2 minutes may be employed without altering the selected value. During the 2-minute interval, the "O_2%" window displays a flashing 100 (unless the selected value is already 100 percent, at which time the displayed 100 is constant). A manual sigh at twice normal V_T or a manual inspiration equal to normal V_T

may be administered by depressing the respective key only; i.e., there is no need to ENTER. End-expiratory pressure (PEEP/CPAP) is adjustable (0–50 cm H_2O) by the only knob on the control panel. Initiation of or changes in PEEP/CPAP does not alter sensitivity for patient-initiated breaths.

Patient data are displayed on an analog meter and three LED windows. Analog display indicates either airway pressure (−20 to 120 cm H_2O) or exhaled minute volume (0–25 L·minute^{-1}). Specific components of airway pressure may be indicated with LEDs. These include mean airway, peak airway and plateau pressures, and PEEP/CPAP. Peak airway and plateau pressures reflect only mechanical breaths. The plateau pressure is averaged over four breaths, whereas peak pressure is displayed breath to breath. Ventilatory rate (mechanical and/or spontaneous) or I:E ratio (mechanical) may be displayed. Tidal volume, minute volume, or spontaneous minute ventilation are also indicated. They are each sampled over 10 breaths, with each new breath (spontaneous or mechanical) becoming the tenth as the oldest one is dropped. Tidal and minute volume sampling does not distinguish mechanical or spontaneous breaths. During SIMV the difference between minute volume and spontaneous minute volume is the mechanical contribution.

Patient data are displayed when the appropriate key is depressed and illuminates the function lamp in the bottom right corner of the key. These are immediate response keys, and therefore the entry protocol is not used.

"Breath type" indicators illuminate, indicating the occurrence of an assisted spontaneous or sigh breath or a plateau. Assist can be either an IMV or CMV breath that was patient-initiated.

Monitored limits for ventilator settings include: high pressure cycle (10–120 cm H_2O), which when reached causes termination of mechanical inspiration; low inspiratory pressure (3–99 cm H_2O), which detects leaks/disconnects during mechanical inspiration; low PEEP/CPAP (0–45 cm H_2O), also detecting leaks/disconnects as well as insufficient demand flow during spontaneous ventilation; low exhaled V_T (0–4 L); low exhaled minute volume (0–60 L·minute^{-1}); and high respiratory rate (0–150 breaths·minute^{-1}). Limits are programmed in a manner similar to that described above. Entered values for any ventilator setting or limit may be displayed in the α-N window by depressing CLEAR followed by the desired function key. When thresholds are exceeded, both audible and visual alarms are activated. Visual indication includes an illuminated red lamp on individual alarm indicators in the "ventilator status" section, and "condition" messages displayed in the α-N window.

Additional alarms include: low O_2 or air inlet pressures, which indicate that the respective source is less than 35 psig; low battery, which indicates an inability to sustain 1 hour of audible alarm operation; exhalation valve leak, showing that more than 10 percent of the V_T or 50 ml passed through the exhalation valve during mechanical inspiration; I:E ratio, which indicates that inspiratory exceeds expiratory time; and apnea, activated when more than 20 seconds has elapsed without a machine or spontaneous exhalation. When apnea occurs, factory-programmed backup ventilation is initiated at a rate of 12 breaths·minute^{-1}, V_T of 500 ml, and PEEP/CPAP at the level present before apnea.

An alarm summary display includes: ALARM, CAUTION, BACKUP VENTILATOR, SAFETY VALVE OPEN, and NORMAL. Alarms are classified as standard and nonstandard. Alarms designated standard include the low limits for exhaled tidal volume, inspiratory pressure, and minute volume; high respiratory rate; and exhalation valve leak. Nonstandard alarms include: high-pressure cycle, low air and oxygen pressure inlet, apnea, I:E ratio, and low battery. When standard alarms activate, a sustained audible tone is emitted and the ALARM (summary) and individual alarm indicator lamps flash. Once the alarm condition is corrected, the steady tone ceases, CAUTION (summary) illuminates, and the individual indicator alarm lamp goes from flashing to steady illumination. These visual indications remain until the alarm reset key is depressed, thus providing evidence that "self-correcting" or automatically reset alarm conditions have occurred.

When nonstandard alarms activate, they evoke an audible and visual indication, except for I:E ratio and low battery, which are indicated only visually. An apnea alarm condition cannot be automatically reset; thus a continuous tone and visual indication of ALARM, BACKUP VENTILATOR, individual alarm indicator, and submode key for square-wave flow pattern all illuminate. As the ventilator switches to backup ventilation, the message displayed in the α-N window as APNEA VENTILATION.

NORMAL is illuminated in alarm summary lights when ventilation is occurring within selected thresholds and design specifications. An individual audible alarm may be deactivated for 2 minutes by depressing ALARM SILENCE and then the ENTER key.

If AC power or both air and oxygen source pressures fail, audible and visual (SAFETY VALVE OPEN) alarms activate as an internal valve opens, permitting spontaneous ventilation from room air. The message in the α-N indicates the specific malfunction.

Operation

Inspiratory (Fig. 10-35) and expiratory (Fig. 10-36) phase gas flows are illustrated. The Bennett 7200 incorporates two main systems comprised of electropneumatic and electrical components. The electropneumatic system requires air and oxygen between 35 and 100 psig. Should air pressure drop below 35 psig, an internal air compressor automatically starts. All ventilator functions are microprocessor-controlled.

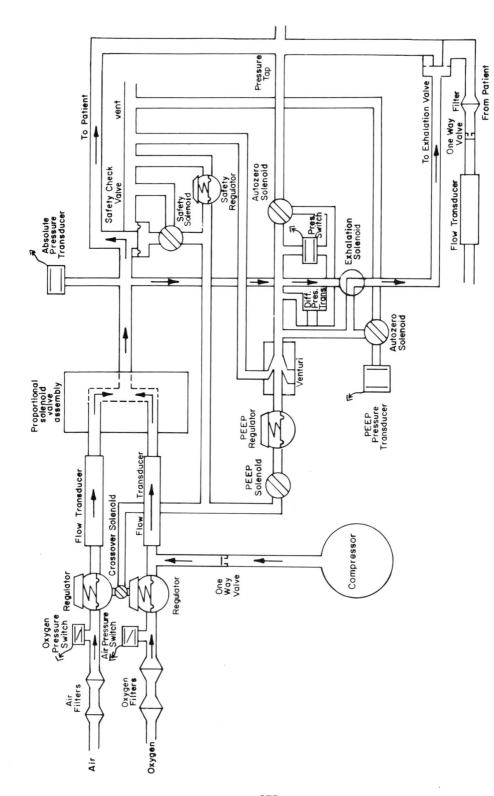

Fig. 10-35. Internal schematic of the Bennett 7200 inspiratory phase gas flows.

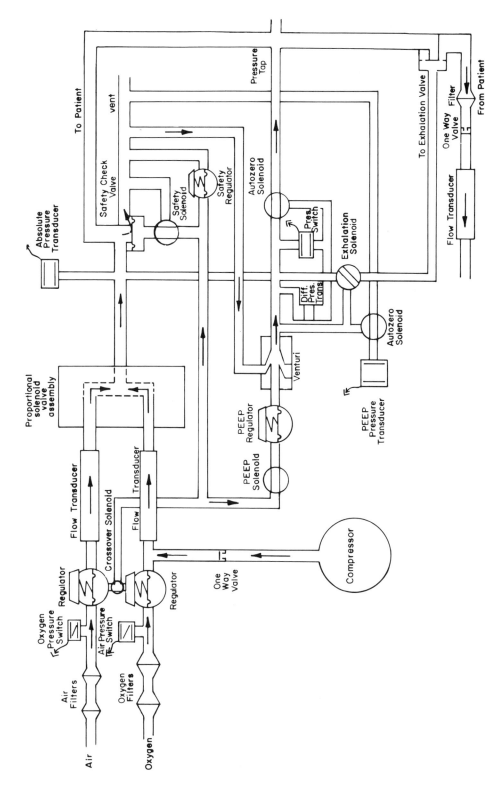

Fig. 10-36. Internal schematic of the Bennett 7200 expiratory phase gas flows.

379

Once air and oxygen enter an external and internal filter, pressure is monitored by respective sensors before the gas enters regulators which decrease the working pressure to 10 psig. A crossover solenoid valve switches to oxygen for pneumatic power should the compressed air source and/or compressor fail. Next, the respective gases enter flow transducers, which measure flow by hot film anemometry. A thermistor is also incorporated in the flow transducer so that the microprocessor can temperature-correct flow measurements. From the transducers the gases flow into a proportional solenoid valve at 10 psig and 180 L·minute^{-1}. The solenoid cycles at a rapid rate to proportion appropriate amounts of each gas for the desired F_{IO_2} and tidal volume. As gas is delivered to the breathing circuit, it passes a barometer and a safety check valve which is normally closed by pressure from the crossover valve system. Should a malfunction of the gas supply system develop, this valve opens, permitting spontaneous ventilation from ambient air. It also serves as a maximum pressure limit device when the system pressure exceeds 120–150 cm H_2O. The safety solenoid and safety regulator also maintain safe pressure levels by monitoring ventilator pressures and adjusting the safety check valve.

PEEP is controlled from a three-way crossover solenoid valve. The PEEP solenoid valve is first activated then the PEEP regulator adjusts pressure to the desired level. Venturi flow generates exhalation system pressure through an exhalation solenoid valve. A differential pressure transducer compares breathing circuit pressure to the baseline pressure at the PEEP venturi outlet port. Pressure in the PEEP flow system is maintained by the microprocessor. The auto-zeroing solenoid is vented to atmospheric pressure hourly by the microprocessor to facilitate zeroing of all pressure transducers.

During exhalation, gas vents through a filter, a one-way valve, and a heated flow transducer similar to that in the inspiratory limb. Expiratory transducer flow is integrated by the microprocessor and referenced to the selected tidal volume and proportioning solenoid.

The backup ventilator (BUV) pressure switch activates backup ventilation should the microprocessor fail. When a microprocessor failure occurs that is not self-correctable within 10 seconds, the ventilator automatically reverts to an F_{IO_2} of 1.0 and delivers a 500 ml tidal volume at 12 breaths·minute^{-1}. The original PEEP level is maintained during backup ventilation. However, a BUV switch terminates mechanical inspiration if the peak inflation pressure exceeds PEEP by more than 20 cm H_2O.

Reference

Model 7200 Operator Manual (Preliminary Copy 03-10-83). Bennett Medical Equipment, Los Angeles, CA

BIO-MED MVP-10 PEDIATRIC/ NEONATAL VENTILATOR

The Bio-Med MVP-10 pediatric/neonatal ventilator (Fig. 10-37) is a pneumatically powered, fluidically controlled, time-cycled, constant-flow generator. It is employed in CMV, IMV, or CPAP modes. Inspiratory pressure plateau and end-expiratory pressure (PEEP/CPAP) may be provided.

Control and Surveillance

A two-position toggle switch located on the control panel (Fig. 10-38) determines the ventilator mode (CPAP or cycle). Continuous circuit flow results from the combined oxygen and air flowmeter output up to 6 L·minute^{-1} each. Oxygen concentration can be read from a nomogram or calculated:

$$[\dot{V}total \times desired\ F_{IO_2}] = [0.21 \times \dot{V}air] + [1.0 \times \dot{V}_{O_2}]$$

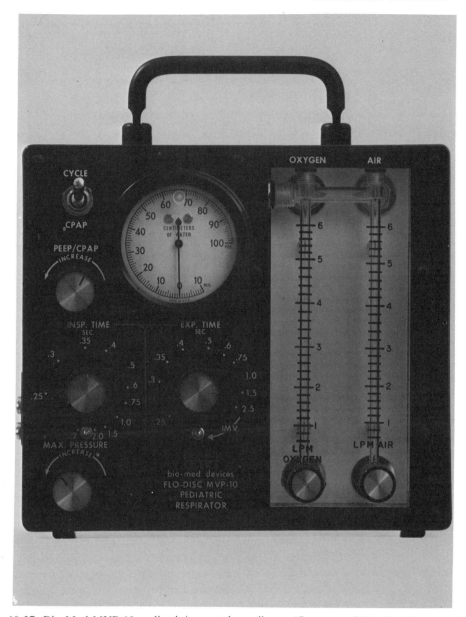

Fig. 10-37. Bio-Med MVP-10 pediatric/neonatal ventilator. (Courtesy of Bio-Med Devices, Inc.)

In the CYCLE mode, mechanical tidal volume (V_T) is determined primarily by the continuous flow rate, inspiratory time (T_I) duration (0.2, 0.25, 0.3, 0.35, 0.4, 0.5, 0.6, 0.75, 1.0, 1.5, and 2.0 seconds), and maximum pressure (up to 70 ± 10 cm H_2O). If maximum pressure is reached, the excess flow is vented to ambient for the remaining T_I, producing an inspiratory pressure plateau. Expiratory time (T_E) is adjustable from 0.25 to 30 seconds duration (0.25, 0.3, 0.35, 0.4, 0.5, 0.6, 0.75, 1.0, 2.5, and 30 seconds). Ventilatory rate (0–120 breaths·minute^{-1}) is dependent on total cycle time (T_I and T_E).

End-expiratory pressure (PEEP/CPAP) is regulated from 0 to 16 ± 4 cm H_2O depending on continuous flow. PEEP/CPAP

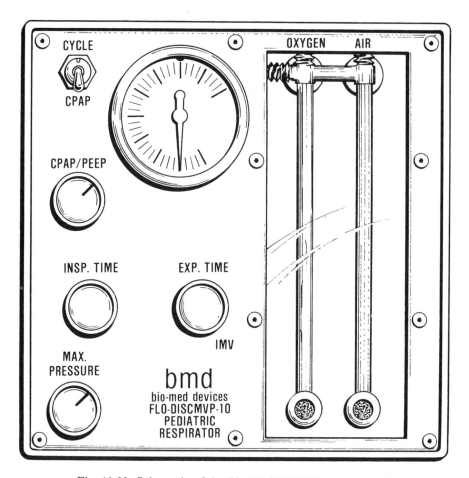

Fig. 10-38. Schematic of the Bio-Med MVP-10 control panel.

may be employed in either ventilatory mode. Circuit pressure is indicated on an anaeroid manometer calibrated from −10 to 100 cm H_2O.

Operation

Inspiratory (Fig. 10-39) and expiratory (Fig. 10-40) phase gas flows are illustrated. The MVP-10 is pneumatically powered by 50 psig air and oxygen. Inlet gases pass through a regulator to their respective air and oxygen flowmeters and are delivered in the desired ratio (F_{IO_2}) as a continuous circuit flow. Mechanical ventilation is con-

trolled by fluidic logic, which is activated when compressed air is shunted through a manual ON/OFF valve. The logic circuit consists of three cartridges which cycle to operate the exhalation valve. During inspiration, shunted compressed air flows into the expiratory cartridge, which is opened to divert gas to a capacitor and the inspiratory cartridge. The inspiratory cartridge directs gas to pressurize the exhalation valve, which diverts the continuous circuit flow into the airway. The capacitor functions as a "buffer" to minimize abrupt exhalation valve closure. When the selected inspiratory time has elapsed, the fluidic cartridges function in reverse, thus depressurizing the

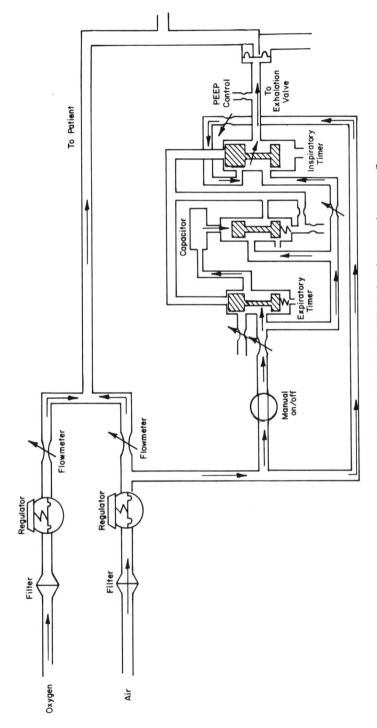

Fig. 10-39. Internal schematic of the Bio-Med MVP-10 inspiratory phase gas flows.

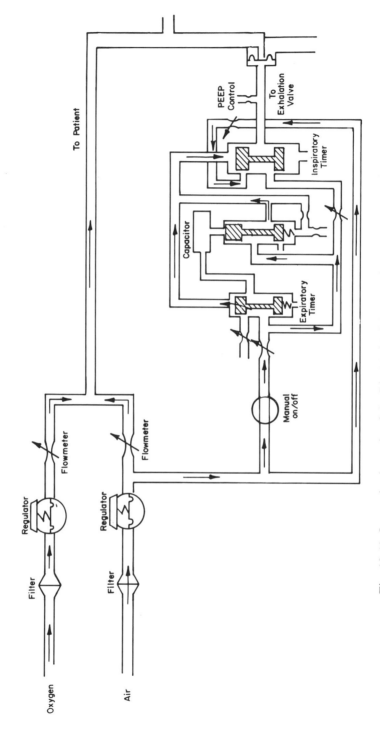

Fig. 10-40. Internal schematic of the Bio-Med MVP-10 expiratory phase gas flows.

exhalation valve, which then opens and allows the ambient venting of gas.

Reference

MVP-10 Instruction Manual. Bio-Med Devices, Inc., Stamford, CT

BIO-MED IC-2 VENTILATOR

The Bio-Med IC-2 ventilator (Fig. 10-41) is a pneumatically powered, fluidically controlled, time-cycled, constant-flow generator. It may be employed in CMV, SIMV, or CPAP modes. Inspiratory pressure plateau and end-expiratory pressure are available.

Control and Surveillance

Pneumatic function is activated by an ON/OFF knob located on the control panel (Fig. 10-42). The ventilator mode (cycle or CPAP) is engaged by a two-position toggle switch. In the cycle position the mechanical tidal volume (V_T) (up to 3000 ml) results from selected inspiratory times (T_I = 0.4, 0.5, 0.75, 1.0, 1.5, or 2.0 seconds) and flow rates ($\dot{V}$ = 20, 30, 40, 50, 60, 70, or 75 L·minute^{-1}). Expiratory time (T_E) is adjustable (0.5, 0.6, 0.75, 1.0, 1.5, and 2.0 seconds; and continuously from 4 to 45 seconds). The ventilatory rate (1.3–66 breaths·minute^{-1}) results from the total cycle duration established by T_I and T_E.

CMV is instituted when the mode selector is in the cycle position and the submode toggle switch is set to normal. CMV may either be controlled, patient-initiated, or a combination of the two. Inspiratory effort for patient-triggered CMV is adjusted by an uncalibrated knob to achieve the desired sensitivity level. When the submode selection is SIMV, spontaneous ventilation (SV) occurs from a demand flow system with periodic mechanical V_T delivery. Upon termination of T_E, the subsequent spontaneous breath initiates SIMV. There is no CMV backup in the event of apnea in the SIMV mode. Inspiratory effort necessary to initiate demand flow and SIMV is also regulated by the "assisted CMV" control. The demand system provides a tidal volume determined by selected and demand $\dot{V}$. If demand $\dot{V}$ exceeds SV, the excess vents to ambient through the exhalation valve. When SV exceeds $\dot{V}$, another inspiratory is sequenced to generate necessary volume.

With the mode selector set to manual/CPAP, the patient breathes completely spontaneously from the demand system. In this mode a manual inspiration may be administered when a pushbutton is depressed. The manual breath is delivered at the prevailing $\dot{V}$.

PEEP/CPAP is regulated from 0 to 25 cm H_2O in all modes. Patient triggering/demand effort must be readjusted when PEEP/CPAP is altered. PIP is regulated from 0 to 100 ± cm H_2O (depending on the type of exhalation valve employed) by a control on the rear panel. When the PIP limit is reached, excess pressure producing flow is vented to ambient for the remaining T_I. A designed PIP limit during T_I permits a relatively consistent inspiratory pressure plateau.

CMV and SIMV/SV breaths are indicated by illuminated cycle and demand indicators, respectively. Circuit pressure is indicated by an anaeroid manometer.

Operation

Inspiratory (Fig. 10-43) and expiratory (Fig 10-44) phase gas flows are illustrated. The IC-2 is powered by 50 psig air and oxygen sources delivered to a blender for selection of the desired F_{IO_2}. Inlet pressure is regulated to 30 psig before entering a pilot valve which is controlled by fluidic logic. The logic circuit directs the pilot valve to

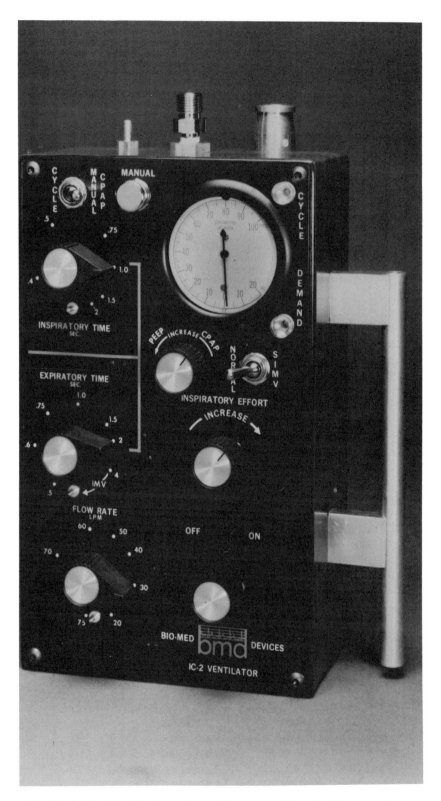

Fig. 10-41. Bio-Med IC-2 ventilator. (Courtesy of Bio-Med Devices, Inc.)

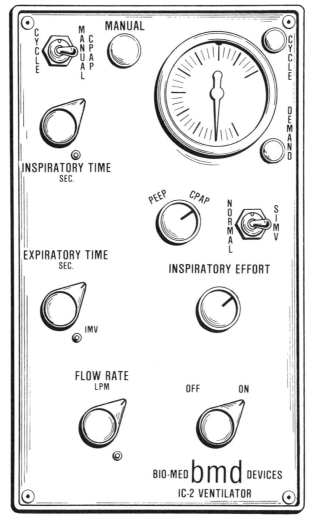

Fig. 10-42. Schematic of the Bio-Med IC-2 control panel.

deliver gas into the breathing circuit through a peak flow control and patient manifold upon spontaneous demand. The patient manifold system regulates the ventilator outflow pressure (driving pressure) up to 100 cm H_2O. When time-controlled ventilation is desired, a manual ON/OFF switch shunts source oxygen regulated to 30 psig to the logic circuit. During mechanical inspiration, gas also pressurizes the exhalation valve for the selected time interval. If the oxygen source pressure decreases below 30 psig, a failsafe cutoff valve interrupts gas pressure to the exhalation valve, thereby preventing occlusion. The ventilator continues to cycle, but the exhalation valve remains depressurized to allow spontaneous breathing and ambient venting. After a normal mechanical inspiratory phase, the valve depressurizes to permit unimpeded exhalation unless selected PEEP/CPAP is generated by fluidic control.

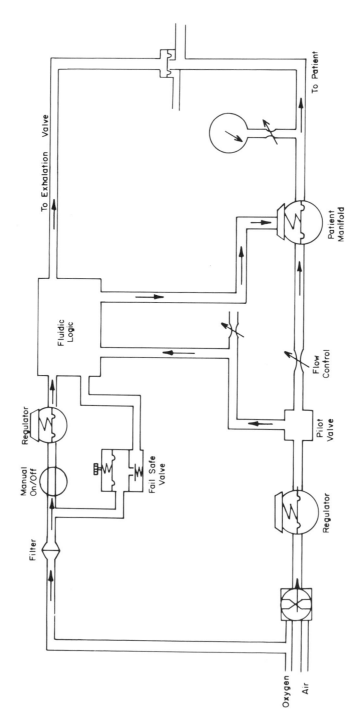

Fig. 10-43. Internal schematic of the Bio-Med IC-2 inspiratory phase gas flows.

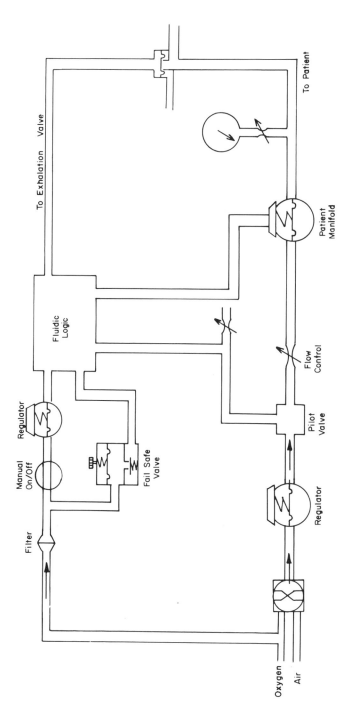

Fig. 10-44. Internal schematic of the Bio-Med IC-2 expiratory phase gas flows.

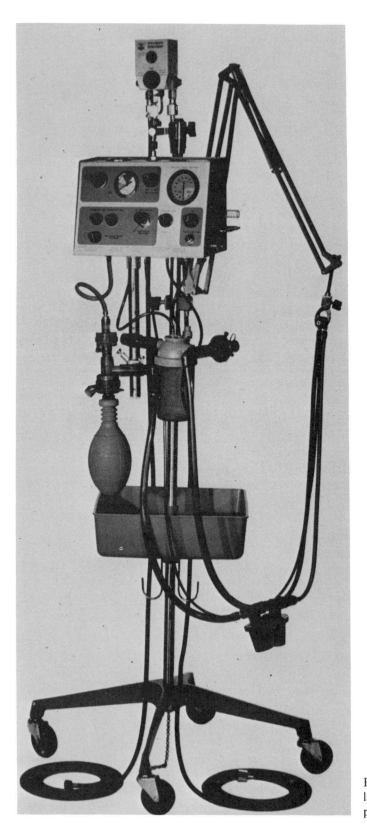

Fig. 10-45. Babybird ventilator. (Courtesy of Bird Corporation/3M.)

Reference

IC-2 Instruction Manual. Bio-Med Devices Inc., Stamford, CT

BABYBIRD VENTILATOR

The Babybird ventilator (Fig. 10-45) is a pneumatically powered and controlled, time-cycled, constant-flow generator. It is employed in IMV and SPONTANEOUS breathing modes. Inspiratory pressure plateau may be administered during IMV, and PEEP/CPAP is available in all modes.

Control and Surveillance

Most of the ventilator parameters are selected by rotary knobs located on the control panel (Fig. 10-46). CPAP is controlled by altering the outflow valve orifice size (flow resistor) on the expiratory circuit limb. Resistance to circuit outflow produced by orifice constriction produces a constant back-pressure (CPAP). CPAP of 0–30 cm H_2O may be developed depending on the continuous circuit flow rate (adjustable from 0 to 30 L·minute^{-1}). Commonly the flow rate is set to approximately 1.5–2.0 times the infant's estimated minute volume to minimize the incidence of rebreathing.

Gas humidification is facilitated by either a 500-ml reservoir nebulizer or a temperature-controlled reservoir-wick humidifier. A maximum of 12 L·minute^{-1} may be diverted to the nebulizer jet to increase the water content of inspiratory gas.

Ventilatory mode control may be positioned on SPONTANEOUS breathing or

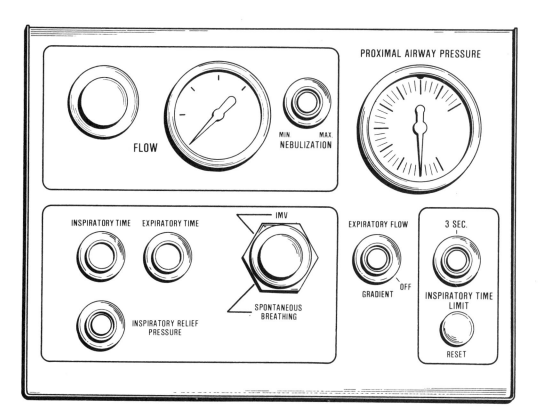

Fig. 10-46. Schematic of the Babybird control panel.

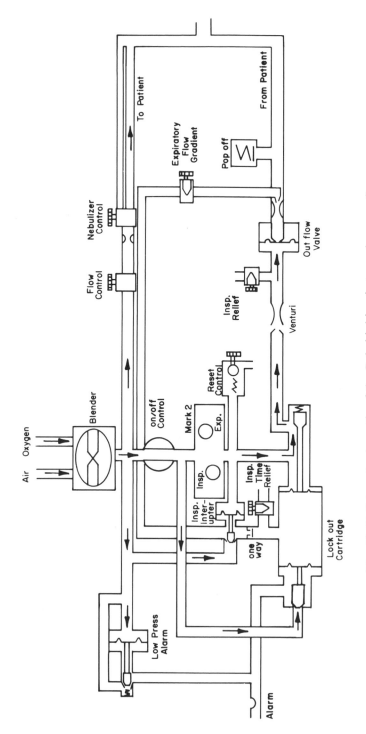

Fig. 10-47. Internal schematic of the Babybird inspiratory phase gas flows.

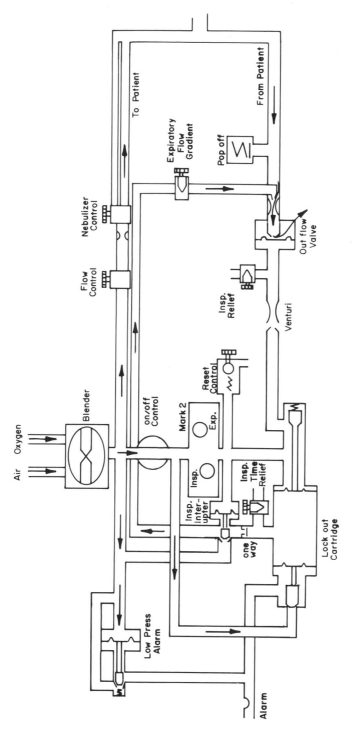

Fig. 10-48. Internal schematic of the Babybird expiratory phase gas flows.

IMV. Spontaneous breathing mode provides gas of a known FIO_2 with or without CPAP. During IMV the cycling frequency is programmed by positioning uncalibrated inspiratory and expiratory time-control knobs. The I:E ratio determines the IMV rate. V_T is primarily dependent on inspiratory time (T_I), flow rate ($\dot{V}$), circuit compliance, and PIP.

PIP control limits the circuit pressure during mechanical V_T delivery. Once the PIP limit is reached, it is held for the duration of the T_I. Thus T_I and PIP limit controls may be used to develop desired inspiratory pressure plateau.

An expiratory flow gradient control powers a venturi device, which decreases expiratory flow resistance by evacuating gas from that limb of the breathing circuit. An inspiratory time limit control prevents sustained mechanical inspiration and usually is set slightly longer than the T_I being utilized. When the T_I limit is exceeded, the ventilator converts to the SPONTANEOUS mode and an audible pneumatic alarm sounds. IMV is reestablished by correcting the T_I limit and depressing a reset button.

Operation

Inspiratory (Fig. 10-47) and expiratory (Fig. 10-48) gas flows are illustrated. Pneumatic power is supplied by compressed air and oxygen sources. If the gradient between air and oxygen pressure exceeds 20 psig, an audible alarm sounds and the blender switches entirely to the higher pressure source gas. Otherwise air and oxygen are equilibrated to the lowest inlet pressure by a two-stage regulator system within the blender. The mixed gas then flows into a manifold which services a "low pressure" alarm, ON/OFF rotary valve, and adjustable pressure gauge which functions as a flow control (0–30 L·minute^{-1}). A portion of the flow (up to 12 L·minute^{-1}) may be diverted by a nebulizer control needle valve to power the jet when a 500-cc reservoir nebulizer is employed. All remaining flow enters an auxiliary port in the nebulizer head. When a nonnebulizer humidification system is utilized, both flow outlets are interfaced at the humidifier inlet port. In either case, a continuous flow of humidified gas is delivered to the inspiratory limb of the breathing circuit. During the spontaneous breathing mode, circuit gas is vented to ambient through an outflow valve with a variable restrictive orifice. Decreasing the orifice size increases resistance to gas outflow and develops a "back-pressure" or CPAP. At high circuit flows, outflow resistance (even with no reduction in orifice size) may produce undesired back-pressure. This pressure can be eliminated by adjusting the "expiratory flow gradient" control needle valve to power a venturi device, which entrains ("evacuates") gas from the expiratory limb gas to decrease flow resistance.

Mechanical ventilation is initiated when the rotary valve control is aligned to interface manifold gas pressure with an internal inspiratory and expiratory timing mechanism (Mark 2 ventilator). During inspiration, gas flow from the Mark 2 is delivered to a venturi device and hence through a needle valve into a chamber on the ambient side of the outflow diaphragm (exhalation valve). Once pressurized, the diaphragm interrupts the venting of continuous flow and diverts it into the airway for the duration of inspiration. The outflow diaphragm occlusion pressure is limited by the needle valve, thereby regulating inspiratory circuit pressure. If circuit pressure exceeds this pressure limit, excess gas flow vents to ambient for the duration of inspiration. During inspiration, gas flow to the expiratory flow gradient control is interrupted. Upon termination of inspiration, gas flow to the expiratory gradient control is reestablished.

A compound lockout cartridge switches the Mark 2 off and activates an audible alarm should the maximum inspiratory time limit to be exceeded. It is normally pressurized during the Mark 2 expiratory phase or continuously in the spontaneous breathing mode. If the pneumatic bleed-down time of the Mark 2 inspiratory timing mechanism exceeds that of the compound lockout cartridge, the ventilator ceases function and switches automatically to the SPONTANEOUS breathing mode while an audible alarm sounds. To reestablish mechanical ventilation, either the inspiratory time or inspiratory time limit must be adjusted for compatibility and a reset button depressed. A low-pressure alarm utilizes the same pneumatic system. When manifold pressure is less than 43 psig, the audible alarm sounds. Adequate Mark 2 function requires a working pressure greater than 43 psig.

A mechanical relief valve in the breathing circuit expiratory limb serves as a backup to the inspiratory pressure relief mechanism during mechanical inflation. It is the *only* potential pressure vent in the SPONTANEOUS mode or during manual inflation with a hand resuscitation bag attached to the breathing circuit.

Reference

Babybird Operators Manual No. L795R1. Bird Corporation/3M, St. Paul, MN

BABYBIRD 2 VENTILATOR

The Babybird 2 ventilator (Fig. 10-49) is an electronically controlled, pneumatically and electronically powered, time-cycled constant-flow generator. It operates in CMV, IMV, or SPONTANEOUS breathing modes with or without PEEP/CPAP.

Control and Surveillance

Electronic circuitry is activated by depressing the main power switch on the control panel (Fig. 10-50). When power is on, an indicator lamp illuminates. If electrical power fails, battery-activated audible and visual alarms engage. Battery competence is established by depressing a pushbutton which initiates an audible alarm and illuminates the power failure indicator light.

Continuous circuit flow is adjusted with a rotary knob and indicated by a calibrated Thorpe tube ($3-25$ L·minute^{-1}). The flow rate is usually set at $1.5-2.0$ times the estimated minute volume or at a level sufficient to minimize spontaneous inspiratory effort as indicated on proximal airway pressure manometer.

Mechanical ventilation is established by engaging the rate control knob (range: OFF, $2-72$ or $4-150$ breaths·minute^{-1} depending on the position of the frequency multiplier). Mechanical tidal volume (V_T) is dependent on inspiratory time T_I ($0.1-2.7$ seconds) and PIP ($0-80$ cm H_2O at 10 L·minute^{-1} circuit flow). If PIP limit is reached, the exhalation valve remains closed while excess gas flow is vented to ambient, creating a pressure plateau for the remaining T_I.

Should cycling frequency and selected T_I result in an expiratory time of less than 0.2 seconds, audible and visual alarms activate. In this condition the ventilator reverts to a T_E of 5 seconds while maintaining a portion of the selected T_I until the situation is corrected. If T_I exceeds 4.25 seconds, usually indicating a timing medium malfunction, the ventilator cycles to exhalation and audible and visual alarms engage. A manual inspiration may be administered in any mode so long as a pushbutton is depressed. Because the manual V_T mechanism is pneumatic, it operates independently of electronic cycling and may be used during electrical power failure.

An electronically controlled pressure relief system is adjustable from 15 to 80 cm H_2O ($\pm$ 10 percent). If the pressure limit is exceeded, gas flow is interrupted, and the circuit pressure is thus reduced to atmospheric pressure. During this condition, audible and visual alarms activate, and spontaneous ventilation is accommodated through an ambient communication provided the inspiratory circuit remains unob-

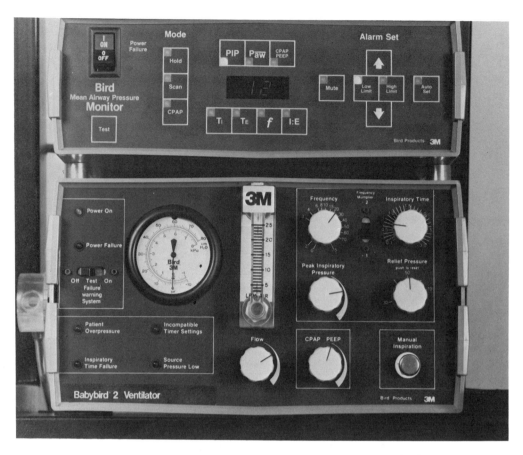

Fig. 10-49. Babybird 2 ventilator. (Courtesy of Bird Corporation/3M.)

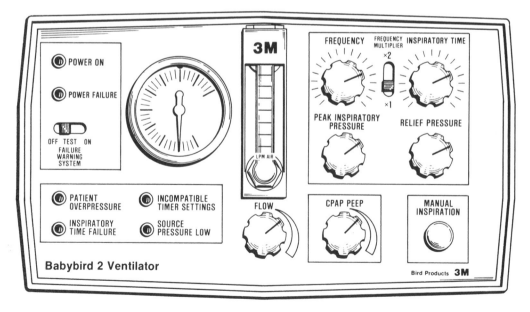

Fig. 10-50. Schematic of the Babybird 2 control panel.

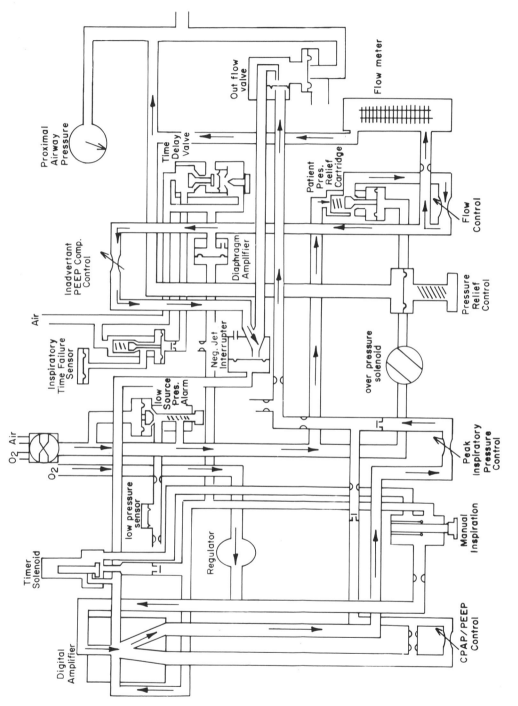

Fig. 10-51. Internal schematic of the Babybird 2 inspiratory phase gas flows.

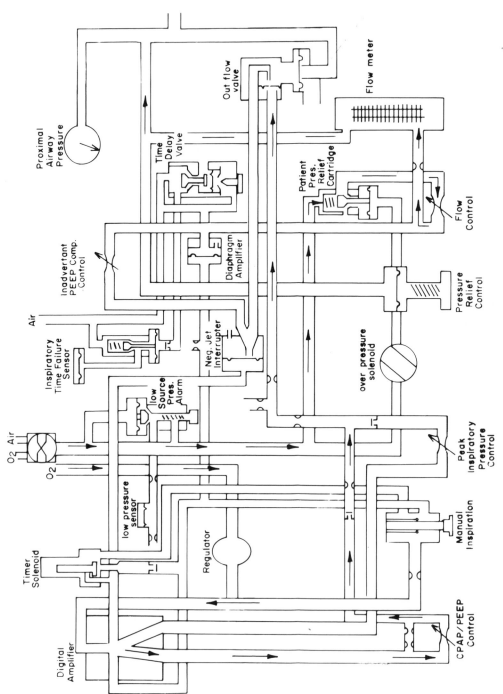

Fig. 10-52. Internal schematic of the Babybird 2 expiratory phase gas flows.

structed. Relief pressure is reset by depressing the control knob.

PEEP/CPAP ranges from 0 to 30 cm H_2O at 10 L·minute^{-1} circuit flow. It is provided by a flow restrictor, and hence baseline expiratory pressure varies directly with the continuous gas flow rate.

If the pressure of the source gas supplying the ventilator falls below 39 psig, audible and visual alarms activate. This condition may adversely affect pneumatic functions.

Operation

Inspiratory (Fig. 10-51) and expiratory (Fig. 10-52) phase gas flows as illustrated. Compressed air and oxygen at 40 ± 5 psig are blended to the desired F_{IO_2}. Pneumatic power is provided by oxygen and air lines interfaced at their respective blender source inlets. Oxygen is delivered to a pressure regulator and diverted to a digital amplifier which supplies the "PEEP" control, "peak inspiratory pressure" control, a timer solenoid, and a "manual inspiration" control. Oxygen flow through the CPAP/PEEP control develops pressure on the outflow (exhalation) valve, creating an elevated breathing circuit baseline pressure. During the mechanical inspiratory phase, oxygen is directed through the peak inspiratory pressure control against the outflow valve. Outflow valve occlusion pressure is thus limited and mechanical inspiratory circuit pressure is regulated. The timer solenoid limits the duration of inspiration. It also serves as the cycle source for the negative jet interrupter.

Compressed air supplies power for the time-delay cartridge, inspiratory time failure lockout cartridge, and diaphragm amplifier. The time-delay cartridge cycles gas to the digital amplifier and timer solenoid. It also activates an inspiratory time failure sensor.

Mixed gas flows through a "low source pressure" alarm, "low pressure" sensor, "overpressure" solenoid, "pressure relief" control, "flow" control, "pressure relief" cartridge, and flowmeter before entering the breathing circuit. The "low source pressure" sensor activates an alarm if the blender outflow pressure is inadequate. The "overpressure" solenoid shuts the ventilator off if system pressure is excessive. The "pressure relief" control regulates the cartridge which vents gas from flow control to ambient if the preselected value is exceeded. Breathing circuit pressure is thereby reduced to zero. Under these conditions spontaneous ventilation occurs with ambient air.

Circuit flow resistance may be minimized by adjusting an "inadvertent PEEP" control (rear panel). It directs gas to a "negative" jet interrupter which evacuates gas from the breathing circuit expiratory limb.

Reference

Babybird 2 Operators Manual No. F-L168. Bird Corporation/3M, St. Paul, MN

IMV BIRD VENTILATOR

The IMV Bird ventilator (Fig. 10-53) is a pneumatically powered and controlled, time-cycled, constant- and nonconstant-flow generator It may be employed in CMV, IMV, or CPAP modes. Inspiratory flow deceleration and PEEP/CPAP are available.

Control and Surveillance

A compact panel (Fig. 10-54) accomodates most of the ventilator control knobs and all breathing circuit service outlets. A master pneumatic ON/OFF rotary switch and auxiliary nebulizer flow control (0–16 L·minute^{-1}) are located on the left side of the ventilator. Tidal volume (V_T) is dependent on the inspiratory time (T_I) (0.5–4.0 seconds) and inspiratory flow rate (up to 72 L·minute^{-1}) at 20 cm H_2O back-pressure).

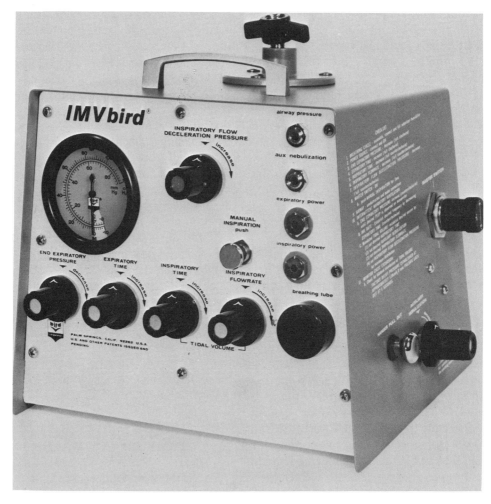

Fig. 10-53. IMV Bird ventilator. (Courtesy of Bird Corporation/3M.)

Because inspiratory flow ($\dot{V}_I$) is generated by a double-jet injector, downstream (circuit) pressure determines total flow; that is, at a given $\dot{V}_I$ and T_I, V_T fluctuates with changing circuit pressure. V_T is also influenced by the adjusted inspiratory flow deceleration pressure (20–65 cm H_2O). At the selected pressure one of the duel injector jets terminates flow, thereby reducing total circuit outflow (inspiratory flow deceleration). A manual inflation for up to 5 seconds may be administered by depressing a pushbutton. An expiratory time (T_E) control (1.5 seconds to infinity), along with T_I regulates cycling frequency (range: OFF, 0.3–30 breaths·minute^{-1}). End-expiratory pressure is adjustable from 0 to 35 cm H_2O (optional adjustment to 60–80 cm H_2O). Proximal airway pressure is indicated with an anaeroid manometer.

Operation

Inspiratory (Fig. 10-55) and expiratory (Fig. 10-56) phase gas flows are illustrated. The IMV bird is pneumatically powered by blended 50 psig air and oxygen, which is

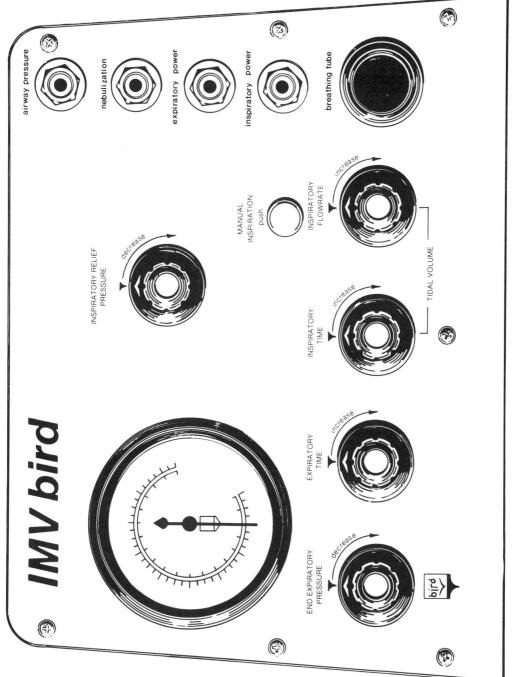

Fig. 10-54. Schematic of the IMV Bird control panel.

401

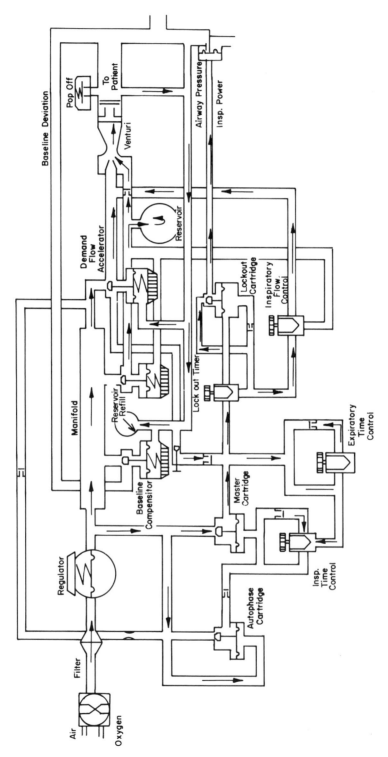

Fig. 10-55. Internal schematic of the IMV Bird inspiratory phase gas flows.

402

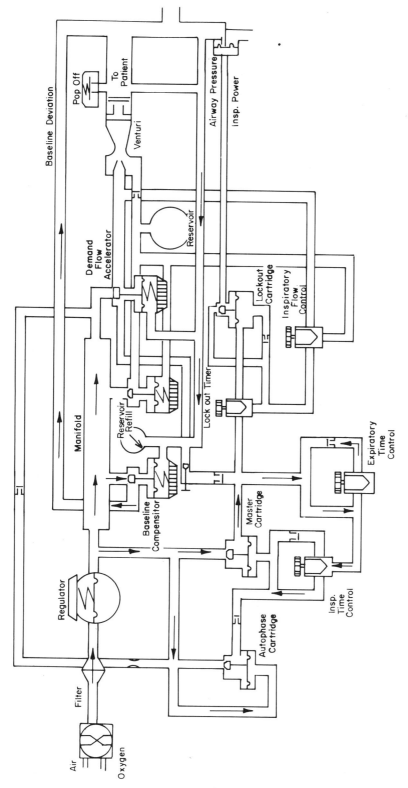

Fig. 10-56. Internal schematic of the IMV Bird expiratory phase gas flows.

403

diverted to the service manifold by a master ON/OFF valve. The service manifold provides gas for all pneumatic functions.

Gas for spontaneous breathing is regulated by a demand-flow accelerator. As spontaneous inspiration is detected by 1–2 cm H_2O decreases in baseline airway pressure, flow is directed to a venturi jet which entrains reservoir gas into the breathing circuit. When baseline circuit pressure is reestablished at the end of inspiration, demand flow ceases. Entrainment reservoir gas volume is maintained by a refill cartridge. It functions similarly to the demand-flow accelerator cartridge in that it maintains reservoir filling pressure (and thus volume). When volume decreases as entrainment occurs, the reservoir pressure declines, initiating flow from the refill cartridge.

A baseline compensator generates PEEP/CPAP through the exhalation valve. It "compensates" the demand-flow accelerator, thereby maintaining "trigger" sensitivity when alterations in PEEP/CPAP caused by spontaneous breathing occur.

Two other cartridges, the master and autophase, are served by the manifold. The master cartridge activates inspiratory and expiratory timing circuits, the "inspiratory lockout" timer, and the "inspiratory flow" control. During mechanical inspiration, gas from the master cartridge is diverted to a venturi device through the "inspiratory flow" control. This gas (plus entrainment) results in volume delivery to the patient circuit. During inspiration the inspiratory power line pressurizes the exhalation valve, and the "inspiratory lockout" timer cartridge is charged through a lockout timer control. If inspiratory time exceeds cartridge filling time, the inspiratory phase is "locked out" and the ventilator cycles to exhalation.

Inspiration is terminated when sufficient gas flow is metered through the inspiratory time control, closing the master cartridge and initiating exhalation. The expiratory timer determines how long it takes a me-

tered gas "bleed" to reopen the master cartridge.

Reference

IMV bird Instruction Manual No. L924. Bird Corporation/3M, St. Paul, MN

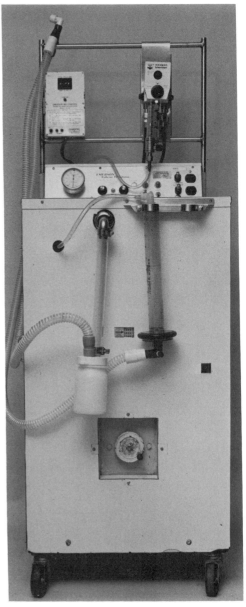

Fig. 10-57. Emerson Volume Ventilator (3PV). (Courtesy of J. H. Emerson Company.)

EMERSON VOLUME VENTILATOR (3PV)

The Emerson volume ventilator (3PV) (Fig. 10-57) is an electronically powered and controlled, time-cycled, nonconstant-flow generator. It delivers ambient air which may be enriched with supplemental oxygen. The 3PV is primarily employed for CMV; however, an optional patient-triggering mechanism is available. IMV also is available as an option, and PEEP may be provided.

Control and Surveillance

The 3PV (Fig. 10-58) is powered by a 115-volt, 60-cycle electrical source. Current to the humidifier heater is controlled by a three-position toggle switch: HI (high), OFF, and LO (low). Heater activation is indicated by an illuminated bulb. The heater usually must be operated in the HI position to ensure adequate humidification when the continuous-flow IMV modification is utilized. The humidity switch should be engaged at least 20 minutes before anticipated use. Mechanical tidal volume delivery is initiated by flipping the two-position pump toggle switch to ON, which illuminates an indicator lamp. Tidal volume is adjusted by a hand crank on the front lower center and is indicated at the middle left of the chassis (as it faces the operator). Mechanical volume ranges up to 2200 ml (adult) and 1000 ml (pediatric) depending on the piston chamber volume. Inspiratory and expiratory times are adjusted independently by continuous rotary knobs. The duration of tidal volume delivery is regulated by IN-HALE. Counterclockwise knob rotation increases the inspiratory time; hence tidal volume delivery is extended but with a reduced flow rate. Clockwise rotation provides the reverse effect. Mechanical expiratory phase length is selected by the EXHALE knob. Counterclockwise and clockwise rotations increase or reduce time periods between inspirations, respectively. Adjusted expiratory time may be accelerated when the assistor toggle switch is ON and the patient makes an inspiratory effort. Baseline cycling frequency is a function of inspiratory and expiratory time adjustments. Additional breaths may be delivered if the patient assist mode is activated. A trim screw permits adjustment of motor speed when unconventional line voltage powers the unit.

Circuit pressure is indicated by an aneroid manometer. Two 110-volt 60-cycle conventional outlets are available and facilitate the use of electrically powered equipment on or about the ventilator.

An optional ventilator cycling control (Fig. 10-59) may be interfaced when IMV is desired. A two-position toggle switch engages the accessory rate function. When it is activated, an indicator lamp illuminates

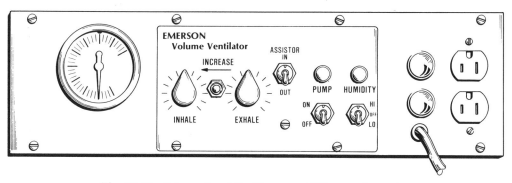

Fig. 10-58. Schematic of the Emerson 3PV control panel.

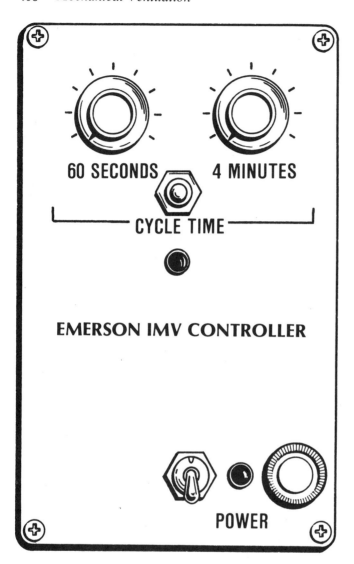

Fig. 10-59. Schematic of the Emerson 3PV IMV control box.

and the exhale time control on the 3PV control panel is overriden. Two continuous rotary knobs—one controlling seconds and the other minutes—permit selection of expiratory time from a few seconds up to 4 minutes.

Operation

Inspiratory (Fig. 10-60) and expiratory (Fig. 10-61) phase gas flows are illustrated. Compressed air and oxygen are mixed and delivered to two reservoir bags. One reservoir system provides gas for spontaneous ventilation. The spontaneous breathing reservoir receives gas either from a continuous-flow or optional demand valve system. Inspiratory gas is warmed and moistened.

A second reservoir provides gas for the ventilator piston, and its filling is regulated by a flowmeter adjusted to a level 4–5 $L \cdot minute^{-1}$ above the desired mechanical minute ventilation (V_T times the IMV rate). Reservoir bag overpressurization is prevented by adjusting a popoff valve so that it opens with minimal pressure. Overdistention of the reservoir can cause inadvert-

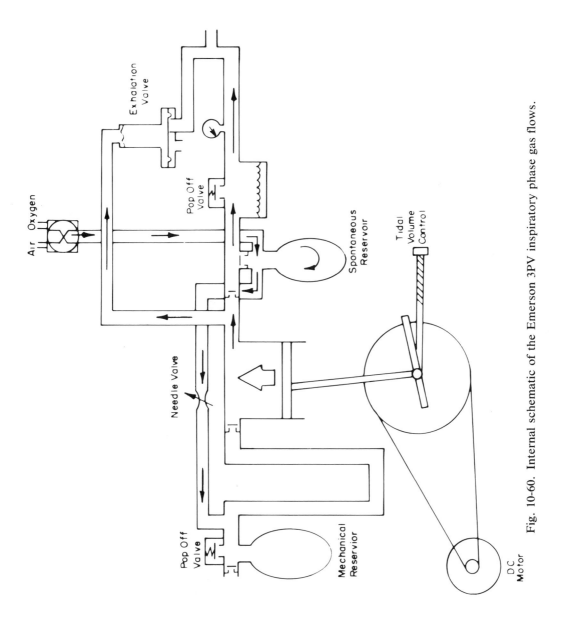

Fig. 10-60. Internal schematic of the Emerson 3PV inspiratory phase gas flows.

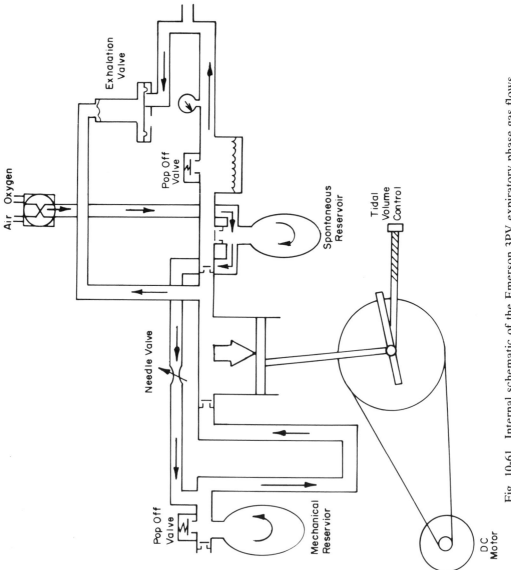

Fig. 10-61. Internal schematic of the Emerson 3PV expiratory phase gas flows.

ent exhalation valve pressure. As the piston descends, gas from the mechanical reservoir bag is drawn into the chamber. Chamber displacement volume is regulated by the tidal volume adjustment crank. When the piston has completed its downward (expiratory) motion and begins its upward stroke (inspiration), its motion is guided by a linkage rod attached to the side of a revolving wheel. This configuration provides a sinusoidal flow contour and a sigmoidal pressure curve. Because this stroke is the same for each breath despite changes in peak airway pressure, the 3PV is classified as a nonconstant-flow generator (compare and contrast with the gear-driven Bear LS 104-150).

The upward stroke of the piston delivers gas through unidirectional valves. As this gas is directed past a pressure relief valve and then through a humidifier to the circuit, a portion is diverted to the exhalation valve, where it prevents any gas leak by "seating" a diaphragm between the patient circuit and ambient surroundings.

Piston displacement is selected with the tidal volume control crank. Inspiratory and expiratory time are regulated with potentiometer assemblies (not illustrated), which convert wall source alternating current (AC) to direct current (DC). This current is then delivered to the motor and piston drive assembly. If a low voltage is relayed from the inspiratory potentiometer, piston upward motion is slow. A faster movement results from a higher voltage. This direct method of influencing motor (piston) speed regulates inspiratory time, flow rate, and pressure.

Inspiratory and expiratory phasing is accomplished by a cam on the wheel which closes a microswitch as the piston moves upward during inspiration. When the microswitch is closed, motor (piston) speed is governed by the inspiratory potentiometer. At the end of the upward motion, the cam opens the microswitch, signaling the start of exhalation. Downward piston motion (motor speed) is determined by the expiratory potentiometer. During the downward

piston stroke, the exhalation is depressurized unless a residual pressure (PEEP) is generated by a water column above the valve diaphragm.

Reference

Model 3-PV Operating Instructions. J. H. Emerson Company, Cambridge, MA

EMERSON IMV VENTILATOR (3MV)

The Emerson IMV ventilator (3MV) (Fig. 10-62) is an electronically powered and controlled, time-cycled, nonconstant-flow generator. It employs CMV and IMV modes. PEEP/CPAP is available.

Control and Surveillance

Most of the ventilator functions are regulated and monitored on a modular control panel (Fig. 10-63). A two-position toggle switch activates all electronic components except the piston motor, which is separately engaged. When the main power is switched ON, an indicator lamp illuminates. Current to the water reservoir heating unit is regulated by a "humidifier output" control. Clockwise knob rotation from OFF turns on an indicator lamp and increases the heating unit temperature.

Tidal volume ranges up to 2200 ml and is adjusted with a hand crank. Selected tidal volume is indicated in 100-ml intervals. Ventilator cycling frequency is determined by a total cycle time control (0.2–22 breaths·minute^{-1}). An "inspiratory time" control regulates the duration of tidal volume delivery (0.5–2.5 seconds). The DC motor is activated by the "pump" switch. Upon completion of tidal volume delivery, the volume pump lamp illuminates. When the pump is on, a mechanical inspiration

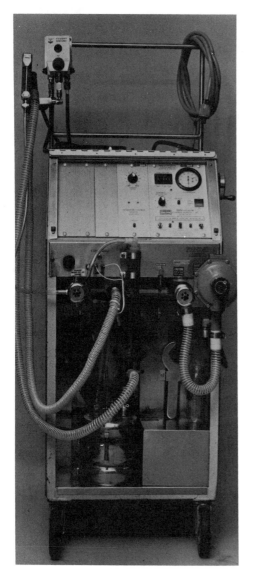

Fig. 10-62. Emerson IMV ventilator (3MV). (Courtesy of J. H. Emerson Company.)

may be administered during expiration by depressing an IMV manual button. Circuit pressure is indicated on an anaeroid manometer.

An optional oxygen analyzer module incorporates a fuel cell oxygen sensor interfaced with the ventilator outflow circuit. Oxygen concentration is displayed by an analog meter. Before use the analyzer is calibrated to a known F_{IO_2}.

Sensitivity adjustment of an optional alarm module permits circuit pressure monitoring. If circuit pressure is not detected at the selected level, an audible and visual alarm becomes operational. Alarm deactivation (up to 120 seconds) may be employed during short periods of ventilator-patient interface disruption. An indicator lamp illuminates during alarm inactivation.

Operation

Inspiratory (Fig. 10-64) and expiratory (Fig. 10-65) phase gas flows are illustrated. Air and oxygen are mixed and delivered to two reservoir bags. One bag provides gas for spontaneous ventilation and is filled by a continuous flow or optional demand valve system.

The second reservoir provides gas for mechanical V_T delivery. Gas to the piston reservoir is regulated by a flowmeter, which should be adjusted to $4-5$ L·minute^{-1} above the desired mechanical minute ventilation (V_T times the IMV rate). Reservoir bag overpressurization is prevented by adjusting a relief valve. Overdistention of the reservoir can cause inadvertent exhalation valve pressure. As the piston descends, gas from the mechanical reservoir is drawn into the chamber. Displacement volume is regulated by the tidal volume adjustment crank. When the piston has completed its full downward (expiratory) motion and begins its upward (inspiratory) stroke, its motion is guided by a linkage rod attached to the side of a revolving wheel. This configuration provides a sinusoidal flow contour and a sigmoidal pressure curve. Upward piston displacement delivers gas volume through unidirectional valves, past a pressure relief valve, and then through a humidifier to the breathing circuit. A small portion of this piston volume is used to pressurize the exhalation valve.

Inspiratory and expiratory time are regulated with potentiometer assemblies (not illustrated) which convert alternating cur-

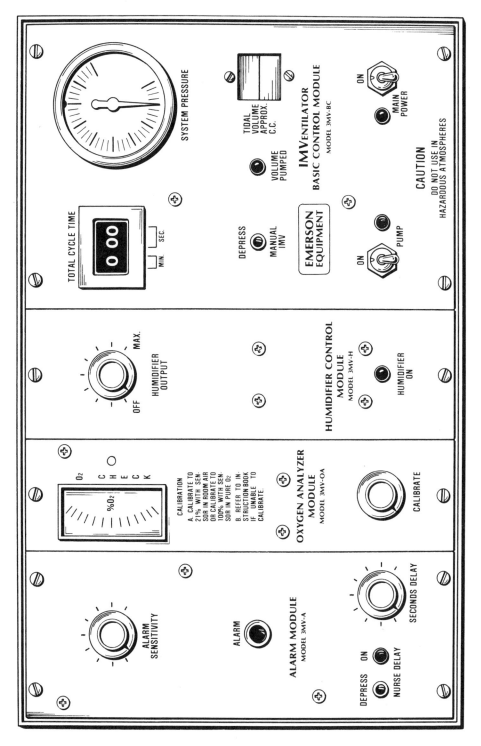

Fig. 10-63. Schematic of the Emerson 3MV control panel.

411

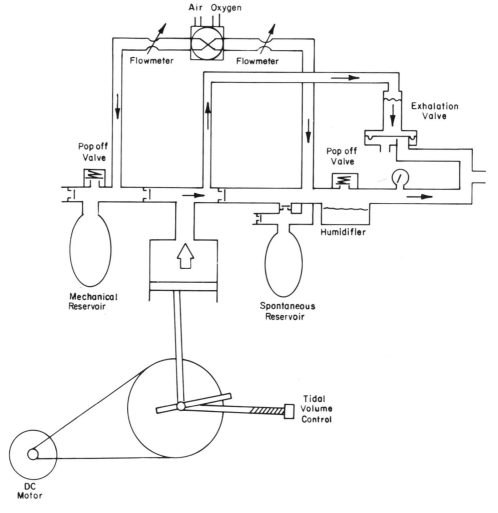

Fig. 10-64. Internal schematic of the Emerson 3MV inspiratory phase gas flows.

rent (AC) to direct current (DC). Current is delivered to the motor and piston-drive assembly. If a low voltage is relayed from the inspiratory potentiometer, upward piston motion is slow. A faster movement results from higher voltage. This direct method of influencing motor (piston) speed regulates inspiratory time, flow rate, and pressure.

Inspiratory and expiratory phasing is accomplished by a cam on the wheel which closes a microswitch as the piston moves upward during inspiration. When the microswitch is closed, motor (piston) speed is governed by the inspiratory potentiometer. At the end of upward motion, the cam opens the microswitch, signaling exhalation. Downward piston motion (motor speed) is determined by the expiratory potentiometer. During the downward piston stroke the exhalation valve is depressurized unless residual pressure (PEEP) is generated by a water column above the valve diaphragm.

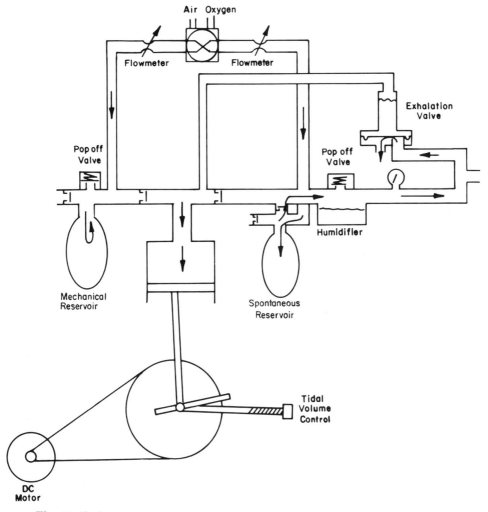

Fig. 10-65. Internal schematic of the Emerson 3MV expiratory phase gas flows.

Reference

Model 3-MV Operating Instructions. J. H. Emerson Co, Cambridge, MA

ENGSTRÖM ER 300 VENTILATOR

The Engström ER 300 ventilator (Fig. 10-66) is an electronically and pneumatically powered, electronically controlled, time-cycled, nonconstant-flow generator. It operates in a CONTROL mode. Expiratory retard and PEEP are available.

Control and Surveillance

Electronic circuits are activated by an ON/OFF switch (Fig. 10-67). Ventilatory frequency is adjustable from 12 to 36 breaths·minute^{-1}. Oxygen concentration is

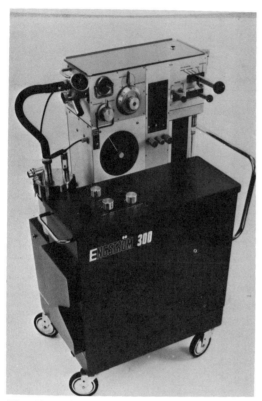

Fig. 10-66. Engström ER 300 ventilator. (Courtesy of LKB Instruments, Inc.)

regulated by a rotameter (for oxygen) and a dose meter which adjusts the ambient air mix. Minute volume is the sum of gas mixtures: oxygen rotameter (0–15, 0–5 L·minute^{-1}), air dose meter (0–30 L·minute^{-1}), and nitrous oxide (N_2O) rotameter (0–10 L·minute^{-1}). Emptying pressure (internal vent to ambient air) is regulated from 50 to 110 cm H_2O at a level higher than the PIP during normal tidal volume (V_T) delivery. The gradient between emptying pressure and PIP determines the slope of the flow curve. When the emptying pressure/PIP gradient is minimal, the flow rate is decreased and V_T delivery consumes the entire inspiratory time (T_I). In contrast, when emptying pressure is adjusted high, the flow rate is increased, facilitating rapid V_T delivery with a postinflation hold (plateau) for the remaining T_I. A submerged pressure vent can be adjusted from 30 to 90 cm H_2O to limit PIP.

PEEP is regulated from 0 to 20 cm H_2O, and flow resistance or retard may be adjusted by a spring-loaded valve control. Circuit pressure is indicated by an aneroid manometer.

Operation

Inspiratory (Fig. 10-68) and expiratory (Fig. 10-69) gas flows are illustrated. An AC electrical motor drives a piston through a clutch control. The clutch mechanism is used to control cycling frequency at a fixed I : E ratio of 1 : 2. A fixed I : E ratio occurs because the AC motor operates at a constant speed. During mechanical inspiration the piston is driven to the right, forcing gas into a rigid plastic cannister (overpressure chamber) containing a reservoir bag. Piston compression is completed within 72–75 percent of inspiratory time. Thus mechanical inspiration normally includes dynamic (75 percent) and static (25 percent) phases. As cannister pressure increases, the reservoir bag is compressed. Gas flows past the underwater pressure relief valve through a humidifier and into the breathing circuit. A portion of this gas flow is shunted to pressurize the exhalation valve.

As the piston returns to its original position during exhalation, a partial vacuum is created in the cannister which facilitates reservoir bag refill and exhalation valve depressurization. Gas flow into the reservoir is regulated by a minute volume control by means of an air-oxygen metering system. Exhaled volume passes through a combined end-expiratory pressure and expiratory resistance valve into a dry gas meter (spirometer). Adjusted spring tension determines the residual pressure (PEEP) maintained in the breathing circuit at end-exhalation.

Reference

Model ER 300 Service Manual. LKB Medical, Solna, Sweden

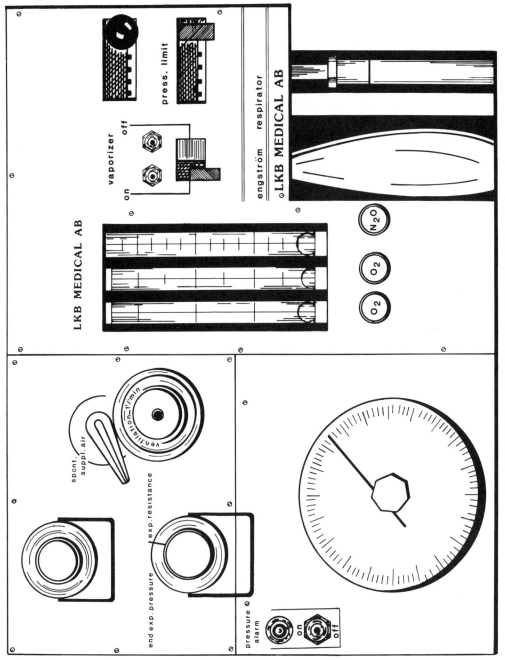

Fig. 10-67. Schematic of the Engström ER 300 control panel.

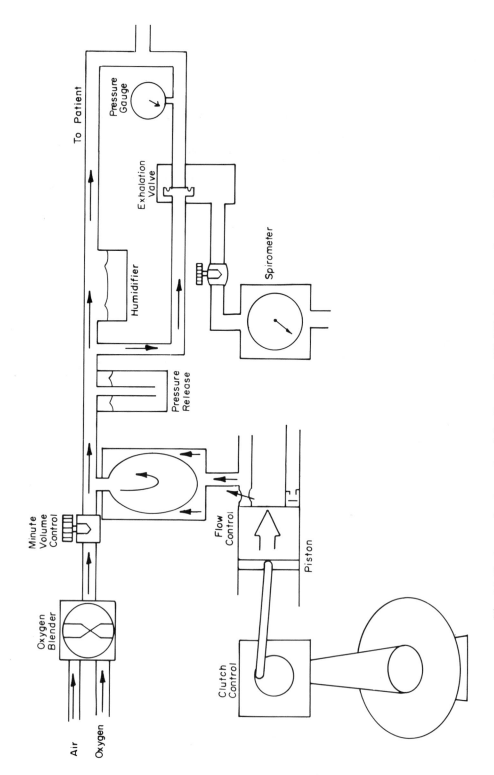

Fig. 10-68. Internal schematic of the Engström ER 300 inspiratory phase gas flows.

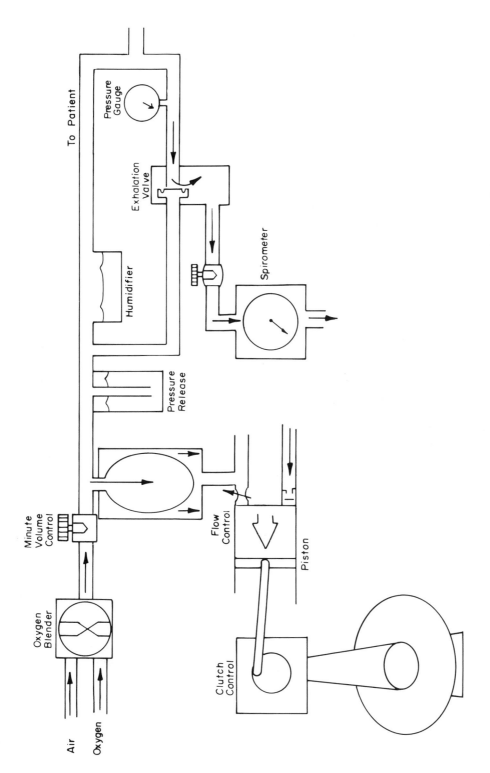

Fig. 10-69. Internal schematic of the Engström ER 300 expiratory phase gas flows.

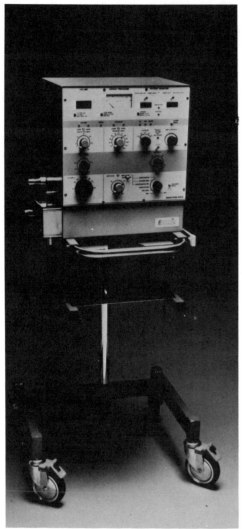

Fig. 10-70. Engström Erica ventilator. (Courtesy of LKB Instruments, Inc.)

ENGSTRÖM ERICA VENTILATOR

The Engström Erica ventilator (Fig. 10-70) is a pneumatically powered, electronically controlled, time-cycled ventilator. Tidal volume is generated by constant, accelerating, or decelerating flow, and spontaneous inspiratory pressure support is available. Ventilatory modes include CMV, ASSIST, SIMV, extended mandatory minute ventilation (EMMV), and SPONTA-

NEOUS. Postinflation pause (plateau) and PEEP/CPAP are available.

Control and Surveillance

Ventilatory parameters are selected and monitored on the control panel (Fig. 10-71). Tidal volume (VT) is continuously adjustable (0.1–2.0 L) at a controlled cycling frequency range (0.4–40 breaths·minute^{-1}). Gas flow may be delivered in accelerating, constant, or decelerating configurations. The desired inspiratory flow wave contour is selected with a three-position toggle switch. The duration of inspiration in CMV and assisted CMV modes depends on the adjusted cycling rate and the I:E ratio (1:3 to 3:1). Inspiration contains both dynamic and static phases. The dynamic time (VT delivery period) is regulated by an inspiratory flow rate control. Subsequently the static phase (end-inspiratory plateau) is held for the remaining inspiratory time and is indicated by a light. During mechanically augmented spontaneous breathing modes (SIMV, EMMV), only a dynamic phase occurs which is primarily regulated by the adjusted flow rate.

A seven-position rotary knob permits ventilatory mode selection, including: OFF, CMV, CMV + SIGH, ASSISTED CMV, SYNCHRONIZED IMV, EXTENDED MMV, and SPONTANEOUS. A depressible safety catch between CMV and OFF minimizes the likelihood of inadvertent ventilator shutdown.

The CMV mode produces constant VT delivery to the circuit at a preselected frequency. In the CMV + SIGH mode, every 100th breath is twice the VT. ASSISTED CMV permits patient-initiated CMV breaths. Flow (>0.1 L·second^{-1}) rather than pressure change initiates inspiration and illuminates the inspiratory effort light. Because the feature is factory-set, no assisted CMV sensitivity control is present.

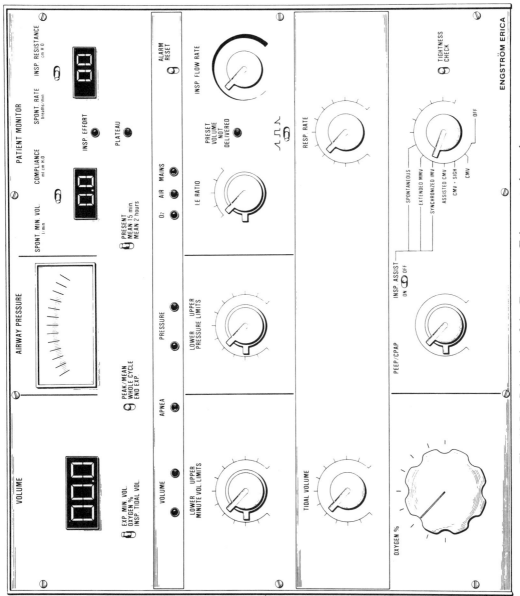

Fig. 10-71. Schematic of the Engström Erica control panel.

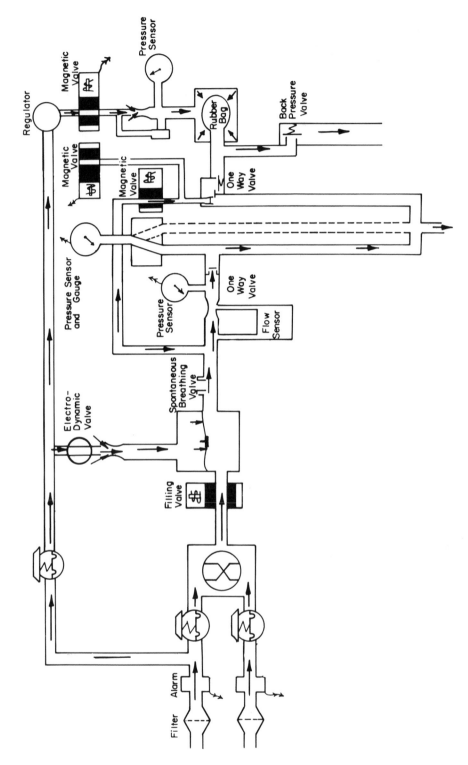

Fig. 10-72. Internal schematic of the Engström Erica inspiratory phase gas flows.

420

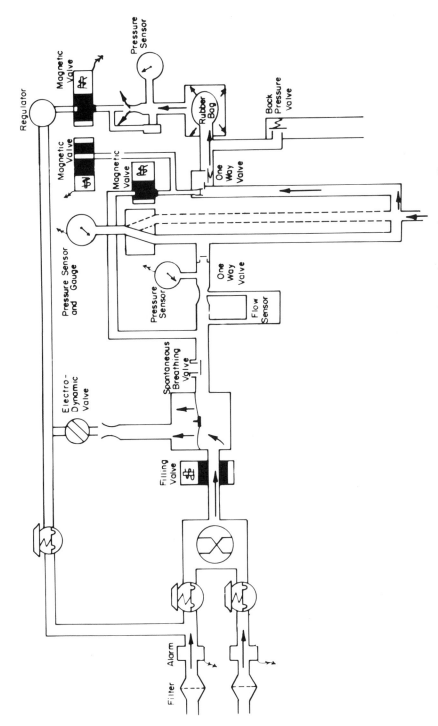

Fig. 10-73. Internal schematic of the Engström Erica expiratory phase gas flows.

SIMV allows mechanical augmentation of spontaneous ventilation. Periodic V_T delivery may be time-controlled or synchronized with spontaneous inspiration. A "synchronization window" is open for the initial 25 percent of time between programmed breaths·minute^{-1}. If a SIMV breath is not initiated during this open window interval (the patient does not generate a spontaneous inspiratory effort), a controlled breath is delivered. Because ventilator cycling frequency is based on the elapsed expiratory time, SIMV breaths may exceed the preselected IMV value by as much as 25 percent. Each inspiratory effort of more than 0.1 L·second^{-1}, spontaneous or SIMV, illuminates the indicator lamp.

EMMV provides a metered, baseline minute volume (MV) which may be mechanical and/or spontaneous. This baseline MV is equal to the product of the preselected V_T and cycling frequency. During EMMV mechanical V_T is delivered whenever spontaneous MV is less than the preselected baseline value. Mechanical MV never exceeds baseline, although spontaneous MV may; thus the mode is called *EXTENDED* MMV. Baseline MV below 2.5 L·minute^{-1} generates an insufficient flow transducer signal to sustain proper function and is not recommended. Mechanical V_T is not delivered during or immediately after spontaneous inspiration, and so synchronization is unnecessary. During EMMV the inspiratory effort lamp functions as in the SIMV mode.

SPONTANEOUS ventilation permits demand breathing at ambient or elevated baseline pressures and is indicated visually. Mechanical V_T is not administered in this mode, even with an alarm condition of apnea. EMMV can be employed as a "mechanical volume backup" for spontaneous breathing.

Inspiratory assist is implemented during SIMV, EMMV, and SPONTANEOUS modes. It is activated by a two-position toggle switch and offers inspiratory pressure assist, continuously adjustable from 0 to 30 cm H_2O above baseline. A safety catch must be depressed to exceed 20 cm H_2O When in use, a constant circuit pressure is maintained throughout spontaneous inspiration (as long as the flow transducer senses more than 0.1 L·second^{-1}). When inspiratory demand falls below 0.1 L·second^{-1}, inspiratory assist terminates and baseline circuit pressure is restored.

Baseline pressure (PEEP/CPAP) is also continuously adjustable from 0 to 30 cm H_2O pressure with a safety catch at 20 cm H_2O. Elevated baseline pressure may be employed in all ventilatory modes.

Ventilator F_{IO_2} is selectable from 0.21 to 1.0. It is monitored by a fuel cell and indicated on a LED when a three-function toggle switch is in the middle position. Expired MV or inspired V_T also is indicated on the LED with appropriate toggle switch positioning. Lower and upper MV limit may be adjusted from 3.0 to 30.0 L·minute^{-1}, respectively. If either limit is reached, audible and visual alarms are activated.

"Apnea" visual and audible alarms function if 30 seconds elapse without a spontaneous or mechanical breath or the inspiratory duration exceeds 7 seconds. If the cycling frequency is more than 10 breaths·minute^{-1}, the alarms engage 15 seconds after two consecutive cycling phases without a breath. Because the apnea monitor input depends on transducer measurements of ventilator outflow, a circuit disconnection does not activate the alarm! Ventilator-patient interface integrity instead is monitored by selected lower MV and pressure limits. In CMV, CMV + SIGH, and ASSISTED CMV modes, each mechanical breath must create a pressure greater than the selected lower limit or a visual and audible alarm activate. Low-pressure surveillance is eliminated during SIMV, EEMV, and SPONTANEOUS modes. PIP may be limited from 0 to 120 cm H_2O, with a depressible safety catch at 75 cm H_2O. When the upper pressure limit is exceeded, audible and visual alarms engage; and in CMV, CMV + SIGH, and AS-

SISTED CMV modes the ventilator switches to a static inspiratory phase (plateau) for the duration of inspiration. A pressure-limited condition during EMMV or SIMV immediately cycles Erica to exhalation. If PIP exceeds the upper limit by $\geq$ 10 cm H_2O or for two consecutive seconds, all circuit pressure (including PEEP/CPAP) is vented.

Circuit pressure is displayed on an analog meter (-10 to 100 cm H_2O). Indicated pressure is determined by positioning a toggle switch in either PEAK/MEAN (intermittent 6 and 2 seconds, respectively), WHOLE CYCLE (real time), or END. EXP. (end-expiratory pressure). Selection of PEAK/MEAN position in the SPONTANEOUS modes registers mean airway pressure continuously.

Pulmonary mechanics during CMV, CMV + SIGH, and ASSISTED CMV, or in SIMV or EMMV mode, spontaneous MV and rate are displayed by LED. In appropriate modes a toggle switch allows each parameter displayed to reflect PRESENT, MEAN over 15 minutes, or MEAN over 2 hours.

Inadequate O_2 (<36 psig) or air (<43 psig) inlet pressure activates audible and visual alarms. Insufficient electrical current engages an audible and visual alert powered by an internal trickle-charged battery.

Audible alarm(s) are silenced and reactivated by downward displacement of a spring-loaded switch. When the audible component is silenced, the appropriate visual alarm indicator flashes.

Operation

Inspiratory (Fig. 10-72) and expiratory (Fig. 10-73) phase gas flows are indicated. Gas mixture is maintained constant by a system of precise needle valves, regardless of system or back-pressure changes. A continuous flow of gas passes through a filling valve which provides the pressure chamber with adequate gas volume. Pressure chamber volume is maintained by an overflow valve which vents excess gas to the atmosphere should the valve reach the chamber top.

When inspiration is initiated, the electrodynamic valve delivers air through an injector into the upper chamber of the cannister. This injector entrains room air to boost cannister flow. Alterations in the electrodynamic valve function facilitate manipulation of inspiratory flow patterns.

Downstream from the pressure chamber (in the patient system) is a spontaneous breathing valve which opens whenever inspiratory flow demand exceeds maximum gas flow from the filling valve (30 L·minute^{-1}) and system cannister volume (1.5 L). Next, gas passes a flow sensor which measures tidal volume and spontaneous minute volume. This sensor, which utilizes a venturi tube and pressure transducer in the calculation of volume, is also used to sense patient effort. Flow detection rather than pressure change initiates the ventilator response to inspiratory effort. The patient system is isolated by a one-way valve into two systems. A pressure sensor and gauge are placed on each side so that independent information can be sent to electronic circuit boards. The insufflation generator side provides information for flow sensors, controls, and ventilator functions, whereas the patient pressure sensor provides a safeguard against excessive pressure and provides signals for the airway pressure meter.

The expiratory side is unique in its configuration and functions. Initially, exhaled gas is prevented from passing beyond the mushroom valve to the one-way valve if the ventilator is in the inspiratory phase. In this case insufflation pressure is shunted to the mushroom valve during inspiration, closing the ventilation loop. Mushroom valve pressurization can be extended beyond dynamic inspiration through closure of magnetic valve No. 1, thus providing a plateau. However, should circuit pressure exceed the preselected limit by 10 cm H_2O or the plateau time limit of 2 seconds, magnetic valve No. 2 opens immediately, venting the mushroom valve to atmospheric pressure. PEEP is maintained by the electrodynamic valve, which maintains an insufflation pressure through the patient system to the mushroom valve. This pressure also is lost when pressure or time limits are exceeded because magnetic valve No. 1 isolates the insufflation pressure system from the mushroom valve during a plateau phase.

During exhalation gas is delivered into a fixed-volume rubber bag. As the bag expands, cannister pressure is vented through the injector throat and mushroom valve side arm. During this period the back-pressure valve is closed and the one-way exhalation valve is open. Once inspiration begins, a measured flow of gas (120 $L \cdot minute^{-1}$) from the injector forces air into the cannister, emptying the bag volume through the back-pressure valve, which has an opening pressure of 8 cm H_2O. This function is meticulously timed until the bag is totally collapsed. Because flow rate and time are known, exhaled volume is calculated by a microprocessor.

Reference

Erica Reference Manual. LKB Medical, Solna, Sweden

HEALTHDYNE 102 INFANT VENTILATOR; HEALTHDYNE 105 INFANT VENTILATOR

The Healthdyne 102 infant ventilator (Fig. 10-74) is an electronically controlled, pneumatically powered, time-cycled, constant-flow generator. It may be utilized in CMV, IMV, or CPAP modes. Inspiratory pressure plateau and PEEP/CPAP are available.

Control and Surveillance

A four-position rotary knob located on the control panel (Fig. 10-75) engages ventilator function: OFF, TEST, CPAP, and IPPB/IMV. To establish battery function, the knob is placed in the TEST position while the ventilator is not attached to an electrical outlet. Adequate battery power is indicated by an audible alarm and illumination of a power failure light in the alarm section. All LED windows display an "8" in the test mode. In CPAP or IPPB/IMV mode positions the appropriate indicator lamp illuminates in the operation section.

Continuous gas flow to the patient circuit (0–10 and/or 0–50 $L \cdot minute^{-1}$) is regulated by a flowmeter for a total flow capability of 60 $L \cdot minute^{-1}$. In CPAP mode, the patient breathes spontaneously from a continuous gas flow at ambient or elevated baseline pressure. Baseline pressure is adjustable from 0 to 20 cm H_2O by a CPAP/PEEP control knob. When mechanical tidal volume (V_T) delivery is desired, the mode selector is placed in IPPB/IMV position. During IPPB/IMV, the exhalation valve closes at a selected rate (1–150 breaths·minute^{-1}) for an adjustable inspiratory time (0.1–4.9 seconds). Mechanical V_T is determined by inspiratory time (T_I) and continuous flow rate. The I : E ratio is indicated by LED display. If the selected expiratory time (T_E) is less than 0.3 second, an audible alarm activates and the insufficient T_E light illuminates, and ventilation continues at a T_E of 0.3 second. A maximum inverse I : E ratio audible and visual alarm occurs if T_E is less than 25 percent of T_I (I : E ≤ 1 : 0.25). Under this condition, the I : E ratio LED indication blinks.

PIP may be regulated from 1 to 70 cm H_2O. Proximal airway pressure is indicated on an aneroid manometer. A manual breath may be administered in either IPPB/IMV or CPAP by depressing a pushbutton. The manual V_T is determined by ventilator settings.

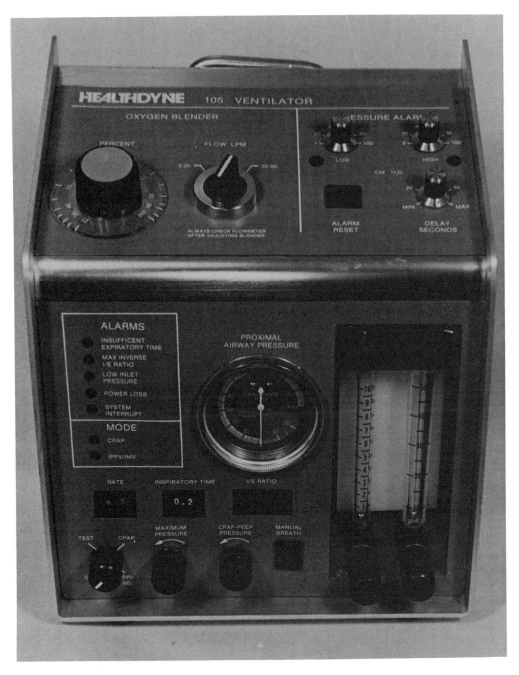

Fig. 10-74. Healthdyne 102 infant ventilator. (Courtesy of Healthdyne, Inc.)

A low inlet pressure audible and visual alarm engage if source gas pressure falls to less than 15–22 psi. Power failure and system failure audible and visual alarms activate if electrical power fails or a malfunction is detected by an internal

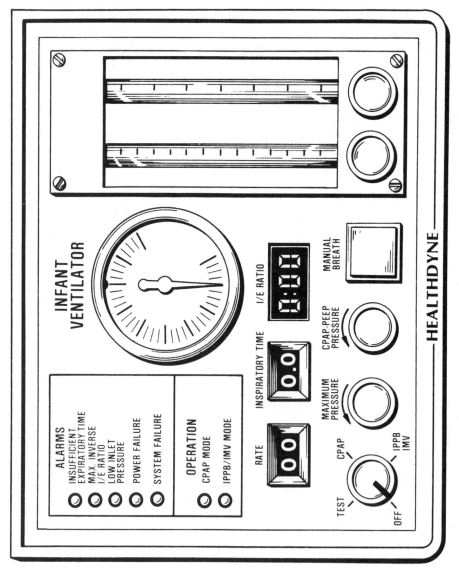

Fig. 10-75. Schematic of the Healthdyne 102 control panel.

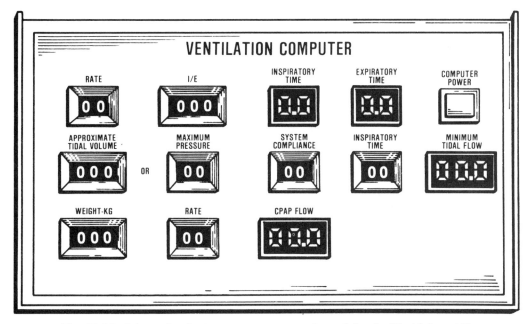

Fig. 10-76. Schematic of microprocessor control panel for the Healthdyne 102.

microprocessor, respectively.

A microprocessor-based ventilation computer (Fig. 10-76) is switched on by depressing a pushbutton. The computer functions independently of the ventilator and may be employed to calculate adjustable parameters or as a bedside teaching device.

Mechanical TE and TI are computed and displayed when the I : E ratio and rate are entered. The minimum total flow for the IPPB/IMV mode is calculated by entering TI, system compliance, and either desired maximum pressure or appropriate VT. System compliance may be determined by di-

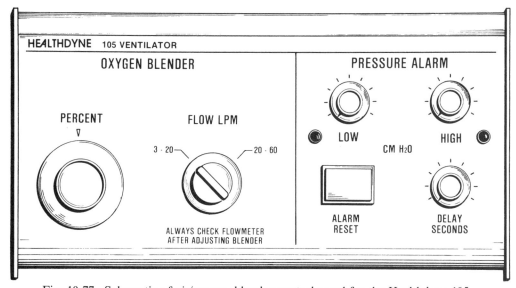

Fig. 10-77. Schematic of air/oxygen blender control panel for the Healthdyne 105.

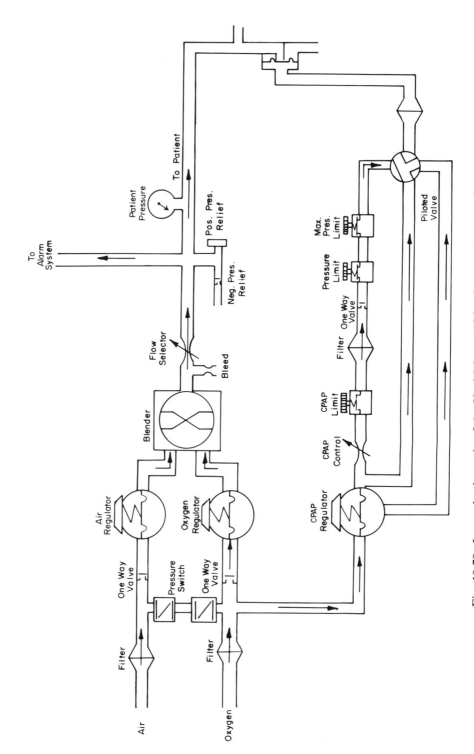

Fig. 10-78. Internal schematic of the Healthdyne 105 inspiratory phase gas flows.

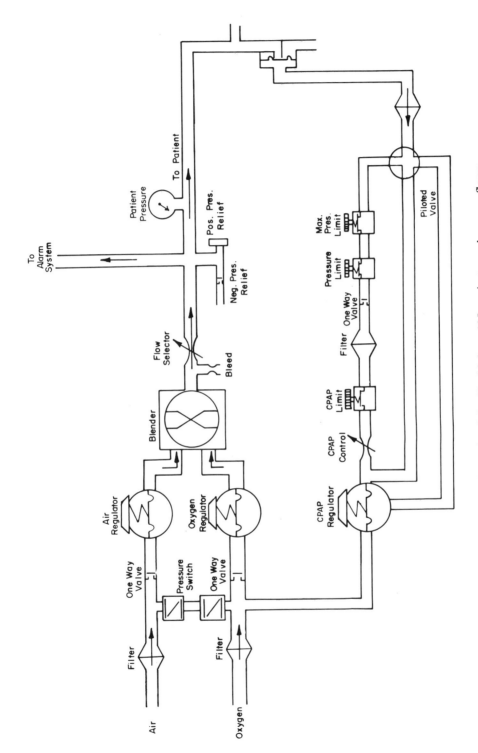

Fig. 10-79. Internal schematic of the Healthdyne 105 expiratory phase gas flows.

viding the product of Tı and total flow (as adjusted by flowmeters) by the PIP generated against an occluded circuit outflow during IPPB/IMV. Adequate circuit flow for CPAP is computed when the spontaneous rate and infant's weight in kilograms are entered.

Healthdyne's model 105 ventilator has virtually the same control panel and operation characteristics but lacks the ventilation computer. Instead it contains an air-oxygen gas blender and pressure alarm module (Fig. 10-77). Desired F_{IO_2} is adjustable from 0.21 to 1.0 at varying flows (3–20 or 20–60 L·minute^{-1}). "Low" and "high" pressure alarms are adjustable from 1 to 100 and 3 to 100 cm H_2O, respectively. A low- or high-pressure alarm condition activates both audible and visual indicators. Activation of the low-pressure alarm may be delayed 0–90 seconds by depressing a pushbutton.

Operation

Inspiratory (Fig. 10-78) and expiratory (Fig. 10-79) phase gas flows are illustrated. Compressed air and oxygen at 50 psig are blended and delivered to a pressure-compensated flowmeter. The flowmeter provides a continuous flow of gas to the patient system, an alarm/monitor system, and subambient (anti-suffocation) and high inspiratory pressure valves.

Gas is also delivered to a CPAP regulator which reduces the pressure to 30 psig. From there it divides into CPAP and exhalation valve systems. Inspiratory pressure is created when an electronic solenoid valve closes. Solenoid valve closure prevents ambient loss of the continuous circuit flow, instead diverting it into the patient's lungs. The solenoid valve remains closed for the duration of Tı or until the pressure limit is attained. Only two moving parts are present, and they are both in the solenoid valve. This valve and all electronic components are controlled by a microprocessor unit.

Once the ventilator is connected to an electrical outlet, a capacitor begins charging. At an appropriate charging level the microprocessor searches the system to find the selected ventilator mode and initiates the appropriate program for operation. Gas from the CPAP regulator goes through CPAP and pressure limit controls and is regulated to maintain pressure on the exhalation valve during the expiratory phase. This system also functions to set a pressure limit during the inspiratory phase. A maximum pressure limit is set independently to maintain safety limits. The intrinsic gas consumption of this pneumatic system is 3 L·minute^{-1}.

Reference

Model 102 and 105 Operators Manual. Healthdyne Inc., Marietta, GA

MONAGHAN 225/SIMV VENTILATOR

The Monaghan 225/SIMV ventilator (Fig. 10-80) is a pneumatically powered, fluidically controlled, constant-flow generator that is volume-, time-, or pressure-cycled. It may be operated in CMV, ASSIST, or SIMV modes with or without PEEP/CPAP.

Control and Surveillance

Most of the ventilatory parameters are selected at the control panel (Fig. 10-81). A notable exception is tidal volume (V_T), which is determined by crank-regulated concertina bag displacement at the base of the bellows cannister. Mechanical V_T is adjustable (100–3300 ml) and delivered at a selected constant flow ranging up to approximately 100 L·minute^{-1}.

The mechanical cycling frequency depends on which method is used to terminate inspiration. A ventilator rate control knob adjusts exhalation time (T_E) (0.5–7.5 seconds) when volume- or pressure-cycling is employed. It determines total cycle duration (1.0–12 seconds) at a preset I:E ratio of 1:1 when time-cycling. In the SIMV mode, a three-position rotary knob selects the range of ventilatory rates (0.3–5 and 4–16 breaths·minute^{-1} or OFF) which deactivates SIMV rate control. A red indicator illuminates during SIMV function but switches off immediately before each mandatory breath to identify the next bellows cycle as a mechanical V$_T$. Spontaneous breathing from circuit gas is provided on demand by bellows compression (exhalation valve occlusion does not occur).

The PIP cycle is continuously adjustable (approximately 10–100 cm H$_2$O) and indicated on an aneroid manometer. When pressure exceeds the selected PIP, mechanical inspiration is terminated and a red indicator is activated. Volume-cycling occurs when the adjusted bellows volume is delivered at a pressure below the PIP cycle or before the programmed inspiratory time (T$_I$). Programmed T$_I$ is determined by the ventilatory rate and a preset I:E ratio of 1:1. For example, if the controlled cycling frequency is 10 breaths·minute^{-1} (1 breath·6 seconds^{-1}), then 3 seconds each is alloted for T$_I$ and T$_E$. If the selected volume or pressure limit is not reached in 3 seconds, inspiration is time-cycled and so designated by a red indicator.

ASSIST, CMV, or SIMV modes may be selected by a three-position knob. Patient effort for initiating mechanical and/or spontaneous demand inspiration is adjusted with an uncalibrated trigger sensitivity control. Spontaneous effort is indicated by needle deflection on the aneroid manometer, and when this is sufficient to initiate inspiration a green indicator flashes. PEEP/CPAP is adjustable (0–20 cm H$_2$O).

A manual inspiration is administered by depressing a pushbutton. After a manual breath, the rate control timer resets T$_E$. Manual exhalation causes immediate depressurization of the exhalation valve (to ambient or PEEP level) and bellows can-

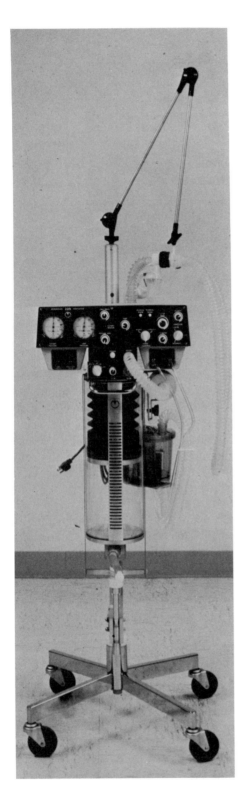

Fig. 10-80. Monaghan 225/SIMV ventilator.

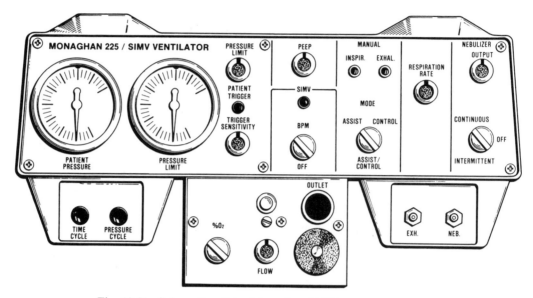

Fig. 10-81. Schematic of the Monaghan 225/SIMV control panel.

nister. This action facilitates refill if the bellows remains in a maximally compressed position either during spontaneous breathing or when a circuit leak/disconnection occurs during SIMV.

Continuous or intermittent (synchronous with mechanical inspiration) nebulization of medication is selected by a three-position rotary knob. Aerosol output is determined by a continuously adjustable nebulizer jet flow control. Nebulizer jet flow comes from the 50-psig oxygen source; therefore it increases both the mechanical V_T and the F_{IO_2}. This effect is appreciable during maximum continuous nebulization.

Operation

Inspiratory (Fig. 10-82) and expiratory (Fig. 10-83) phase gas flows are illustrated. The Monaghan 225 is a fluidic ventilator powered by a 50-psig oxygen source. The desired F_{IO_2} is achieved by a fluidic air entrainment device. A bellows is utilized to deliver the gas mixture to the patient. After compression the bellows descends within the cannister, drawing in the requisite volume of air to produce the desired F_{IO_2}. The

source pressure is regulated at 5–7 psig before entry into the fluidic logic circuit. Should the internal regulator malfunction, a 10-psig pressure relief valve prevents significant overpressurization of the logic circuit. Initially gas at the reduced pressure is delivered to a ventilator mode selector. A manual trigger switch can override the mode selector at any time to initiate inspiration or exhalation.

Gas then flows to a fluidic element timing module. This is a flip-flop unit which serves as the main valve. It cycles the ventilator into inspiratory and expiratory phases as the elapsed times dictate and controls gas flow to the bellows. An "or/nor" gate controls gas flow to the exhalation valve.

Tidal volume is set to the appropriate cannister displacement level by adjusting the bellows with a movable platform. As inspiration begins, flow is delivered into the cannister, compressing the bellows at a rate adjusted by the flow control valve. As the bellows reaches the top of the cannister, a fluidic touch sensor terminates inspiration.

The ventilator may be pressure-cycled by means of a pressure cut-off system incorporating a fluidic positive-pressure com-

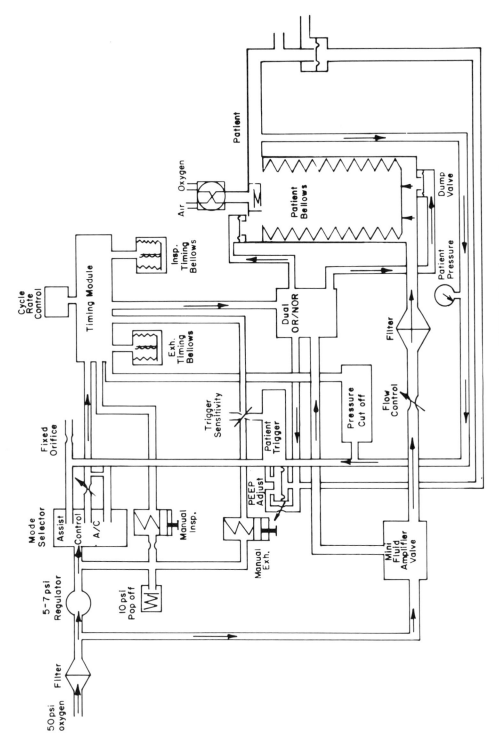

Fig. 10-82. Internal schematic of the Monaghan 225/SIMV inspiratory phase gas flows.

433

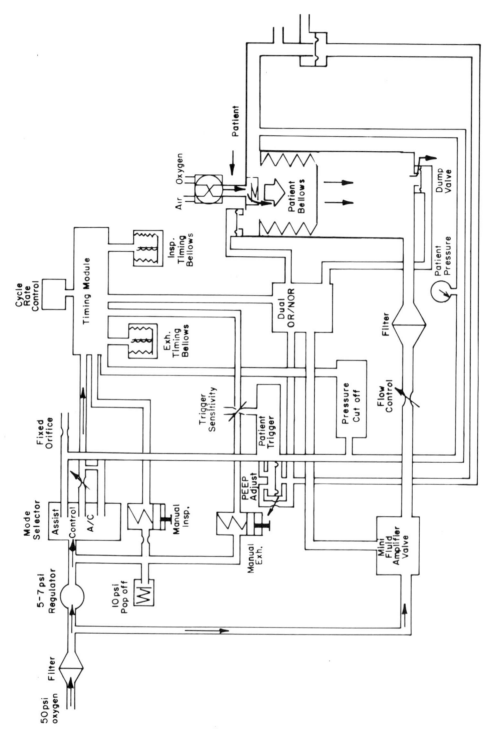

Fig. 10-83. Internal schematic of the Monaghan 225/SIMV expiratory phase gas flows.

434

parator. This comparator is connected to the patient circuit to maximize sensitivity for pressure cycling as well as the response to patient-initiated mechanical or demand breaths. Also connected within this system is the PEEP adjustment control.

Fluidic logic oxygen consumption is only 8–10 L·minute^{-1}, making the Monaghan 225 a reasonable choice for a transport ventilator.

Reference

Model 225 Operators Manual No. 13837B. Monaghan, Inc., Littleton, CO

NEWPORT VENTILATOR E-100

The Newport E-100 ventilator (Fig. 10-84) is a pneumatically powered, electronically controlled, constant-flow generator when time-cycled and a nonconstant-pressure generator when pressure-cycled. It may be employed in CMV, IMV, or CPAP modes. Inspiratory pressure plateau and PEEP/CPAP are available.

Control and Surveillance

Electronic circuitry is activated by a master switch (not illustrated) on the rear panel of the ventilator chassis (Fig. 10-85). If electrical power failure occurs, a battery-activated audible alarm engages.

Pressure- and time-cycled modes are available. During pressure cycling, inspiration is terminated when a selected inspiratory pressure (P_I) is reached. P_I is adjusted by a rotary knob and indicated by a red arrow on the aneroid manometer. If P_I is not reached, the selected inspiratory time (T_I) terminates the mechanical breath. In a time-cycled mode, T_I ranges from 0.1 to 3.0 seconds.

Mechanical tidal volume (V_T) in the pressure-cycled mode is primarily dependent on P_I and inspiratory flow ($\dot{V}$ = 0.1–0.8 L·second^{-1}). In the time-cycled mode, V_T is dependent on adjusted T_I and $\dot{V}$. Mechanical inspiration may be patient-initiated or controlled. The inspiratory effort necessary to initiate a mechanical V_T in either mode is regulated by a trigger level control (-10 to 20 cm H_2O), which also is indicated by a red arrow on the aneroid manometer. The CMV rate is adjustable (1–60 breaths·minute^{-1}). A manual inspiration is administered when a pushbutton is depressed. A manual breath may be given in any mode and recycles the timing circuit.

PEEP/CPAP (0–25 cm H_2O) is regulated by an uncalibrated knob. The trigger level is *not* PEEP/CPAP-compensated; thus it

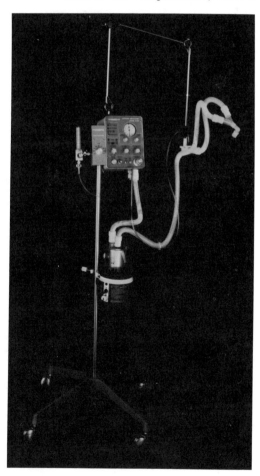

Fig. 10-84. Newport E-100 ventilator. (Courtesy of Newport Medical Instrumentation.)

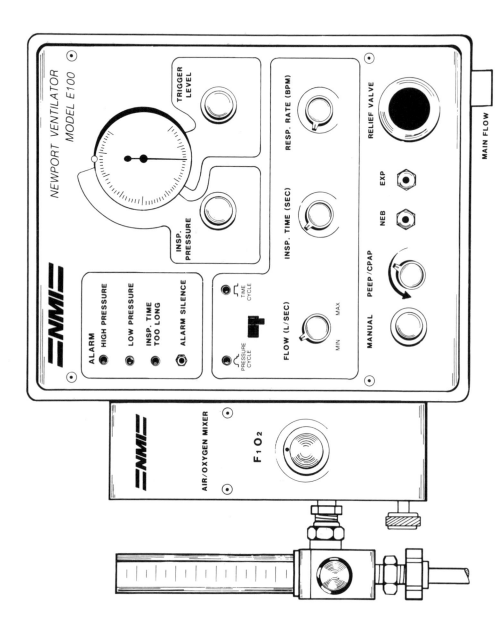

Fig. 10-85. Schematic of the Newport E-100 control panel.

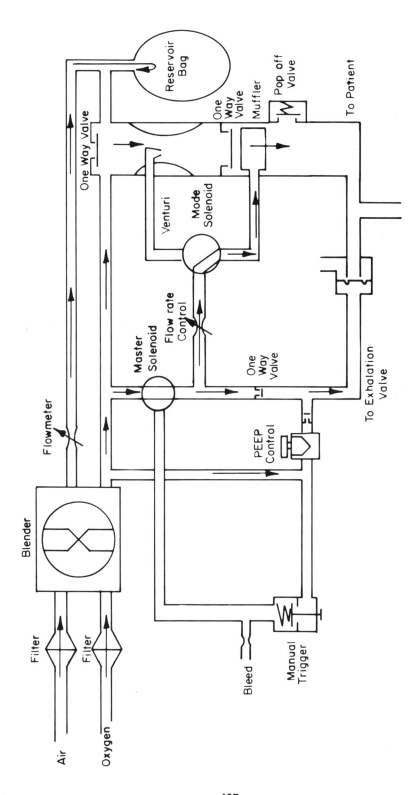

Fig. 10-86. Internal schematic of the Newport E-100 inspiratory phase gas flows.

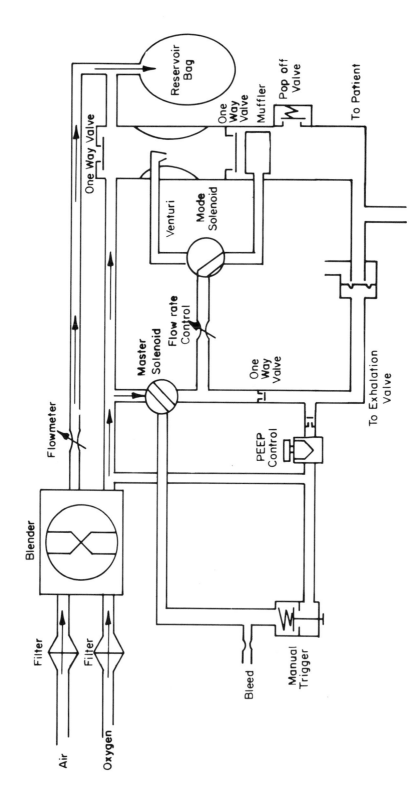

Fig. 10-87. Internal schematic of the Newport E-100 expiratory phase gas flows.

must be adjusted when PEEP/CPAP is altered. A mechanical relief valve may be regulated (0–80 cm H_2O). Generally this is set slightly above the operational P_I. In the time-cycled mode, the relief pressure may be adjusted to provide a postinflation hold (plateau) for a given T_I.

F_{IO_2} is regulated from 0.21 to 1.0. An auxiliary metered flow (0–15 L·minute^{-1}) may be interfaced with the breathing circuit (proximal to the humidifier) to provide continuous flow for spontaneous breathing with IMV and/or CPAP. Breathing circuit connections for the main flow, nebulizer, and exhalation valve are located on the control panel.

"High" and "low" pressure audible and visual alarms and a visual "prolonged inspiratory time" alarm are present. Audible alarms may be silenced for 55 seconds by depressing a pushbutton. The "low pressure" alarm is activated when the adjusted P_I level is not reached during CMV or IMV. The "high pressure" alarm is activated and the inspiratory phase terminated in the time-cycled mode when airway pressure exceeds the selected P_I by 20 cm H_2O. When the selected T_I exceeds 50 percent of total cycle time, the prolonged T_I amber lamp illuminates, indicating an internal T_I override.

Operation

Inspiratory (Fig 10-86) and expiratory (Fig. 10-87) phase gas flows are illustrated. Compressed air and oxygen at 50 psig are blended to the desired F_{IO_2}. Blended gas is metered (7–10 L·minute^{-1}) to a reservoir bag, a master solenoid, and a PEEP control needle valve.

The mode selector diverts gas through a flow rate control to a venturi device. The latter entrains reservoir gas and delivers it to the patient circuit. When the selected pressure or time interval is reached, the ventilator is cycled to the exhalation phase. During time-cycled ventilation, the mode selector delivers gas directly into the breathing circuit at a selected flow rate. A spring-loaded valve vents excess pressure to ambient air. When the master solenoid is open during mechanical inspiration, the exhalation valve is pressurized. After pressure- or time-cycled inspiration, the master solenoid interrupts flow to the mode selector solenoid and depressurizes the exhalation valve to ambient pressure or the PEEP/CPAP level. During the expiratory phase, a manual breath may be administered by depressing a pushbutton.

Reference

Newport Ventilator E-100 Instruction Manual. Newport Medical Instrumentation, Inc., Newport Beach, CA

OHIO 550 VENTILATOR

The Ohio 550 ventilator (Fig. 10-88) is a pneumatically powered, fluidically controlled, volume-cycled, constant-flow generator. It may be used in CMV or ASSIST modes.

Control and Surveillance

Pneumatic power to the fluidic circuitry is controlled by a two-position rotary knob located on the control panel (Fig. 10-89). Tidal volume (V_T) is selected by adjusting bellows displacement (200–2000 ml). Mechanical V_T at a preselected F_{IO_2} (0.21–1.0) is delivered by an inspiratory flow control (30–90 L·minute^{-1}) against a compressed gas source 20 cm H_2O circuit pressure. Maximal attainable circuit pressure is 100 cm H_2O (70 cm H_2O on models before 1976). A spring tension pressure relief valve located at the ventilator outflow port is continuously adjustable (10–100 cm H_2O). Relief pressure is selected by occluding the circuit outflow during V_T delivery and rotating

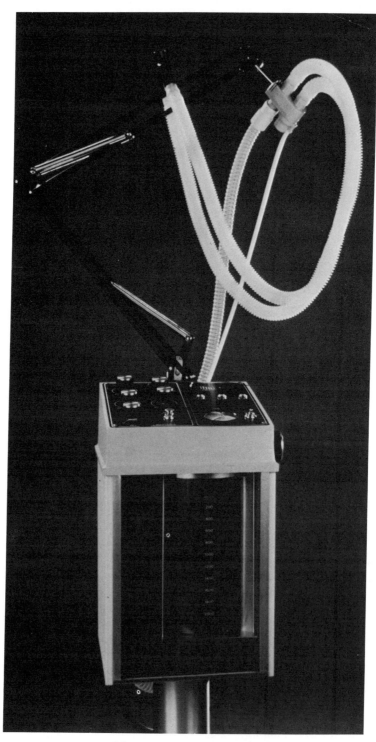

Fig. 10-88. Ohio 550 ventilator.

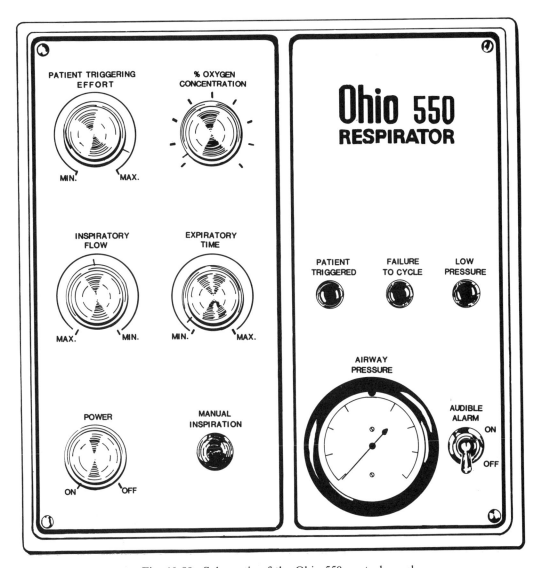

Fig. 10-89. Schematic of the Ohio 550 control panel.

the spring-tension control knob while observing the aneroid manometer.

Controlled cycling frequency is determined by adjusting an uncalibrated expiratory time (TE) control (1–15 seconds). At a given TE, cycling frequency fluctuates with changes in the duration of inspiration. Effort necessary for patient-initiated breaths is adjustable (-0.5 to -5.0 cm H_2O). A manual VT may be delivered during TE by depressing a button. Sustained button depression permits an inflation hold (up to 15 seconds).

Patient-initiated VT flashes a green indicator. A "failure-to-cycle" or "low pressure" condition flashes a red indicator and sounds an audible alarm when activated by a toggle switch. The "failure-to-cycle" alarm functions if the programmed TE elapses without a mechanical breath. A "low pressure" condition presents when a minimum pressure of 8 cm H_2O fails to develop in the patient circuit during VT delivery.

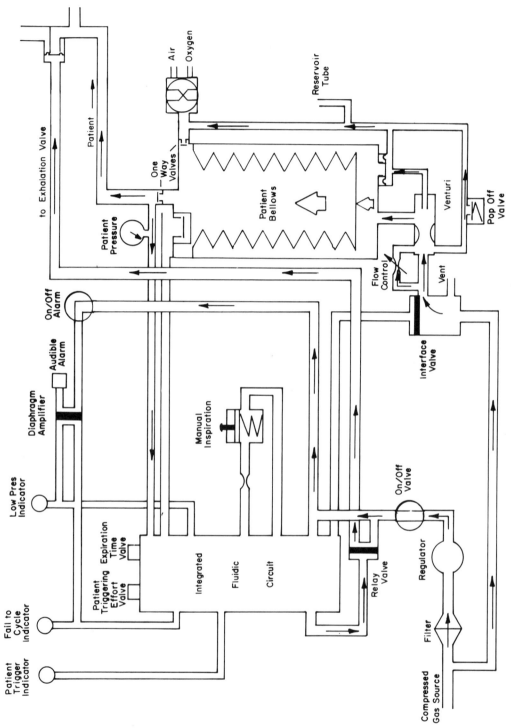

Fig. 10-90. Internal schematic of the Ohio 550 inspiratory phase gas flows.

442

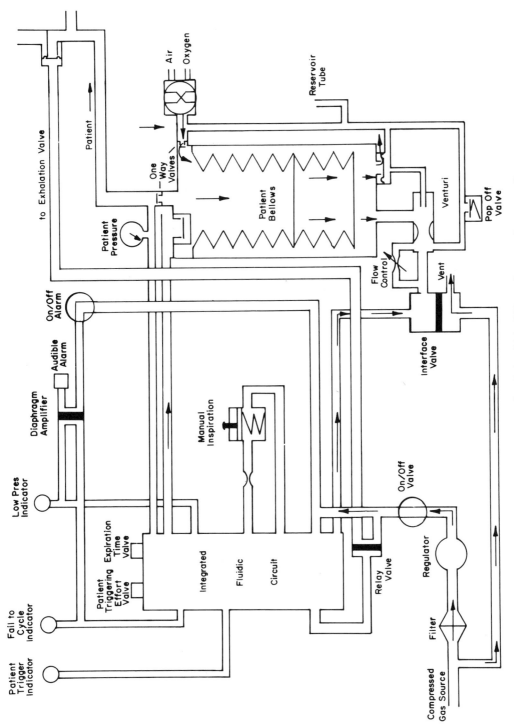

Fig. 10-91. Internal schematic of the Ohio 550 expiratory phase gas flows.

Operation

Inspiratory (Fig. 10-90) and expiratory (Fig. 10-91) phase gas flows are illustrated. The Ohio 550 is a fluidic ventilator that may be powered by compressed air (for a desired F_{IO_2} of 0.21). For a higher F_{IO_2} pressurized oxygen must be diluted with ambient air.

Compressed gas is filtered, regulated to 3.0 psig, and directed to the fluidic control circuit by an ON/OFF valve. During inspiration the fluidic control output opens a relay valve and delivers compressed gas to close the exhalation valve. Simultaneous output through the interface valve directs the compressed source gas by means of an inspiratory flow control to a venturi jet. Venturi jet flow plus entrained air pressurizes the rigid plastic cannister, compressing the bellows and directing its gas volume into the breathing circuit. At the same time, a portion of the venturi output is diverted to seat the cannister dump valve. Maximum inspiratory pressure is limited by a facotry preset 70 cm H_2O relief valve (100 cm H_2O since 1976). When the bellows is completely compressed against the top of the cannister, a spring-loaded plunger closes, signaling the beginning of exhalation. The fluidic logic circuit closes both relay and interface valves, depressuring the exhalation valve and interrupting venturi jet flow, respectively. Mechanical inspiration may then be initiated again by a fluidic timer, patient inspiratory effort, or manually.

Reference

Model 550 Operation/Maintenance Manual No. 1936. Ohio Medical Products, Madison WI

OHIO 560 VENTILATOR

The Ohio 560 ventilator (Fig. 10-92) is an electronically powered and controlled, volume-cycled, constant-flow generator. It

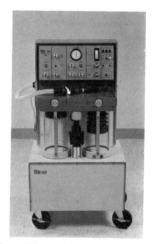

Fig. 10-92. Ohio 560 ventilator.

may be used in CMV or ASSIST modes. Mechanical inspiration may be extended by a postinflation pause (plateau), and PEEP or optional negative end-expiratory pressure (NEEP) are available.

Control and Surveillance

All electronic circuits are activated by the power ON/OFF toggle switch on the control panel (Fig. 10-93). Normal tidal volume (V_T) is adjustable (0–2000 ml) at an inspiratory flow rate ($\dot{V}$) up to 180 L·minute^{-1}. Mechanical inspiration may be extended by a plateau (0.2–2.0 seconds). Manual inspiratory and expiratory phases are initiated by depressing respective pushbuttons. A manual exhalation terminates mechanical inspiration and/or plateau. Controlled cycling frequency is determined by the duration of inspiration ($V_T \times \dot{V}$ + plateau) and the selected expiratory time (0.5–7.0 seconds). The resultant ventilatory rate is displayed. Mechanical V_T may be patient-initiated at a regulated triggering effort (which is *not* PEEP-compensated). An assisted breath is indicated by lamp illumination. A deep breath volume (0–2000 ml) superimposed on a normal V_T may be automatically delivered at an interval of 1, 2, 4, 6, 8, or

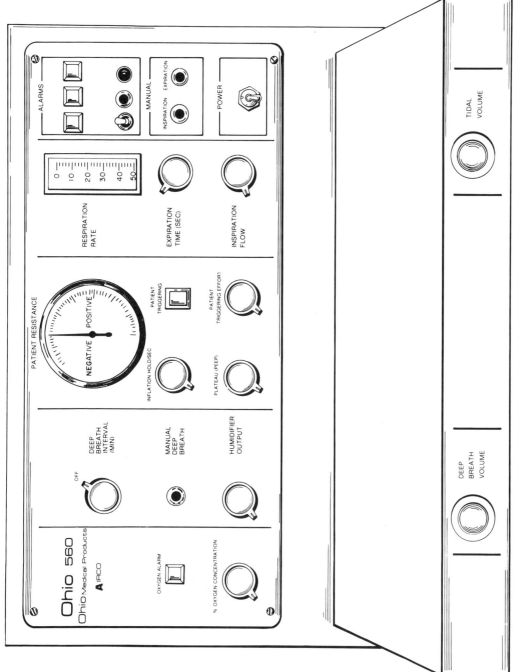

Fig. 10-93. Schematic of the Ohio 560 control panel.

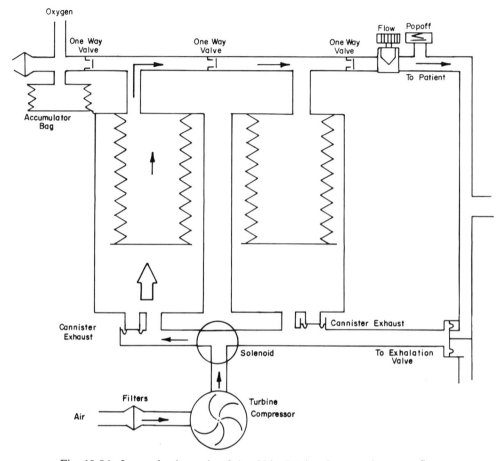

Fig. 10-94. Internal schematic of the Ohio 560 inspiratory phase gas flows.

10 minutes. A manual deep breath may be administered by depressing a pushbutton. Expiratory time is doubled following either an automatic or a manual deep breath.

Circuit pressure is indicated by an aneroid manometer and is limited with an adjustable spring-loaded pressure relief valve (beneath the panel tray) which vents excess pressure (10–100 cm H_2O) to ambient air. PEEP is adjustable (0–12 cm H_2O).

F_{IO_2} is adjustable from 0.21 to 1.0. When the control is set above 0.21 and the ventilator demand exceeds the internal reservoir capacity, audible and visual alarms activate. Other alarms include "fail-to-cycle" and "low" and "high pressure," each of

which can be silenced or reset. The "failure-to-cycle" alarm activates if inspiration or expiration exceeds 8 to 14 seconds, respectively. If a minimum of 8 cm H_2O pressure is not developed during mechanical inspiration, the "low pressure" alarm engages. The "high pressure" alarm threshold is adjustable and should be set to engage at a level equal to or slightly less than the relief pressure.

Operation

Inspiratory (Fig. 10-94) and expiratory (Fig. 10-95) phase gas flows are illustrated.

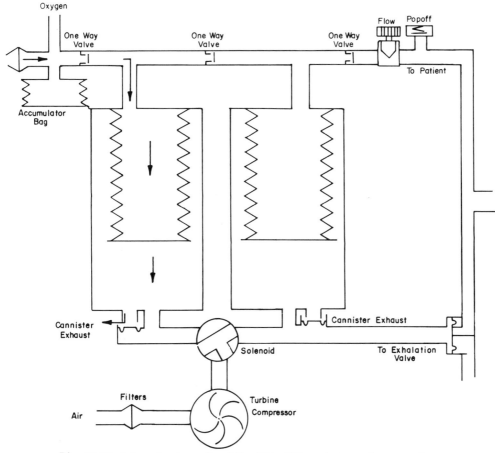

Fig. 10-95. Internal schematic of the Ohio 560 expiratory phase gas flows.

The Ohio 560 utilizes a venturi blending mechanism that delivers gas to an accumulator bag at ambient pressure. This accumulator bag stores mixed gas (O_2 and air) for tidal volume delivery. Once inspiration terminates, the bellows descends, filling with gas from the accumulator bag until it reaches the tidal volume position for the next breath (both bellows in the case of a sigh volume). One-way check valves ensure correct directional flow.

The turbine compressor circuit is open to the bellows cannister when the main solenoid valve opens. As cannister pressure increases, the bellows is compressed, forcing gas through a flow control into the breathing circuit. An adjustable spring-loaded relief valve prevents excessive circuit pressure. During exhalation the circuit exhalation valve and cannister dump valve(s) depressurize. As the dump valve(s) open, cannister pressure decreases to ambient pressure, thereby facilitating bellows refill.

Reference

Model 560 Operation/Maintenance Manual. Ohio Medical Products, Madison, WI

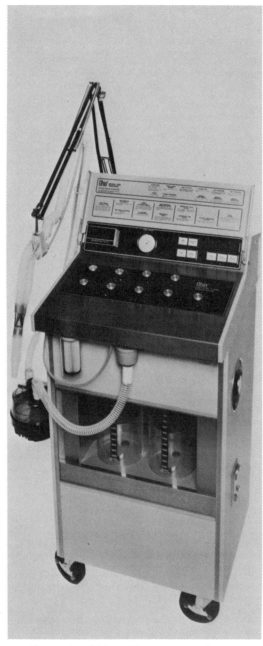

Fig. 10-96. Ohio critical care ventilator-2 (CCV-2).

OHIO CRITICAL CARE VENTILATOR-2 (CCV-2)

The Ohio CCV-2 ventilator (Fig. 10-96) is an electronically powered and controlled, volume-cycled, constant-flow generator. It may be operated in CMV, ASSIST, IMV/SIMV, or CPAP modes. Mechanical inspiration is extended by a postinflation hold (plateau), and PEEP/CPAP is available.

Control and Surveillance

Electrical circuitry is activated by depressing an illuminated pushbutton on the CCV-2 control panel (Fig. 10-97). Mechanical tidal volume (V_T = 200–2000 ml) is selected with a rotary control knob located on the ventilator chassis. This maneuver positions the concertina bag within the compression cannister to an appropriate volume displacement. CMV cycling frequency is primarily dependent on four factors: V_T, inspiratory flow rate ($\dot{V}_I$), plateau time, and expiratory time. $\dot{V}_I$ determines the duration of dynamic inspiration. After V_T delivery, exhalation valve opening may be delayed (0–2 seconds) by the inspiratory plateau control knob.

Expiratory time (T_E) is programmable (1–10 seconds). The resultant average breath-to-breath cycling frequency, or $I:E$ ratio, is indicated on a LED display when respective illuminating switch caps are depressed. Manual inspiration and expiration may be activated independently of automatic cycling functions by depressing appropriate pushbuttons. Manual inspiration may be used at any time during exhalation to deliver the selected V_T and delays exhalation valve opening (plateau) for as long as the pushbutton is depressed. If manual inspiration exceeds 5 seconds, "fail-to-cycle" audible and visual alarms activate. Manual expiration immediately terminates and prevents further mechanical inspirations while this pushbutton is depressed. After 22 seconds of manual expiration, the "fail-to-cycle" audible and visual alarms engage.

The inspiratory effort required for patient-initiated mechanical breaths may be set from 8 to 0.5 cm H_2O below baseline

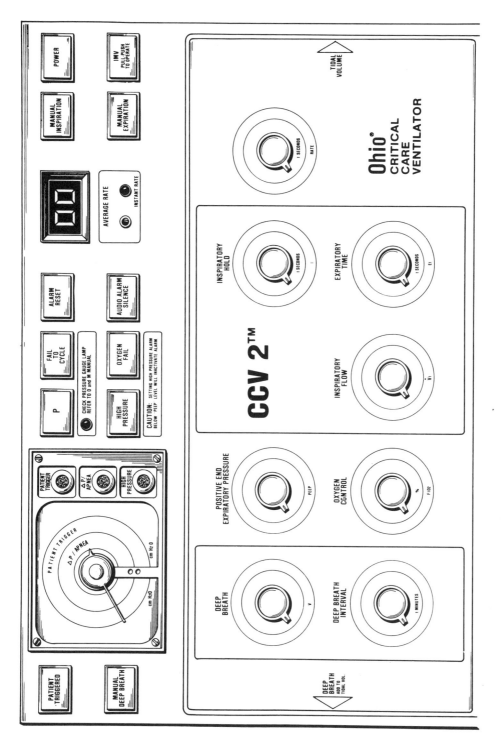

Fig. 10-97. Schematic of the Ohio CCV-2 control panel.

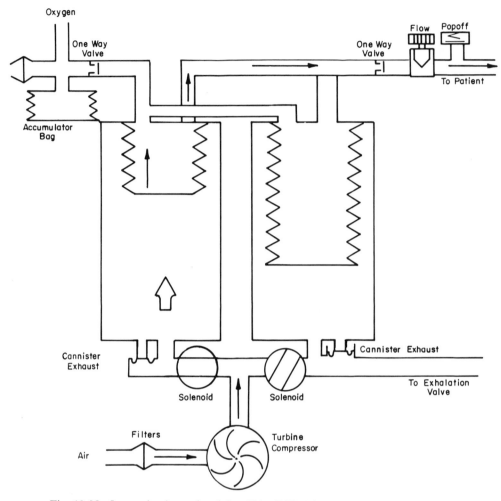

Fig. 10-98. Internal schematic of the Ohio CCV-2 inspiratory phase gas flows.

pressure and is indicated by an arrow on the appropriate portion of the aneroid manometer. Each patient-triggered breath illuminates a green light.

A volume (200–2000 ml) may be superimposed on the VT to provide a deep breath (sigh). Desired additional sigh volume is adjusted with a hand crank. Deep breaths may be administered singly in lieu of a normal VT at 3-, 5-, 7.5-, or 15-minute intervals or in multiples of two or three. A manual sigh is engaged by depressing a pushbutton and is delivered at the subsequent mechanical breath. After programmed or manual sighs,

controlled mechanical TE is doubled. Subsequent patient-initiated breaths may occur at any time.

IMV/SIMV mode is activated by pulling out and then depressing an illuminating switch cap. In the IMV/SIMV mode, all ventilator parameters except TE, patient trigger, and deep breath controls are functional. The IMV rate is determined by the adjusted minimum interval (4–120 seconds) and the synchronous period (0–10 seconds). The IMV timer activates a synchronous period light and internal sensitivity control permitting patient-initiated IMV (SIMV). If

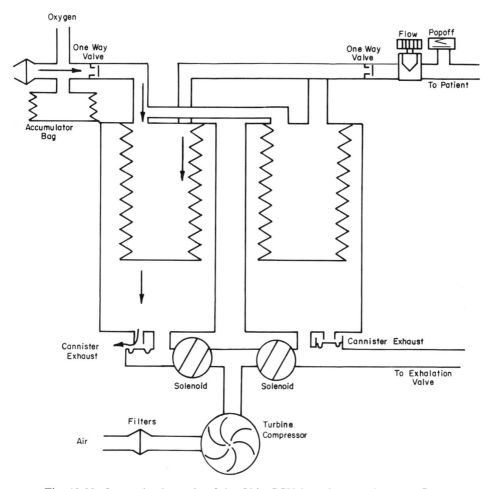

Fig. 10-99. Internal schematic of the Ohio CCV-2 expiratory phase gas flows.

the patient fails to generate sufficient effort, a mandatory V_T is delivered at the end of the synchronous period.

Photosensor-activated change of pressure (ΔP), high pressure alarm, and patient-triggering effort controls are all located in the aneroid pressure module. Patient-triggered effort is adjustable (-10 to 40 cm H_2O) and when achieved is indicated by an illuminated lamp. ΔP is adjusted (-10 to 50 cm H_2O pressure). If circuit pressure does not reach the ΔP point within 15 seconds, audible and visual alarms engage. The ΔP control functions as an apnea alarm during IMV/SIMV and switches ventilation to CMV when activated. The "high pressure"

(30–100 cm H_2O) cycles the ventilator to exhalation and engages audible and visual alarms when activated.

Proper photosensor alarm system function is indicated by a blinking light. Continuous illumination occurs when ΔP and high-pressure points are very near baseline and should be adjusted to monitor respective conditions adequately. "Fail-to-cycle" audible and visual alarms occur if T_I or T_E exceed approximately 5 and 22 seconds, respectively. "Oxygen failure" visual and audible alarms signify failure of the oxygen source to meet ventilator demand. Audible alarms may be deactivated for approximately 2 minutes by depressing a pushbutton, which is illuminated during the silence period. Alarm functions, except "high pressure alert," may be reset by depressing a pushbutton. If the condition remains uncorrected, alarm activation recurs.

Operation

Inspiratory (Fig. 10-98) and expiratory (Fig. 10-99) phase gas flows are illustrated. The CCV-2 utilizes a venturi blending mechanism to fill a reservoir with desired FIO_2 at ambient pressure. When inspiration terminates, the bellows descends, filling with reservoir gas through a unidirectional valve until it reaches the V_T position for the next breath (both bellows in case of a sigh volume).

During inspiration, compressed gas from the turbine is directed into the rigid plastic cannister (both for a sigh breath), and a portion is used to pressurize the cannister dump valve(s) and exhalation valve in the breathing circuit. As cannister pressure rises, the bellows is compressed, forcing mixed gas through a peak flow control into the breathing circuit. A spring-loaded relief valve is adjusted to regulate maximum circuit pressure. During exhalation, circuit exhalation and cannister dump valve(s) depressurize. As the dump valve(s) open, cannister pressure decreases to ambient level and bellows refill occurs.

Reference

CCV2 Operation/Maintenance Manual No. 4928. Ohio Medical Products, Madison WI

SEARLE VVA VENTILATOR

The Searle VVA ventilator (Fig. 10-100) is an electronically powered and controlled, volume-cycled, constant- and nonconstant-flow generator. It may be operated in CMV, ASSIST, or INTERMITTENT DEMAND VENTILATION (IDV) modes.

Control and Surveillance

A power button, when depressed, becomes illuminated and activates all ventilator electronic circuits (Fig. 10-101). Tidal volume (V_T) is adjustable (300–2200 ml). Ventilatory rate (5–60 breaths·minute^{-1}) is displayed. The inspiratory effort required to initiate a mechanical breath is adjustable (minimum to -20 cm H_2O); no patient-initiated breaths can occur in the OFF position. Each patient-initiated breath is indicated by an illuminated lamp. An optional IDV module (not illustrated) permits delivery of a mechanical breath to augment spontaneous ventilation. IDV differs from IMV/SIMV in that it is adjusted to administer a mechanical V_T after a selected number of spontaneous breaths rather than a per-minute frequency. Mechanical minute ventilation may change from minute to minute with IDV.

Inspiratory flow rate is regulated (up to 200 L·minute^{-1} at 90 ± 10 cm H_2O backpressure). The flow contour may be constant (square wave) or decelerating (tapered). As the flow taper control is moved toward maximum, deceleration increases and the inspiratory duration increases to facilitate V_T delivery. In the maximum taper position, only the initial 25 percent of inspiration is at the preselected flow rate. Deceleration then occurs until flow is approximately 33 percent of the original value. The I : E time ratio is displayed.

Inspiration may be extended by a time-cycled plateau period (0–5 seconds). PEEP is adjustable (0–20 cm H_2O). The PEEP control knob locks at 0, 5, and 10 cm H_2O positions. Patient-triggering effort is PEEP-compensated; thus adjustments in PEEP require no change in patient effort to initiate assisted ventilation.

A deep breath (300–2200 ml) may be administered singly or in multiples of two or

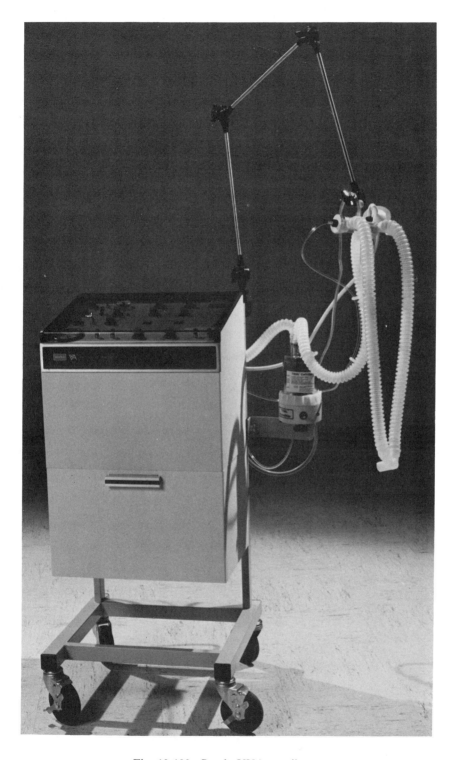

Fig. 10-100. Searle VVA ventilator.

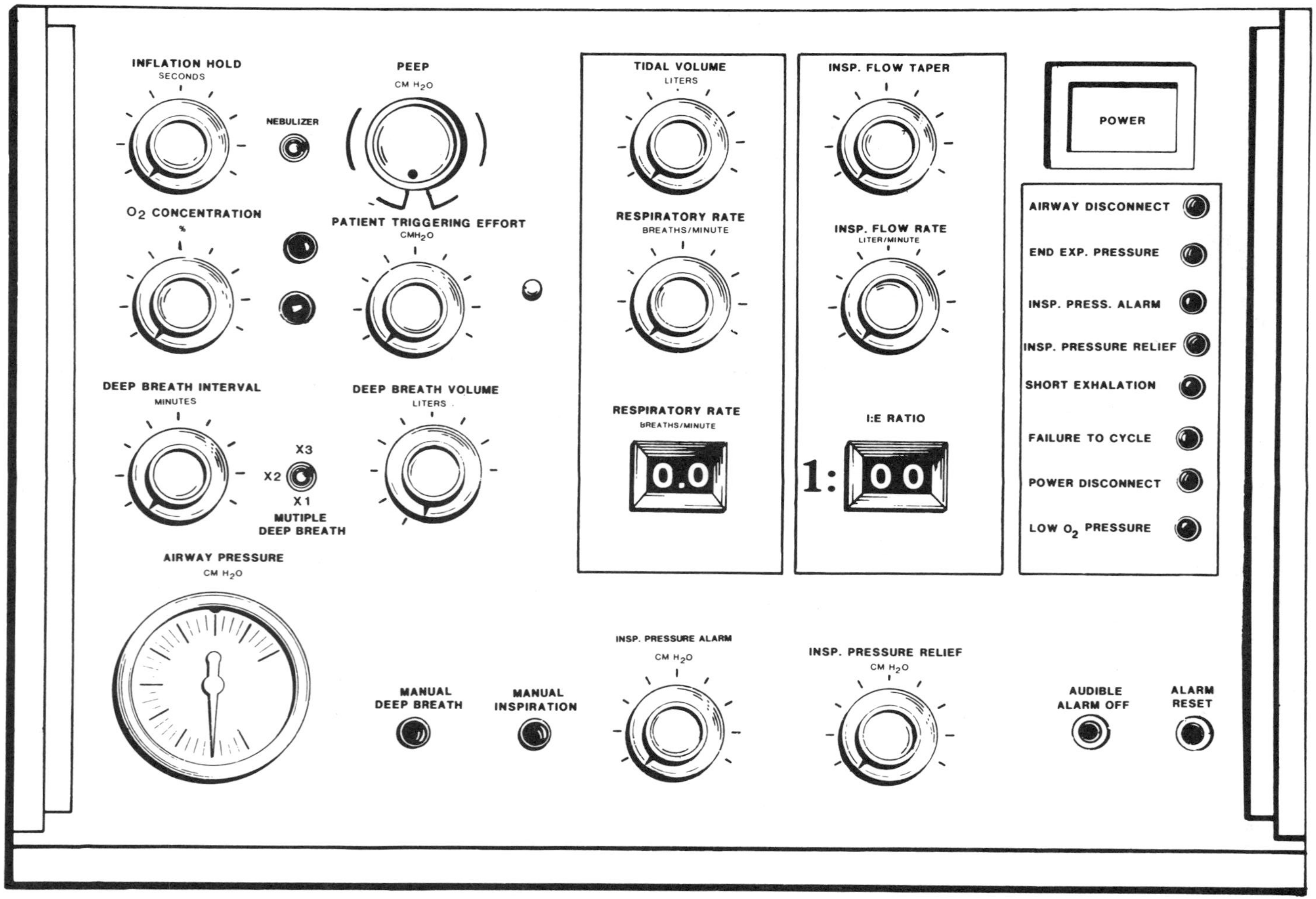

Fig. 10-101. Schematic of the Searle VVA control panel.

454

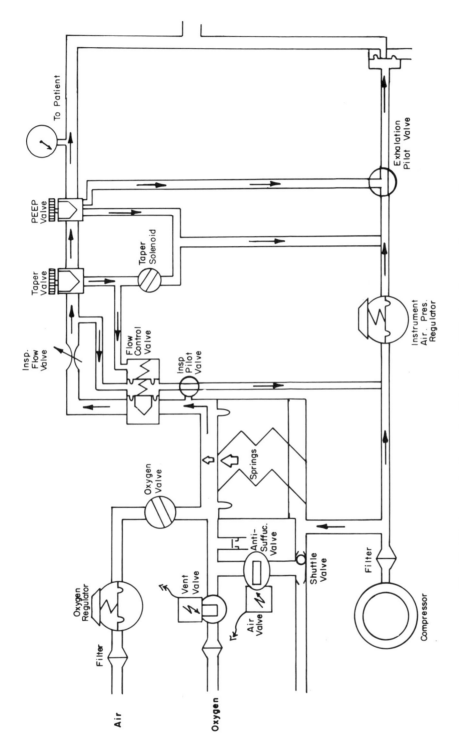

Fig. 10-102. Internal schematic of the Searle VVA inspiratory phase gas flows.

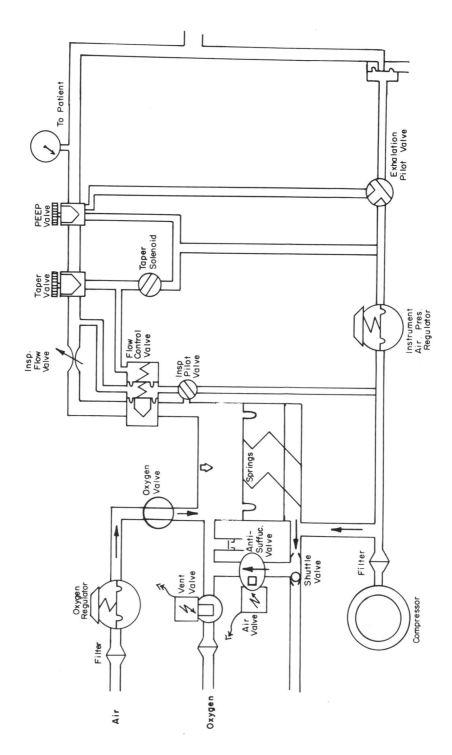

Fig. 10-103. Internal schematic of the Searle VVA expiratory phase gas flows.

three at intervals of 0–10 minutes. A manual
V_T and deep breath may be administered by
depressing respective pushbuttons. When
depressed, a manual deep breath occurs at
the next mechanical inspiration and resets
the automatic deep breath timer. It may not
be delivered when the deep breath interval
control is OFF.

FIO_2 is variable from 0.21 to 1.0. A pushbutton may be depressed to deliver 100 percent oxygen for 2 minutes. During this time
period an audible "chirp" sounds every 10
seconds and an indicator lamp illuminates.

Circuit pressure is indicated on an aneroid manometer (-30 to 100 cm H_2O). PIP
ranges from 0 to 100 cm H_2O. If the PIP
is exceeded, audible and visual alarms engage, and mechanical inspiration is terminated. An inspiratory pressure alarm may
be adjusted (0–100 cm H_2O). When the preset PIP is exceeded, audible and visual
alarms engage, but mechanical inspiration
is not terminated.

Other audible and/or visual alarms include: "airway disconnect" (if at least 3 cm
H_2O PIP above PEEP is not generated);
"end-expiratory pressure" (if 5 cm H_2O or
greater pressure above PEEP is in the circuit immediately before a mechanical
breath, exhalation is not complete; "short
exhalation," visual only (if inspiratory exceeds expiratory time); "failure to cycle"
(when 15 seconds elapse without void of a
mechanical breath); "power disconnect"
(no wall current when main power button
is on); and "low oxygen pressure" (if supply pressure falls below 10–15 psig when
oxygen concentration control is above 21
percent).

Audible alarms may be silenced by depressing a pushbutton. Visual indicators remain illuminated, and a "chirp" is heard
every 10 seconds until the alarm reset button is depressed.

Operation

Inspiratory (Fig. 10-102) and expiratory
(Fig. 10-103) gas flows are illustrated. During inspiration, the inspiratory pilot valve
(solenoid) interrupts compressed air pressure to the flow control valve, thus allowing
it to open by spring action. The piston is
driven upward by spring tension (120–200
cm H_2O), forcing gas contained in the cylinder through the inspiratory flow rate valve
and flow taper control into the breathing circuit. When flow taper is employed, the
taper solenoid opens the taper valve inter-
facing with the compressed air and flow
control valve, thus limiting the degree to
which it can freely open and permit outflow
from the piston during mechanical inspiration. As circuit pressure approaches the
flow control valve opening pressure (i.e.,
functional driving pressure), inspiratory
flow decreases. The exhalation pilot valve
(solenoid) also opens to pressurize the exhalation valve. If the selected PIP is
reached, the cylinder vent valve opens to
exhaust any remaining volume to ambient.
Should pneumatic or electronic failure
occur, the patient can breathe spontaneously through an antisuffocation valve.

During exhalation the cylinder is filled
with air or an air-oxygen mixture as the piston moves downward. If oxygen is required, it is regulated and passed through a
solenoid that remains open until sufficient
piston displacement occurs to provide the
selected FIO_2. The oxygen solenoid then
closes and the air valve opens, delivering
compressed air to the chamber until total
displacement equals the selected tidal volume. The exhalation pilot valve also closes,
permitting depressurization of the exhalation valve to ambient or PEEP levels.

Reference

Searle VVA Operating Manual. Searle Cardiopulmonary Systems Inc., Emeryville, CA

SECHRIST IV-100B INFANT VENTILATOR

The Sechrist IV-100B infant ventilator
(Fig. 10-104) is a pneumatically and elec-

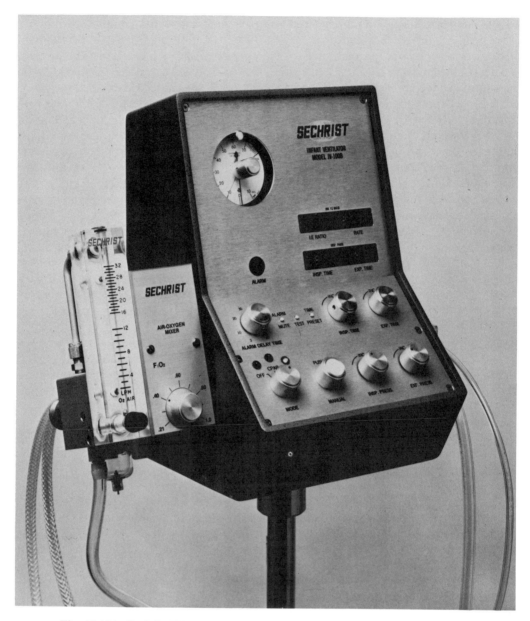

Fig. 10-104. Sechrist IV-100B ventilator. (Courtesy of Sechrist Industries, Inc.)

tronically powered, electronically and FLUIDICALLY controlled, time-cycled, constant- and nonconstant-flow generator. It may be operated in CMV, IMV, or SPONTANEOUS breathing modes. Dynamic inspiratory and expiratory pressure wave contours are variable. Negative and positive end-expiratory pressure (NEEP, PEEP) are available.

Control and Surveillance

Most of the ventilator functions are controlled on the front panel (Fig. 10-105) An

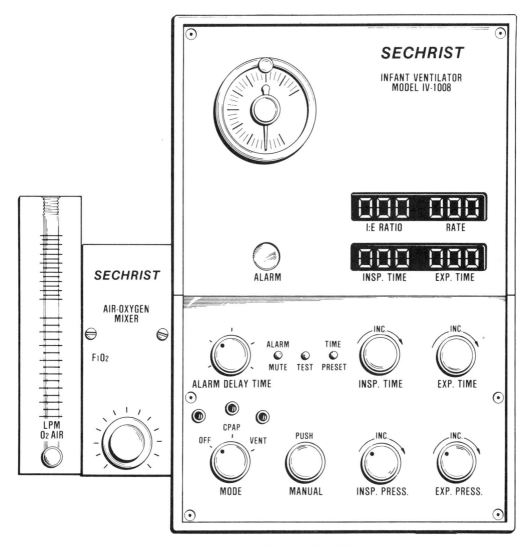

Fig. 10-105. Schematic of the Sechrist IV-100B control panel.

AC power switch (rear panel) must be engaged for ventilator operation. Ventilatory mode is selected by a three-position rotary switch. Each position illuminates its respective pilot lamp.

Continuous flow is adjusted with a rotary knob and is indicated on a calibrated Thorpe tube (0–32 L·minute^{-1}). A flow rate of 1.5–2.0 times the estimated minute volume, or enough to prevent inordinate spontaneous inspiratory deflection of the proximal airway pressure manometer, generally is selected.

IMV is initiated by placing the mode selector in VENT position. The IMV rate is determined by the inspiratory (T_I) and expiratory (T_E) times and is indicated on LED display. T_I is adjustable from 0.10 to 2.9 seconds (0.10–1.0 and 1.0–2.9 in increments of 0.01 and 0.1 seconds, respectively). Mechanical T_I is indicated by LED display. T_E is adjustable from 0.2 to 60 seconds (0.3–1.5, 1.5–10, 10–20, and 20–60 in increments of 0.01, 0.1, 1.0, and 5.0 seconds, respectively). The resultant T_E and I:E ratio are indicated via respective LED displays.

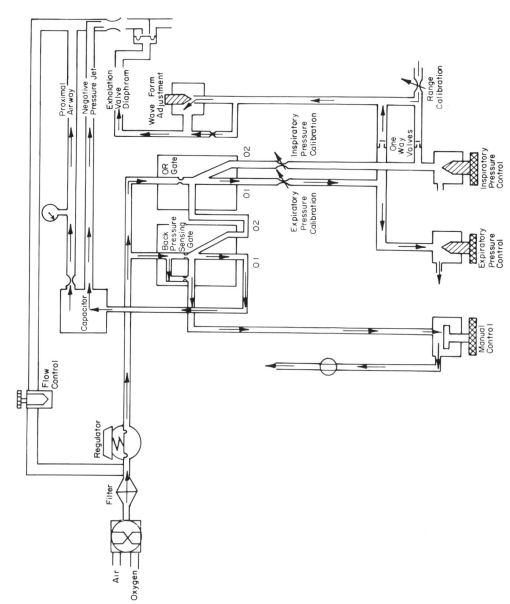

Fig. 10-106. Internal schematic of the Sechrist IV-100B inspiratory phase gas flows.

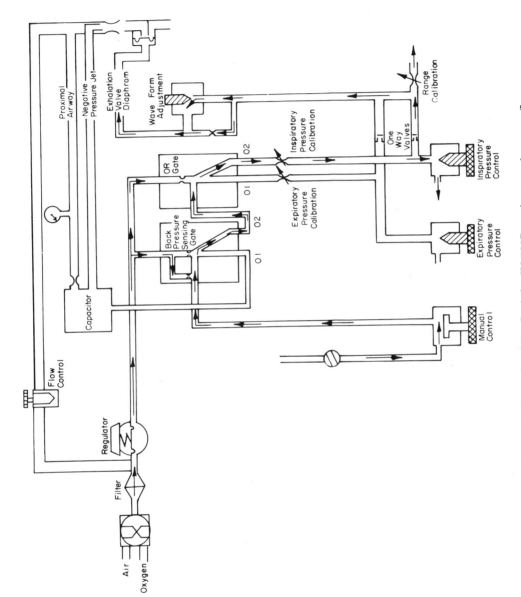

Fig. 10-107. Internal schematic of the Sechrist IV-100B expiratory phase gas flows.

In the CPAP mode, all LED displays are deactivated. The T_I and T_E display may be reactivated by depressing a pushbutton. This maneuver facilitates appropriate adjustment of the timing mechanism in the CPAP mode before engaging IMV.

Mechanical tidal volume (V_T) is determined by the continuous flow rate, T_I, and PIP limit control (7–70 cm H_2O). If the PIP limit is exceeded, the exhalation valve remains closed while the continuous flow is vented, thereby creating a pressure plateau for the remaining T_I. Mechanical inspiratory and expiratory pressure contours are selected by a control in the exhalation valve assembly. A full range of square-wave to sine-wave flow curves are available. A manual inspiration limited to the selected PIP may be administered for as long as the pushbutton is depressed. T_E is not reset after manual inspiration.

NEEP and PEEP/CPAP are continuously adjustable (−2 to 15 cm H_2O). NEEP cannot be generated when the continuous flow exceeds 10–12 L·minute^{-1}.

Audible and visual alarm and LED functions are tested by depressing a pushbutton. A "minimum pressure" alarm is selected by adjusting a red marker on the aneroid gauge. The manometer needle must cross the marker within an interval selected by the delay control (3–60 seconds) or audible and visual alarms activate. This feature acts as a disconnect alarm and may be adjusted to monitor apnea during CPAP or low IMV rates.

Audible alarms are silenced by depressing a pushbutton. This alarm mute lasts approximately 25 seconds then resets.

Operation

Inspiratory (Fig. 10-106) and expiratory (Fig. 10-107) phase gas flows are illustrated. The Sechrist IV-100B is pneumatically powered by 50 psig air and oxygen blended to the desired F_{IO_2}. Continuous circuit flow is provided by a flowmeter interfaced with the blender. The microprocessor control circuit switches the solenoid valve to ON or OFF positions in response to operator-selected inspiratory and expiratory times. These time units are referenced to a time base generator incorporated in the ventilator. Once the solenoid valve is closed, back-pressure trips two fluidic valves (the back-pressure sensing gate and the "or" gate) from the 01 to 02 positions and, in the process, turns off the negative pressure jet. In this configuration gas travels from the fluidic gates to an "inspiratory pressure" control and bleeds out to the appropriate pressure level. Simultaneously, gas passes through one-way valves to a factory preset range calibration valve, then into a waveform adjustment valve, and finally to the exhalation valve diaphragm. As pressure is applied to the exhalation valve diaphragm, continuous circuit flow to ambient is interrupted, and gas is diverted into the lungs. Exhalation valve pressurization is regulated by a turn screw (waveform modifier) located on the exhalation manifold. Abrupt pressurization produces a square-wave flow pattern. Graded or dampened flow to the exhalation diaphragm facilitates a slower interruption of circuit flow, thus approximating a sinusoidal delivery of the tidal volume.

Reference

Model IV-100B Operational Instructions. Sechrist Industries, Inc., Anaheim, CA

SIEMENS-ELEMA SERVO VENTILATOR 900B

The Siemens-Elema Servo ventilator 900B (Fig. 10-108) is a pneumatically and electronically powered, electronically controlled, time-cycled ventilator. It can be utilized as a constant or nonconstant (accelerating or decelerating) flow generator or a constant-pressure generator. CMV, AS-

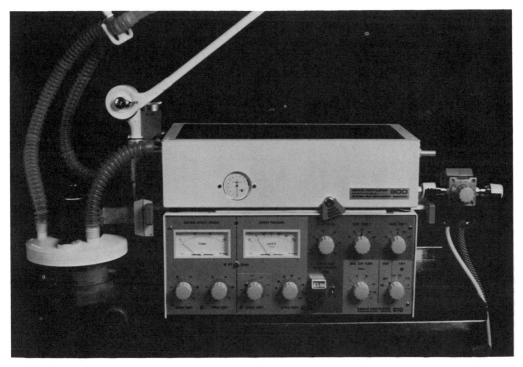

Fig. 10-108. Siemens-Elema servo ventilator 900B. (Courtesy of Siemens-Elema.)

SIST, SIMV, or SPONTANEOUS modes are available. Mechanical inspiration may be extended by a postinflation hold (plateau). Flow retardation and PEEP/CPAP are available.

Control and Surveillance

Ventilator functions are adjusted and monitored on the control panel (Fig. 10-109). Rather than selecting a tidal volume (V_T) directly, one adjusts a minute volume (MV = 0.5–30.0 L·minute^{-1}) and cycling frequency (6–60 breaths·minute^{-1}). Inspiratory and plateau times are adjusted as a percentage of the total ventilator cycle time. The inspiratory time (T_I) control is calibrated at 15, 20, 25, 33, and 50 percent. Inspiration may be extended by a plateau beyond the dynamic phase (0, 5, 10, 20, or 30 percent).

Internal working pressure is continuously adjustable (10–100 cm H_2O). The selected value is indicated on an aneroid manometer. Various inspiratory flow configurations are attainable with the 900B ventilator. A toggle switch permits use of either a constant or accelerating inspiratory pattern. A working pressure of 30–40 cm H_2O greater than the PIP facilitates selection of the desired flow contour. Decelerating flow is available when the working pressure and PIP gradient is narrow. Maximum deceleration is effected when PIP equals working pressure. Under these conditions, the ventilator is pressure-limited and V_T-variable.

The 900B ventilator may be operated as a constant-pressure generator by selecting a maximum minute volume, cycling frequency, inspiratory time, and constant pressure (i.e., working pressure). The inspiratory servo mechanism provides maximum flow to maintain the selected working pressure in the breathing circuit throughout the entire inspiratory phase. The ventilator also provides an inspiratory pressure pla-

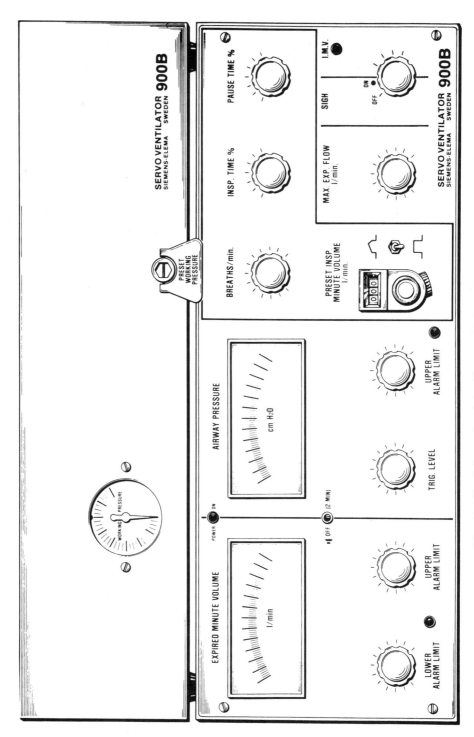

Fig. 10-109. Schematic of the Siemens-Elema 900B control panel.

teau during which spontaneous breathing may occur.

Expiratory flow is adjustable (1.0 to ∞ L·minute^{-1}). Retardation is added by decreasing the maximum expiratory flow rate until a desired effect is achieved (simulated "purse lip" breathing). A deep breath equal to twice the VT is delivered every 100 cycles when the control knob is placed in the ON position.

IMV is activated by the sigh-IMV knob. IMV rate may be selected at $f/2$, $f/5$, $f/10$, or $f/0$; where f is ventilator cycling frequency and $f/0$ is total spontaneous breathing. When IMV function is switched on, spontaneous breathing effort is sensed by a pressure transducer, and an electronic circuit regulates demand flow to the patient. When the patient exhales, a positive pressure above baseline is sensed by the transducer, causing the inspiratory valve to close and the expiratory valve to open. IMV is synchronized with the inspiratory effort (SIMV) in spontaneously breathing patients. If an IMV breath is not patient-initiated, subsequent cycling intervals provide CMV until SIMV resumes.

Expired minute volume (MVE) is indicated on an analog meter calibrated to 0–30 L·minute^{-1}. MVE includes both mechanical and spontaneous exhaled volume. Proximal airway pressure is indicated by an analog meter (-10 to 100 cm H$_2$O). A lower and upper MVE and upper Paw alarm control with audible and visual signals are selected to monitor the ventilatory status. The trigger level knob serves as an inspiratory effort control for patient-initiated mechanical VT and/or demand flow for spontaneous breathing.

An indicator lamp illuminates when the patient initiates either a spontaneous or a mechanical breath. If the preselected PIP is exceeded, visual and audible alarms activate and inspiration is terminated. When the main power switch (rear of ventilator) is on, a green lamp glows continuously. If the ventilator becomes unplugged or a power failure occurs, the "power-on" light

flashes, an audible alarm sounds, and inspiratory and expiratory valves open. Power for the "electrical failure" alarm is derived from a storage capacitor.

All alarms may be silenced for 2 minutes by depressing a pushbutton. Dissipation of storage capacitor voltage is accelerated by depressing the button for several seconds. This action prevents continuous audible alarming when the ventilator is disconnected from the patient.

Operation

Inspiratory (Fig. 10-110) and expiratory (Fig. 10-111) phase gas flows are illustrated. An air/oxygen blender provides gas at the prescribed FIO_2. Metered gas may be added via a low-pressure auxiliary inlet. Upon demand, a lever-activated valve opens, permitting blended gas to flow through a bacterial filter into a pressurized concertina bag (reservoir). Concertina bag pressure is generated by spring tension, which itself is regulated by the "working pressure" control. During inspiration gas from the concertina bag is directed to the breathing circuit by the inspiratory servo system, which consists of a flow transducer, servo valve, and pressure transducer interfaced with the electronic circuitry. Mixed gas passes through a flow transducer which is divided into two channels; a large channel contains a mesh screen which creates resistance, diverting a specific amount of gas through a smaller measuring channel. Gas flowing through the measuring channel presses against a flag which applies force to a strain gauge. This electronic flow signal is integrated and referenced to the selected volume, rate, and inspiratory time control. Inspiratory valve opening is modulated to facilitate volume delivery at selected flow patterns in the alloted time. During spontaneous breathing (IMV or CPAP), inspiratory effort sensed by the pressure transducer initiates demand flow through the

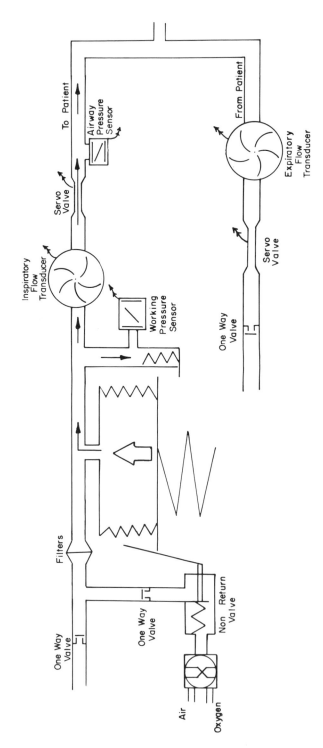

Fig. 10-110. Internal schematic of the Siemens-Elema 900B inspiratory phase gas flows.

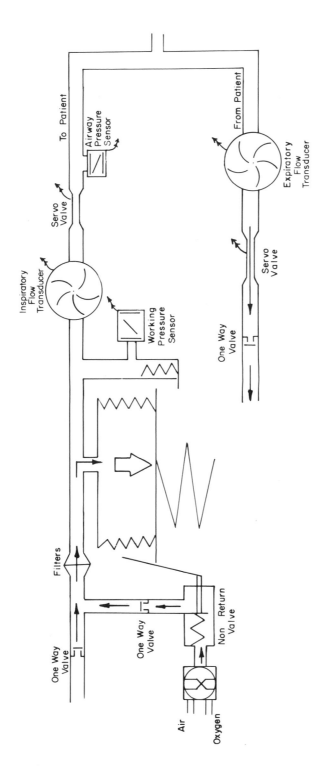

Fig. 10-111. Internal schematic of the Siemens-Elema 900B expiratory phase gas flows.

servo system. When baseline pressure is reestablished, servo flow ceases.

The servo valves are scissors type, opening and closing similarly to solenoid valves. During inspiration, the servo valve is activated by a stepping motor which cycles a lever at a rapid rate against a fixed lever in scissor-like fashion. The motor operates at about 500 steps·second^{-1}, facilitating instantaneous servo valve adjustments of flow. During spontaneous or mechanical exhalation, the inspiratory servo valve closes as the expiratory valve opens. The expiratory servo system consists of a flow transducer and valve. Valve action is directed by electronically referencing the expiratory flow transducer signal and maximum expiratory flow (retardation) control.

Inspiratory flow and pressure and expiratory flow signal output plugs are located on the rear panel of the ventilator. These may be used with recording equipment or connected to optional lung mechanics monitors designed for the 900B ventilator.

Reference

Model 900/900B Operating Manual No. 6887525E037E. Siemens-Elema Solna, Sweden

SIEMENS-ELEMA SERVO VENTILATOR 900C

The Siemens-Elema Servo 900C ventilator (Fig. 10-112) is a pneumatically and electronically powered, electronically controlled, time-cycled ventilator. It can be utilized as a constant or nonconstant (accelerating or decelerating) flow generator or constant-pressure generator. It may be employed in CMV, ASSIST, SIMV, or SPONTANEOUS modes. Mechanical inspiration may be extended by a postinflation hold (plateau). PEEP/CPAP are available.

Control and Surveillance

Selection and monitoring of ventilation parameters are confined to the control panel (Fig. 10-113). A main power switch, which activates the electronic circuitry, is situated on the rear panel. Mechanical breath size is determined by the adjusted minute volume (0.5–40 L·minute^{-1}) and cycling frequency (5–120 cycles·minute^{-1}). Inspiratory time and plateau time cumulatively regulate the inspiratory phase as a percent of the total ventilatory cycle. Inspiratory time (T$_I$) is adjustable at 20, 25, 33, 50, 67, or 80 percent of total cycle time, and may be extended by a static plateau of 0, 5, 10, 20, and 30 percent. If T$_I$ plus plateau time exceed 80 percent of the cycling period, the plateau time is automatically reduced, permitting a minimum exhalation period equal to 20 percent of total cycle time.

An accelerating or constant inspiratory flow pattern may be selected. A decelerating inspiratory flow occurs when the waveform toggle switch is set to square wave and the working pressure is adjusted to a value equal to or only slightly greater than the PIP during tidal volume (V$_T$) delivery. When PIP and ventilator working pressures equalize, flow ceases, even through the programmed inspiratory time might not have lapsed. Under decelerating flow conditions, the ventilator is pressure-limited and V$_T$-variable.

Ventilatory mode is determined by an eight-position rotary knob. Available modes are: PRESSURE SUPPORT, PRESSURE CONTROL, VOLUME CONTROL PLUS SIGH, VOLUME CONTROL, SIMV WITH PRESSURE SUPPORT, SIMV, CPAP, and MANUAL.

Pressure-supported ventilation (PRESS. SUPPORT) is a spontaneous breathing mode in which the ventilator functions as a constant-pressure generator. The level of constant pressure is adjustable (0–100 cm H$_2$O) above the baseline pressure (maximum 120 cm H$_2$O). A safety catch must be depressed to advance beyond 30 cm H$_2$O.

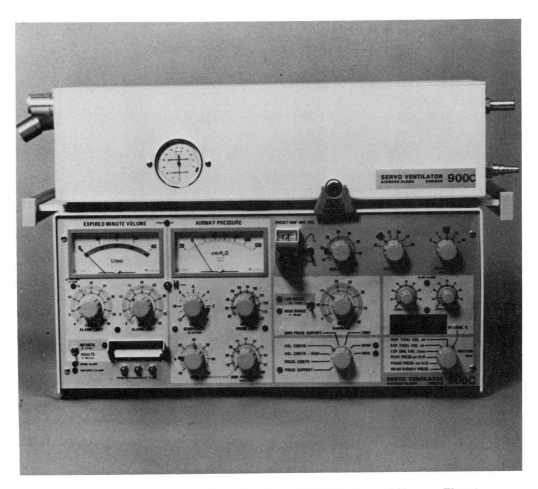

Fig. 10-112. Siemens-Elema Servo Ventilator 900C (Courtesy of Siemens-Elema).

If pressurized inspiration surpasses 80 percent of cycle time (based on cycle·minute^{-1} control), circuit pressure is vented to the baseline level. Normal termination of pressure support occurs when the inspiratory flow transducer senses little or no flow, or the pressure transducer registers a higher than selected level.

Pressure-controlled ventilation (PRESS. CONTR.) permits patient-initiated or controlled exposure to constant pressure for a selected inspiratory time. Constant pressure is adjusted similarly as in the pressure support mode. Resultant tidal volume depends on inspiratory time and pressure, cy-

cling frequency, and lung-thorax compliance, and circuit and airway resistance.

Volume control and sigh ventilation (VOL. CONTR. + SIGH) generates uniform V_T delivery to the circuit with a double-volume sigh every 100th breath. V_T depends on the selected minute volume and cycling frequency. When the inspiratory flow deceleration technique is employed, inspired volume fluctuates with changes in lung-thorax compliance. Volume-controlled mode (VOL. CONTR.) provides tidal ventilation without periodic sighs.

Synchronized intermittent mandatory ventilation with pressure support (SIMV +

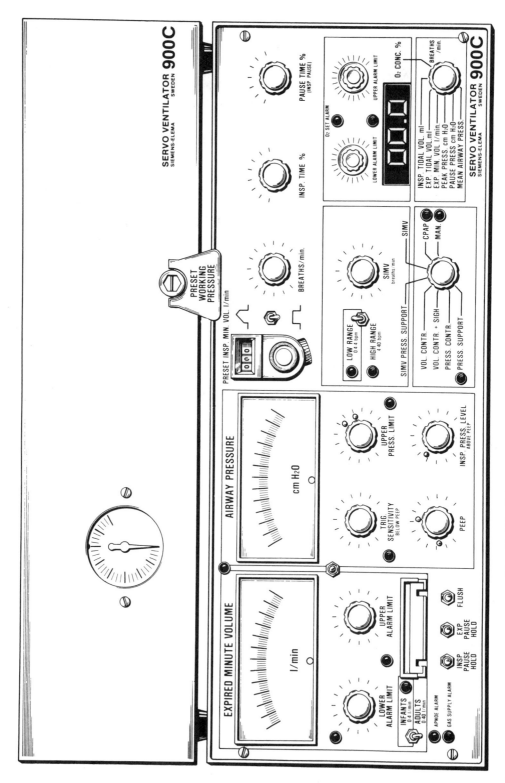

Fig. 10-113. Schematic of the Siemens-Elema 900C control panel.

PRESS. SUPPORT) permits pressurized spontaneous inspiration augmented by periodic mechanical tidal volumes. During spontaneous breathing, inspiratory pressure support is adjusted as previously described. SIMV cycling frequency is selected from two ranges: low rate (0.4–4.0 breaths·minute^{-1}) and high rate (4.0–40 breaths·minute^{-1}). SIMV cycling frequency cannot exceed the rate selected on the breaths·minute^{-1} control; thus it must be adjusted to a value higher than the desired SIMV rate. SIMV breaths are either controlled or patient-triggered. In SIMV spontaneous breathing occurs at baseline pressure (ambient pressure or PEEP/CPAP). Mechanical tidal volume in either SIMV mode is determined by the adjusted minute volume and the breath·minute^{-1} control, not the SIMV rate. CPAP allows spontaneous ventilation at ambient pressure or PEEP/CPAP, with no mechanical tidal volumes.

Manual mode (MAN.) is employed in conjunction with a reservoir bag and manual ventilation valve (accessory equipment) interfaced between the ventilator outflow port and inspiratory limb of the breathing circuit. Manual compression of the reservoir bag drives gas into the circuit causing a pressure rise. When the circuit pressure equals 4 cm H_2O, the expiratory valve closes, diverting the manual volume to the patient. When manual bag compression is terminated, circuit pressure decreases to less than 4 cm H_2O, allowing the exhalation valve to open. As circuit pressure approaches 2 cm H_2O, demand flow from an inspiratory servo mechanism refills the reservoir bag. In the MANUAL mode, the "apnea" alarm is deactivated.

Inspiratory effort necessary for patient-initiated ventilator functions is determined by a trigger sensitivity (TRIG, SENSITIVITY BELOW PEEP) control (0–20 cm H_2O below baseline PEEP/CPAP). Each patient-triggered ventilator response is indicated by an illuminated lamp. If the selected PIP (18–120 cm H_2O) is reached during timed mechanical inspiration, the ventilator cycles to exhalation and visual and audible alarms activate.

PEEP/CPAP is adjustable (0–50 cm H_2O). During spontaneous ventilation modes, if the adjusted sensitivity requires an inspiratory effort greater than the end-expiratory pressure, the patient is breathing with spontaneous PEEP. If the sensitivity is adjusted so as to prevent ambient or subambient pressure inspiratory efforts, CPAP is employed. The inherent flexibility of this demand system allows easy manipulation of end-expiratory to end-inspiratory pressure gradients.

Encased beneath the UPPER ALARM LIMIT control are three pushbuttons for the following functions: inspiratory pause hold (INSP. PAUSE HOLD), expiratory pause hold (EXP. PAUSE HOLD), and GAS CHANGE. Inspiratory pause hold extends inspiration as a static plateau for as long as the button is depressed, theoretically enhancing alveolar gas mixing. Precise quantitation of the end-expiratory pressure may be determined by extending the exhalation phase with the expiratory pause hold pushbutton. Rapid alteration of the inspired gas mixture is effected when the GAS EXCHANGE button is depressed. This maneuver causes simultaneous opening of inspiratory and expiratory valves, permitting internal and external circuits to be "washed out" with the new gas mixture. During this procedure, the exhaled volume meter automatically zeros.

Exhaled minute volume (MVE) is measured by the expiratory flow transducer and displayed on an analog meter in one of two ranges: infant (0–4.0 L·minute^{-1}) or adult (1–40 L·minute^{-1}). A lower and upper MVE limit is adjustable. If either limit is reached, visual and audible alarms are triggered.

Operation

Inspiratory (Fig. 10-114) and expiratory (Fig. 10-115) phase gas flows are illustrated.

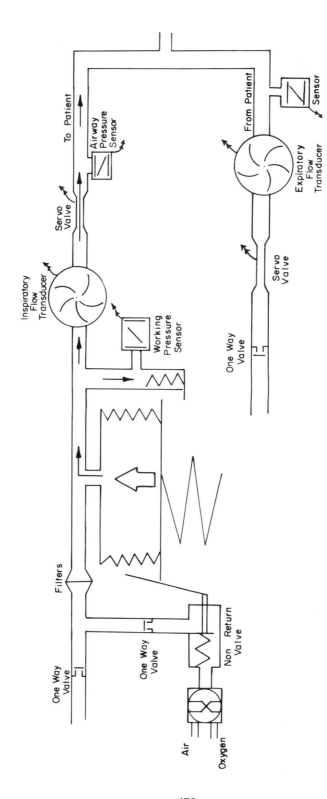

Fig. 10-114. Internal schematic of the Siemens-Elema 900C inspiratory phase gas flows.

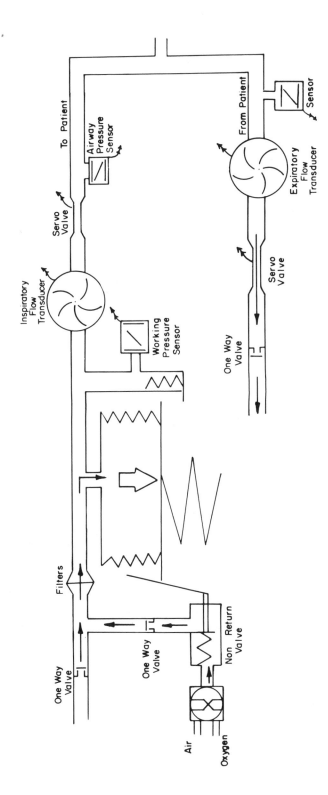

Fig. 10-115. Internal schematic of the Siemens-Elema 900C expiratory phase gas flows.

An air/oxygen blender provides gas at the prescribed F_{IO_2}. Metered gas may be added through a low-pressure auxiliary inlet. Upon demand, a lever-activated valve opens, permitting blended gas to flow through a bacterial filter into a pressurized concertina bag (reservoir). Concertina bag pressure is generated by spring tension, which is regulated by the "working pressure" control. During inspiration, gas from the concertina bag is directed to the breathing circuit by the inspiratory servo system consisting of a flow transducer, servo valve, and pressure transducer interfaced with the electronic circuitry. Mixed gas passes through the flow transducer, which is divided into two channels; a large channel contains a mesh screen which creates resistance and diverts a specific amount of gas through a smaller measuring channel. Gas flowing through the measuring channel presses against a flag, which creates force on a strain gauge. This electronic flow signal is integrated and referenced to the selected volume, rate, and inspiratory time control. The inspiratory valve opening is modulated to facilitate volume delivery at the selected flow pattern during the alloted time. During spontaneous breathing (IMV or CPAP), inspiratory effort sensed by the pressure transducer initiates demand flow through the servo system. When baseline pressure is reestablished, servo flow ceases.

The servo valves are scissor type, opening and closing similarly to solenoid valves. During inspiration, the servo valve is activated by a stepping motor, which cycles a lever at a rapid rate against a fixed lever in a scissor-like fashion. The motor operates at about 500 steps·second^{-1}, facilitating instantaneous servo valve adjustments of flow. During spontaneous or mechanical exhalation, the inspiratory servo valve closes as the expiratory valve opens.

If a patient-initiated or CMV breath does not occur for more than 15 seconds, visual and audible "apnea" alarms activate. Visual and audible alarms also occur if the gas supply maintains inadequate internal reservoir (concertina bag) pressure. Lower and upper F_{IO_2} limits are continuously adjustable (0.21–1.0). If either is reached, visual and audible alarms engage.

An eight-position rotary knob selects one of the following parameters to be digitally displayed: mean airway pressure, pause (plateau) pressure, peak airway pressure, expired minute volume, inspired tidal volume, oxygen concentration, and breaths per minute.

Reference

Model 900C Operating Manual No. 6978761E313E. Siemens-Elema, Solna, Sweden

ACKNOWLEDGMENTS

Representatives of ventilator manufacturers were exceedingly helpful and Ms. Sue Heine (Shands Hospital, University of Florida) provided graphics.

Index